A Textbook of BIOCHEMISTRY *for* DENTAL STUDENTS

Fourth Edition

Revised As Per New Syllabus

Other Books by The Same Author

- A Textbook of Biochemistry
- Biochemistry for B.Sc. Nursing Students, 2nd edition
- Food & Nutrition (for Medical, Nursing & Allied Sciences)

A Textbook of

BIOCHEMISTRY

for

DENTAL STUDENTS

Fourth Edition

Revised As Per New Syllabus

HARBANS LAL
Senior Professor, Department of Biochemistry,
Postgraduate Institute of Medical Sciences,
Pt. B.D. Sharma University of Health Sciences,
Rohtak (Haryana)

CBS

CBS PUBLISHERS & DISTRIBUTORS PVT. LTD.

NEW DELHI • BANGALORE • PUNE • COCHIN • CHENNAI

ISBN : 978-81-239-1806-8

First Edition : 1997
Reprint : 1999
Second Edition : 2000
Reprint : 2000
Reprint : 2003
Reprint : 2004
Third Edition : 2006
Reprint : 2006
Reprint : 2008
Fourth Edition : 2010
Reprint : 2011

Published by Satish Kumar Jain and produced by V.K. Jain for
CBS Publishers & Distributors Pvt. Ltd.,
CBS Plaza, 4819/XI Prahlad Street, 24 Ansari Road, Daryaganj,
New Delhi - 110002, India. • Website: www.cbspd.com
e-mail: delhi@cbspd.com, cbspubs@vsnl.com, cbspubs@airtelmail.in
Ph.: 23289259, 23266861, 23266867 • Fax: 011-23243014

Branches:

- ***Bengaluru:*** Seema House, 2975, 17th Cross, K.R. Road,
  Bansankari 2nd Stage, Bangalore - 560070 Ph.: 26771678/79
  Fax: 080-26771680 • e-mail: bangalore@cbspd.com
- ***Pune:*** Bhuruk Prestige, Sr. No. 52/12/2+1+3/2,
  Narhe, Haveli (Near Katraj-Dehu Road by Pass), Pune-411051
  Ph.: +91-20-32404169 • Fax: 020-24464059
  e-mail: pune@cbspd.com
- ***Kochi:*** 36/14, Kalluvilakam, Lissie Hospital Road,
  Cochin - 682018, Kerala • e-mail: cochin@cbspd.com
  Ph.: 0484-4059061-65 • Fax: 0484-4059065
- ***Chennai:*** 20, West Park Road, Shenoy Nagar, Chennai - 600030
  e-mail: chennai@cbspd.com Ph.: 044-26260666-26202620
  Fax: 044-45530020

Printed at :
India Binding House, Noida (India)

PREFACE

Preface to the Fourth Edition

Recently, Dental Council of India has revised syllabi for various subjects, including Biochemistry, being taught to B.D.S. Students. Accordingly, there was a need for the revision of this book. Keeping in view the new syllabus of the subject, I am happy to present Fourth Edition of the Book on "Biochemistry for Dental Students". All the chapters have been thoroughly rewritten in a very lucid manner and several new chapters have been added. Various new topics, such as Integration of Metabolism, Oxygen Toxicity, Cancer, Acid-Base Regulation, Electrolyte Balance, Connective Tissue, Cytoskeleton, Hemoglobin Metabolism, and Immunoglobulins have been introduced. The practical exercises have been put separately at the end, for better understanding. Even in this chapter all the exercises have been rewritten and a new exercise on milk has been added. Several new questions have also been included at the end of each chapter.

I am sure, the new edition of the book will be appreciated, like the previous ones, by the Faculty as well as Students of the various Dental Colleges of the Country.

Several persons have helped me in bringing out this edition of the book and I am highly thankful to each one of them individually. I am also thankful to Mr. Satish Kumar Jain and the entire staff of CBS Publishers & Distributors Pvt. Ltd., Delhi, for its publication in a short time.

Suggestions and comments for its improvement are welcome.

July 2009 **HARBANS LAL**
Rohtak (Haryana)

PREFACE

Preface to the First Edition

In the past few years, a number of textbooks in biochemistry have been published primarily for students of medicine, but none for students of dentistry. This textbook "A Textbook of Biochemistry for Dental Students" has been written to meet the needs of dental students. While compiling this book the author has consulted several syllabi so as to cover all the topics prescribed for the B.D.S. students of various universities. However, though concise, this textbook provides sufficient upto-date material for learners of biochemistry even in Pharmacy, Nursing and other allied disciplines at the undergraduate level. The quantum of knowledge that is to be imparted to these students, in this period of ever-growing interdisciplinary speciality, has been presented in a simple and easily understandable language. Wherever necessary, the text has been illustrated with the help of self-explanatory reactions, diagrams, and tables. Some important questions have also been given at the end of each chapter for the benefit of students.

The text consists of 14 chapters and begins with an introduction to the subject. After a note on the cell and functions of the various organelles, is a chapter covering some aspects of enzymes. In the next 3 chapters the chemistry of carbohydrates, lipids, amino acids and proteins has been discussed. Various metabolic pathways have been given with an emphasis on those reactions that have particular relevance for health. Bone and teeth metabolism has also been included, briefly. Following this, is a description of nutrients considered regulatory in nature, namely, the minerals and trace elements, and vitamins. A chapter has also been written about nucleic acids to give an idea regarding the brief chemistry and functions of the macromolecules which form the chemical basis of heredity and are involved in the process of protein synthesis. After a focus on nutrition, there is mention about the regulatory molecules (hormones) which act as messengers for the various metabolic processes which occur within the cell. To cover the practicals, details of the various qualitative tests of carbohydrates, lipids and proteins, besides the analysis of urine, gastric juice and bile, have been given.

I wish to express my gratitude of my colleague, Dr. S.K. Aggarwal, Associate Professor of Biochemistry for numerous helpful suggestions and comments. I also wish to express my appreciation to my daughter Anubha and son Ashish who renered consistent help in the completion of this book. I am also thankful to my wife Veena for her patience. The anthusiastic cooperation received from Mr. S.K. Jain and the staff members of CBS Publishers and Distributors, New Delhi is acknowledged.

Suggestions and comments for its improvement are welcome.

May, 1997
Rohtak (Haryana)

HARBANS LAL

CONTENTS

Contents

CHAPTER

1

Chemistry of Carbohydrates

Carbohydrates, also called **saccharides** (Greek: *Sakcharon*, sugar), are most abundant biological molecules containing C, H, and O, which are combined in the ratio as $(CH_2O)_n$, where n is 3 or more. They may be defined as the **aldehyde or the ketone derivatives of the higher polyhydroxyalcohols or their anhydrides.**

BIOLOGICAL IMPORTANCE OF CARBOHYDRATES

1. Carbohydrates **provide a significant fraction of the energy in a diet** of most of the organisms.
2. They also **act as the storage form of energy in the body.**
3. Carbohydrates also serve as **components of the cell membrane** that mediates intracellular communication.
4. They also serve as the **structural components** of many organisms, including the cell wall of the bacteria, the exoskeleton of many insects, and the fibrous cellulose portion of the plants.

CLASSIFICATION OF CARBOHYDRATES

Depending upon the number of the monomer units present in the molecule, carbohydrates are classified as **monosaccharides, disaccharides,** and **polysaccharides** (Fig. 1.1).

MONOSACCHARIDES

Monosaccharides are the **simple sugars,** which join in several ways to form various di and polysaccharides. Monosaccharides are the aldehyde or the ketone derivatives of the straight chain polyhydroxyalcohols, which contain 3 or more carbons.

Different monosaccharides can be separated from a mixture by the technique known as chromatography.

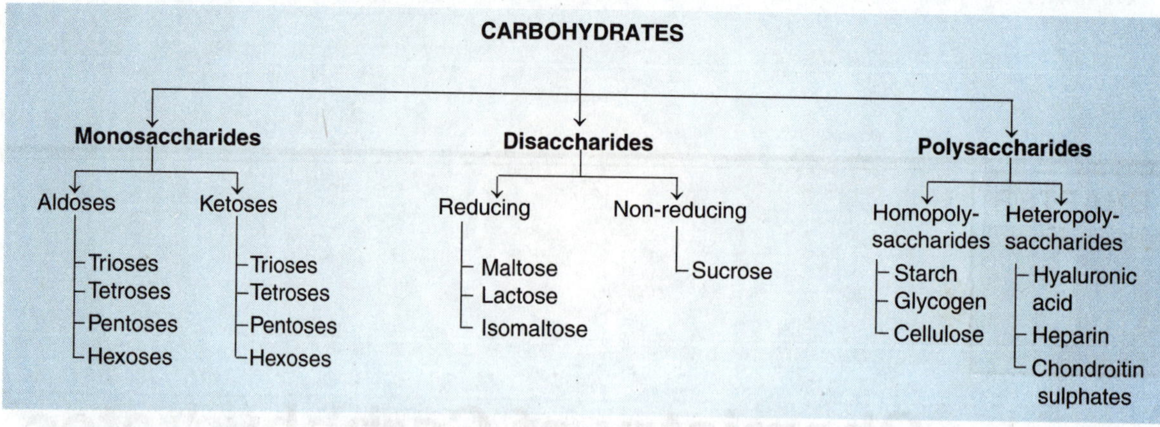

Fig. 1.1. Classification of carbohydrates.

CLASSIFICATION OF THE MONOSACCHARIDES

Classification of the monosaccharides is given in Table 1.1.

Monosaccharides are divided into different groups, according to:

- **Chemical nature** of their carbonyl group, or
- **Number of carbon atoms** in the chain

Table 1.1. Classifications of monosaccharide

Monosaccharides	*Number of carbons*	*Aldoses*	*Ketoses*
Trioses	3	Glyceraldehyde	Dihydroxyacetone
Tetroses	4	Erythrose	Erythrulose
Pentoses	5	Ribose	Ribulose
Hexoses	6	Glucose	Fructose

According to chemical nature of the carbonyl group

According to chemical nature of the carbonyl group, monosaccharides are divided into two groups as, aldoses **and** ketoses:

Aldoses: The sugar is an aldose when it has an **aldehyde (–CHO) group** on carbon-l, e.g. glucose.

Ketoses: The sugar is a ketose when it has a **ketone (–CO)** group at carbon-2, e.g. fructose.

Some of the ketoses are named by inserting **'-ul'** before the suffix **'-ose'**, in the name of the corresponding aldose, e.g. **erythrulose**. It is a ketose corresponding to erythrose, which is an aldose.

According to number of the carbon atoms

According to number of the carbon atoms, monosaccharides are designated as trioses, tetroses, pentoses**, etc.**

Trioses: Trioses are the smallest monosaccharides with **three carbon atoms,** e.g. **glyceraldehyde** (an aldotriose) and **dihydroxyacetone** (a ketotriose). Both of these molecules are of physiological significance, as phosphate esters of these sugars; i.e. glyceraldehyde-3-phosphate and dihydroxyacetonephosphate, are intermediates in the process of glycolysis.

Tetroses: Tetroses have **four carbon atoms,** e.g. **erythrose** (an aldotetrose) and **erythrulose** (a ketotetrose). Erythrose, as erythrose-4-phosphate, is an intermediate in the hexosemonophosphate (HMP) shunt.

Pentoses: Pentoses are the sugars containing **five carbon atoms**, such as **ribose** (an aldopentose) and **xylulose** (a ketopentose). Both of them are the intermediates of the HMP shunt. Ribose is also an important constituent of nucleotides, in RNA.

Hexoses: Hexoses contain **six carbon atoms**, e.g. **glucose** (an aldohexose) and **fructose** (a ketohexose). Glucose, commonly known as dextrose, is used as a source of energy, in the body. Galactose is a constituent of the milk sugar, lactose. Fructose is a constituent of the common sugar, sucrose.

Some of the monosaccharides of biological importance are shown in Fig. 1.2.

Isomerism

Monosaccharides are **optically active** compounds and can rotate plane of the polarized light either to right or to left. Such a property is a characteristic of the substances having a tetrahedral carbon (asymmetric carbon), that has four different atoms or groups attached to the same carbon atom.

Stereoisomerism

Simple sugars contain a center of asymmetry and thus, are the chiral molecules. A compound having one asymmetric carbon may occur in two forms, both of which are the **non-super-imposable mirror images of**

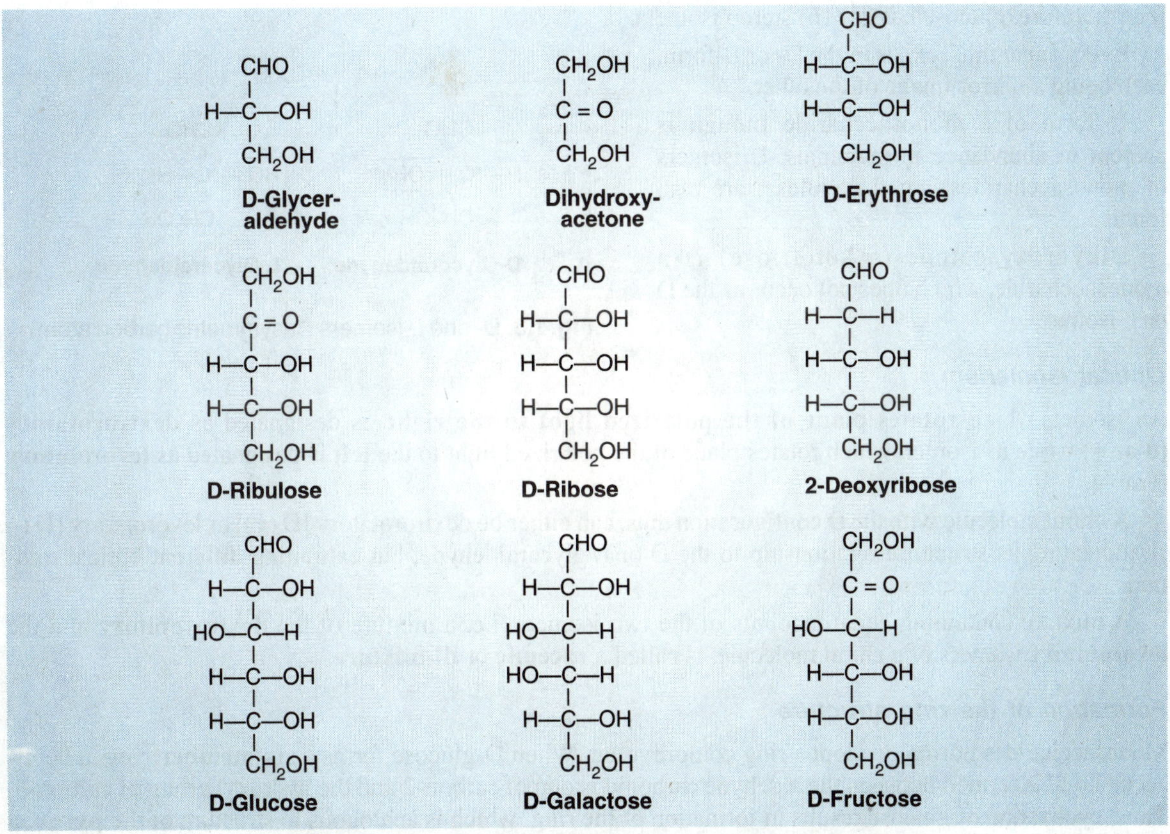

Fig. 1.2. Some monosaccharides of biological significance.

each other. These two molecules are referred as the spatial isomers or stereoisomers (enantiomers). Both the enantiomers rotate plane of the polarized light to the same degree but in the opposite directions.

D- and L-Isomerism

According to Fischer, two isomers of the parent compound of the carbohydrate family, i.e. the glyceraldehyde, are designated as **D-glyceraldehyde** and **L-glyceraldehyde.** D or L form of the monosaccharide is determined with respect to its spatial relationship with the glyceraldehyde.

In the Fischer projection, glyceraldehyde, with an **–OH group** around the asymmetric center (i.e. the α carbon atom or the carbon atom adjacent to the carbon atom with the terminal primary alcoholic group) **on the right hand side** when the –CHO group is at the top, is designated as **D-glyceraldehyde**. Its nonsuperimposable mirror image, which has **–OH group** around the asymmetric center **on the left**, is designated as **L-glyceraldehyde** (Fig. 1.3).

An addition of the successive carbon atom, in the form of –CHOH (the secondary alcoholic group), to the parent compound (D-glyceraldehyde) gives rise to the family of the D sugars. Thus, D sugars have same absolute configuration at the asymmetric center (farthest from their carbonyl group) as does D-glyceraldehyde (e.g. the –OH at carbon 5 of D-glucose on the right hand, similar to the –OH at carbon 2 of D-glyceraldehyde). Since each of new carbon atoms (as a secondary alcoholic group) is added as an asymmetric center, number of the isomers increase with the increasing number of the carbon atoms, as the asymmetric centers. Number of the isomers so formed thus, depends upon the number of the asymmetric centers in the molecule. It is represented by the formula 2^n since number of the asymmetric carbon atoms (n) in a glucose molecule is four therefore, glucose has 2^4 (16) stereo isomers.

Every sugar thus, exists in the D- or L-form, each being a mirror image of the other.

D form of a monosaccharide though is present in abundance in mammals, L isomers of monosaccharides, e.g. L-xylulose, are also found.

Dihydroxyacetone (a ketotriose) is a monosaccharide, which does not occur as the D or L isomer.

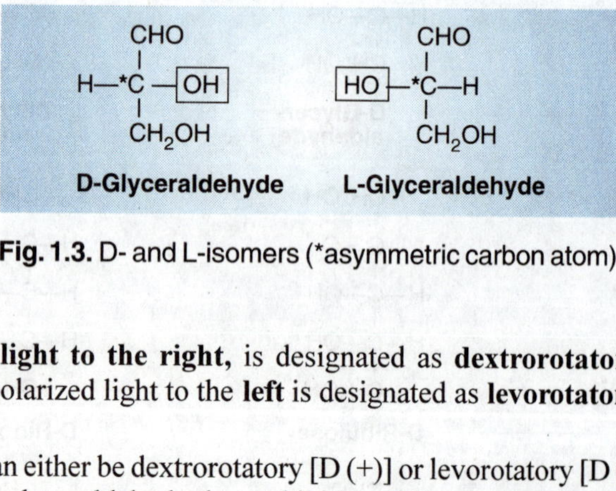

Fig. 1.3. D- and L-isomers (*asymmetric carbon atom).

Optical Isomerism

An isomer, which **rotates plane of the polarized light to the right,** is designated as **dextrorotatory (d or +)** while its isomer, which rotates plane of the polarized light to the **left** is designated as **levorotatory (l or –).**

A chiral molecule with the D configuration thus, can either be dextrorotatory [D (+)] or levorotatory [D (–)], indicating its structural relationship to the D or L glyceraldehyde, but exhibiting different optical rotations.

A mixture containing equal amounts of the two isomers, i.e. a mixture of the **dextrorotatory** and the **levorotatory** isomers of a chiral molecule, is called a **racemic** or **dl-mixture.**

Formation of the ring structure

Monosaccharides normally adopt a ring conformation. When D-glucose forms a **six-member ring**, a hemiacetal bond is formed between the aldehyde carbonyl group of carbon-2 and the hydroxyl group of carbon-5. Thus, cyclization of glucose results in formation of the ring, which is analogous to structure of the **pyran,** a six-member ring containing **five carbons** and **oxygen** (Fig. 1.4).

Sugars with a six-member ring (pyran ring) are designated as pyranoses and cyclization of **D-glucose** yields a cyclic hemiacetal, referred as **glucopyranose.**

A five-member ring with **four carbons** and **oxygen** is called **furan**. Smallest monosaccharide having a furan ring is called ribose.

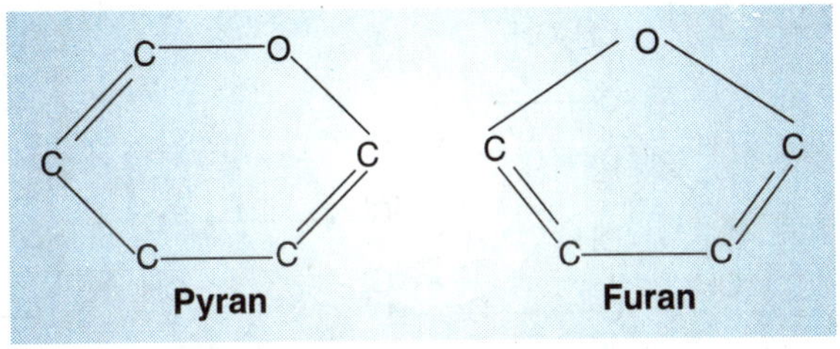

Fig. 1.4. Pyran and Furan rings.

Linear form of D-**fructose** cyclizes between the carbonyl group of carbon 2 and the alcoholic group of carbon 5 to yield a hemiketal that is referred to as **fructofuranose.**

Ring structures of the sugars were proposed by Haworth and are called **Haworth structures**.

Anomerism

When a monosaccharide cyclizes, its **carbonyl carbon,** called **anomeric carbon,** also becomes asymmetric and exhibits two configurations, which are referred as the α- form and the β-form. Such **stereoisomers** that differ in configuration at the anomeric carbon, i.e. at **carbon-1 in an aldose**, e.g. glucopyranose, or **carbon-2 in a ketose**, e.g. fructofuranose, are called **anomers** (Fig. 1.5).

Both the anomers have different physical and chemical properties, including the optical rotation.

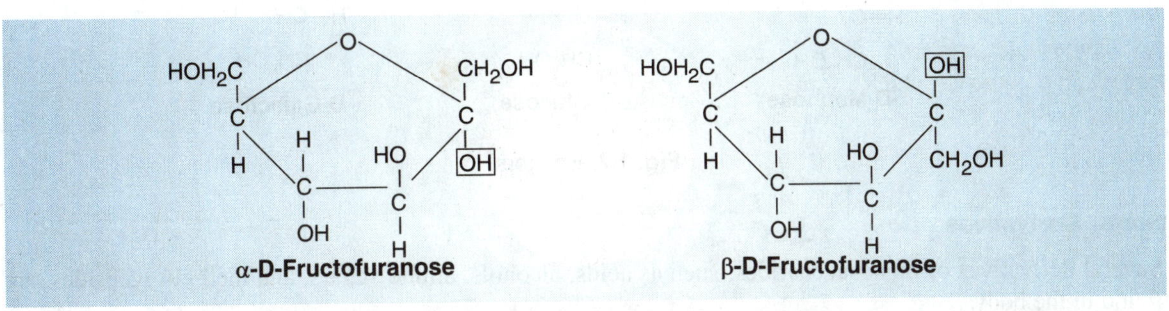

Fig. 1.5. Anomers.

Two anomers of glucose are freely interconvertible in an aqueous solution. At equilibrium, D glucose is a mixture of β-anomer (63.6°) and α-anomer (36.4°), in a ratio of nearly 2:1.

Interconversion of the two anomers also results in change in optical rotation of glucose. During equilibrium, **optical rotation of D (+) glucose slowly changes** with time and reaches a **constant value of 52.5°**. This phenomenon of change in optical rotation of D (+) glucose, in an aqueous solution, and reaching a constant value, due to interconversion of the two anomers, is called **mutarotation** (Fig. 1.6).

Epimerism

Sugars that differ in configuration of its **–H** and **–OH groups around** only **one of the optically active carbons** are known as **epimers.**

D-Mannose differs in configuration around carbon 2, with respect to D glucose. Similarly, D galactose has different configuration than D glucose around carbon 4. **D Mannose** and **D galactose,** therefore, are two **epimers of D glucose** (Fig. 1.7).

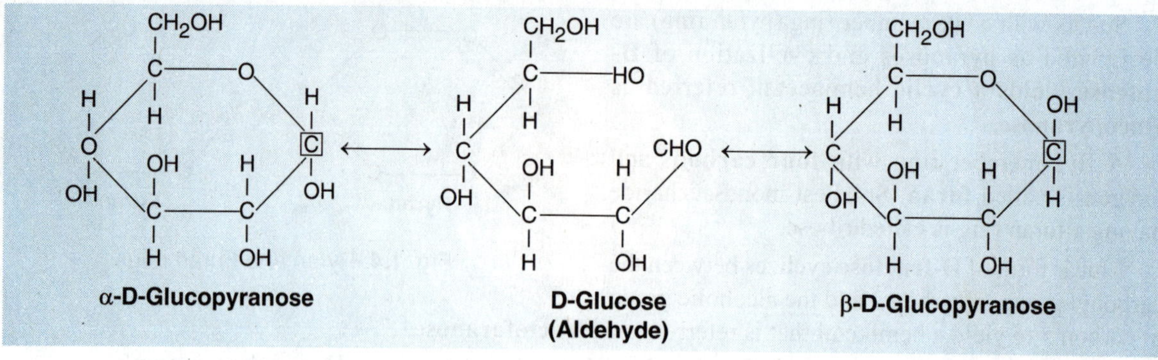

Fig. 1.6. Mutarotation.

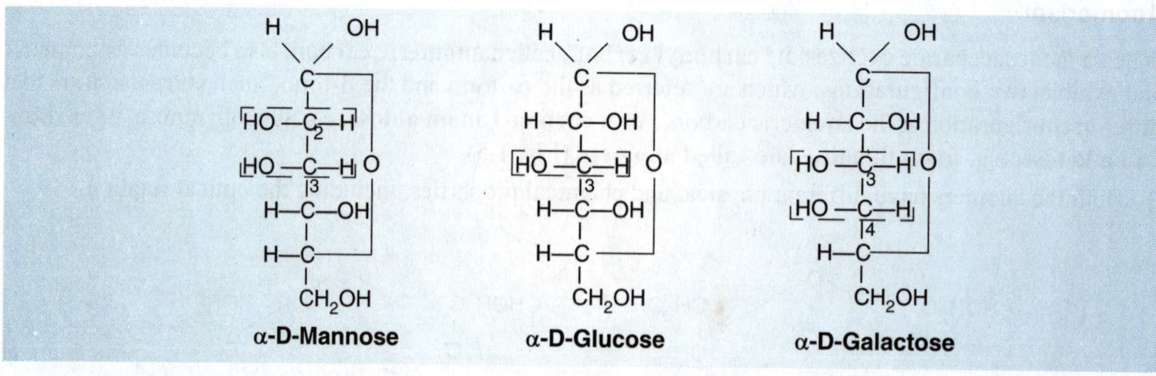

Fig. 1.7. Epimers.

Sugar Derivatives

Several derivatives of monosaccharides, such as acids, alcohols, amino sugars, and methyl-glycosides, are found in the body.

Sugar Acids

Oxidation of carbon 1 of an aldose **converts** its **aldehyde group to the carboxyl group** and **forms an acid,** called **aldonic acid,** such as D-gluconic acid.

On the other hand, **oxidation of the primary alcoholic group at carbon 6** of an aldose produces **uronic acid,** such as D-glucuronic acid (Fig. 1.8).

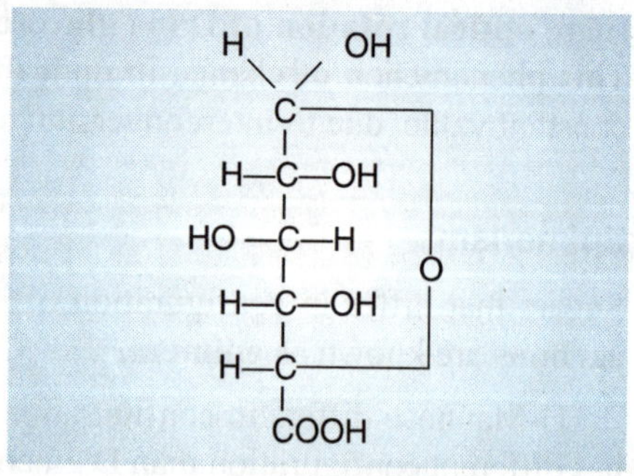

Fig. 1.8. D-Glucuronic acid.

Sugar Alcohols

Sugars reduce under mild conditions and produce cyclic polyhydroxyalcohols called **alditols,** e.g. **ribitol** (a component of FMN and FAD) and **xylitol** (a sweetener used in formation of gums and candies).

Amino Sugars

Amino sugars, such as **glucosamine** and **galactosamine,** are formed **when –NH2 group substitutes -OH group at carbon-2 (Fig. 1.9).**

Some amino sugars also occur as their acetylated derivatives.

Several derivatives of the amino sugars are found in glycosaminoglycans, such as hyaluronic acid, chondroitin sulfates, erythromycin, etc.

N-acetylneuraminic acid and its derivatives are called **sialic acids.** They are important constituents of **glycoproteins** and **glycolipids**.

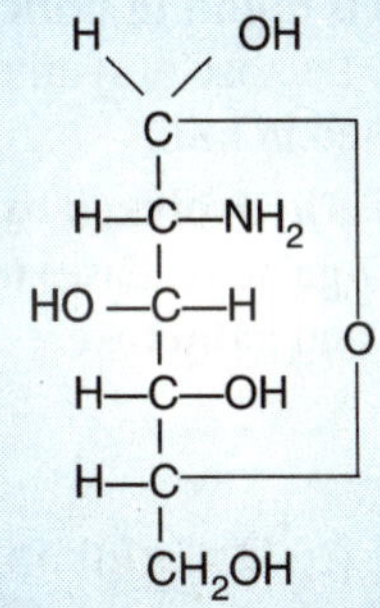

Fig. 1.9. D-Glucosamine.

Methylglycosides

When **carbon-1 of the sugar reacts with an alcohol**, such as methanol, it **yields** a **methylglycoside.** Methylglycosides are **found in glycosaminoglycans.**

DISACCHARIDES

Disaccharide consists of **two** similar or dissimilar **monosaccharides,** which are **linked** together **by a glycosidic bond**. **Maltose, lactose,** and **sucrose** are the disaccharides, which have biological significance.

Maltose

Maltose, [α-D glucopyranosyl-(1, 4)-α-D glucopyranosyl], **consists of two α-D glucopyran units,** which are linked together by **α-1,4-glycosidic linkage.** The **glycosidic bond links carbon-l of glucose to carbon-4 of the other glucose molecule**. Accordingly, in maltose, the -OH group at carbon 4 of a glucose molecule is linked to the –OH group at the carbon l (the anomeric carbon) of the other glucose molecule. This in turn leaves **–OH,** which **is free at** the anomeric carbon, i.e. **carbon-l** of the first glucose molecule, suggesting that **maltose is a reducing disaccharide** (Fig. 1.10).

Maltose is usually obtained as one of the hydrolyzed product of some polysaccharides, such as starch and glycogen.

Maltose can be **hydrolyzed** to its monosaccharides, i.e. **two glucose units,** by the enzyme **maltase,** in the intestinal lumen.

Isomaltose: Partial hydrolysis of glycogen and starch produces isomaltose. This is also a reducing sugar and contains **two glucose units, which are linked by the α-1,6 glycosidic linkage.**

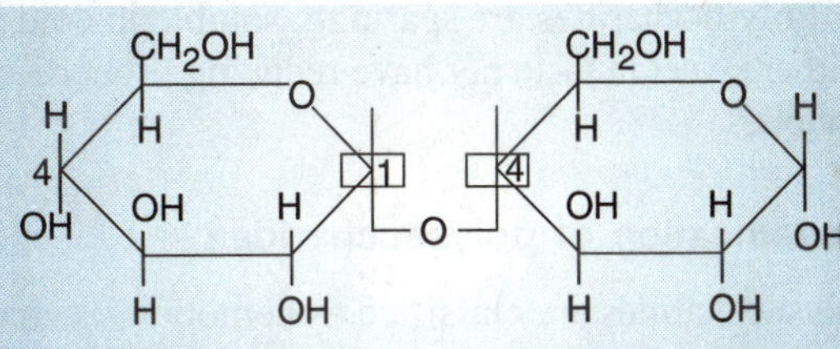

Fig. 1.10. Maltose.

Lactose

Lactose, [β-D galactopyranosyl-(1,4)-β-D glucopyranose)], consists of a molecule each of **β-D galactopyranose** and **β-D-glucopyranose,** which are **linked together by the β-1,4-glycosidic linkage.** The glycoside bond links **carbon 1 of galactose to carbon 4 of glucose**. This in turn, leaves a **free anomeric carbon on the glucose residue**. Thus, **lactose is a reducing disaccharide** (Fig.1.11).

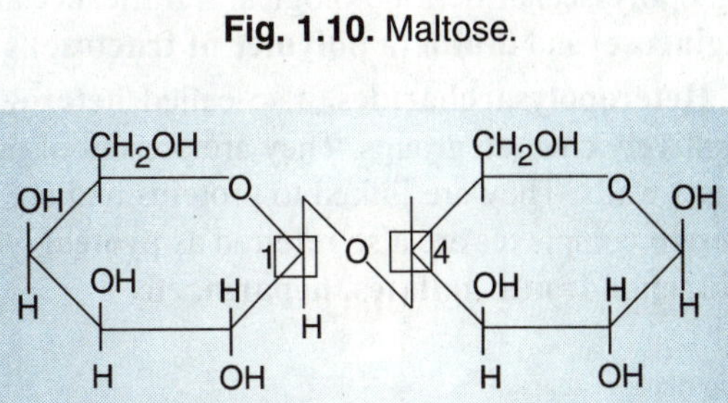

Fig. 1.11. Lactose.

Lactose is found in milk, hence it is also called **milk sugar**. Lactose is synthesized during lactation and is secreted in milk.

Lactose is hydrolyzed by the intestinal enzyme **lactase** (β-D-galactosidase) **to** its monosaccharides, i.e. **glucose** and **galactose.**

Sucrose

Sucrose, [α-D glucopyranosyl-(1,2)-β-D fructofuranose], consists of one molecule each of **α-D glucopyranose** and **β-D fructofuranose,** which are linked by the **β-1,2-glycosidic linkage** (Fig. 1.12).

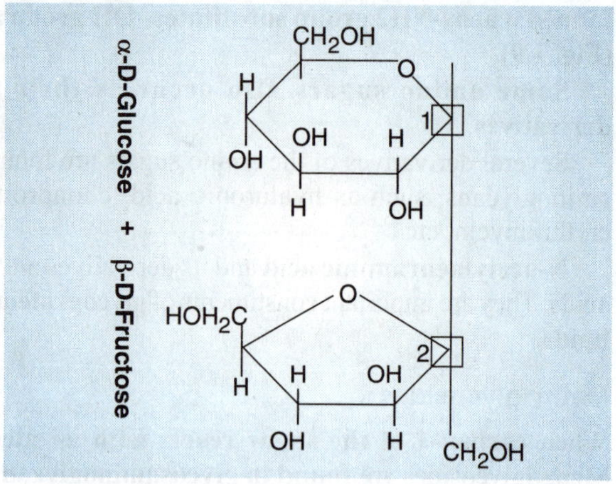

Fig. 1.12. Sucrose.

Since the carbonyl groups of both the monosaccharides, i.e. **carbon 1 of glucose and carbon 2 of fructose, participate in formation of the glycosidic bond** and that as such **there is no free carbonyl carbon on any of its monosaccharides,** hence **sucrose is a nonreducing sugar.**

Sucrose, also known as **invert sugar,** is most abundant disaccharide, which is **found in plants.** It is also referred as **table sugar** or **cane sugar.** It is **hydrolyzed to** two monosaccharides, i.e. **glucose** and **fructose, by** the intestinal enzyme **sucrase,** which is also referred as **invertase.**

POLYSACCHARIDES

Polysaccharides, also called **glycans,** are **polymers** of a large number of **monosaccharides**, which are linked together by glycosidic bonds. When the number of monosaccharides is small, such compounds are referred as **oligosaccharides.**

Polysaccharides are sparingly soluble in cold water but form a colloidal solution in hot water. They are neither sweet in taste nor have reducing properties. Polysaccharides are the linear molecules as well as have branches.

Classification of polysaccharides

Polysaccharides are classified as homopolysaccharides and heteropolysaccharides.

Homopolysaccharides or **homoglycans** are polymers of the **identical** monosaccharide units. Common homopolysaccharides of biological significance are **starch, glycogen** and **cellulose** (which are the **polymers of glucose)** and **inulin (a polymer of fructose).**

Heteropolysaccharides, also called **heteroglycans,** contain repeating disaccharide units, which bear negatively charged groups. They are present in the connective tissue, e.g. cartilage, tendon, skin, and blood vessel walls. They are linked to proteins and are also called as glycosaminoglycans. **Glycosaminoglycan-protein** complexes are also referred as **proteoglycans.** Most important glycosaminoglycans are **hyaluronic acid, chondroitin sulfates, heparin,** etc.

Starch

Starch is stored as a reservoir of food in cereals (wheat, maize, etc.) and tubers (potato, etc.), in **plants.** Starch consists of two polysaccharides units, called **α-amylose** and **amylopectin.**

α-Amylose is a **linear** polymer of glucose. In amylose, glucose residues are linked together by **α-(1→4)-glycosidic bonds.**

Amylopectin is a **branched polymer of glucose.** It has both **α-1→4** linkages (in the straight chain) as well as **α-1→6** linkages (at the branching points). Branching occurs after every 24 to 30 glucose residues (Fig. 1.13).

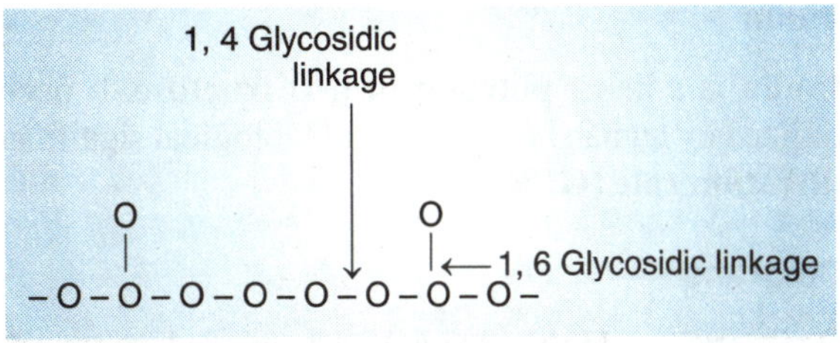

Fig. 1.13. Starch (–O– A glucose unit).

Starch is a main source of **carbohydrate** in the **human diet. Amylase,** present in the saliva and the pancreatic juice, randomly hydrolyses **α-1→4 glycosidic bonds** of starch and degrades it to a mixture of **maltose, maltotriose, and dextrins.**

Glycogen

Glycogen is a polysaccharide that is found in animals. It is also called as **animal starch.** Though, glycogen is found in all the cells but is most prevalent in muscles and the liver.

Glycogen has both, α-**1→4** glycosidic bonds as well as **α-1→6 linkages,** at the branch points. It is a highly branched structure and branching occurs more frequently, i.e. after every 10-12 glucose residues (Fig. 1.14)

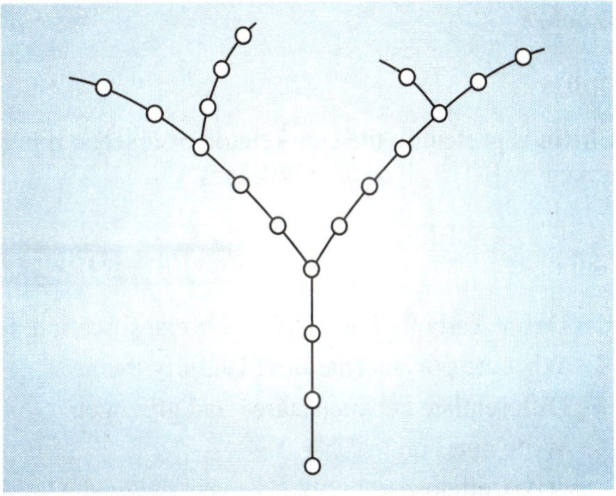

Fig. 1.14. Structure of glycogen

In the liver, glycogen is used as a readily available source of glucose during starvation.

Table 1.2 lists various differences between starch and glycogen.

Table 1.2. Differences between starch and glycogen

Starch	*Glycogen*
It is a plant reserve food, mostly stored in seeds	It is an animal reserve food, stored in the liver and muscle
It is less branched. Branching occurs after nearly 20-30 glucose units.	It is highly branched. Branching occurs after nearly 10-12 glucose units.
It consists of amylose and amylopectin	No such structures are present
It is sparingly soluble in cold water and forms a paste in hot water.	It forms an opalescent solution in water.
It gives violet color with iodine	It gives brown to red color with iodine

Cellulose

Cellulose is a component of **plant cell wall.** It is a linear polymer having β-D glucosyl-(1→4)-α-D glucosyl repeating units. Cellulose thus **has β-(1→4)** glycosidic **linkages.**

Cellulose can not be digested by human beings because they lack cellulases, enzymes that are capable of hydrolyzing β-(1→4) linkages. Cellulose, though can not be utilized by human beings, it forms a considerable part of the vegetarian food and adds to bulk of the feces.

Inulin

Inulin is a linear **polymer of β-D fructose**. It occurs in bulbs of dahalia, onion, and garlic. Inulin is not utilized by human beings but is of biological significance since **it is used in determination of the glomerular filtration rate (GFR).**

Dextrans

Dextrans are **highly branched homopolymers of glucose** having 1→6, 1→4, as well as1→3 linkages. Various microorganisms grown in a sucrose media produce dextrans. They have molecular weights between 1-4 millions. They are used for intravenous infusion, as volume expanders, in the treatment of a **hypovolemic shock.**

Chitin

Chitin is present in the exoskeleton of insects. It is composed of **N-acetylglucosamine residues**, which are linked by β-1 **4**-glycosidic **linkages.**

SOME IMPORTANT QUESTIONS

1. Define carbohydrate. Give their classification. Explain stereoisomerism of carbohydrates.
2. What are polysaccharides? Classify them.
3. Differentiate between starch and glycogen.
4. Write notes on :
   (i) Cellulose
   (ii) Anomerism
   (iii) Epimerism
   (iv) Inulin
   (v) Homopolysaccharides
   (vi) Heteropolysaccharides

CHAPTER

2

Chemistry of Lipids

Lipids (Greek: *lipos,* fat) is a heterogeneous group of **hydrophobic organic molecules** found in cells. They are **sparingly soluble in water** but **soluble in organic solvents,** such as acetone, ether, alcohol, and chloroform. Lipids, therefore, can be easily separated from other biological material by their extraction into an organic solvent.

BIOLOGICAL IMPORTANCE OF LIPIDS

1. Lipids are important dietary constituents of food, due to their **high calorific value.**
2. Dietary lipids are also sources of the **fat-soluble vitamins** and **essential fatty acids.**
3. Lipids also serve as **energy stores,** e.g. fat stored in the adipose tissue.
4. Fat, present in the subcutaneous tissue, acts as an **insulating material.**
5. Lipids, in the form of a bilayer, together with proteins are important **components of biological membranes.**
6. Lipids are also involved in **signaling events.**

CLASSIFICATION OF LIPIDS

Lipids exhibit greater structural variability and constitute a category of the substances that are similar only in that they are largely hydrophobic and soluble in nonpolar solvents. They are classified into three groups, as **simple lipids, compound lipids,** and **derived lipids** (Fig. 2.1).

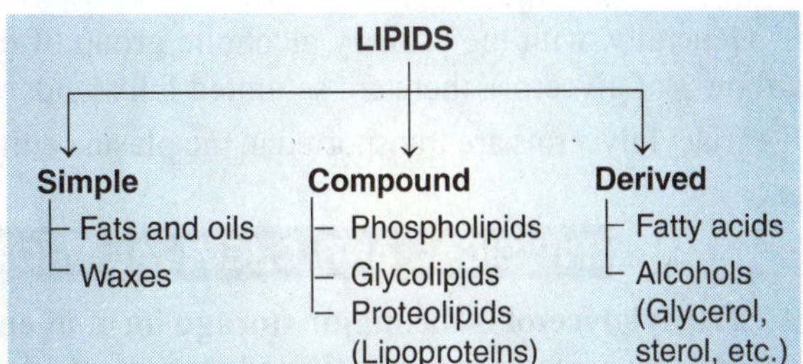

Fig. 2.1. Classification of lipids.

SIMPLE LIPIDS

Simple lipids are **esters of fatty acids** with various types of **alcohols.** They include fats, oils and waxes.

Fats and oils are mixtures of triacylglycerols (triglycerides) whose fatty acid composition may vary with source. They differ only in that **fats** are **solid** while **oils** are **liquid** at room temperature.

Fats are obtained from animal sources. They have, comparatively, more number of saturated fatty acids. They also have higher melting points.

On the other hand, **oils** are obtained from the plant seeds. They are usually rich in unsaturated fatty acids and have low melting points.

Esters of long chain fatty acids with high molecular weight mono-hydroxy aliphatic alcohols are called **waxes**. They are used in manufacturing of wax-polish.

COMPOUND LIPIDS

In addition to **fatty acids** and **alcohol, compound lipids** also contain an **amphipathic group.** For example, lipids conjugated with phosphoric acid are called **phospholipids.**

DERIVED LIPIDS

They are derived after the hydrolysis of simple and compound lipids. They include **fatty acids, glycerol,** etc.

TRIACYLGLYCEROLS

Triacylglycerols (also called **triglycerides**) or *neutral fats* are the **fatty acid tri-esters of glycerol** (glycerin), which is a tri-hydric alcohol.

Glycerol with one molecule of fatty acid is called **monoacylglycerol,** with two molecules of fatty acids as **diacylglycerol** and with three molecules of fatty acids as **triacylglycerol** (Fig. 2.2).

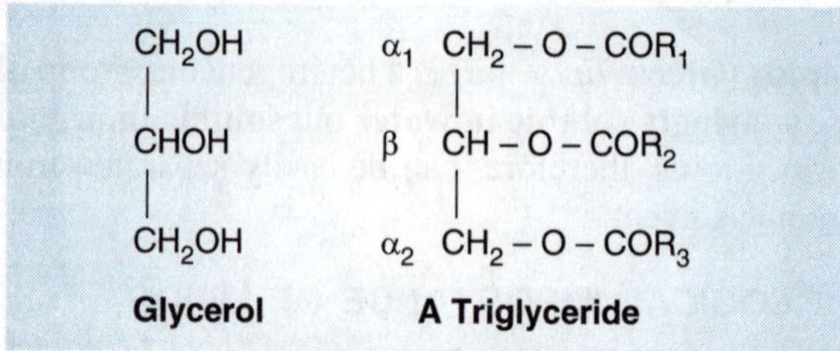

Fig. 2.2. Structure of Glycerol and a Triglyceride.

A molecule of the triacylglycerol may contain three similar or dissimilar fatty acids, which may be saturated and/or unsaturated. Most of the triacylglycerols contain different types of fatty acids.

Triglycerides are named according to presence of the fatty acid residues attached to glycerol, e.g. 1-palmitoyl-2-arachidonoyl-3-stearoylglycerol has palmitic acid at carbon 1, arachidonic acid at carbon 2, and stearic acid at carbon 3 of glycerol.

All natural fats and oils invariably, are the mixed triacylglycerols. Plant oils are usually rich in unsaturated fatty acids.

Generally, with the primary alcoholic group of the triacylglycerol, i.e. at α-positions (at carbon-1 and carbon-3 of glycerol), there are saturated fatty acids while at carbon-2 there is an unsaturated fatty acid.

Triacylglycerols are transported in the plasma either as chylomicrons or as very low-density lipoproteins.

PHYSICAL AND CHEMICAL PROPERTIES OF TRIACYLGLYCEROLS

1. **Triacylglycerol** is the **major storage form of energy** in the body. In animals, the fat cells (adipocytes) are specialized for synthesis and storage of triacylglycerols. Average fat content of a normal human being is about 21% in men and 26% in women. This allows them to survive for 2-3 months.
2. They can be **hydrolyzed** by **lipases,** to **free fatty acids** and **glycerol** (Fig. 2.3).
3. Naturally occurring fats, particularly from animal source, develop unpleasant odor and taste, if stored

under moist conditions. This is called **rancidity**. Antioxidants, e.g. vitamin E, can prevent development of rancidity.

4. **Unsaturated fatty acids,** found in triacylglycerols, can **accept halogen,** such as iodine at the double bond. This process is termed as **halogenation**. It is a measure of degree of unsaturation.

$$\begin{array}{lcll} CH_2OCOC_{15}H_{31} & & CH_2OH & \\ | & & | & \\ CHOCOC_{15}H_{31} & \xrightarrow{\text{Lipase}} & CHOH & + 3\,C_{15}H_{31}COOH \\ | & & | & \\ CH_2OCOC_{15}H_{31} & & CH_2OH & \\ \textbf{Tripalmitin} & & \textbf{Glycerol} & \textbf{Palmitic acid} \end{array}$$

Fig. 2.3. Hydrolysis of a Triglyceride.

FATTY ACIDS

Fatty acids are **the carboxylic acids** with a **long hydrocarbon side chain.** The hydrocarbon chain may be **saturated or unsaturated**, with one or more double bonds.

Major source of the circulating free fatty acids is adipose tissue. Free fatty acids also enter plasma during intra-plasmic hydrolysis of triacylglycerols in chylomicrons and very low-density lipoproteins. Although plasma concentration of free fatty acids is low, they have very rapid turnover and are important source of energy for many tissues. Since they have limited solubility in water, they are bound to plasma albumin, which has specific binding sites for free fatty acids.

Nomenclature of fatty acids

Nomenclature of fatty acids may be either according to the **delta (δ) system** or the **omega (ω) system.**

Delta System of Nomenclature

In this system of nomenclature, **carbon atoms** in a fatty acid are **numbered** beginning with the **carboxyl carbon** (–COOH) as **carbon number 1**. The next carbon, to which the carboxyl group is attached, is designated as **carbon number 2**. This is also called **α-carbon atom**. Accordingly, carbon 3 is referred as the β carbon, and so on. This system of numbering the carbons is called **delta (δ) system** of nomenclature.

Omega System of Nomenclature

In this system of nomenclature, **carbon atoms** are **counted,** beginning with the **methyl terminal (CH_3^-) end** of the chain, where a double bond first encounters. This carbon atom, i.e. the carbon atom of the terminal CH_3 group is called **omega (ω) carbon** and this system of nomenclature is called **omega (ω) system**. Recently, replacement of the symbol ω, by the letter "n" has been recommended (Fig. 2.4).

Most of the naturally occurring fatty acids have even number of carbon atoms because they are synthesized from acetyl CoA, i. e. by combination of the two carbon units. They are divided into three groups as **short chain fatty acids** containing 4-8 carbons, **medium chain fatty acids** with 10-14 carbons, and **long chain fatty acids** having 16 or more carbons. They have different physico-chemical properties and are metabolized in the body, in different ways.

In plants and higher animals, predominant fatty acids are those containing 16 or 18 carbon atoms, such as palmitic acid, oleic acid, linoleic acid, and stearic acid.

$$\begin{array}{cccccccccc} & & & & & \gamma & \beta & (\alpha\text{– carbon}) & & \\ CH_3 - & CH_2 - & CH_2 - & CH_2 - & CH_2 - & CH_2 - & CH_2 - & CH_2 - & CH_2 - & COOH \\ (\omega\text{-carbon}) & & & & & & 4 & 3 & 2 & 1 \quad \text{Carbon atom number} \end{array}$$

Fig. 2.4. Nomenclature of a fatty acid.

PHYSICAL AND CHEMICAL PROPERTIES OF FATTY ACIDS

1. Generally, **short chain fatty acids** are **liquid** while **long chain fatty acids** are **solid** at room temperature.
2. Fatty acids present in various oils, react with **alkali** and form **salts.** Salts of various fatty acids are used as **soaps** and **emulsifying agents.**
3. **Unsaturated fatty acids** undergo reduction and are **converted to saturated fat,** such as hydrogenation of vegetable oil results in the formation of ghee.
4. **Unsaturated fatty acids** exhibit **cis-trans isomerism** due to presence of double bonds.
5. Various fatty acids can be **separated** from a mixture **by gas liquid chromatography.**

Saturated Fatty Acids

Saturated fatty acids end in **"-anoic"**, e.g. octadecanoic acid (stearic acid) that is a fatty acid with 18 carbon atoms. Saturated fatty acids are highly flexible molecules and can assume wide range of conformations because there is relatively free rotation around each of their C-C bonds. These are obtained from animal fats, e.g. butter.

Saturated fatty acids of common biological significance are listed in Table 2.1.

Table 2.1. Saturated fatty acids

Fatty acids	*No. of carbons*	*Formula*	*Sources*
Acetic acid	2	CH_3-COOH	Fermentation of carbohydrates
Butyric acid	4	CH_3-$(CH_2)_2$-COOH	Butter
Caproic acid	6	CH_3-$(CH_2)_4$-COOH	Butter, some fats from plants
Caprylic acid	8	CH_3-$(CH_2)_6$-COOH	- do -
Capric acid	10	CH_3-$(CH_2)_8$-COOH	- do -
Lauric acid	12	CH_3-$(CH_2)_{10}$-COOH	Coconut oil
Myristic acid	14	CH_3-$(CH_2)_{12}$-COOH	- do -
Palmitic acid	16	CH_3-$(CH_2)_{14}$-COOH	Animal and plant fats
Stearic acid	18	CH_3-$(CH_2)_{16}$-COOH	- do -
Arachidic acid	20	CH_3-$(CH_2)_{18}$-COOH	Peanut oil

Unsaturated Fatty Acids

Unsaturated fatty acids end with **"-enoic"**, e.g. octadecenoic acid (oleic acid) that is a fatty acid with 18 carbon atoms with one double bond.

Widely used convention to name an unsaturated fatty acid is to indicate number of carbon atoms. This is followed by the number of double bonds with their positions in the chain, such as octadecenoic acid (18:1; 9) that is a fatty acid with 18 carbons with one double bond at carbon 9, i.e. between carbon-9 and -10 (Fig. 2.5).

$$\overset{18}{CH_3} - (CH_2)_7 - \overset{10}{CH} = \overset{9}{CH} - (CH_2)_7 - \overset{1}{COOH}$$

Fig. 2.5. Oleic acid (18 : 1; 9).

The number followed by the symbol Δ also indicates number of double bonds. This is followed by a superscript, which indicates number of carbons. For example, linoleic acid that has 18 carbons and two double bonds at carbons 9 and 12 can be written as 18: 2 $\Delta^{9,\,12}$ (Fig. 2.6).

According to ω system of nomenclature, linoleic acid is designated as ω-6 fatty acid because the double bond that is close to the ω-end is present on the sixth carbon (from the ω-end).

Double bonds may be present in cis- or trans-orientation. Naturally occurring fatty acids predominantly, have cis-double bonds. Unsaturated fatty acids are chemically more reactive than the saturated fatty acids and are more prone to alterations, such as lipid peroxidation. Fluidity of the lipid also increases with the degree of unsaturation.

18 13 12 10 9 1

$$CH_3-(CH_2)_4-CH=CH-CH_2-CH=CH-(CH_2)_7-COOH$$

C18; 2 $\Delta^{9,12}$

OR

1(ω) 6 18

$$CH_3-(CH_2)_4-CH=CH-CH_2-CH=CH-(CH_2)_7-COOH$$

An ω-6 fatty acid

Fig. 2.6. Linoleic acid.

Polyunsaturated Fatty Acids

Fatty acids obtained from the plant seeds usually contain **two or more double bonds.** These fatty acids are called **polyunsaturated fatty acids (PUFA)**. In these fatty acids double bonds generally occur after every three carbons. They are mainly obtained from plants oils, e.g. soybean oil, sunflower oil, groundnut oil, etc.

Physiological Significance of PUFA

1. Three PUFAs, i.e. linoleic acid, linolenic acid, and arachidonic acid, form an **essential** component of a human diet since they are necessary for **growth** as well as **normal health**. Hence, they are called as essential fatty acids.
2. They are also important constituents of a biological **membrane.**
3. They are also used for **esterification of cholesterol** and thus help in its transport and metabolism. Particularly, consumption of the fat containing **ω-6 fatty acids** helps in **lowering plasma cholesterol.**
4. Diet rich in **ω-3 fatty acids** promotes **reduction in plasma triacylglycerols.**
5. **Arachidonic acid** also acts as **precursor of eicosanoids,** such as **prostaglandins, thromboxanes,** and **leukotrienes.**

PHOSPHOLIPIDS

Phospholipids are a heterogeneous group of compounds, which contain one or more phosphoric acid residues and a polar group that may be a nitrogenous base, an amino acid, or a polyhydroxyalcohol. In addition, they also contain one or two long chain fatty acids.

They are **amphipathic in nature,** i.e. they contain both a **hydrophilic head** and a long **hydrophobic tail**.

The **hydrophilic domain** interacts with the aqueous environment and contains phosphate group plus the attached alcohol, e.g. serine, choline, etc.

The **hydrophobic domain** forms the nonaqueous environment and contains a long chain fatty acid or fatty acid-derived hydrocarbon.

Physiological Significance of Phospholipids

1. Phospholipids are the predominant lipids of a **cell membrane**. Membrane phospholipids also function as a reservoir for intracellular messengers. They also serve as anchor for some proteins in a cell membrane.
2. Phospholipids are also **components of the lung surfactants**.
3. They are also **essential component of bile** and help in the regulation of cholesterol.

Classification of Phospholipids

Phospholipids are classified into several groups (Table 2.2):

Table 2.2. Classification of phospholipids

Glycerophospholipids
• Lecithin (Phosphatidylcholine)
• Cephalins (Phosphatidylethanolamine and phosphatidylserine)
• Phosphatidylinositols
• Cardiolipin and plasmalogens
Sphingolipids
• Sphingomyelins
• Cerebrosides
• Gangliosides

Glycerophospholipids

Phospholipids, which are **derivatives of glycerol**, are called glycerophospholipids or phosphoglycerides. They are major components of a biological membrane. They are derivatives of phosphatidic acid.

Phosphatidic acid consists of a molecule of glycerol, two residues of fatty acids, and a molecule of phosphoric acid (Fig. 2.7).

When phosphoric acid is attached at carbon 3 of glycerol, it is referred to as glycerol-3-phosphate. Its carbon-1 and -2 are esterified with two fatty acids. Usually, a saturated fatty acid is attached at carbon-1 (α -carbon) while commonly a polyunsaturated fatty acid is attached at carbon-2 (β-carbon) of glycerol.

The phosphoryl group of phosphatidic acid may be linked either to a nitrogenous compound, such as ethanolamine, choline, serine; or to some other group like inositol. Various glycerophospholipids include phosphatidylethanolamine (cephalin), phosphatidylcholine (lecithin), phosphatidylinositol, etc.

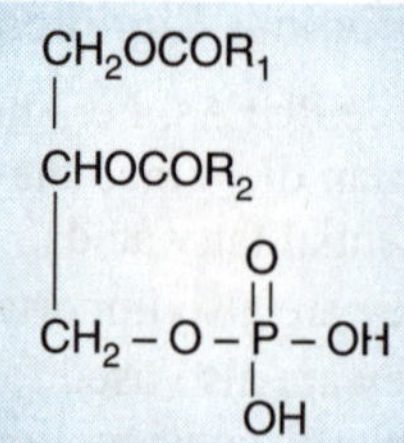

Fig. 2.7. Phosphatidic acid.

Lecithins

Lecithins contain **choline** (a nitrogenous base) at carbon 3 in phosphatidic acid. They are surface active agents and help in emulsification of fat. They are widely distributed in the brain, nerve cells, sperm, and egg yolk. Various hydrolytic enzymes, known as phospholipases, act at different sites of glycerophospholipids and hydrolyze them. For example, phospholipase A_2 removes a fatty acid from carbon 2 and forms lysophospholipid (Fig. 2.8).

Cephalins

Cephalins are glycerophospholipids where instead of choline present in the lecithin either **ethanolamine** or **serine** is present as a nitrogenous base. Cephalins are present in erythrocyte membrane, brain, and many other tissues.

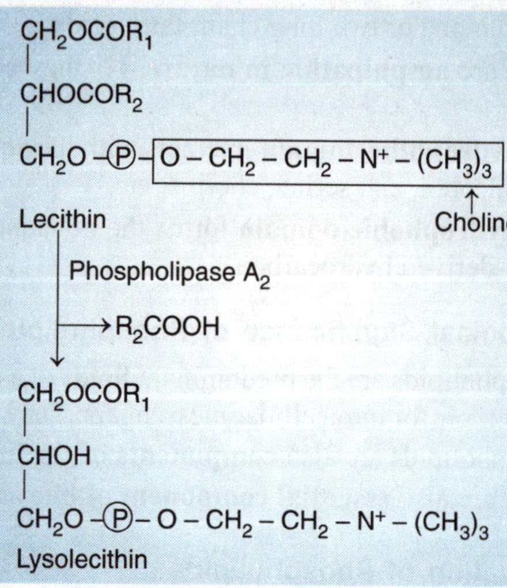

Fig. 2.8. Lecithins.

Phosphatidylinositols

Phosphatidylinositols are the glycerophospholipids containing inositol instead of a nitrogenous base. They are found, mainly, in the brain.

Plasmalogens

Plasmalogens are the glycerophospholipids in which carbon 1 of **glycerol** is linked to **an unsaturated fatty acid,** by an ether linkage (in the cis configuration), rather than with a saturated fatty acid, which is linked by the ester linkage. Plasmalogens are present in cardiac and skeletal muscles and semen. Because of their large concentration in the cardiac muscle, these are also called cardiolipin.

Sphingolipids

Sphingolipids do not contain glycerol but are derivatives of an unsaturated amino alcohol, which is referred to as **sphingosine**. Sphingolipids have 18 carbon atoms and one double bond.

N-Acyl derivatives of sphingosine are called **ceramides**. They are the parent compounds of most of the sphingolipids, e.g. sphingomyelins, cerebrosides, and gangliosides.

Sphingomyelin

Sphingomycelins are the **ceramides, which contain** either **phosphocholine** or **phosphoethanolamine** and are called **sphingophospholipids.** Myelin sheath, that surrounds and electrically insulates many nerve cell axons, is rich in sphingomyelin.

Cerebrosides

Cerebrosides are glycosphingolipids. They contain **ceramide that is attached to a sugar residue,** such as galactose or glucose. Hence, cerebrosides are ceramide-monosaccharides. Most prevalent cerebrosides are **galactocerebrosides** and **glucocerebrosides.**

A number of the cerebrosides are found in white matter of the brain and in the myelin sheath of nerves. They are named with respect to the presence of fatty acid, e.g. a galactosylceramide called **cerebron** contains cerebronic acid. Similarly, **nervon** has an unsaturated derivative of lignoceric acid, called nervonic acid.

Gangliosides

Gangliosides are the most complex glycosphingolipids. They are **ceramides that contain oligosaccharides,** including those containing **hexosamines** (glucosamine or galactosamine) and at least one molecule of **N-acetylneuraminic acid** (NANA or sialic acid).

Gangliosides are present in large amount in ganglion cells of the central nervous system, particularly, in the nerve endings. More than 60 gangliosides are known to occur. Each one of it has different oligosaccharide head-groups. Gangliosides are designated as GM_1, GM_2, GM_3, etc.

CHOLESTEROL

Cholesterol is a steroid, a derivative of **the cyclopentanoperhydrophenanthrene ring,** also called the **steroid nucleus,** that consists of four-fused, non polar rings, which are labeled as A, B, C, and D (Fig. 2.9).

Cholesterol is a most abundant steroid in animals. It has **27 carbons,** a **hydroxyl group** at **carbon 3,** a **double bond** between **carbons 5 and 6, two methyl groups at carbons 18 and 19,** and a **side chain at carbon 17** (Fig. 2.10).

Because of presence of an OH group, cholesterol is a steroid alcohol (sterol). Due to the presence of this group, cholesterol gets esterified with a long-chain fatty acid and forms ester.

An adult man contains about 1g of cholesterol/kg body weight. Nearly 25% of it is present in membrane of the nervous system, as a major component of the myelin sheath. Cholesterol is also a major component of plasma membrane. **Cholesterol** is also a metabolic **precursor** of various substances, such as **steroid hormones** (glucocorticoids, and mineralocorticoids (androgens and estrogens), **vitamin D**, and **bile acids and salts**.

Normal serum cholesterol level is 140-220 mg/dl.

Egg, meat, and milk are important dietary sources of cholesterol. It is also synthesized in the body by nearly all the cells. The amount of cholesterol synthesized, each day, in man is at least twice that of what is ingested in diet.

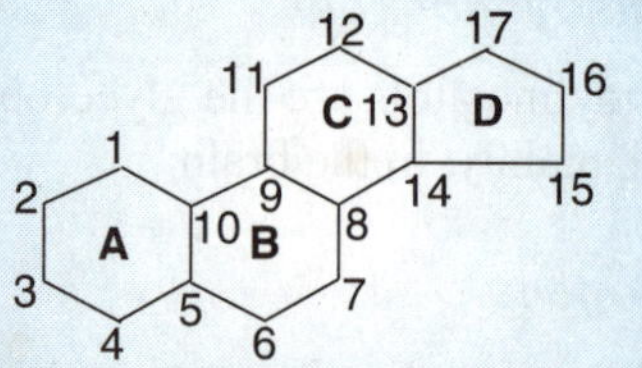

Fig. 2.9. Steroid nucleus (cyclopentanoperhydrophenanthrene ring).

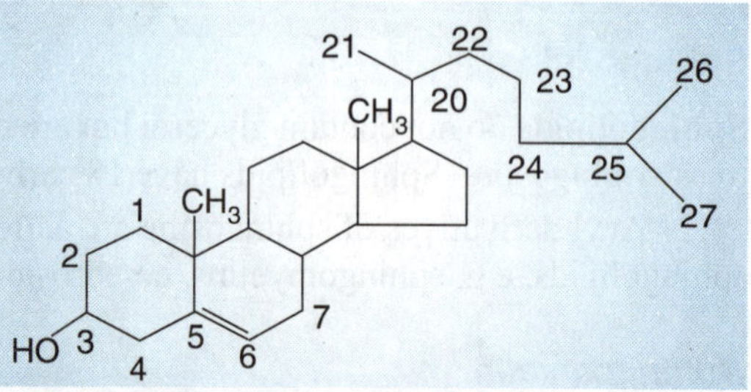

Fig. 2.10. Cholesterol.

BILE SALTS

Bile salts are **glycine or taurine conjugates of bile acids**. Bile acids contain 24 carbons with two or three hydroxyl groups and a side chain that has a carboxyl group, which is not fully ionized at physiological pH. They are amphipathic in nature.

Primary Bile Acids

Bile acids are synthesized in the liver from cholesterol. The most common compounds that are synthesized in the liver are **cholic acid and chenodeoxycholic acid**, called **primary bile acids.** Before they leave the liver, they are conjugated to a molecule of either glycine or taurine (derived from cystine) by an amide bond, which is formed between the carboxyl group of the bile acid and the amino group of the added glycine or taurine. These conjugates, i.e. **glycocholate and glycochenodeoxycholate** as well as **taurocholate and taurochenodeoxycholate** are referred to as **bile salts**. Normally, the ratio of glycine to taurine conjugates is approximately 3:1. Because of their enhanced amphipathic nature, bile salts are more effective detergents than bile acids.

Secondary Bile Acids

Bacteria in the intestine remove glycine and taurine from bile salts and regenerate bile acids. These bacteria also remove a hydroxyl group from the primary bile acids, producing **deoxycholic acid** (from cholic acid) and **lithocholic acid** (from chenodeoxycholic acid). These compounds are called **secondary bile acids.**

The mixture of primary and secondary bile acids and salts is observed primarily, in the ileum. They are actively transported from the intestinal mucosal cells into the portal blood and are removed by the liver parenchymal cells. The liver converts both primary and secondary bile acids into bile salts by conjugation with glycine or taurine and secrets them into the bile.

The continuous process of secretion of bile salts into the bile, their passage through the duodenum where some are converted to bile acids, and their subsequent return to the liver as a mixture of bile acids and salts is termed ***enterohepatic circulation***.

Bile salts have detergent properties and are essential for the digestion and absorption of dietary lipids.

MICELLES AND BIMOLECULAR LEAFLET

In living systems, lipids are rarely found as free molecules but are generally associated with other molecules, usually other lipids. The basic structural characteristic of membrane is due to the physiochemical properties of the glycerophosphate lipids and sphingolipids. These amphipathic compounds have a **hydrophobic head** and **hydrophilic tail**, which interact in aqueous system, to form spheres termed **micelles**. Their changed polar head groups are on the outside of the sphere while the hydrophobic tails interact to exclude water.

Micelles are the spheroid globules of up to several thousand amphiphilic molecules arranged so that the hydrophilic groups at the globule surface can interact with the aqueous solvent while the hydrophobic groups associate at the center, away from the solvent. Micelles have only one polar surface, which is the side presented to the aqueous phase. Micelles can be prepared that contain a single lipid or a mixture of lipids. Formation of micelles also depends on the temperature and ratio of concentration of the different lipids. The structure of a micelle is very stable because of hydrophobic interactions between hydrocarbon chains and attraction of the polar head groups to water.

Micelles are important in intestinal digestion and absorption of lipids. The approximate size and shape of a micelle can vary. For example, the single tailed amphiphiles, such as soap anions because of their tapered shapes, form spheroidal or ellipsoidal micelles. On the other hand, the two hydrocarbon tails of glycerophospholipids and sphingolipids because of the cylindrical van der Walls envelope causes them to form large disk like micelles that look similar to the extended ***bimolecular leaflet***, as in a **lipid bilayer**.

A ***lipid bilayer*** has two layers of lipids, forming a structure in which there is minimal contact of hydrocarbon chains with water. The polar head groups are at the interface between the aqueous medium and the lipid and the hydrophobic tails interact, creating an interior hydrophobic environment that excludes water. Lipid bilayers are extremely stable, being held together by hydrophobic forces of hydrocarbon chains and ionic interaction of charged head groups with water. This bilayer configuration is the basic lipid structure of all biological membranes (Fig. 2.11).

LIPOPROTEINS

Various lipids such as triacylglycerols, cholesterol, and phospholipids are sparingly soluble in aqueous solution (plasma) hence they are transported in blood in association with proteins. These protein-lipid complexes are

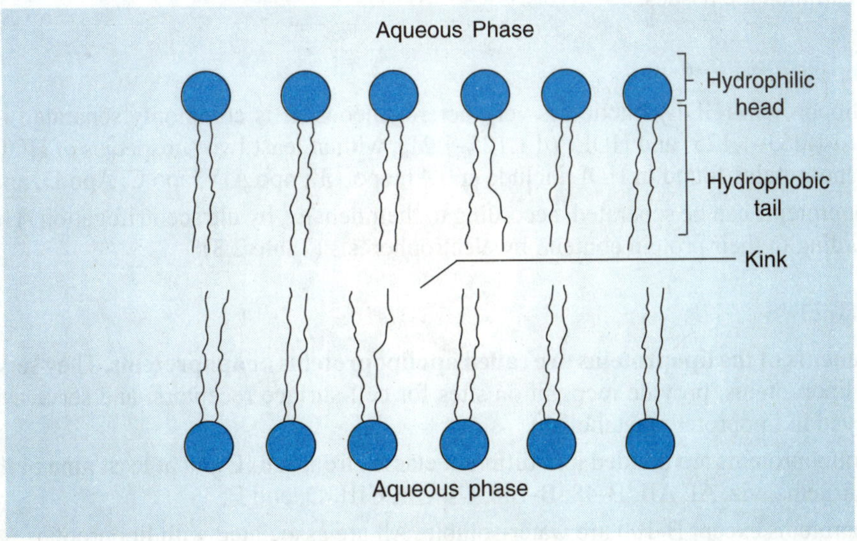

Fig. 2.11. The lipid bilayer.

called **lipoproteins** or proteolipids. They **are globular, micelle-like particles consisting of** nonpolar core of **triacylglycerols** and **cholesterol esters,** which are surrounded by the amphiphilic coat of **proteins, cholesterol, and phospholipids.**

Classification of Lipoproteins

Lipoproteins are classified into different groups as follows:

Chylomicrons

They are very large particles, which are secreted into intestinal lymphatics by mucosal cells of the small intestine. About 90% of its mass is triglycerides, which together with cholesterol esters and fat soluble vitamins form core of the particle. The surface layer is made of free cholesterol, phospholipids, and apoproteins (apo B48, Apo AI, and Apo AIV).

Very Low Density Lipoproteins

Very low density lipoproteins (VLDL) are large particles, which are secreted into blood stream by hepatocytes. Fifty to sixty percent of their mass is triacylglycerols. They contain relatively more cholesterol esters than chylomicrons. Their surface coat contains free cholesterol and phospholipids, a single molecule of Apo B-100 and other apoproteins. Eventually, VLDL is transformed into intermediate density lipoproteins (IDL).

Intermediate Density Lipoproteins

Intermediate density lipoproteins (IDL) are derived from catabolism of VLDL. They are referred to as IDL (also called LDL_1) since their density as well as lipid composition is in between VLDL and LDL. Major apoproteins of IDL is apo C and apo B–100. IDL is either removed by the liver or converted to LDL_2, also called low-density lipoproteins (LDL).

Low Density Lipoproteins

Low-density lipoprotein (LDL) has a density range of 1.019–1.063. It contains a single molecule of apo B–100 and carries about 75% of the total cholesterol in human plasma. Its major function is to transport cholesterol to extrahepatic tissues.

High Density Lipoproteins

High-density lipoprotein (HDL) fraction is very heterogeneous. It is commonly separated into two major classes HDL_2 (d 1.063–1.125) and HDL_3 (d 1.125–1.21), with at least two subspecies of HDL_2 and three of HDL_3. Major apoproteins found in HDL include apo AI, apo AII, apo AIV, apo C, Apo D, and Apo E.

Various lipoproteins can be separated, according to their density, by ultracentrifugation. They can also be separated according to their protein content, by electrophoresis (Table 2.3).

APOLIPOPROTEINS

Protein components of the lipoproteins are called apolipoproteins or **apoproteins.** They serve as structural component of lipoproteins, provide recognition sites for cell-surface receptors, and serve as activators for enzymes involved in lipoprotein metabolism.

Various apolipoproteins are divided into different classes from A to E and at least nine of them are found in human lipoproteins, viz. AI, AII, B-48, B-100, CI, CII, CIII, D, and E.

All the apoproteins except B-100 are water-soluble. All are associated with lipoproteins.

Table 2.3. Physical properties and chemical composition of human serum lipoproteins

	Chylomicrons	*VLDL*	*LDL_1(IDL)*	*LDL_2*	*HDL_2*	*HDL_3*
Density (g/ml)	<1.006	<1.006	1.006-1.019	1.019-1.063	1.063-1.125	1.125-1.210
S_f	>400	20-400	12-20	0-12	3.6-9.0	0-3.5
Electrophoretic mobility	Origin	Pre-β	Fast–β	β	α	α
Fasting plasma concentration (mg %)	—	20-300	10-20	200-400	40-100	120-300
Protein concentration (%)	2-4	8-12	15-20	20-25	40-45	50-55
Free cholesterol (%)	1-3	5-10	7-8	7-10	5	3-4
Cholesterol esters (%)	2-4	10-15	18-22	35-40	12-18	10-12
Triacylglycerols (%)	85-90	50-65	25-30	6-10	4-6	3-5
Phospholipids (%)	8-10	16-20	18-22	20-24	25-30	22-25

Apolipoprotein B–100 (apo B-100) is one of the largest monomeric proteins that is synthesized by the liver and is present in LDL.

SOME IMPORTANT QUESTIONS

1. What are lipids? Classify them. Give biological significance of lipids.
2. What are fatty acids? Classify them. Write biological significance of polyunsaturated fatty acids.
3. Describe briefly:
   (i) Classification of lipids with suitable examples
   (ii) Plasmalogens
   (iii) Sphingolipids
   (iv) Chemistry and functions of cholesterol
   (v) Cerebrosides.
4. Write notes on :
   (i) PUFA
   (ii) Triacylglycerol
   (iii) Lecithins
   (iv) Cardiolipin
   (v) Phospholipids
   (vi) Bile salts
   (vii) Micelles
   (viii) Bimolecular leaflet
   (ix) Lipid bilayer
   (x) Lipoproteins
   (xi) Apoproteins

CHAPTER

3

Chemistry of Proteins

Protein (Greek: *proteios*, means primary) is the class of natural products, which **contain nitrogen**. It is **essential for life**. It is now well known that proteins are at the center of action in biological processes and are **essential structural components of a cell**. They are most abundant and functionally diverse molecules present in living systems.

BIOLOGICAL IMPORTANCE OF PROTEINS

Proteins play several important roles in the body (Table 3.1).

Table 3.1. Biological importance of proteins

Biological role	*Examples*
As structural proteins	Collagen, keratins, etc.
As enzymes	Pepsin, amylase, etc.
As hormones	Insulin
As transport proteins	Hemoglobin
As receptors	Hormone receptors
For storage	Ferritin
In immune response	γ-Globulins

With respect to their biological importance, proteins are divided into different groups:

1. **Structural proteins:** Some proteins , e.g. **collagen** (found in bone and cartilage), **keratins** (found in hair and nail), etc., form an essential part of the particular structure with in the body
2. **Enzymes:** Proteins, such as **pepsin**, catalyze biological reactions.
3. **Hormones:** Some proteins act as hormones, e.g. **insulin**. They regulate metabolic processes within the body.

4. **Transport proteins:** These proteins, e.g. **hemoglobin** (for transport of O_2), **ceruloplasmin** (for Cu), etc., serve as carriers for transport of substances with in the body.
5. **Protein receptors:** Proteins, such as **hormone receptors**, act as receptors and play an important role in signal transduction.
6. **Storage proteins:** Some proteins bind a substance for its storage in different tissues, e.g. **ferritin** for storage of Fe^{3+}.
7. **Antibodies:** Proteins, such as **γ-globulins**, act as antibodies and provide immunity to the body.

AMINO ACIDS

All proteins, from whatever source it may be, are polymers of small units called **amino acids**. Although a large number of amino acids have been described in nature, only **20** are commonly found as constituents of mammalian proteins. Since amino acids are hydrolyzed products of proteins, they are also called building blocks of proteins. Commonly occurring amino acids are designated as **α-amino acids** because each amino acid has a **carboxylic group (–COOH), a primary amino group (–NH_2), and a distinctive side chain (R-group)**, which is present on the α-carbon atom.

General structure of an amino acid is shown in Fig. 3.1.

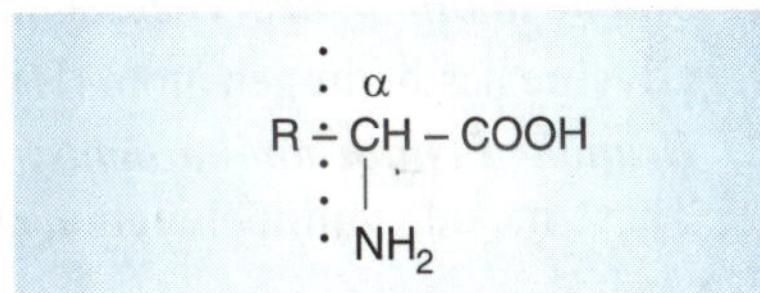

Fig. 3.1. General structure of an α-amino acid.

BIOLOGICAL SIGNIFICANCE OF AMINO ACIDS

1. Amino acids are important **dietary source of nitrogen.**
2. They are used in protein biosynthesis.
3. **Glucogenic amino acids**, e.g. alanine, serve **as a source of energy**.
4. Some of the **amino acids are also used in the biosynthesis** of various **specialized products. For example**
   (i) **Glycine** is a precursor for **creatine, glutathione, heme, bile acids,** and **purines.**
   (ii) **Sulphur-containing amino acids** are **source of sulphur** for the body.
   Cysteine is also used in the biosynthesis of glutathione while **methionine** is important in **one-carbon metabolism**.
   (iii) **Aromatic amino acids** are precursors **of thyroid hormones, catecholamines** (hormones of the adrenal medulla, i.e. dopamine, norepinephrine, and epinephrine), and **melanin** (a brown-black pigment present in skin).
   (iv) **Aspartate** and **glutamate** participate in **transamination reactions.**
   (v) **Aspartate and glutamine** are used **in the biosynthesis of purines** and **pyrimidines.**

CLASSIFICATION OF AMINO ACIDS

Amino acids may be classified according to the properties of their side chain. They are also classified according to the nutritional requirement.

Classification of Amino Acids Based on the Properties of Their Side Chain

According to the Charge of their Side Chain

According to the charges of their side chain (R-group attached to α-carbon atom), amino acids may be electrically neutral, have positive charge, or negative charge. Thus, based on the presence of the ionic charge, amino acids are classified as:

Neutral Amino Acids

These amino acids are neutral in reaction and have **one amino group ($-NH_2$)** and **one carboxylic group (–COOH)**. These amino acids are also referred as **monoamino-monocarboxylic acids.**

According to presence of the R group, these amino acids are further subdivided as aliphatic amino acids and aromatic amino acids:

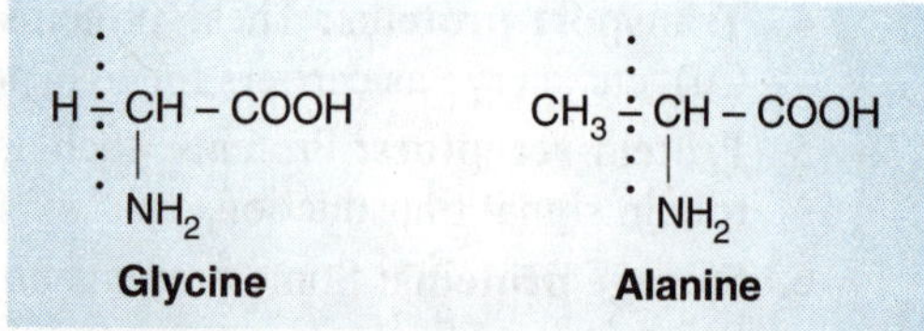

Fig. 3.2. Simple aliphatic amino acids.

Aliphatic Amino Acid

Aliphatic amino acids are further classified as:

1. ***Simple amino acids:*** These amino acids have either hydrogen or a simple aliphatic chain. **Glycine** has hydrogen atom (H) whereas **alanine** has a methyl group ($-CH_3$) (Fig. 3.2).
2. ***Branched chain amino acids*:** These amino acids have an aliphatic side chain, which has a branch. These include **valine, leucine,** and **isoleucine** (Fig. 3.3).

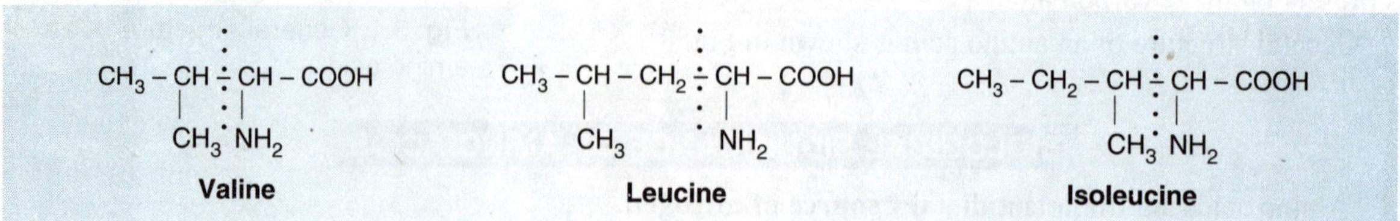

Fig. 3.3. Branched chain amino acids.

3. ***Hydroxy amino acids*:** These amino acids have a hydroxyl (–OH) group in its aliphatic side chain. These include **serine** and **threonine** (Fig. 3.4).
4. ***Sulphur containing amino acids*:** In addition to C, H, O, and N, these amino acids also contain sulphur (S) in the side chain. These include **cysteine** and **methionine.**

   Cysteine has a thiol group (–SH). It can combine with another cysteine residue and form **dicysteine,** which has a disulfide bond (–S–S–). **Dicysteine is also referred as cystine.**

   Methionine has a methyl group, which is attached to sulphur (CH_3–S–) in its side chain (Fig. 3.5).

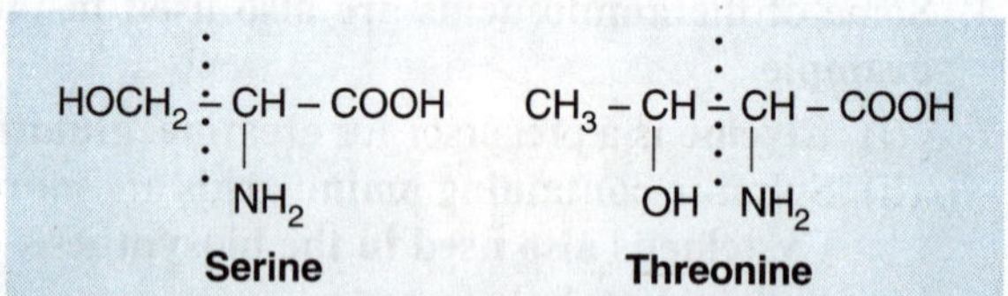

Fig. 3.4. Hydroxy amino acids.

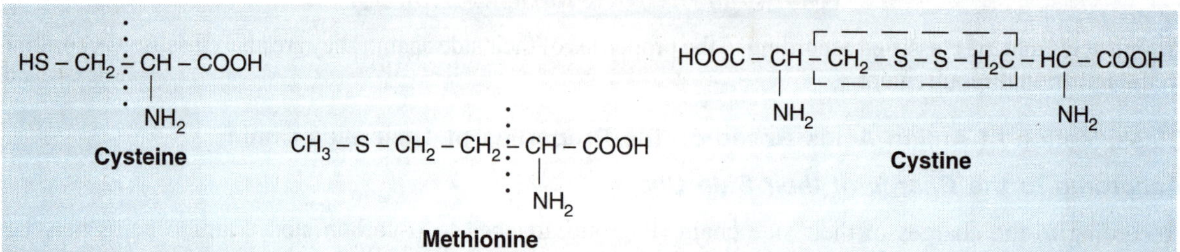

Fig. 3.5. Sulphur containing amino acids.

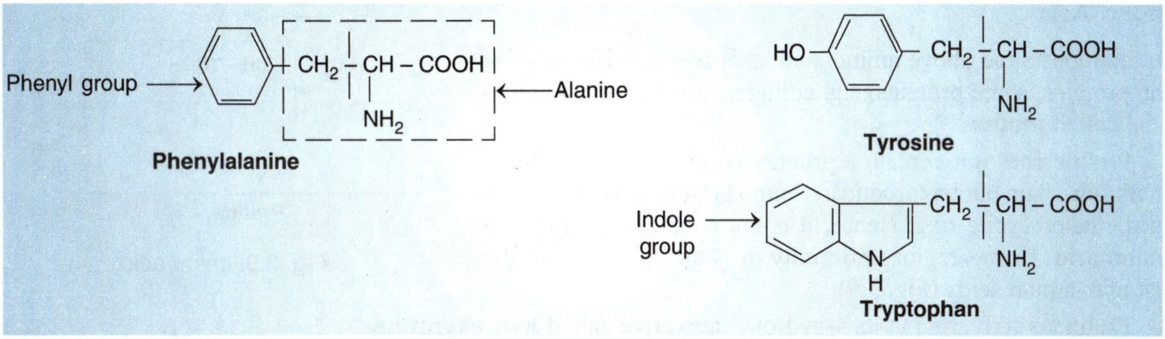

Fig. 3.6. Aromatic amino acids.

Aromatic Amino Acids

These amino acids have an **aromatic ring.** They include **phenylalanine** (alanine with a phenyl group), tyrosine (4-hydroxyphenylalanine), and **tryptophan** (alanine with an indole ring), as shown in Fig. 3.6.

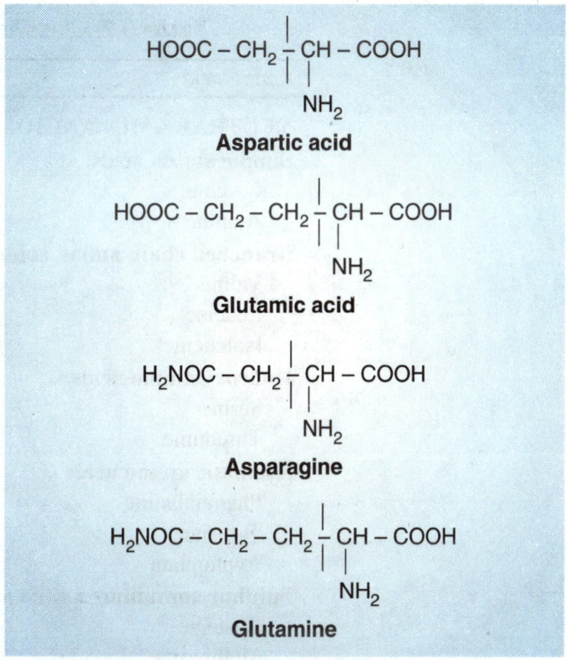

Fig. 3.7. Acidic amino acids and their amides.

Acidic Amino Acids

An acidic amino acid has **one amino group** but **more than one** (generally two) **carboxylic acid groups.** These amino acids are also referred as monoaminodicarboxylic acids. These are **aspartic acid** and **glutamic acid** (Fig. 3.7).

Besides, there are two amino acids, which occur as **amides** of these two amino acids.

Amide of aspartic acid is called **asparagine** while that of glutamic acid is called **glutamine** (Fig. 3.7).

Basic Amino Acids

Basic amino acids have **one carboxylic group** with either **more than one amino group** in its aliphatic side chain **or a heterocyclic ring,** which is basic in reaction. These are **lysine, arginine,** and **histidine.**

Lysine has **two $-NH_2$** groups while **arginine** has a **guanidino group** in the aliphatic side chain.

Histidine has a **heterocyclic ring** called imidazole ring, which is alkaline in reaction (Fig. 3.8).

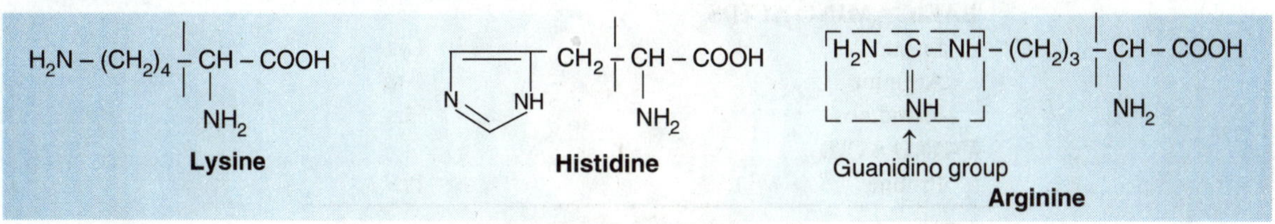

Fig. 3.8. Basic amino acids.

Imino Acid

In addition to the above amino acids that are found in most of the proteins, some proteins, e.g. collagen, are rich in an amino acid called **proline**.

Proline does not contain a primary α-amino group ($-NH_2$) in its side chain but has secondary imino group (–NH–) as a part of the heterocyclic ring. Hence, it is not an amino acid but an imino acid. However, for uniformity, it is also included in the list of α-amino acids (Fig. 3.9).

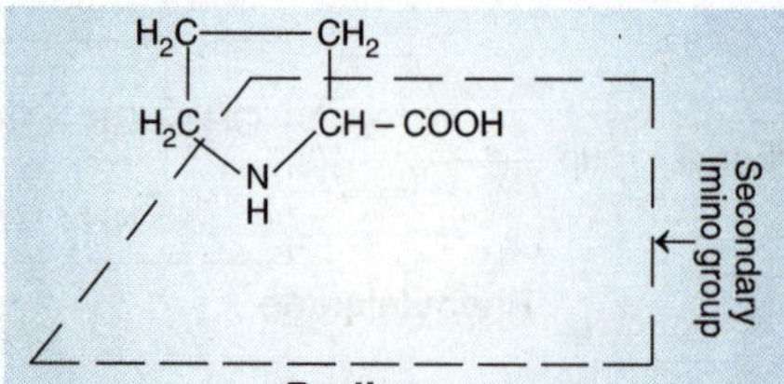

Fig. 3.9. Imino acid.

Proline is converted to its 4-hydroxy derivative called **hydroxyproline**.

Various naturally occurring amino acids, with their commonly used three-letter abbreviations, are shown in Table 3.2.

Table 3.2. Classification of amino acids

Amino acid	*Abbreviation**
NEUTRAL AMINO ACIDS	
Simple amino acids	
Glycine	Gly
Alanine	Ala
Branched chain amino acids	
Valine	Val
Leucine	Leu
Isoleucine	Ile
Hydroxy amino acids	
Serine	Ser
Threonine	Thr
Aromatic amino acids	
Phenylalanine	Phe
Tyrosine	Tyr
Tryptophan	Trp
Sulphur containing amino acids	
Cysteine	Cys
Methionine	Met
ACIDIC AMINO ACIDS	
Aspartic acid	Asp
Glutamic acid	Glu
Amides of the acidic amino acids	
Asparagine	Asn
Glutamine	Gln
BASIC AMINO ACIDS	
Lysine	Lys
Arginine	Arg
Histidine	His
IMINO ACID	
Proline	Pro

* Three-letter abbreviation is widely used. This, generally, includes first three letters of the amino acid.

Classification of Amino Acids According to Polarity of Side Chain

According to polarity of side chain, amino acids are classified as nonpolar or polar amino acids.

Amino Acids with a Non-polar Side Chain

Each such amino acid has a nonpolar side chain, which neither gives-off protons nor participates in hydrogen/ionic bonds, e.g. glycine, alanine, valine, leucine, isoleucine, methionine, phenylalanine, tryptophan, and proline.

Amino Acids with a Polar Side Chain

These amino acids have an uncharged polar side chain and have zero net charge at neutral pH. For example, serine, threonine, and tyrosine, each has a hydroxyl group that can participate in hydrogen bond formation. The hydroxyl group serves as a site of attachment for a phosphate group or an oligosaccharide.

Asparagine and glutamine contain a carboxyl group as well as an amide group both, of which also participate in a reaction.

Classification of Amino Acids Based on Their Nutritional Requirement

According to their nutritional requirement, amino acids are divided into two groups, referred as **essential amino acids and nonessential amino acids** (Table 3.3).

Table 3.3. Classification of amino acids according to nutritional requirement

Essential	*Semiessential*	*Nonessential*
Methionine	Arginine	Glycine
Threonine	Histidine	Alanine
Tryptophan		Serine
Valine		Cysteine
Isoleucine		Tyrosine
Leucine		Aspartate
Phenylalanine		Glutamate
Lysine		Asparagine
		Glutamine
		Proline

Essential Amino Acids

Among various amino acids that are found in proteins, all cannot be synthesized in the body. Some of them are to be essentially included in the diet. These are called indispensable or **essential amino acids.**

There are eight amino acids, which are essential for adult human beings. These are **methionine, threonine, tryptophan, valine, isoleucine, leucine, phenylalanine,** and **lysine.**

Semi essential Amino Acids

Arginine and **histidine** though are not essential for a normal adult human being but their synthesis is not sufficient during growth, pregnancy, and lactation, or during conditions, such as a high-grade fever and chronic infections, when their requirements are increased. Under these conditions, arginine and histidine also become dietary essential. Hence, these two amino acids are called **semi essential amino acids.**

Nonessential Amino Acids

The **remaining amino acids** can be synthesized by a normal human being. Hence they **are not dietary essential.** These amino acids are called **nonessential amino acids.**

GENERAL PROPERTIES OF AMINO ACIDS

Isomerism

All naturally occurring **amino acids** except glycine **have at least one asymmetric carbon atom** and **are optically active compounds. They have L-configuration.**

Acid Base Properties

Amino acids exhibit acid base properties. An amino acid may have either a positive charge or a negative charge. **At low pH, an amino acid exists in the cationic form** as its amino group is protonated and is present as $-NH_3^+$. As pH rises, carboxyl group loses its proton and the ampholyte form appears. With the further increase in pH, amino group is deprotonated and the anionic form is formed. At physiological pH (pH 7.4), their carboxyl groups are dissociated ($R-COO^-$) while the amino groups are protonated ($R-NH_3^+$).

Such an ionized molecule, which has both negative as well as positive charges, is called **ampholyte. Molecules with equal number of ionizable groups,** i.e. when the number of cations is equal to the number of anions, **are called zwitter ions.**

The pH at which molecules exist as a zwitter ion is called isoelectric pH or isolectric point (pI).

At pH more than its pI, the amino acid is negatively charged while at pH less than its pI, it is positively charged (Fig. 3.10).

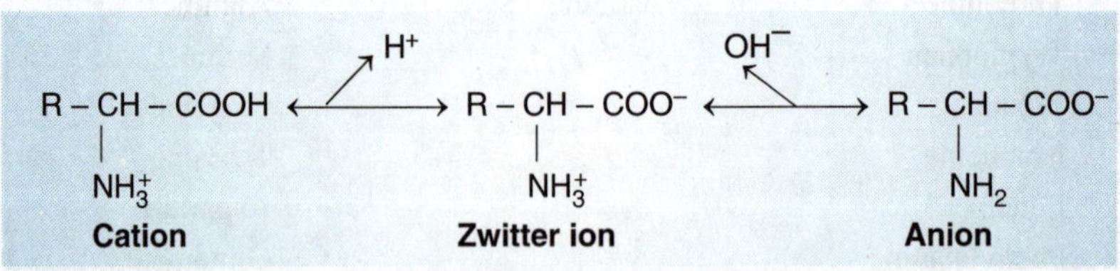

Fig. 3.10. Ionic forms of an amino acid.

Buffer Action

Amino acids in aqueous solution contain weakly acidic α-carboxyl groups and weakly basic α-amino groups. In addition, each of the acidic and basic amino acids contains an ionizable group in its side chain. Hence, **both free amino acids and some amino acids combined in peptide linkages can act as buffers.**

BUFFERS

A buffer is a solution, which **resists change in pH**; i.e. it minimizes a change in the H^+ concentration **following the addition of an acid or a base**. A buffer can be prepared by mixing a weak acid, e.g. HA, with its conjugate base (A^-). When a strong acid, such as HCl, is added to such a solution, A^- can neutralize it and in this process, it gets converted to HA. On the other hand, if a base is added HA gives its H^+ and gets converted to A^-.

$$\underset{\text{(Weak acid)}}{HA} \rightleftharpoons \underset{\text{(Proton)}}{H^+} + \underset{\text{(Salt or conjugate base)}}{A^-}$$

The dissociation constant (Ka) of the acid can be expressed as:

$$Ka = \frac{[H^+][A^-]}{[HA]}$$

The larger the Ka, the stronger is the acid because most of the HA has been converted into H^+ and A^-. Similarly, the smaller the Ka, the less acid has dissociated and therefore, the weaker is the acid.

A buffer has maximum buffering capacity at its pKa (–log Ka), when acidic and basic forms are present in equal concentrations. The acid, (protonated) form reacts with the added base while the basic (unprotonated) form neutralizes the added acid.

An amino acid, e.g. alanine, contains two ionizable groups, i.e. a α-carboxyl group (α-COOH) and a α-amino group (α-NH_3). While titrating the alanine solution from pH 0 to pH 12 with NaOH, these two groups are titrated. The pKa of the α-COOH group (pKa1) is 2.4 while that of the α-NH_3 group (pKa2) is 9.0. In the first stage of titration, i.e. at very low pH, the predominant ion species of alanine is the fully protonated form.

At the mid point in this first stage of titration (pH 2.4) or pKa1, equimolar concentrations of proton-donor and proton-acceptor species are present, proving good buffering power. The second stage of titration corresponds to the removal of a proton from the –NH_3^+ of alanine. The pH at mid point of this stage is 9.8, equal to the pKa for the –NH_3^+ group, again providing good buffering capacity. At about pH 12, the predominant form of alanine is the proton acceptor form.

When dissolved in water, alanine exists as a dipolar ion, or **zwitterion**, in which the carboxyl group is unprotonated (–COO^-) and the amino group is protonated (–NH_3^+). The pH of this solution is 6.2, i.e. the pI, which is halfway between the pKa of the carboxyl group (2.4) and the amino group (9.8).

The quantitative relationship between the concentration of a weak acid, e.g. HA and its conjugate base, i.e. A^- is described by the **Henderson-Hasselbalch equation.**

Henderson-Hasselbalch Equation

The general dissociation of a weak acid, such as a carboxylic acid, is given, by the euqation 1:

$$HA \rightleftharpoons H^+ + A^- \qquad ....1$$

Where, HA is the protonated form or the conjugate acid (associated form) and A^- is the unprotonated form or the conjugate base (the dissociated form)

The dissociation constant (Ka) for such a weak acid is defined as the equilibrium constant for the dissociation reaction of the acid, by equation 2:

$$Ka = \frac{[H^+][A^-]}{[HA]} \qquad ....2$$

The hydrogen ion concentration $[H^+]$ of a solution of a weak acid then can be calculated by rearranging this equation, to equation 3:

$$[H^+] = Ka \times \frac{[HA]}{[A^-]} \qquad ....3$$

A negative logarithm of the above can be expressed, as equation 4:

$$-\log [H^+] = -\log Ka - \log \frac{[HA]}{[A^-]} \qquad ....4$$

Since pH is the negative logarithm of $[H^+]$, multiplying to equation 4 by -1 arrives at the equation 5, which is referred as the Henderson-Hasselbalch equation:

$$pH = pKa + \log \frac{[A^-]}{[HA]} \quad ....5$$

Where pH is the negative logarithm of $[H^+]$, i.e. $-\log [H^+]$, pKa is equal to the negative logarithm of dissociation constant (Ka), i.e. as $-\log Ka$.

Henderson-Hasselbalch equation can be used for analysis of acid base equilibrium systems. The extent of protonation, of acidic and basic functional groups and therefore the net charge will vary with the pKa of the functional group and the pH of the solution. For example, for alanine, which has two functional groups with pKa1 of 2.4 and pKa2 of 9.8, the net charge varies with pH, from –1 to +1. At a point intermediate between the two pKa values (6.2), it has a net zero charge. This pH is called its **isoelectric point** (pI).

Formation of the Peptide Bond

Most important property of amino acids is formation of the **peptide bond (-CO-NH-)**. During this process, the carboxyl group of one amino acid reacts with the amino group of the next amino acid. The process is a condensation reaction and results in formation of an **amide linkage** (Fig. 3.11)

When several amino acids are linked together, a **polypeptide** is formed.

Each polypeptide has a **free α-amino group** on the first amino acid that is present on **left-hand** side of the peptide chain. This end of the protein chain is referred as **amino terminal (N-terminal) end.** A protein chain also has a free **α-carboxylic group** on the last amino acid that is present on the **right hand** side of the peptide chain. This end of the protein chain is referred as **carboxyl terminal (C-terminal) end** (Fig. 3.12).

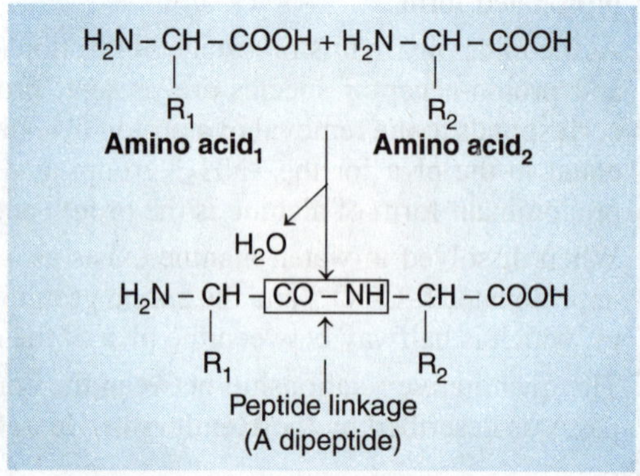

Fig. 3.11. Formation of the peptide bond.

$$H_2NAA_1 - AA_2 - AA_3 \text{-------------------} AA_{n-1} - AA_nCOOH$$

N-terminal end ... C-terminal end

Fig. 3.12. A polypeptide.

PROTEINS

Depending upon their **solubility** and **physical properties**, proteins are classified into three classes (Table 3.4).

Simple Proteins

Based on their solubility, simple proteins are further **subdivided** as follows:

1. ***Albumins:*** Albumins are present in serum, milk, egg, etc. They are soluble in water as well as in a salt solution.
2. ***Globulins:*** Globulins are present in serum, milk, and egg. They are sparingly soluble in water but soluble in a neutral salt solution.

3. ***Prolamines:*** Prolamines, e.g. gliadin of wheat or zein of maize, are insoluble in water but soluble in 60-80% of alcohol.
4. ***Glutelins:*** Glutelins, e.g. glutin of wheat or oryzenin of rice, are soluble in dilute acids and alkalies.
5. ***Scleroproteins:*** They are highly insoluble. Scleroproteins are present in supporting tissues, such as bone, cartilage, etc. They are also found in protective tissues like skin, hair, nail, etc.
6. ***Histones:*** Histones, e.g. nucleohistones, are rich in basic amino acids. They are soluble in water.

Conjugated Proteins

Proteins conjugated **with** a **nonprotein substance,** called prosthetic group, are referred as conjugated proteins. For example, **nucleoproteins** (histones conjugated with nucleic acids), **glycoproteins** (proteins conjugated with carbohydrates), **phosphoproteins** (phosphoric acid attached through the serine or threonine moieties of the protein, such as casein present in milk), **metalloproteins** (metal containing proteins, such as ceruloplasmin, a cuproprotein), and **lipoproteins** (lipid-associated proteins).

Derived Proteins

These are the derivatives of simple proteins such as denatured and coagulated proteins, called **primary derived proteins,** or those produced by the cleavage of the peptide bonds, called **secondary derived proteins**.

Table 3.4. Classification of proteins

Simple proteins	*Conjugated proteins*	*Derived proteins*
Albumins	Nucleoproteins	Primary derived proteins
Globulins	Glycoproteins	Secondary derived proteins
Prolamines	Phosphoproteins	
Glutelins	Metalloproteins	
Scleroproteins	Lipoproteins	
Histones		

PROTEIN CONFORMATION

Variations in number and order of amino acids, i.e. the manner in which various amino acids are arranged in a polypeptide chain, reflects protein conformation. There are four levels of protein conformation, referred as the primary, secondary, tertiary, and quaternary levels of protein structure.

Primary Structure of Protein

Primary structure of protein refers to the **order and sequence of amino acid residues in a protein chain** (Fig. 3.13).

Some proteins, such as insulin, are synthesized as a single polypeptide and are later cleaved into two or more chains. These proteins have intrachain as well as interchain disulfide linkages.

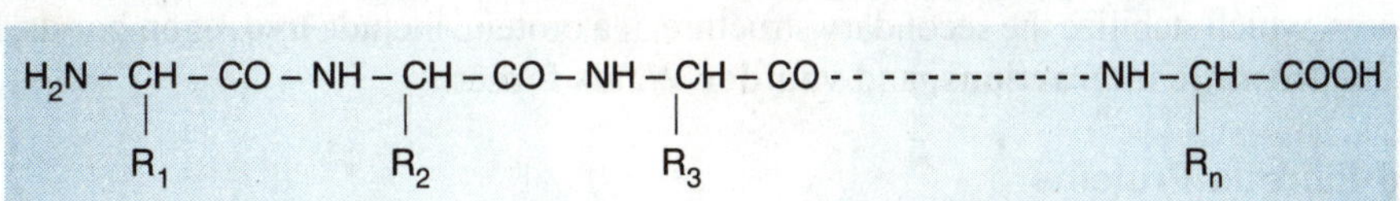

Fig. 3.13. Primary structure of a protein.

Secondary Structure of Protein

Secondary structure of a protein **refers to folding and twisting patterns of the polypeptide chain,** i.e. the spatial arrangements of the polypeptides. Secondary structures include α-helix and β-sheets.

α-Helix

Twisting the backbone of a polypeptide chain forms a coil or helix. As a result of its folding, hydrogen bonds may also be formed between the –CO and the –NH groups, with in the polypeptide chain. These types of linkages are called intrachain peptide linkages.

The helix may be a α-helix or a β-helix.

α-Helix refers to the **right-handed folding** of the protein chain. It is the most stable conformation of a polypeptide chain, e.g. α-keratin. There are 3.6 amino acid residues per turn of a helix (Fig. 3.14).

Left-handed helix generally does not occur in proteins.

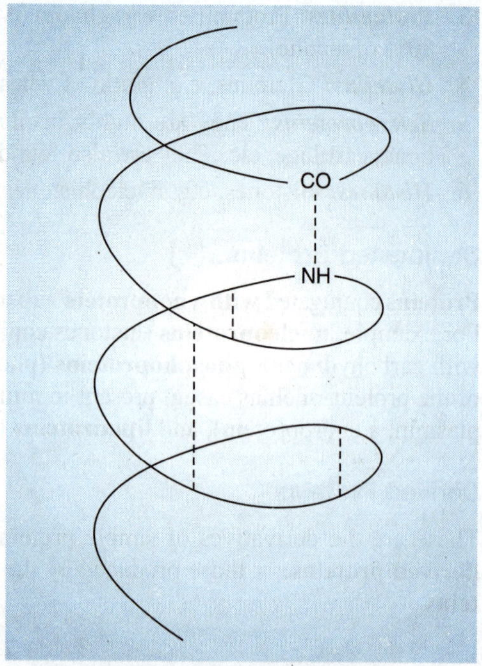

Fig. 3.14. The α-helix structure.

β-Sheets

The second regular conformation present in proteins is referred to as **β-structure.** β-Denotes that it is the second regular structure described after α-helix. The conformation, in which the β-structure is optimally hydrogen-bonded, has rippled or pleated-edge, on appearance. Therefore, this conformation is also called as the **pleated sheet** like structure.

Such proteins, e.g. wool, may contain 2 to 12 polypeptides in β-strand conformation. Each strand may contain up to 15 residues. The β-sheet orientation is formed due to **stretching of the polypeptide chains,** as a result of formation of hydrogen bonds between the –CO and the –NH groups of the neighboring polypeptides. These types of linkages are called **interchain peptide linkages** (Fig. 3.15).

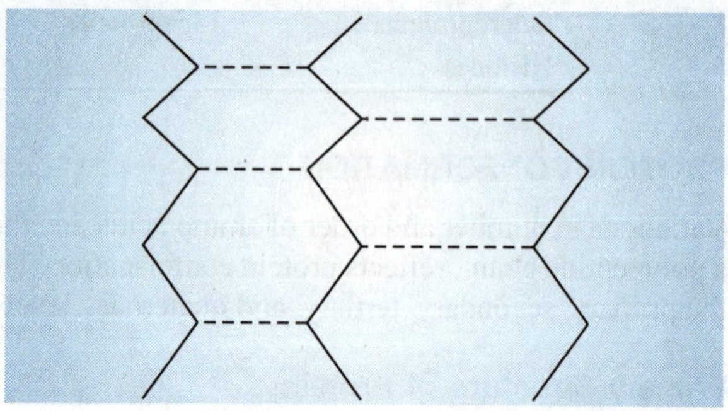

Fig. 3.15. β-structure.

In these types of proteins, the polypeptide chains may run either in antiparallel or parallel directions.

Antiparallel β-Sheet: It is formed when two polypeptide chains run in **opposite directions.**

Parallel β-sheet: It is formed when two chains run in **same direction.**

Various **forces,** which stabilize the secondary structure of a protein, include **hydrogen bonds, hydrophobic interactions, electrostatic interactions,** and **van der Waals forces.**

Globular and Fibrous Proteins

Depending on their overall morphology, proteins have been classified as either globular or fibrous.

Globular Proteins

Globular proteins have a spheroidal shape and vary in size. They have relatively high water solubility and function as catalysts, transporters, and regulators of metabolic pathways and gene expression. Their shapes are result of complex interactions between the secondary, tertiary, and some times quaternary structural elements. The major types of the secondary structural elements, i.e. the α-helices and β-sheets, occur in globular proteins, in varying proportions and combinations. Certain groupings of secondary structural elements, called super-secondary structures or motifs, also occur in many unrelated globular proteins. Some proteins, such as cytochromes, consist of only α-helices, spanned by short connecting links. Others, such as immunoglobulin folds, have a large proportion of β-sheets and are devoid of the α-helices. Most of the proteins, such as lactate dehydrogenase, however, have significant amounts of both types of secondary structures. The most common globular proteins are hemoproteins, such as hemoglobin, myoglobin, cytochromes, and catalase.

Fibrous Proteins

Fibrous Proteins exhibit special mechanical properties. They characteristically contain larger amounts of the regular secondary structures and have long cylindrical (rod-like) shape. They have low solubility in water. Rather than a dynamic role, fibrous proteins have a protective, connective, or supportive role in living organisms. For example, collagen, keratin, and tropomyosin, etc., which are found as components of skin, connective tissue, blood vessel walls, and sclera and cornea of the eyes.

Tertiary Structure of Protein

Tertiary structure involves **intramolecular folding** of the polypeptide chain, forming a compact three-dimensional structure, with a specific shape (Fig. 3.16).

Electrovalent linkages, hydrogen bonds, disulfide bridges, van der Waals forces, and hydrophobic interactions maintain tertiary structure of a protein.

Quaternary Structure of Protein

Multisubunit proteins contain several identical and/or different chains, where each one of the peptide chains is referred as a **subunit**. These polypeptide subunits are associated with a specific geometry. Spatial arrangement of these subunits is referred as the quaternary structure of protein (Fig. 3.17).

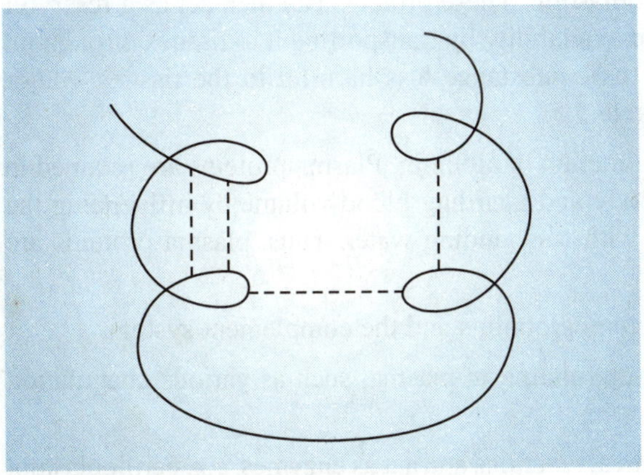

Fig. 3.16. Tertiary level of protein structure.

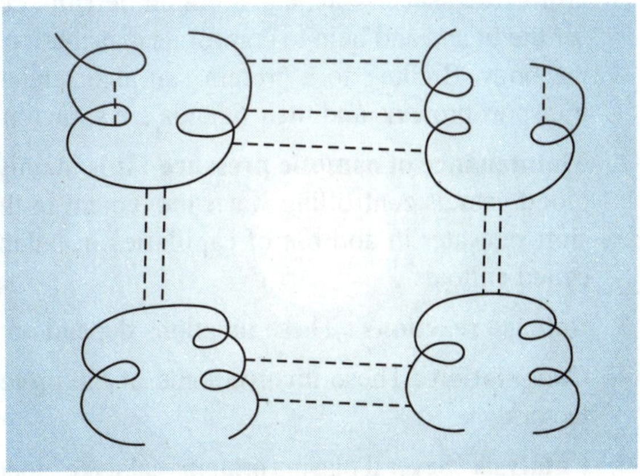

Fig. 3.17. Quaternary structure of proteins.

Proteins with **more than one subunit** are called **oligomeric** proteins. For example **hemoglobin,** it is an oligomeric protein with **four subunits** ($\alpha_2\beta_2$).

Disintegration of the monomer subunits of a multimeric protein results **in loss of its biological activity**.

DENATURATION OF PROTEIN

Denaturation of proteins results in unfolding and disorganization of the secondary and tertiary structures. This is not accompanied by the hydrolysis of the peptide bonds.

Denaturing agents include heat, mechanical mixing, detergents, strong acids or bases, and the ions of heavy metals, such as lead and mercury. Under ideal conditions, denaturation may be reversible. However, most proteins, once denatured remain permanently disordered. Denatured proteins are often insoluble and therefore precipitate from solution.

PLASMA PROTEINS

Plasma contains over 300 proteins. Many of these have a specific role but albumin and globulins predominate. Total plasma proteins concentration varies from 6.3 to 8.0 g/dl. Out of which albumin may be approximately 3.7 to 5.3 g/dl while globulins are nearly 1.8 to 3.7 g/dl. This in turn gives an albumin to globulin ration nearly 2:1. An increase in total proteins may occur in **dehydration.** Because of hemoconcentration, both albumin and globulin are increased, and albumin to globulin ratio remains unaltered.

A decrease in total proteins is mostly due to a fall in albumin level, which may be accompanied either by no increase in globulin, or by an increase that is less than the fall in albumin, resulting in reduced albumin to globulin ratio. A reduction in the total protein is one of the causes of **edema**.

The ranges for the various globulin fractions are approximately :

α_1 plus α_2	0.4 to 1.4 g/dl
β	0.5 to 1.3 g/dl
γ	0.6 to 1.5 g/dl

FUNCTIONS OF PLASMA PROTEINS

Many proteins in plasma have a specific role to play and carry out a wide range of functions including

1. **Transport functions** : A number of plasma proteins have the ability to bind certain ligands with a high affinity and specificity, e.g. albumin, ferritin, ceruloplasmin. These proteins can then act as a reservoir for the ligand and help to control its distribution and availability by transporting it to tissues throughout the body. Binding to a protein can also render a toxic substance less harmful to the tissues. Major transport proteins and their ligands are shown in Table 3.5.
2. **Maintenance of osmotic pressure** : It is mainly a function of albumin. Plasma proteins are retained in blood vessels controlling water movement in the body and guarding blood volume by influencing the shift of water in and out of capillaries in balance with surrounding water. Thus, plasma proteins are called colloids.
3. **Defense reactions** : These functions depend on immunoglobulins and the complement system.
4. **Coagulation** : These involve some of the proteins circulating in plasma, such as various coagulation factors.
5. **Catalysis** : Several plasma proteins catalyze biochemical reactions and act as enzymes, e.g. ceruloplasmin and all protein enzymes.

6. **Hormones** : Several proteins bind to their receptors and catalyze signal transduction such as insulin, prolactin, etc.

Table 3.5. Transport proteins and their ligands

Protein	*Ligand*
Albumin	Divalent and trivalent cations, such as Cu^{2+}, Fe^{3+}, heme, bilirubin, steroids and nonesterified fatty acids
Ceruloplasmin	Copper
Transferrin, ferritin, and hemosiderin	Iron
Thyroid binding globulin	Thyroid hormones
Cortisol binding globulin	Cortisol
Sex hormone binding globulin	Androgens, estrogens
Haptoglobin	Hemoglobin

ALBUMIN

Albumin accounts for approximately 50% of the protein found in human plasma and is present normally at a concentration of 3.5–4.5 g/dl. Its molecular weight is about 66 kD. It is highly polar and dissolves easily in water. Its rate of synthesis is dependent on nutritional status. The half life of albumin is about 20 days.

Albumin performs several functions:

1. It functions as a protein reserve in nutritional depletion.
2. Albumin acts as an osmotic regulator. It exerts colloidal osmotic pressure to maintain integrity of the blood volume. Thus, it helps to maintain normal circulation of tissue fluids and capillary blood flow. Infact, albumin is quantitatively the most important contributor towards maintaining the colloid oncotic pressure of plasma. Accordingly, hypoalbuminemia may lead to the development of edema whereas increased albumin concentration is found in dehydration.
3. It is the primary plasma protein responsible for the transport of a large number of substances, which include the long chain fatty acids, steroids, unconjugated bilirubin and several drugs including salicylates, barbiturates, sulfonamides, penicillin and warfarin. Proteins also act as the vehicle in which nutrients are carried throughout the body. Lipoproteins are necessary to transport fats in the blood.

Hypoalbuminemia

Hypoalbuminemia may arise due to a number of reasons which include:

1. *Impaired synthesis* : Severe and prolonged liver disease, malnutrition and intestinal malabsorption may result in reduced synthesis of albumin in the liver.
2. *Excessive losses* : Hypoalbuminemia may occur in increased albumin losses, such as in urine, e.g. in nephrotic syndrome, a gastrointestinal disease, burns or certain skin diseases.
3. *Increased capillary Permeability* : Reduction in plasma albumin may be observed due to increased capillary permeability, which enables plasma to leak into the extra-vascular compartment, e.g. in severe burns, or effusion, such as in ascitis
4. *Increased catabolism* : Hypoalbuminemia may be a result of increased catabolism of albumin, such as in injury due to major surgery or trauma, sepsis (infection), or malignancy.

5. Overhydration – artifact causes:
   Dilution of sample due to taking a blood sample from a site close to an intravenous infusion.
   Physiological causes – such as pregnancy
   Pathological causes

Analbuminemia

Analbuminemia refers to a condition in which plasma albumin concentration is almost completely absent (usually less than 100 mg/dl). There may be compensatory increase in plasma globulins concentrations.

Hyperglobulinemia

Increase in globulin occurs most commonly in advanced liver disease, in multiple myeloma, and in a number of chronic infections.

An increase in globulins may also be observed in many chronic infections and other conditions such as tuberculosis, rheumatoid arthritis etc.

Liver disease, infection or an autoimmune disease gives rise to stimulation of B lymphocytes and an increased production of γ-globulin, which on serum protein electrophoresis is revealed as a broad (diffused) band.

Paraproteinemia

Discrete immunoglobulins bands, visible on electrophoresis of serum, are known as paraproteins or monoclonal components. They are commonly associated with multiple myeloma and malignant lymphoid tumors. They are due to production of a single immunoglobulin or immunoglobulin fragment, e.g. light chain or heavy chain fragments, by a single class of B cells. Malignant paraproteinemia occurs in multiple myeloma.

MULTIPLE MYELOMA

Multiple myeloma is a disease in which there is proliferation of plasma cells and plasma cell precursors. Most myelomas produce complete immunoglobulin molecules, usually IgA or IgG, and the amount produced is often proportional to the tumor mass. The most characteristic finding on serum protein electrophoresis in multiple myeloma is the presence of a band of abnormal protein, which has been termed as M protein. It occurs as an intense, narrow band most often found with the γ-globulin.

In some of these patients dimmers of light chains are also found in urine. These are called Bence Jones Proteins.

SOME IMPORTANT QUESTIONS

1. What are proteins? Classify proteins, based on their solubility.
2. What are amino acids? Classify them.
3. Name plasma proteins. What is the biological importance of plasma proteins?
4. Discuss briefly:
   (i) α-helix
   (ii) β-sheets
   (iii) Quaternary structure of protein

(iv) Protein conformation
(v) Biological significance of amino acids
(vi) Aromatic amino acids
(vii) Sulfur-containing amino acids
(viii) Essential amino acids
(ix) Branched chain amino acid
(x) Basic amino acids
(xi) Classification of amino acids according to nutritional requirement

5. Write notes on:
(i) Zwitter ion
(ii) Fibrous proteins
(iii) Globular proteins
(iv) Protein denaturation

CHAPTER 4

Chemistry of Nucleic Acids

Nucleic acids are the macromolecules, which occur in a cell in association with the basic proteins, such as histones and protamines. They are strongly acidic in nature and are negatively charged at the physiological pH.

The repeated monomer units, called **nucleotides**, are the **building units** of nucleic acids, as amino acids to proteins or monosaccharides to polysaccharides.

A **nucleotide** has 3 constituents and consists of **phosphoric acid,** a **pentose sugar,** and a **nitrogenous base.**

PENTOSE SUGARS

Presence of the pentose sugar defines type of the nucleic acid. There are two classes of nucleic acids, called **deoxyribonucleic acid (DNA)** and **ribonucleic acid (RNA)**. As the name suggests, **deoxyribonucleic acid** contains **deoxyribose** whereas **ribonucleic acid** contains **ribose.**

Ribose

Ribose has three –OH groups, one each at carbon atom numbers 1, 2, and 3 of the pentose sugar.

Deoxyribose

Deoxyribose does not contain oxygen at the second carbon atom and has only two –OH groups, one each at carbon atom numbers 1 and 3. Deoxyribose thus, is also called as 2-deoxyribose (Fig. 4.1).

Sugar molecule is linked to **nitrogenous base** on one side, through **carbon atom number one (C-1)**, and to **phosphoric acid** on the other side through carbon number five (**C-5**).

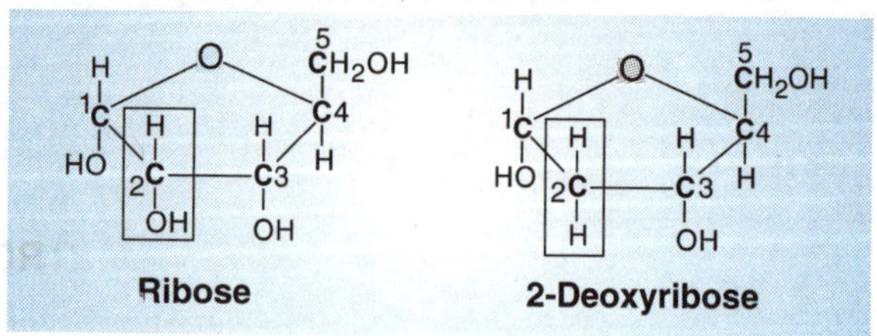

Fig. 4.1. Sugars present in nucleic acids.

NITROGENOUS BASES

Nitrogenous bases found in the nucleotides, are derivatives of either a **purine** or a **pyrimidine**.

Purine is a **nine-member ring,** containing **5 carbons** and **4 nitrogens**. On the other hand, pyrimidine is a **six-member ring** with **4 carbons** and **2 nitrogens** (Fig. 4.2).

Various nitrogenous bases have appropriate substitutions on the parent heterocyclic rings.

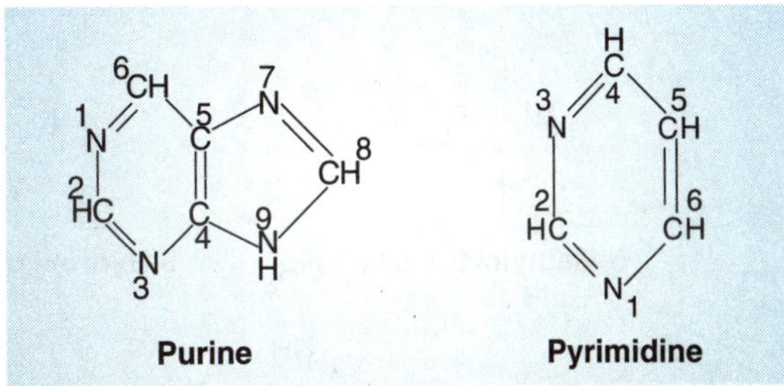

Fig. 4.2. A purine and a pyrimidine ring.

Purines

There are two types of **purine** bases, found in nucleic acids. These are referred as **adenine** (6-aminopurine) and **guanine** (2-amino, 6-oxypurine).

Pyrimidines

Pyrimidine bases found in nucleic acids are designated as **cytosine** (2-oxy, 4-amino pyrimidine), **uracil** (2, 4-dioxypyrimidine), and **thymine** (2, 4-dioxy, 5-methylpyrimidine). Thymine is also referred as 5-methyluracil (Fig. 4.3).

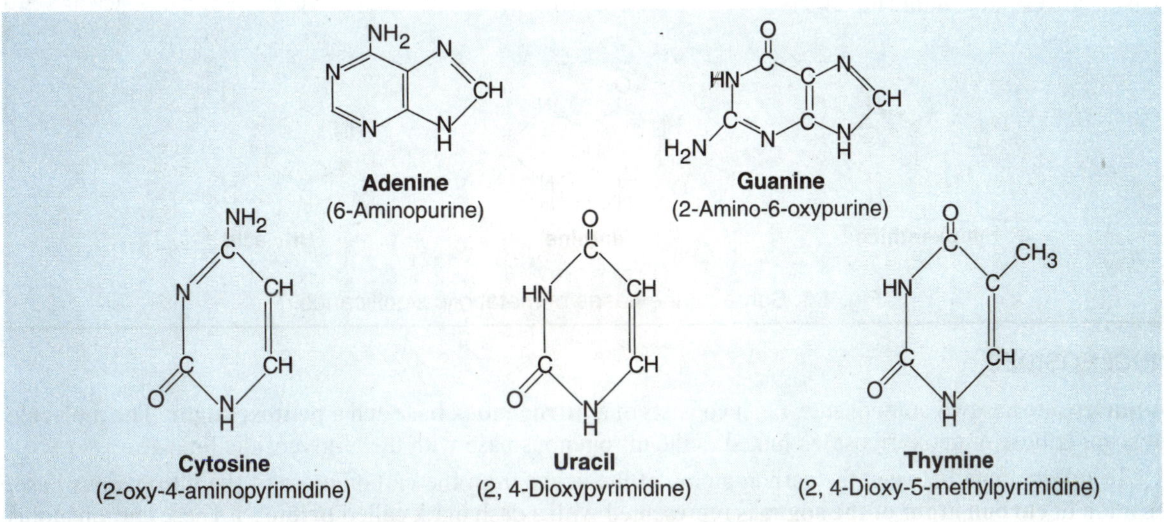

Fig. 4.3. Nitrogenous bases found in nucleic acids.

Out of the three-pyrimidine bases, only two are found in a nucleic acid. Usually, **cytosine** and **uracil** are found in **RNA,** while **cytosine** and **thymine** are found in **DNA**.

UNUSUAL NITROGENOUS BASES

Besides four nitrogenous bases (2 purines and 2 pyrimidines), that commonly occur in nucleic acids, few others are also found in some of the nucleic acids. For example, **5-methylcytosine, 5-hydroxymethylcytosine, pseudo-uracil** (where structural positions of N-1 and C-5 of the uracil molecule are interchanged), **N^6-methyladenine, N^7-methylguanine**, etc., are found in some RNAs (Fig. 4.4)

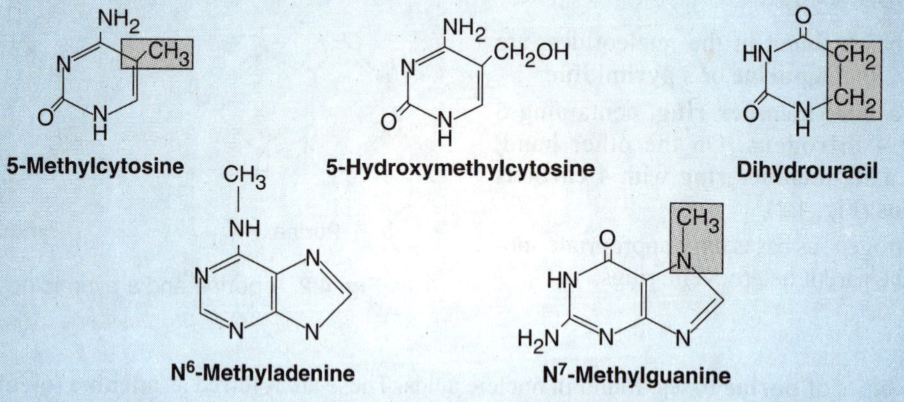

Fig. 4.4. Some unusual nitrogenous bases found in nucleic acids.

These nitrogenous bases are referred to as **unusual nitrogenous bases,** as they are not usually found in nucleic acids.

Certain other purine derivatives of metabolic significance are also found either as intermediates during purine biosynthesis, such as **hypoxanthine** and **xanthine**, or occur as end product of purine catabolism, such as **uric acid** (Fig. 4.5).

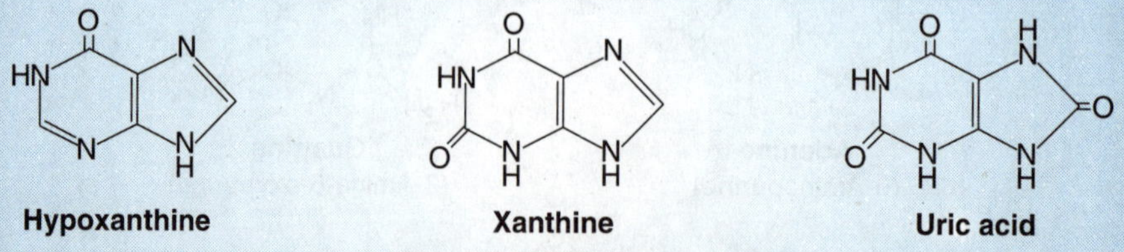

Fig. 4.5. Some purine bases of metabolic significance.

NUCLEOSIDES

A nucleoside has two components, i.e. it consists of a **nitrogenous base** and a **pentose sugar**. The molecule of sugar (ribose or deoxyribose) is linked to the nitrogenous base with the N-glycosidic linkage.

To differentiate between the carbon atoms of the sugar from the carbon atom of the nitrogenous base, position of **carbon atom of the sugar** is represented with a dash mark called **prime** (′). These carbon atoms are represented as **C-1′, C-5′**, etc. On the other hand, carbon and nitrogen atoms of the **nitrogenous bases** are represented without the prime sign, i.e. as **N-1, C-2**, etc.

First carbon atom of the sugar (C-1′) is mostly linked to N-1 of a pyrimidine or N-9 of a purine:

Base–N–(1/9)–C-1′-Sugar

Nucleosides, which contain **ribose,** are called **ribonucleosides.** Accordingly, the ribonucleosides of adenine, guanine, cytosine, and uracil are designated as **adenosine, guanosine, cytidine,** and **uridine,** respectively (Fig. 4.6).

Nucleosides containing **deoxyribose** are designated as deoxy-ribonucleosides and are written with deoxy-(d), as a prefix. Thus, **deoxy-adenosine, deoxy-guanosine, deoxy-cytidine,** and **deoxy-thymidine** are the

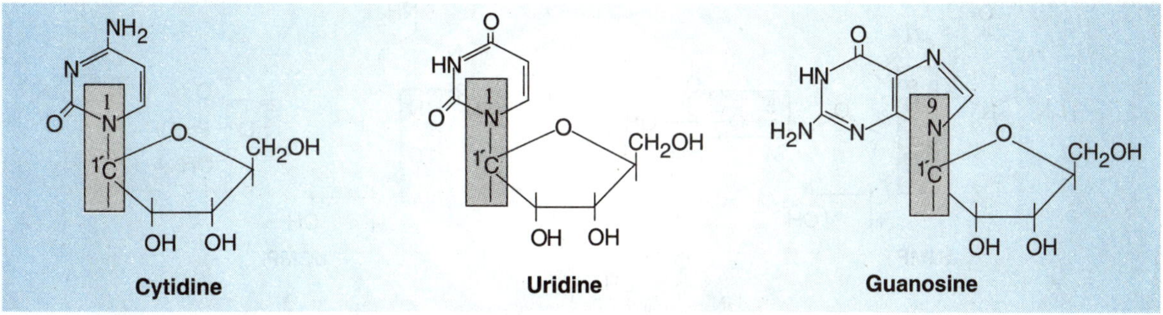

Fig. 4.6. Ribonucleosides.

nucleosides containing deoxy-ribose with adenine, guanine, cytosine, and thymine, respectively. Since thymine is usually found in DNA only and is linked to deoxyribose, its nucleoside is commonly referred to as **thymidine,** and not as deoxythymidine (Fig 4.7).

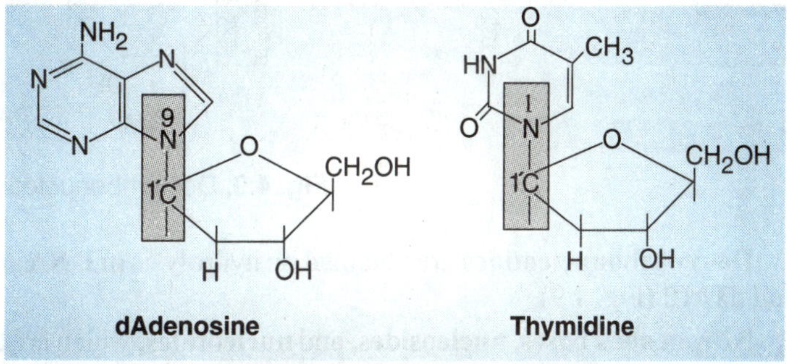

Fig. 4.7. Deoxyribonucleosides.

NUCLEOTIDES

A **nucleotide** has 3 constituents and consists of a **nitrogenous base**, a **pentose sugar,** and **phosphoric acid.**

The sugar molecule (ribose or deoxy-ribose) is linked to a nitrogenous base on one side and to phosphoric acid on the other.

The **C-1′** of the **sugar** is linked to a **nitrogenous base** through **N-1 of pyrimidine** or **N-9 of purine.** Although any of the hydroxyl groups (-OH) of the sugar may get esterified with phosphoric acid but commonly, C-5′ of the sugar is linked to phosphate.

Base–N–(1/9)–C-1′-Sugar C-5′–P

Nucleotides containing **ribose** are called **ribonucleotides.** Four ribonucleotides are generally obtained on hydrolysis of RNA. These are designated as **adenosine monophosphate** or **adenylate (AMP), guanylate (GMP), cytidylate (CMP),** and **uridylate (UMP)**. Some of these are shown in Fig. 4.8

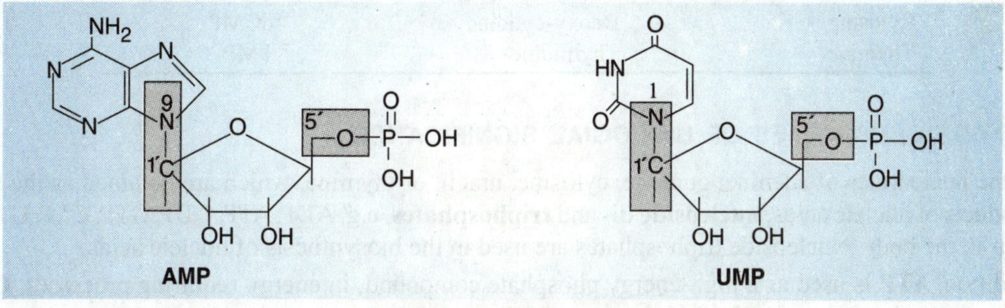

Fig. 4.8. Ribonucleotides.

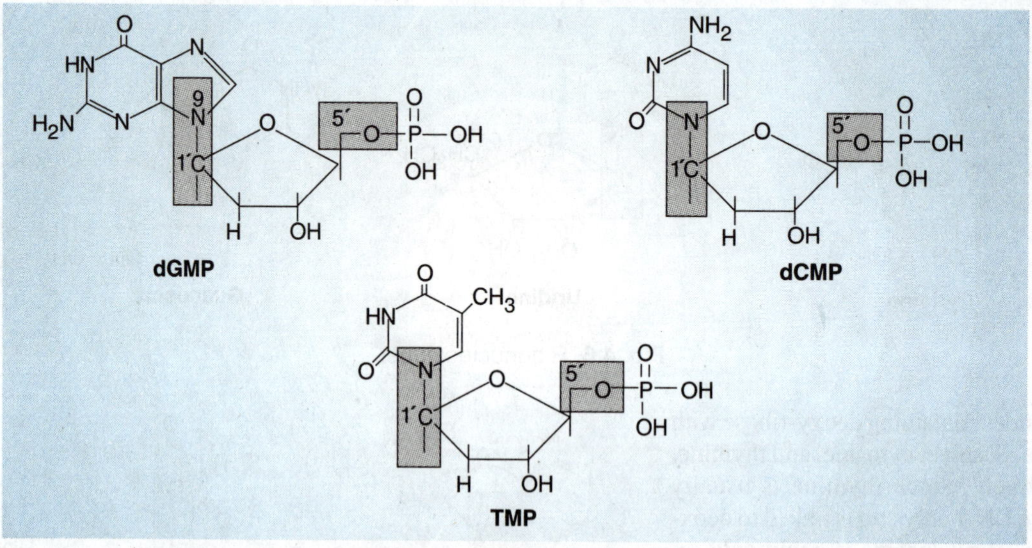

Fig. 4.9. Deoxyribonucleotides.

Deoxy-ribonucleotides are obtained on hydrolysis of **DNA** and are designated as **dAMP, dGMP, dCMP,** and d**TMP** (Fig. 4.9).

Nitrogenous bases, nucleosides, and **nucleotides,** which are commonly obtained on hydrolysis of nucleic acids, are shown in Table 4.1.

Table 4.1. Nitrogenous bases, nucleosides, and nucleotides commonly obtained on hydrolysis of nucleic acids

Nitrogenous bases	*Nucleosides (base + sugar)*	*Nucleotides (base + sugar + P)*
RNA		
Adenine	Adenosine	AMP
Guanine	Guanosine	GMP
Cytosine	Cytidine	CMP
Uracil	Uridine	UMP
DNA		
Adenine	Deoxy-adenosine	dAMP
Guanine	Deoxy-guanosine	dGMP
Cytosine	Deoxy-cytidine	dCMP
Thymine	Thymidine	TMP

NUCLEOTIDE DERIVATIVES OF BIOLOGIAL SIGNIFICANCE

Besides the nucleotides of adenine, guanine, cytosine, uracil, or thymine, which are obtained as the hydrolyzed products of nucleic acids, **nucleoside di-** and **triphosphates**, e.g. ADP, ATP, GDP, GTP, CTP, UTP, etc, also occur in the body. Nucleoside triphosphates are used in the biosynthesis of nucleic acids.

In addition, **ATP** is used as a high-energy phosphate compound, in energy requiring processes. **CTP** is used in biosynthesis of phosphoglycerides.

Several sugar derivatives of UDP, such as **UDP-glucose** and **UDP-galactose,** are important in the inter conversion of glucose and galactose. **UDP-glucuronic acid** is used in conjugation reactions.

Cyclic nucleoside monophosphates of adenine and guanine, i.e. **cyclic-3′, 5′- AMP** (cAMP) and **cyclic-3′, 5′- GMP** (cGMP), mediate a series of reactions and act as intracellular signals.

Other important derivatives of AMP include **S-adenosylmethionine** (active methionine), which serves as a methyl donor, and as several coenzymes, such as **NAD⁺, NADP⁺, FAD,** etc.

Inosinemonophosphate (IMP) is also found in the body. It is a nucleotide of hypoxanthine. It is formed by deaminatoin of AMP.

Some nucleotide derivatives of biological significance are shown in Fig. 4.10.

Polymerization of the monomeric units, i.e. the nucleotides, results in the formation of a polynucleotide.

Nucleotides are linked together by 3′, 5′-phosphodiester linkage, where hydroxyl group of the sugar molecule of one nucleotide is linked to the hydroxyl group of the sugar moiety of the next nucleotide.

One end of the polynucleotide has a 5′-hydroxy (or 5′-phosphate) terminus while the other end has a 3′-phosphate (or 3′-hydroxy) terminus. These are referred to as the 5-end, and the 3-end, respectively.

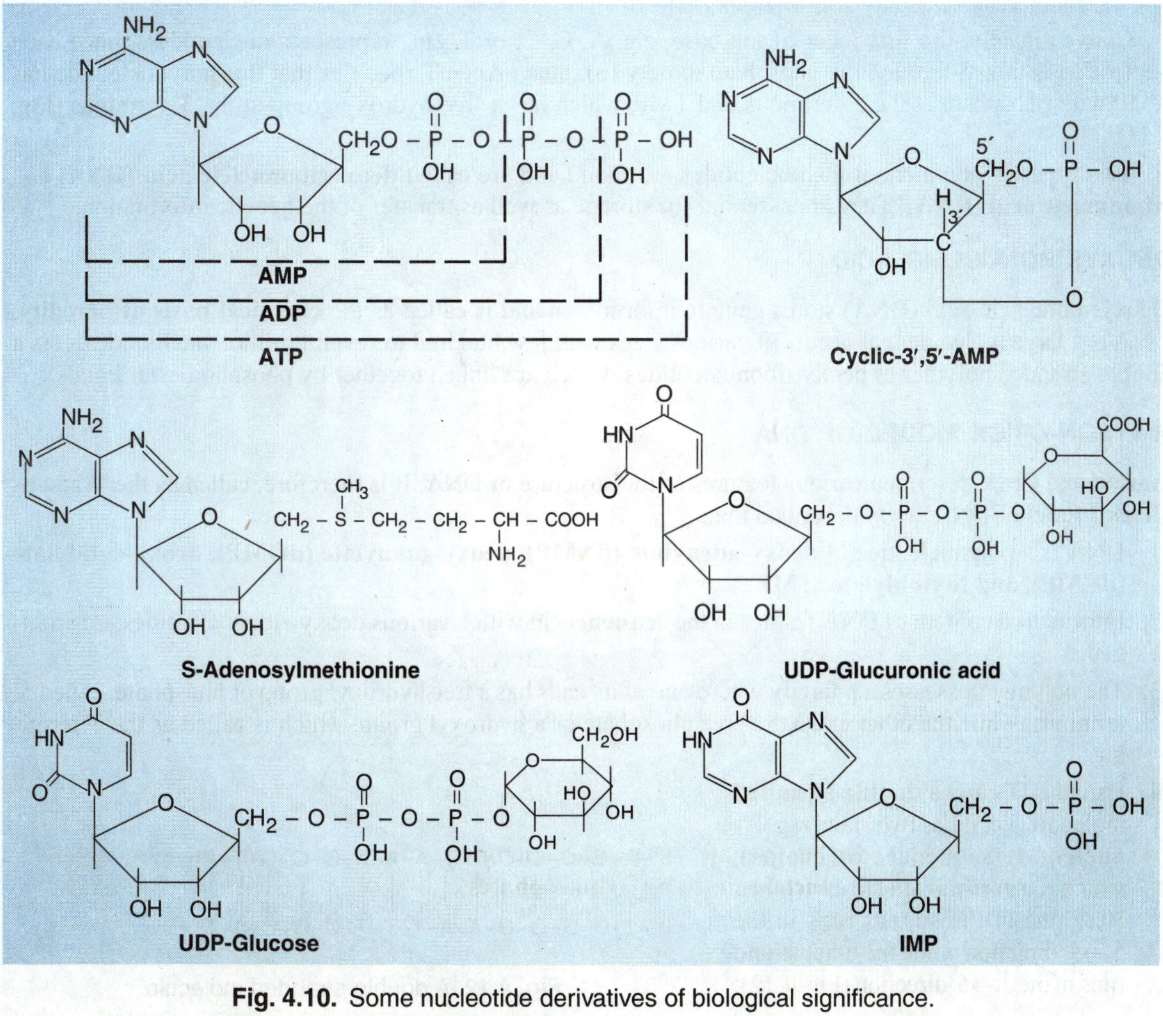

Fig. 4.10. Some nucleotide derivatives of biological significance.

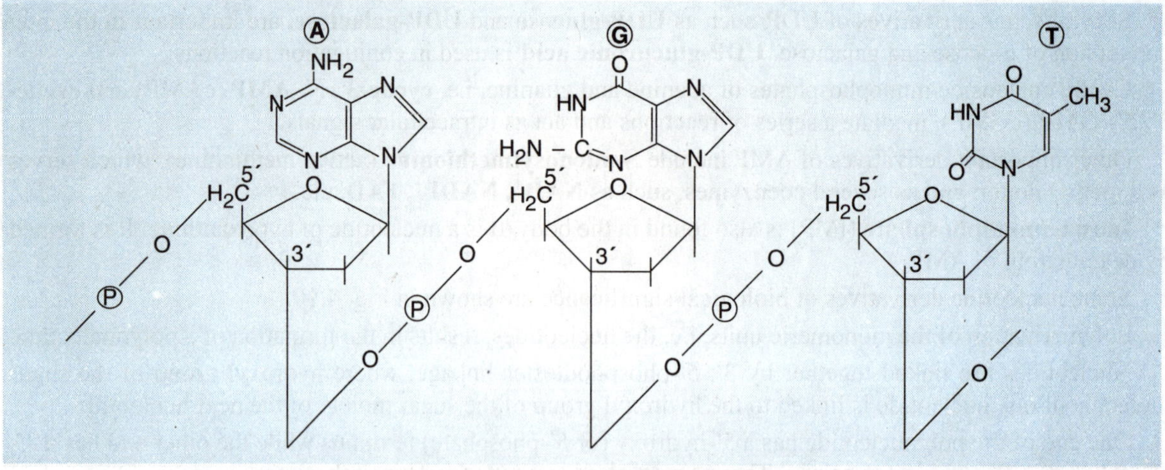

Fig. 4.11. A polynucleotide (deoxypolynucleotide).

Conventionally, the first letter of the base, e.g. A, G, C, or T, etc., represents nucleotides. Since each nucleotide is linked through the phosphate moiety (p), thus pApGpT specifies that this polynucleotide has AMP with phosphate at the 5′ terminus and TMP, which has a free hydroxy group at the 3′ terminus (Fig. 4.11).

Two types of polymers of the nucleotides are found and are called **deoxyribonucleic acid (DNA)** and **ribonucleic acid (RNA)**. They are essential for storage as well as transfer of the genetic information.

DEOXYRIBONUCLEIC ACID

Deoxyribonucleic acid (**DNA**) stores genetic information and is called as the **chemical basis of heredity**. DNA is a large molecule that occurs in various sizes with few hundred to several million nucleotides. It is a double-stranded polymer of deoxy-ribonucleotides, which are linked together by phosphodiester bonds.

WATSON-CRICK MODEL OF DNA

Watson and Crick described various features of the structure of DNA. It is therefore, called as the **Watson-Crick Model** of DNA. They described that:

1. DNA is a polynucleotide of **deoxy-adenylate (dAMP), deoxy-guanylate (dGMP), deoxy-cytidylate (dCMP), and thymidylate (TMP).**
2. Information content of DNA resides in the **sequence**, in which various deoxy-ribonucleotides are arranged.
3. The polymer possesses a **polarity** where one of its ends has a free hydroxyl group or phosphate, called 5′ terminus, while the other end has a free phosphate or a hydroxyl group, which is called as the 3′ terminus.
4. Usually, DNA is a **double-stranded** molecule, i.e. it has two stands (polynucleotide sequences or chains), which run **anti-parallel** to each other. Here one of the strands runs in the 5′→3′ direction while the other strand runs in the 3′→5′ direction (Fig. 4.12).

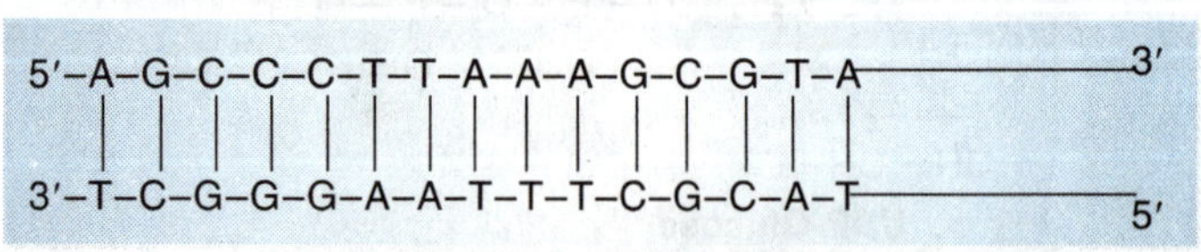

Fig. 4.12. A double-stranded molecule.

5. Both the polynucleotide chains are wound around a common axis, forming a **right-handed helix,** which is nearly 20Å in diameter.
6. The helix has a **pitch of 34 Å** and has10 base pairs per turn.
7. Two strands of the double-stranded molecule are held together by **hydrogen bonds** between a purine and a pyrimidine. This base pairing is very specific, as A is always linked to T with two hydrogen bonds while G is linked to C with three hydrogen bonds (Fig. 4.13).

   DNA molecule thus, has equal number of adenine and thymine residues as well as guanine and cytosine residues. This relationship is known as **Chargaff's rule.**
8. The base occupies core of the helix while sugar-phosphate chain runs along the periphery. This in turn forms two grooves, of unequal width. These are called as the **major groove** and the **minor groove** (Fig. 4.14).

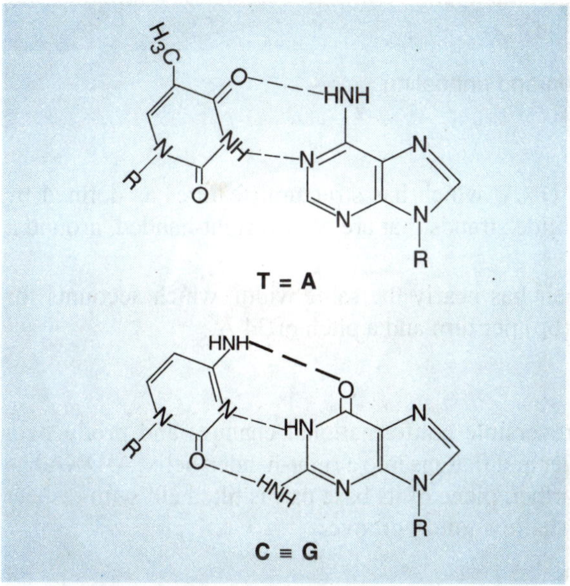

Fig. 4.13. Hydrogen bonding in a DNA molecule.

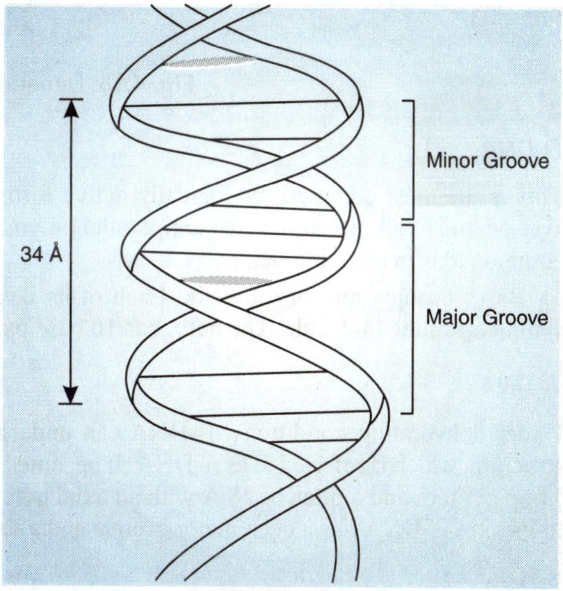

Fig. 4.14. DNA helix.

DNA Denaturation

Two strands of the DNA double helix get separated (melted), when DNA solution is heated above certain temperature. This process of separation (unwinding) of the two stands is called **denaturation.**

Denaturation results in breakage of hydrogen bonds and separation of the base pairs. It also changes physical properties of DNA, such as a decrease in viscosity and increase in ultraviolet absorbance.

The temperature at which DNA is half-denatured is called as **melting temperature (Tm)**. When melted DNA is slowly cooled to temperature below Tm, it results in reformation of double helix DNA, i.e. renaturation, due to formation of the complementary base pairs. This process is called as **annealing** (Fig. 4.15).

Formation of the RNA-DNA hybrid, with the complimentary strands of RNA and DNA, is called **hybridization.**

Different Types of DNA

There are 3 different structural forms of DNA. These are referred to as B-DNA, A-DNA, and Z-DNA.

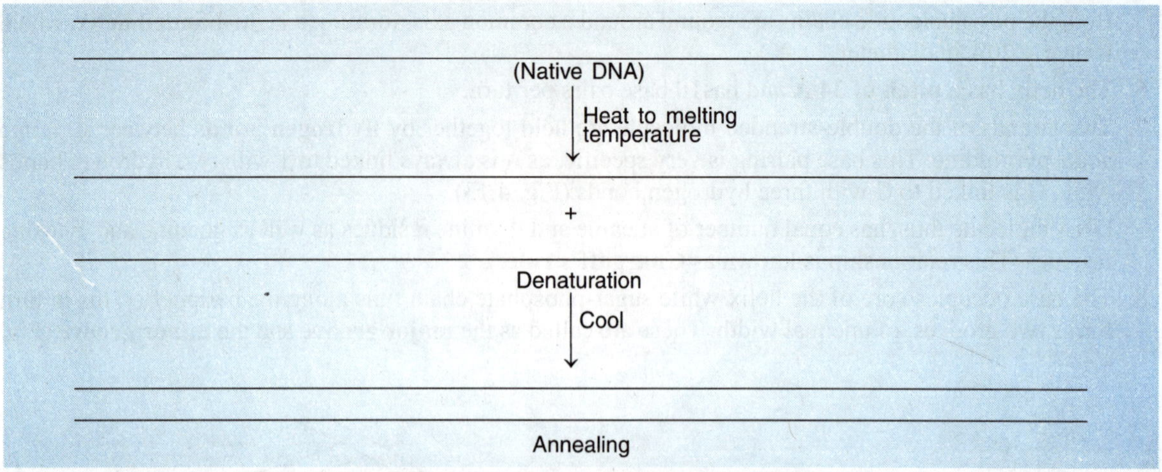

Fig. 4.15. Denaturation and annealing.

B-DNA

This is the most common, biologically active form of DNA, which has structural features as defined by Watson and Crick, i.e. it has two antiparallel polynucleotide strands that are wound right-handed, around a common axis in a double-helix.

Bases occupy core of the helix. Each of its base pair has nearly the same width, which accounts for symmetry of the molecule. The helix has 10 base pairs (bp) per turn and a pitch of 34 Å.

A-DNA

Under dehydrating conditions, B-DNA can undergo reversible conformational changes and produces a structure, which is referred to as A-DNA. It becomes wider and flattens into a right-handed helix. A-DNA has 11 bp per turn and a pitch of 28 Å with an axial hole. Further, plane of its base pair is tilted 20° with respect to its axis. A-DNA has a deep major groove and a very shallow minor groove.

Z-DNA

Z-DNA has 12 bp per turn, a pitch of 45 Å, and a deep major groove but no identifiable minor groove. It has complementary polynucleotides with alternating purines and pyrimidines, such as poly d (GC).d(AT) or poly d(AC).d(GT), assuming a Z (zigzag) conformation.

CELLULAR FUNCTIONS OF DNA

DNA performs various functions, such as that:

- It makes copies of itself and thus, transfers genetic information from one generation to next. This process is known as **replication.**
- DNA also determines properties of the living cell and regulates biological information by controlling protein synthesis.

Biological information passes from one class of the nucleic acid to another, i.e. from DNA to RNA. This process is referred to as **transcription.**

The sequence of bases in RNA is then translated into the sequence of amino acids in a protein. This process is referred to as **translation**.

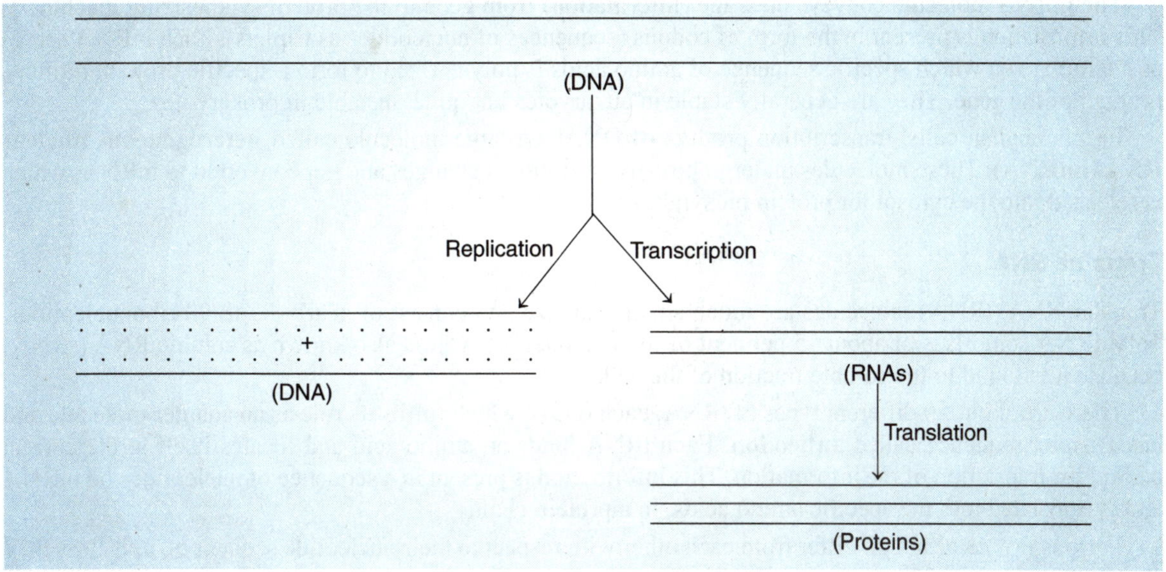

Fig. 4.16. Cellular functions of DNA.

DNA molecule thus serves as a template both for replication of information into the daughter DNA as well as for transcription of this information into RNA and its subsequent translation into protein (Fig. 4.16).

RIBONUCLEIC ACIDS

Three main classes of the RNA are found to occur in all types of cells. These are referred to as **messenger RNA, ribosomal RNA,** and **transfer RNA.** Though all the three types of the RNA are involved in protein biosynthesis, they differ from each other with respect to size, composition, and location with in the cell as well as their functions.

TYPES OF RNA

Messenger RNA

Messenger RNA (mRNA) is a group of RNAs, which is most heterogeneous. They are highly elongated and short-lived molecules. They are synthesized with in the nucleus as a result of transcription.

The mRNA transcript has $5' \rightarrow 3'$ polarity, which is complementary to the coding strand of the gene (DNA molecule) with a difference that mRNA contains uracil in place of thymine (Fig. 4.17).

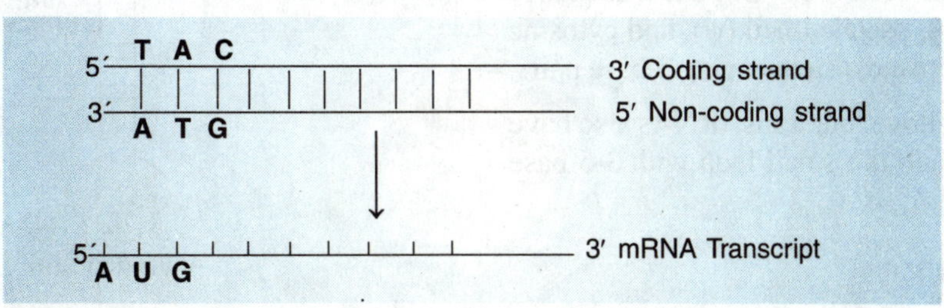

Fig. 4.17. Formation of the mRNA transcript from a DNA molecule.

The mRNA molecule conveys message (information) from gene to the protein synthesizing machinery. This information is present in the form of codons (sequences of nucleotides as triplets). Each mRNA serves as a template on which specific sequence of amino acids is polymerized to form a specific protein, ultimate product of the gene. They are generally stable in eukaryotes but quite unstable in prokaryotes.

In mammalian cells, transcription product of DNA is a large molecule called **heterogeneous nuclear RNA (hnRNA)**. These molecules undergo post-transcriptional changes and get converted to mRNA, which is released into the cytosol for protein biosynthesis.

Transfer RNA

Transfer RNA (tRNA) molecules are much smaller in size and consist of nearly 75 to 90 ribonucleotides. Total tRNA comprises of about 15 per cent of total cellular RNA. It is also known as soluble RNA (sRNA) because it is found in the soluble fraction of the cell.

There are about 50 different types of tRNA, each one of which fulfils its role as an adapter molecule and has a triplet sequence called **anticodon**. Each tRNA binds an amino acid and locates itself at the correct codon, for translation of the information. This information is present in a sequence of nucleotides on mRNA and is translated into the specific amino acids, in a protein chain.

Various tRNAs although differ from each other with respect to their nucleotide sequences, as a class they have many common features:

1. The nucleotide sequence (the primary structure) allows extensive folding and intramolecular base pairing, to form a secondary structure, giving it a cloverleaf like appearance.
2. All the tRNA molecules, in addition to 4 usual bases (A, G, C, and U), have several unusual (modified) bases, e.g. 7-methylguanine, thymine, dihydrouracil, pseudouracil, hypoxanthine, etc.
3. All the tRNA molecules have 4 arms, which are referred as the amino acid acceptor arm, the anticodon arm, the DHU arm, and the TψC arm.

- **The amino acid acceptor arm:** The amino acid acceptor arm has 7 base-paired stem, which terminates in CCA ($5' \rightarrow 3'$ sequence) whose A (the adenosyl-moiety) accepts an amino acid. The carboxyl group of amino acid forms an ester linkage with the 3′-hydroxyl group of the adenosyl moiety.
- **The anticodon arm:** The anticodon arm has 5 base pairs and a loop, which has a triplet, three nucleotides sequence (the anticodon) that is complementary to the codon. This anticodon is responsible for specificity of the **tRNA** molecule.
- **The DHU arm:** The DHU arm has dihydrouracil (DHU or UH_2) in its loop along with 3 or 4 base-paired stem.
- **The TψC arm: The** TψC arm has a sequence of thymine (T), pseudouracil (ψ), and cytosine (C), in the loop and a stem having 5 base pairs.

In addition to above four arms, tRNAs also have an **extra arm**, which is a small loop with 3-5 base pairs (Fig.4.18).

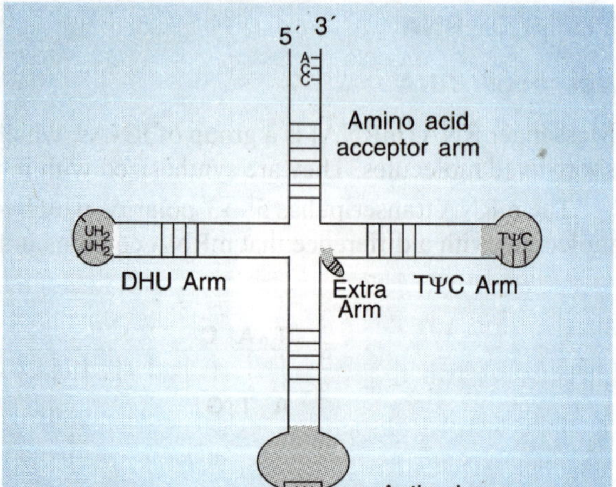

Fig. 4.18. tRNA.

Ribosomal RNA

Ribosomal RNA (rRNA) molecules are present in

ribosomes, in association with several polypeptides (Fig. 4.19).

Ribosomes are found in cytosol of the cell and contain nearly 80% of the total RNA that is found in a cell. Both, mRNA and tRNA interact on ribosomes to translate the information, which is transcribed from gene into a specific protein.

Mammalian ribosomes are very complex in nature with a sedimentation velocity of 80S. Each ribosome has 2 subunits, which are referred to as the large subunit (60S) and the small subunit (40S).

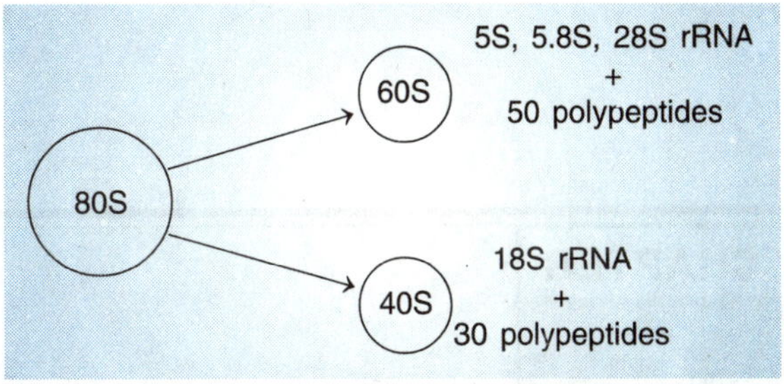

Fig. 4.19. Mammalian ribosomes.

The large subunit contains 3 different types of rRNA, which are designated as 5S, 5.8S, and 28S rRNA and more than 50 polypeptides. The small subunit has an RNA, which is referred to as 18S rRNA and nearly 30 polypeptides.

DIFFEENCES BETWEEN DNA AND RNA

1. In RNA, the sugar moiety is ribose while it is deoxy-ribose in DNA.
2. RNA does not contain thymine, which is present in DNA. Instead of thymine, RNA contains uracil.
3. RNA is normally a single-stranded molecule. Its purines content, therefore, may not be equal to pyrimidines.

SOME IMPORTANT QUESTIONS

1. Describe various features of the Watson - Crick Model of DNA.
2. Describe various types of RNA, with their functions.
3. What is a nucleotide? Name different nucleotides found in DNA. Describe in brief various nucleotides of biological significance.
4. Write notes on :
   (i) Structure and functions of tRNA
   (ii) Differences between DNA and RNA
   (iii) Various nitrogenous bases found in nucleic acids
   (iv) Unusual nitrogenous bases
   (v) DNA Denaturation
   (vi) B-DNA
   (vii) A-DNA
   (viii) Z-DNA
   (ix) Nucleoside
   (x) Nucleotide
   (xi) hnRNA
   (xii) Different types of DNA
   (xiii) Structural features of tRNA
   (xiv) Messenger RNA

CHAPTER

5

High Energy Compounds

There are several **compounds**, such as the phosphate esters and mixed anhydrides, **which have** a bond, called **high-energy bond,** hydrolysis of which yields large amount of energy. These compounds are referred to as **high-energy compounds.** Some of these compounds have a high energy phosphate bond, called **high-energy phosphate compounds** while others are **thioesters.**

HIGH-ENERGY PHOSPHATE COMPOUNDS

High-energy phosphate compounds include active phosphate carriers, such as various **nucleoside-triphosphates (ATP, GTP, CTP, UTP**, etc.); phosphorylamidines, e.g. **creatine-phosphate;** and enol-phosphates, like **1, 3-bisphosphoglycerate, phosphoenolpyruvate, etc.**

ADENOSINE-5′-TRIPHOSPHATE

Adenosine-5′-triphosphate (ATP) is a **nucleoside-triphosphate** in which **adenine** is attached, in a glycosidic linkage, to **D-ribose. Three phosphoryl groups** are sequentially linked to the fifth carbon of the ribose moiety via a phosphoester bond, followed by two phospho-anhydride bonds. **The terminal two phosphoryl- groups,** called γ- and β-phosphoryl- groups are attached as phosphoric acid anhydride bonds, which are designated as the **energy-rich bonds** or **high-energy bonds** and are symbolized by the squiggle (~). ATP can therefore, be represented as A-R-P~P~P (Fig. 5.1).

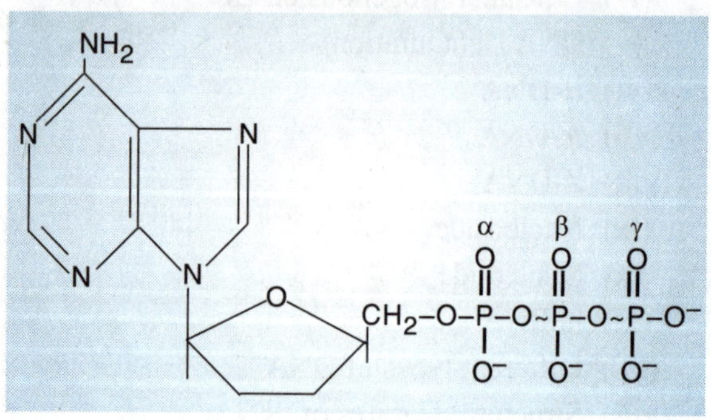

Fig. 5.1. ATP.

ATP is a high-energy compound, which occurs in all forms of life. It is said to be a **primary cellular energy currency** since its synthesis (as a result of catabolic processes) or utilization (in the energy-dependent cellular functions) involves formation, and either **hydrolysis or transfer of the terminal phosphate (γ) group**. When this terminal phosphate group is removed, the **reaction is** said to be **exothermic**. Hydrolysis of this high-energy bond yields 7.3 Kcal of energy and the products of this hydrolysis are ADP and inorganic phosphate (Pi):

$$\text{ATP} \xrightarrow[\searrow \text{ 7.3 Kcal}]{} \text{ADP} + \text{Pi}$$

Various **nucleoside triphosphates other than ATP**, such as CTP, GTP, and UTP, or their deoxynucleoside triphosphates, which are required for the synthesis of nucleic acids, are also synthesized from ATP and the corresponding nucleoside diphosphates.

COUPLED REACTIONS

The exergonic reactions of high-energy compounds can be coupled to the endergonic processes, to drive them to completion. For example, ATP can be regenerated from ADP and Pi, by coupling its synthesis, to the exergonic cleavage of phosphoenol-pyruvate. This reaction is catalyzed by the enzyme pyruvate kinase, which transfers a phosphoryl- group from phosphoenol-pyruvate to ADP, to regenerate ATP.

$$\text{Phosphoenol-pyruvate} + \text{ADP} \xrightleftharpoons{\text{Pyruvate kinase}} \text{Pyruvate} + \text{ATP}$$

$$(\Delta G^{o'} = -14.8 \text{ kcal/mol})$$

Since an exergonic reaction of a high-energy compound is usually coupled to an endergonic process, to drive it to completion, and as long as the overall pathway is exergonic, the reaction operates in the forward direction.

Thus, there is a flow of energy from the high-energy phosphate compound, such as 1, 3-bisphosphoglycerate towards ADP, and from ATP to some low-energy compound, such as glucose-6-phosphate and glycerol-3-phosphate whose free energy of hydrolysis is lower than the preceding high-energy compound.

PYROPHOSPHATE CLEAVAGE

In some of the reactions, such as attachment of amino acids to tRNA molecules during protein synthesis, hydrolysis of ATP results in the pyrophosphate cleavage and yields AMP and PPi (pyrophosphate). Thereafter, pyrophosphate is rapidly hydrolyzed to 2 molecules of Pi. Thus pyrophosphate cleavage of ATP ultimately consumes two high-energy phospho-anhydride bonds. These types of reactions are the two step reactions where both the steps are readily reversible. The overall reaction is driven to completion by the irreversible hydrolysis of PPi:

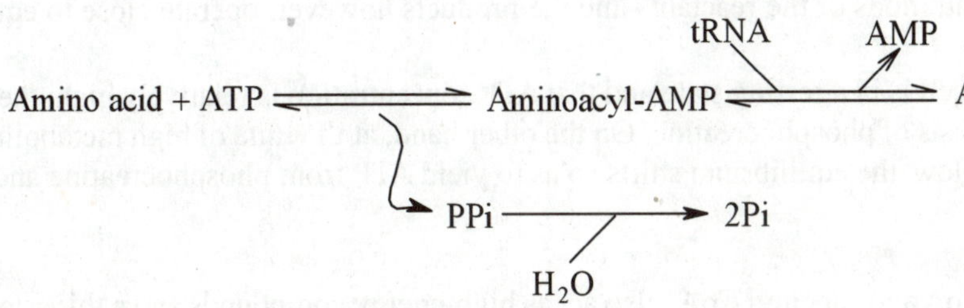

$$(\Delta G^{o'} = -4.5 \text{ kcal/mol})$$

ENOL PHOSPHATES

Several phospho-anhydrides (enol-phosphates), such as 1,3-bisphosphoglycerate, and acyl-phosphates, also have phosphoryl-group transfer potentials. ATP can therefore, be regenerated from ADP, by direct transfer of the phosphoryl-group from such a high-energy compound. This type of reaction is referred to as the **substrate level phosphorylation**. Such compounds rank above ATP and are referred to as **high-energy phosphate donors.**

On the other hand, there are other compounds, such as glucose-6-phosphate and glycerol-3-phosphate, whose free-energy of hydrolysis is much less than the high-energy compounds, mentioned above. Such compounds are referred to as the **low-energy phosphate acceptors** and rank below ATP in position.

ATP thus occupies a middle rank with respect to the standard free-energy of the phosphate hydrolysis of various high-energy phosphorylated compounds, since it is continuously hydrolyzed as well as regenerated.

Standard free energy of phosphate hydrolysis of some of the phosphorylated compounds of biological significance is listed in Table 5.1.

Table 5.1. Some high-energy phosphate compounds

High-energy phosphate compound	*Free-energy of hydrolysis ($-\Delta G^{o'}$/Kcal/mol)*
Phosphoenol-pyruvate	14.8
1,3-Bisphosphoglycerate	11.8
Creatine-phosphate	10.5
ATP	7.3*
Glucose-1-phosphate	5.0
Glucose-6-phosphate	3.3
AMP	2.2

* ATP since occupies a central position, it is called as the universal energy currency of the cell.

PHOSPHORYLAMIDINES

Phosphorylamidines **or** phospho-guanidines, **such as** phospho-creatine and phospho-arginine, **called phosphogens, also have phosphoryl-group transfer potentials.**

Phosphocreatine acts as an ATP buffer in cells that contain creatine kinase, such as muscle and nerve cells, which have a high ATP turnover:

$$\text{ATP + Creatine} \xrightleftharpoons{\text{Creatine kinase}} \text{Phosphocreatine + ADP}$$

The intracellular concentrations of the reactants and the products however, operate close to equilibrium ($\Delta G = 0$).

Accordingly, when the cell is in a resting state and that ATP concentration is relatively high, the reaction proceeds towards the synthesis of phosphocreatine. On the other hand, at the time of high metabolic activity when ATP concentration is low, the equilibrium shifts so as to yield ATP from phosphocreatine and ADP.

THIOESTERS

Thioesters, such as acetyl CoA and succinyl CoA, also act as high-energy compounds and a thioester bond is also involved in **substrate-level phosphorylation.**

Coenzyme A

Coenzyme A (HSCoA or CoA) consists of a β-mercapto-ethylamine group, which is linked through an amide linkage to the vitamin pantothenic acid that in turn is attached to the 3′-phospho-adenosine moiety, via a pyrophosphate bridge. CoA functions as a carrier of the acetyl and other acyl groups. The formation of the thio-ester bond in a metabolic intermediate conserves a portion of the free-energy of oxidation of a metabolic fuel and that free energy is used to drive the exergonic process.

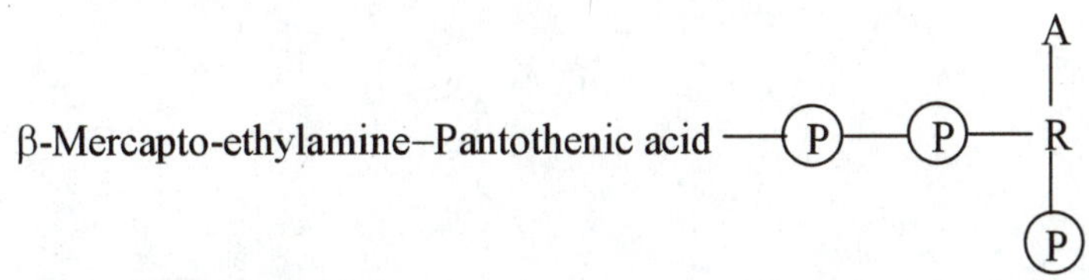

Coenzyme A (Adenosine-3′-phosphate)

The acetyl group in acetyl CoA bound as a thioester to the sulfhydral portion of the β-mercapto-ethylamine. Thus, acetyl CoA is also a high-energy compound. $\Delta G^{o'}$ for the hydrolysis of its thioester bond is –7.8 kcal/mol, which makes this reaction slightly more exergonic than the hydrolysis of ATP.

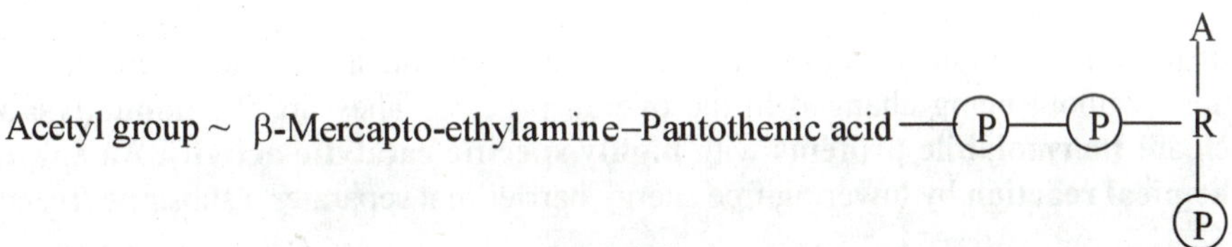

Acetyl CoA

Succinyl CoA

Cleavage of succinyl CoA also releases sufficient free-energy to synthesize GTP from GDP and Pi, in the citric acid cycle.

SOME IMPORTANT QUESTIONS

1. Discuss various high-energy compounds.
2. Write notes on:
   (i) ATP
   (ii) Phosphocreatine
   (iii) Thioesters
   (iv) Enol phosphates
   (v) ATP as cellular currency of energy

CHAPTER

6

Enzymes

Enzymes are **organic** macromolecules produced in the living organisms, which increase the rate of biochemical reactions without being changed in the overall process. They are the **nondialysable, colloidal particles,** which are **thermolabile proteins** with **highly specific catalytic activity.** An enzyme **increases the rate of a chemical reaction** by lowering free energy barrier that separates a substrate (reactant) from the product.

Most of the enzymes are produced with in the cell of a particular tissue and function there only. Such enzymes are called **intracellular enzymes,** e.g. **enzymes of the glycolysis, citric acid cycle, fatty acid synthesis**, etc. On the other hand, there are certain enzymes, which are produced by the cells of a particular tissue, from where they are liberated but function in some other tissue. Such enzymes are called **extracellular enzymes**, e.g. proteolytic enzymes, such as **trypsin, chymotrypsin, etc.** They are secreted in pancreatic juice for their action in the small intestine.

CLASSIFICATION OF ENZYMES

Enzymes are usually named by **the suffix "-ase"** with the **name of the substrate** or with the **catalytic action** of the enzyme, e.g. lipase that catalyzes hydrolysis of lipids, fatty acid synthase that catalyzes synthesis of fatty acids, etc. These names are called as the **trivial names**. However, while assigning a trivial name to an enzyme, no systematic rules are followed.

International Union of Biochemistry and Molecular Biology (IUBMB) adopted a scheme for the rational naming of each enzyme and suggested a **functional classification**. According to IUBMB, **each enzyme is assigned a four-digit systematic code**, commonly known as the **Enzyme Commission number (E.C. number).**

The **first digit of the code denotes the main class of the enzyme**, which is according to general type of the chemical reaction enzyme catalyses.

Its **second digit** characterizes the **sub-class,** which may be based on the nature of the chemical group removed or transferred, or any bond spliced or formed.

Its **third digit** indicates the **sub-sub-class** and describes detailed subdivision of the each subclass.

The **last digit** of the E.C. number indicates a **serial number** of the particular enzyme in the sub-sub-class. For example, 1.1.1.1 is the enzyme code for alcohol dehydrogenase, which is the first enzyme of the sub-sub-class 1, of the sub-class 1, of the class 1.

According to the enzyme commission, enzymes are classified into six classes, as follow:

1. Oxido-reductase

Oxido-reductases are involved in **oxidation and/or reduction of the substrate,** i.e. they catalyze addition of oxygen, or removal of hydrogen or electrons. Their sub-classes include dehydrogenase, oxidase, oxygenase, etc.

Examples of the class oxido-reductase are alcohol dehydrogenase, xanthine oxidase, glutathione reductase, etc.

2. Transferase

Transferases catalyze **transfer of a particular group from one substrate to another**. On the basis of the group being transferred, transferases are sub-classified as aminotransferases, phosphotransferases, etc.

Glutamate oxaloacetate transaminase, hexokinase, glucose-1-phosphate uridyltransferase, etc., are the examples of the class transferase.

3. Hydrolase

Hydrolases bring about **hydrolysis of a substrate with the addition of a molecule of water**. According to nature of the group or bond hydrolyzed, hydrolases are sub-classified as peptidases, glycosidases, etc.

Examples of the class hydrolase include glucose-6-phosphatase, amylase, pepsin, etc.

4. Lyase

Lyases catalyze **removal of a small molecule from the substrate without addition of water**. They are sub-classified on the basis of the linkage splitted. Various sub-classes of lyases include the lyases catalyzing breakdown of the C–C, C–N, or C–S bond.

Examples of the class lyase include fumarase, pyruvate decarboxylase, histidase, etc.

5. Isomerase

Isomerases are involved in **isomerisation of the substrate.** This in turn **catalyses the interconversion of one isomeric form of the substrate to another**. Racemases, epimerases, and mutases, etc., are some of the sub-classes of the isomerases.

Examples of the class isomerase include phosphohexose isomerase, phosphoglucomutase, alanine racemase, etc.

6. Ligase

Ligases are involved in **synthesis of a molecule from two substrates**. This joining of the two substrates requires energy, which is coupled with the hydrolysis of some high-energy bond. Its various sub-classes include ligases that can form a C–C, C–N, or C–S bond.

Examples of the class ligase are glutamine synthetase, acetyl CoA carboxylase, glutathione synthetase, etc.

Table 6.1 lists different classes of enzymes, with examples.

Table 6.1. Classification of enzymes with examples

Class of Enzyme	*Examples*
Oxido-reductase	Alcohol dehydrogenase, xanthine oxidase, catalase
Transferase	Glutamate pyruvate transaminase, serine hydroxymethyl transferase, hexokinase
Hydrolase	Glucose-6-phosphatase, carboxypeptidase, pepsin
Lyase	Pyruvate decarboxylase, aldolase, histidase
Isomerase	Phosphotriose isomerase, phosphoglucomutase, alanine racemase
Ligase	Glutamine synthetase, acetyl CoA carboxylase, glutathione synthetase

ENZYME SPECIFICITY

Enzymes are highly specific, interacting with one or a few substrates and catalyzing only one type of chemical reaction. They exhibit several types of specificities, such as stereo-specificity, reaction specificity, etc.

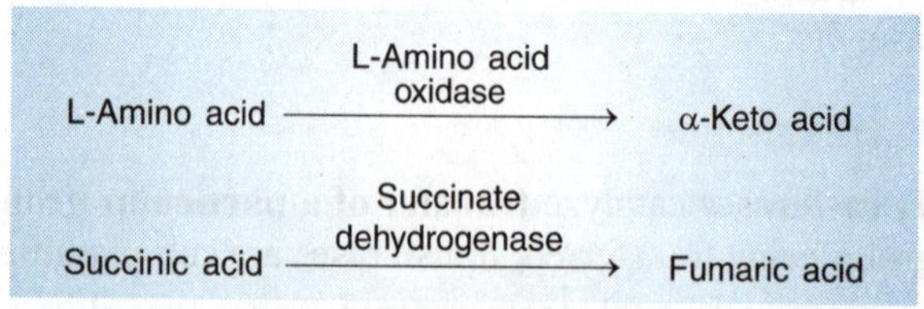

Fig. 6.1. Stereospecificity.

STEREOSPECIFICITY

There can be many optical isomers of a compound but it is only one of the isomers, which acts as a substrate for the enzyme. For example, L-amino acid oxidase will oxidize only L-amino acids. Similarly, succinate dehydrogenase acts only on succinate and not on malate (Fig. 6.1).

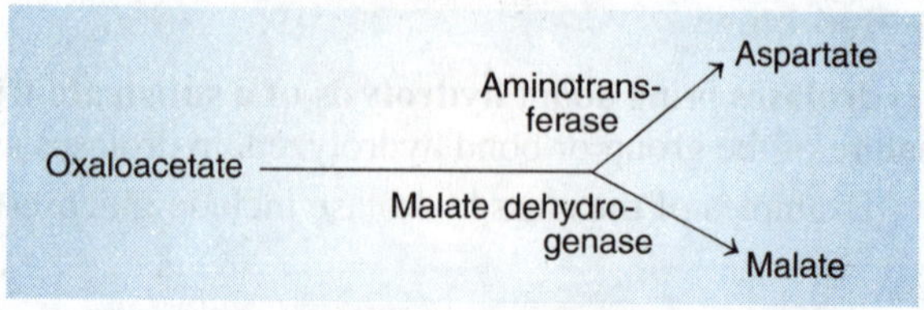

Fig. 6.2. Reaction specificity.

REACTION SPECIFICITY

A substrate though can be used in several reactions but a particular enzyme will catalyze only one of these reactions. For example, oxaloacetate can be converted to aspartate as well as to malate but the two reactions are catalyzed by two separate enzymes and not by the same enzyme (Fig. 6.2).

SUBSTRATE SPECIFICITY

The extent of substrate specificity varies from enzyme to enzyme. An enzyme may have either an absolute specificity or a relative specificity, for the substrate:

Absolute Specificity

An enzyme has an absolute specificity for its substrate and does not bind with any other substrate, e.g. urease. It has absolute specificity for urea.

Relative Specificity

The specificity of the enzyme may be group-dependent or bond-dependent:

Group specificity: It refers to the action of highly group specific enzymes, such as pepsin. It hydrolyses aromatic amino acid residues while trypsin hydrolyses basic amino acid residues in a peptide chain.

Bond specificity: It refers to the action of protease, glycosidase, or lipase, which specifically hydrolyzes a particular bond, such as peptide bonds in proteins, glycosidic bonds in polysaccharides, or ester bonds in lipids, respectively.

CHEMICAL NATURE OF ENZYMES

All enzymes are **protein** in nature with a large molecular weight although certain RNA molecules, called **ribozymes,** also show high substrate-specific catalytic activity.

> **RIBOZYMES**
>
> A ribozyme is an **RNA molecule,** which exhibits highly substrate-specific catalytic activity. They catalyze hydrolysis of a phosphodiester bond with in the RNA molecule and play a key role in **intron splicing**, which is essential in the conversion of pre-mRNA to mature mRNA, e.g. RNase P from *E.coli*.

Most of the enzymes though are simple proteins with a single polypeptide chain, there are several **enzymes** which have more than one polypeptide. Such enzymes **(multimeric proteins)** may be found either as **oligomeric enzymes** or as **multi-enzyme complexes.**

OLIGOMERIC ENZYMES

Enzymes with two or more subunits are called **oligomeric enzymes**, e.g. phosphorylase, hexokinase, lactate dehydrogenase, etc. These enzymes are tetramers, i.e. each enzyme has four protein subunits. On the other hand, phosphofructokinase, fructose-1, 6-bisphosphatase, creatine phosphokinase, etc., are dimmers, i.e. each one of these enzymes has two protein subunits.

MULTIENZYME COMPLEXES

Several enzymes occur in the form of a **multienzyme complex, which** catalyzes conversion of a substrate, in a sequential series of reactions, to different products, e.g. pyruvate dehydrogenase complex, α-ketoglutarate dehydrogenase complex, etc. Each of these enzyme complexes contains three enzymes. Fatty acid synthetase has seven enzyme activities.

ACTIVE SITE OF ENZYME

Enzyme molecules contain a special pocket or cleft, called the active site. The active site contains amino acids side chains that create a three-dimensional surface, complementary to the substrate. The active site on the **enzyme (E)** binds the substrate **(S),** forming an **enzyme-substrate (ES) complex.** This complex is subsequently converted to the enzyme-product complex, which subsequently dissociates to enzyme and **product (P)**.

$$E + S \longrightarrow ES \longrightarrow P + E$$

Various models have been proposed to explain this binding of the substrate with the enzyme. These include lock and key model, and induced-fit model.

LOCK AND KEY MODEL

Complementarity between the enzyme and the substrate, is the basis of the lock and key model of enzyme-substrate binding. In this model, during the process of formation of the enzyme-substrate complex, **the substrate attaches itself on the active sites**, having specific groups on the enzyme, **as a key fits into its lock**. This model was proposed by Emil Fischer and is called as the **lock and key model** or the rigid template model.

The active site may be a free hydroxyl group of serine, phenol group of tyrosine, SH-group of cysteine, or an imidazole group of histidine. Formation of the specific ionic pair contributes to recognition of the substrate. Various groups, which are important in substrate binding, are brought together at the active center. Thereafter, activation and transformation of the substrate takes place.

INDUCED-FIT MODEL

Induced-fit model explains that though the **substrate-binding sites** on the enzyme are preformed but these sites **undergo conformational changes after binding of the enzyme with the substrate.**

During its binding with the enzyme, a **substrate induces configurational changes in the active site of the enzyme,** so as to attain the desired shape in such a way that the substrate can fit the active site, conveniently. This was proposed by Koshland and is called as the **induced-fit model** (Fig. 6.3).

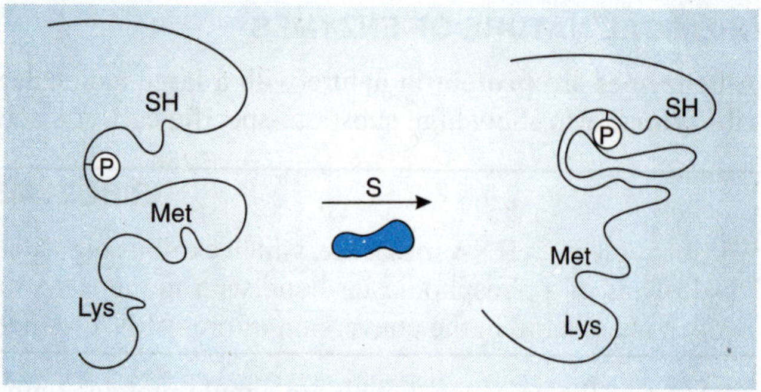

Fig. 6.3. Induced-fit model.

Functional groups, which are present on the active site, are arranged in a definite spatial configuration. The enzyme-substrate complex is formed by multiple bonding of the substrate with the enzyme, such as by covalent bonds, hydrogen bonds, and electrostatic bonds.

An enzyme, which also requires a coenzyme for its activity, possesses a site for the attachment of a coenzyme, as well.

COFACTORS AND COENZYMES

Most of the enzymes require presence of certain organic or inorganic substances for their activity. These enzymes are referred to as conjugated proteins. The protein part of such an enzyme is called as **apo-enzyme** (apo-protein) while these enzymes are called **holo-enzymes**. The nonprotein component of the holoenzyme is called a **prosthetic group.**

Apo-enzyme (protein) + Coenzyme (prosthetic group) = Holo-enzyme

If prosthetic group is removed, the enzyme loses its biological activity. The prosthetic group may be an organic compound, which is called as coenzyme or some inorganic ions, which is referred to as cofactor.

COENZYMES

A coenzyme is a **dialyzable, thermostable, low-molecular weight, organic substance**, which may be referred to as a co-substrate or the second substrate. It is required with the enzyme to catalyze a highly specific group/type of reaction.

Generally, coenzymes are **derivatives of the B complex** group of **vitamins,** e.g. **TPP** (coenzyme form of vitamin B_1), FMN and **FAD** (derivatives of B_2), **pyridoxal-5-phosphate** (coenzyme form of vitamin B_6), etc.

An enzyme, which catalyses transfer of hydrogen from one substrate to another may require FMN, FAD, NAD^+, or $NADP^+$ while the enzyme that catalyzes the transfer of a group may require TPP, pyridoxal-5-phosphate, or tetrahydrofolic acid.

Table 6.2 lists various B complex vitamins, their coenzyme forms, and some of the reactions where they are used as coenzymes.

Besides, certain other compounds, such as cytochromes, coenzyme Q, biopterin, S-adenosylmethionine, or certain nucleotide derivatives like ATP, GTP, UDP, etc., also act as coenzymes (Table 6.3).

Table 6.2. Vitamins, their coenzymes, and type of the reaction where they are used

Vitamin	*Coenzyme form*	*Reaction catalyzed*
Thiamin	TPP	Pyruvate ⟶ Acetyl CoA
		α-Ketoglutarate ⟶ Succinyl CoA
Riboflavin	FMN, FAD	α-Amino acids ⟶ α-Keto acids
		Succinate ⟶ Fumarate
Niacin	NAD^+, $NADP^+$	Lactate ⟶ Pyruvate
		Glucose-6-P ⟶ 6-P-Gluconolactone
Pyridoxine	Pyridoxal-5-P	Alanine + α-Ketoglutarate ⟶ Pyruvate + Glutamate
		Tyrosine ⟶ Tyramine
Pantothenic acid	CoA	Pyruvate ⟶ Acetyl CoA
		Fatty acid ⟶ Fatty acyl CoA
Biotin	Active biotin	Acetyl CoA ⟶ Malonyl CoA
		Pyruvate ⟶ Oxaloacetate
Folate	Tetrahydrofolic acid	Glycine ⟶ Serine
		Homocysteine ⟶ Methionine
B_{12}	Deoxyadenosylcobalamin/ Methylcobalamin	Methylmalonyl CoA ⟶ Succinyl CoA
		Homocystenine ⟶ Methionine
Lipoic acid	Lipoic acid	Pyruvate ⟶ Acetyl CoA
		α -Ketoglutarate ⟶ Succinyl CoA

Table 6.3. Coenzymes and the reactions catalyzed by them

Coenzyme	*Apo-enzyme*	*Reaction catalyzed*
Oxidation-Reduction Reactions		
Tetrahydrobiopterin	Phenylalanine hydroxylase	Phenylalanine ⟶ Tyrosine
Group Transfer		
ATP	Hexokinase	Glucose ⟶ Glucose-6-P
S-Adenosyl-methionine	Methyltransferase	Homocysteine ⟶ Methionine
Tetrahydrofolic acid	Glutamate- formiminotransferase	N-Formiminoglutamate ⟶ Glutamate
Isomerisation		
UDP	Epimerase	UDP-Galactose ⟶ UDP-Glucose
Covalent bond formation		
UDP	Lactose synthase	UDP-Galactose + Glucose ⟶ Lactose
ATP	Glutamine synthetase	Glutamate + NH_3 ⟶ Glutamine

COFACTORS

Several enzymes require certain **metal ions**, such as Mg^{2+}, Zn^{2+}, or Cl^-, for their activity. Such metal ions **are called as cofactors.**

A metal ion may be bound to the enzyme either tightly or loosely. These enzymes are referred to as metalloenzymes and metal-activated enzymes, respectively.

The metal ion may **form an integral part of the enzyme**. Such enzymes are referred to as **metalloenzymes**, e.g. zinc is an essential component of superoxide dismutase.

Some of the metalloenzymes are shown in Table 6.4.

In certain enzymes, a **metal ion** may be **loosely associated with the apo-enzyme** and forms a **metal-enzyme complex.** Such enzymes are called as **the metal-activated enzymes**. They require presence of the particular ions for their activity, e.g. Cl^- (as NaCl) acts as activator for salivary amylase.

Table 6.5 lists metal ions as activators of some enzymes.

Table 6.4. Some important metallo-enzymes

Metallo-enzyme	*Associated metal*
Cytochromes, peroxidases, catalase	Fe
Ascorbic acid oxidase, cytochrome oxidase, tyrosinase	Cu
Aldehyde oxidase, xanthine oxidase, nitrate reductase	Mo
Carbonic anhydrase, lactate dehydrogenase, carboxypeptidase	Zn
Glutathione peroxidase	Se

Table 6.5. Role of metal ions as enzyme activators

Metal ion	*Enzyme*
Ca	Lipase, ATPase, succinate dehydrogenase
Co	Lecithinase, peptidases
Mg	Phosphorylase, enolase, DNA polymerase
Mn	Arginase, phosphoglucomutase, choline esterase
Cl	Salivary amylase
K	Pyruvate kinase

FACTORS AFFECTING ENZYME ACTIVITY

An enzyme exhibits maximum activity only under optimal conditions. Enzyme activity is markedly affected by several factors, such as temperature, pH, concentration of the enzyme or the substrate, or by the presence of some activator or inhibitor.

EFFECT OF TEMPERATURE

Rate of an enzyme catalyzed reaction increases with increase in temperature of the reaction mixture. It is due to the reason that an increase of temperature, increases **energy of activation** of the chemical system, which in turn increases reaction velocity. It is, however, possible only up to **optimum temperature** that is defined as the temperature at which enzyme activity is maximum.

For most of the enzymes, optimum temperature is near the body temperature, i.e. about 37°C.

With **rise in temperature** of the reaction mixture, beyond the optimum temperature, **enzyme (protein) is denatured** and looses its biological activity.

Relationship of the enzyme activity to the change in temperature is usually represented by a bell-shaped curve, peak of which represents **optimum temperature** (Fig. 6.4).

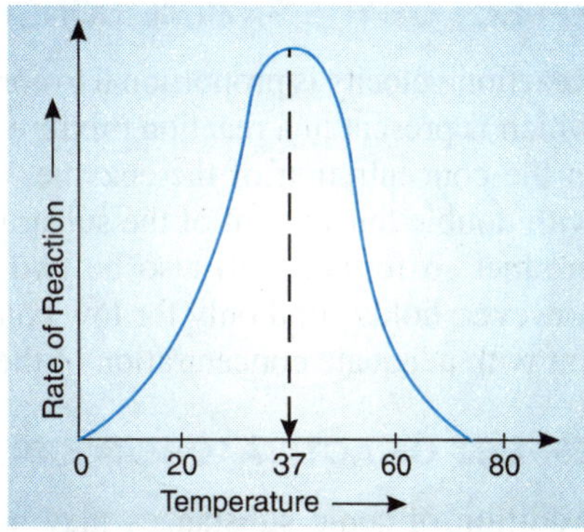

Fig. 6.4. Effect of temperature on enzyme activity.

EFFECT OF PH

The pH of the reaction medium also affects reaction velocity. The relationship of enzyme activity to the pH is represented by a bell-shaped curve, which has its peak at **optimum pH**. Optimum pH for most of the enzymes is in the neutral range, i.e. around 7.0 (Fig. 6.5).

Optimum pH of an enzyme depends upon ionization of the enzyme as well as the substrate. Change in pH affects **ionization of the enzyme (protein),** thereby **decreasing the number of the active sites**. Hence, at extremely low or high pH, enzyme gets denatured. For pepsin, optimum pH is about 2.0 while for enzymes of the pancreatic juice optimum pH is near 8.0.

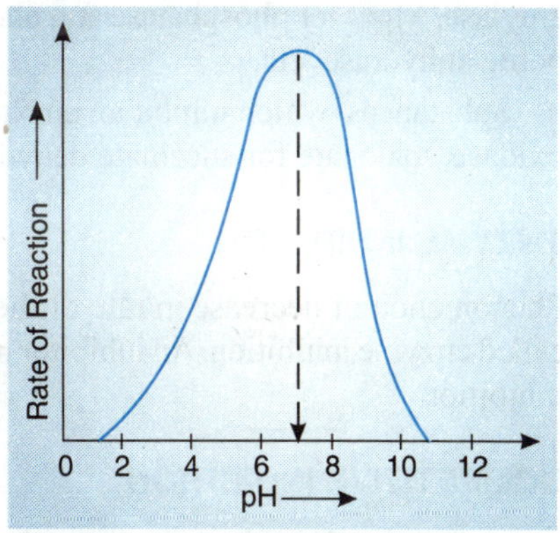

Fig. 6.5. Effect of pH on enzyme activity.

EFFECT OF SUBSTRATE CONCENTRATION

With a fixed quantity of the enzyme, reaction rate is proportional to substrate concentration. This is, however, true only up to a certain point when its velocity is maximum (V_{max}). Further increase in substrate concentration does not increase rate of the reaction (Fig. 6.6).

Michaelis and Menten derived a relationship between the substrate concentration and the reaction velocity and described an equation called **Michaelis-Menten equation**, which is as follows:

$$V_0 = \frac{V\max\,[S]}{Km + [S]}$$

where, V_0 is the initial reaction velocity, Vmax is the maximum velocity of a reaction, [S] is concentration of the substrate, and **Km** is a constant, which is referred to as **Michaelis Constant**.

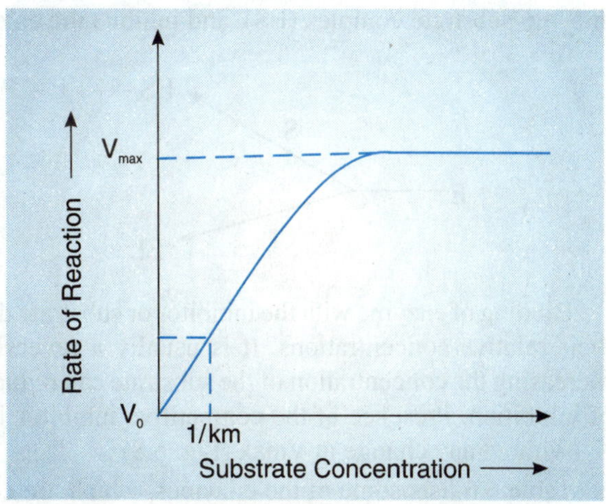

Fig. 6.6. Effect of substrate concentration on enzyme activity.

EFFECT OF THE ENZYME CONCENTRATION

Reaction velocity is proportional to concentration of the enzyme, which is present in a reaction mixture. With a two-fold increase in the concentration of the enzyme, the enzyme will combine with double the amount of the substrate, and the amount of the product so formed will also be two folds. This relationship, however, holds good only for low concentration of the enzyme but with adequate concentration of the substrate (Fig. 6.7).

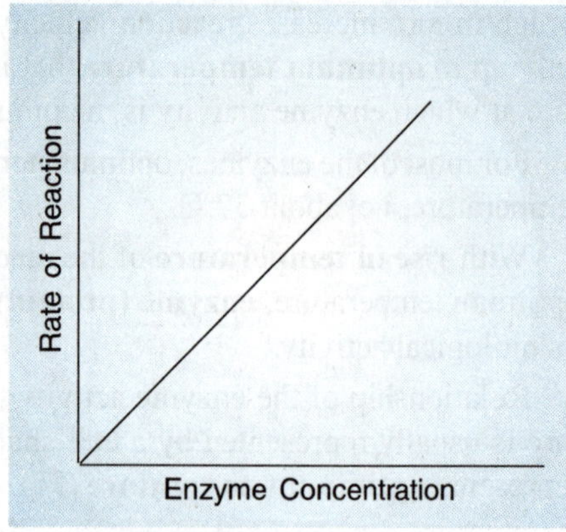

Fig. 6.7. Effect of enzyme concentration on enzyme activity.

EFFECT OF ACTIVATORS/INHIBITORS

Addition of some substances may activate while others may inhibit enzyme activity. As discussed earlier, **certain inorganic ions** are required for the activity of various enzymes. These substances are referred to as **activators,** such as Cl^- for salivary amylase, Mg^{2+} for phosphatase and phosphorylase, Zn^{2+} for carbonic anhydrase, etc.

Substances, which inhibit an enzymatic reaction, are referred as **inhibitors**, e.g. cyanide for cytochrome oxidase, malonate for succinate dehydrogenase, etc.

ENZYME INHIBITION

Phenomenon of decrease in rate of the enzymatic reaction, brought about by the addition of a substance, is called enzyme inhibition. An inhibitor may affect enzyme activity by competitive inhibition, or noncompetitive inhibition

COMPETITIVE INHIBITION

A competitive **inhibitor competes with the substrate,** for its binding at the active site of the enzyme. **Chemical structure** of such an inhibitor closely **resembles the substrate,** e.g. malonate inhibits action of succinate dehydrogenase.

The inhibitor forms a complex with the enzyme, called **enzyme-inhibitor complex** (EI), instead of the enzyme-substrate complex (ES), and inhibits the enzyme of its action on the substrate.

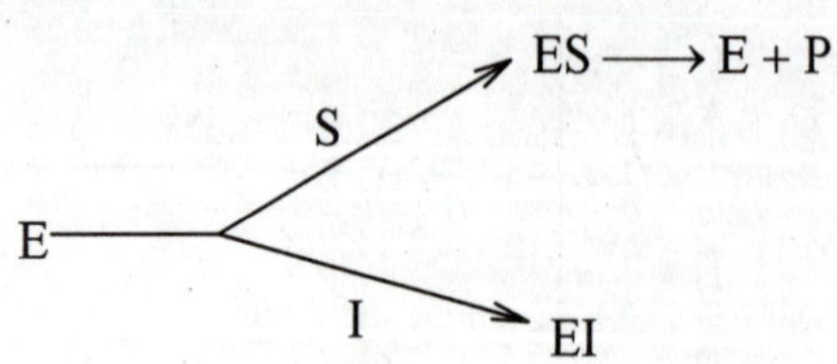

Binding of enzyme with the inhibitor or substrate depends upon their relative concentrations. It is usually a reversible process. Increasing the concentration of the substrate can reduce the degree of inhibition. Presence of the competitive inhibitor increases the K_m without any change in Vmax (Fig. 6.8)

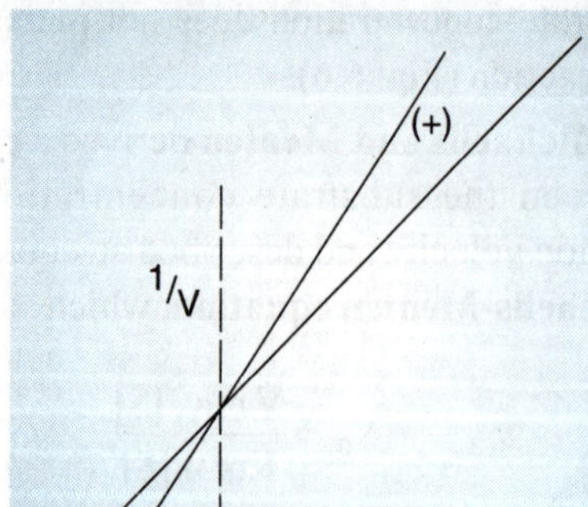

Fig. 6.8. The Lineweaver-Burk plot for a competitive inhibitor (+).

Table 6.6 lists some of the enzymes, which are competitively inhibited.

Due to their inhibitory effects, several drugs are used as

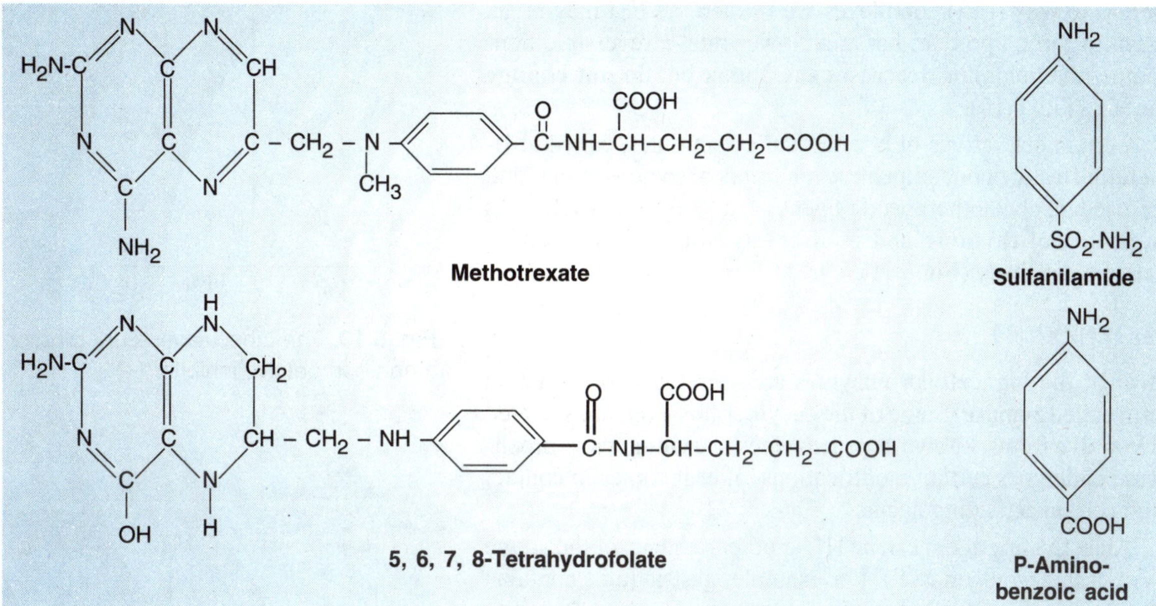

Fig. 6.9. Some competitive inhibitors.

inhibitors of some of the specific enzymes in a metabolic pathway. For example, **sulfanilamide (**a sulfa drug) is an antibacterial agent and resembles **p-aminobenzoic acid**, structurally. It is a **competitive inhibitor of** the enzyme, **dihydropteroic acid synthase**, in bacteria.

Similarly, **methotrexate, a structural analog of folate, competitively inhibits dihydrofolate reductase** and is used in the treatment of childhood leukemia (Fig. 6.9).

Table 6.6. Some enzymes, their substrates, and competitive inhibitors

Enzyme	*Substrate*	*Competitive inhibitor*
Succinate dehydrogenase	Succinate	Malonate
Carbonic anhydrase	Carbonate	Acetazolamide
Dihydrofolate reductase	Dihydrofolate	Amethopterin (methotrexate)
L-Histidase	L-Histidine	D-Histidine
Xanthine oxidase	Hypoxanthine	Allopurinol
HMG CoA reductase	HMG CoA	HMG

NONCOMPETITIVE INHIBITION

Certain chemical **substances react covalently with the functional groups that** are present on the active sites **of the enzymes** and thus inactivate enzymes, non-competitively. For example, many enzymes have free SH-groups in their molecules, and substances like iodoacetate or p-chloromercurobenzoate combines with these SH-groups and inactivate the enzyme. Heavy metals, like Hg^{2+} and Ag^{+}, also inactivate some enzymes. This type of inhibition is usually irreversible and makes the active sites of the enzyme ineffective.

A **noncompetitive inhibitor** may also **bind at a site other than the substrate-binding site.** In such cases either the enzyme or the enzyme-substrate complex binds the inhibitor. As a result, both binary (EI) as well as ternary (ESI) complexes are formed. As ESI may break down to form a product but at a slower rate, a reversible non-competitive inhibitor **decreases the Vmax** but **do not change the K_m** (Fig. 6.10).

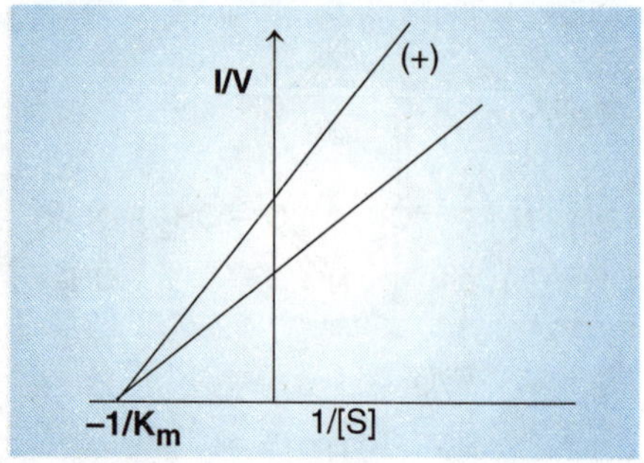

Fig. 6.10. The Lineweaver-Burk plot for a non-competitive inhibitor (+).

Certain derivatives of purines and pyrimidines, called **anti-metabolites**, are noncompetitive inhibitors of some enzymes and are used as chemotherapeutic agents, e.g. **5-fluorouracil**. It is an analog of **thymine** and inhibits **thymidylate synthetase, noncompetitively** (Fig.6.11).

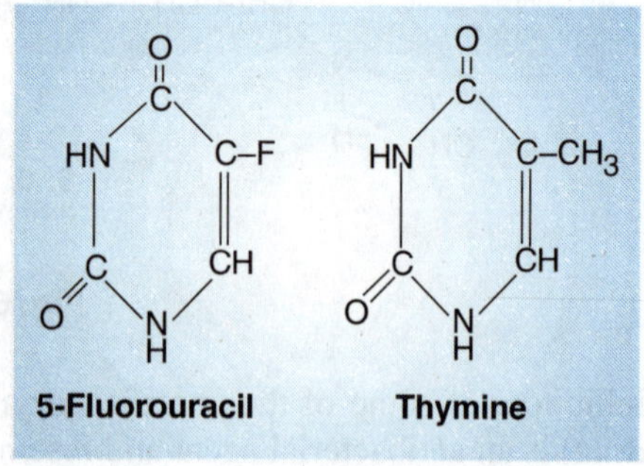

Fig. 6.11. A non-competitive inhibitor.

PROENZYMES

Most of the intracellular enzymes are secreted in their active form called **zymase**. Some of the enzymes however, are secreted in **inactive** forms, known as proenzymes or **zymogens**. A proenzyme undergoes certain modifications, after it comes in contact with certain activating agents.

An activating agent can be H^+, another enzyme, or the active form of the zymogen itself. For example, gastric juice contains **pepsin**, which is secreted as **pepsinogen** (a zymogen). Pepsinogen is transformed to its active form pepsin by H^+ of the gastric juice. Once formed, pepsin can act on pepsinogen and catalyse its conversion to pepsin. This process is referred as **autocatalysis** (Fig. 6.12).

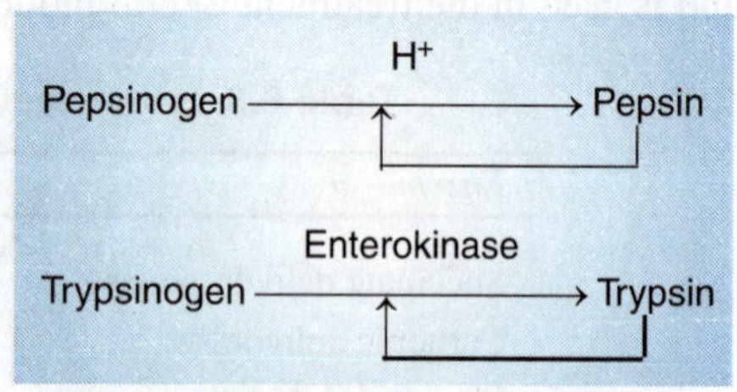

Fig. 6.12. Conversion of a zymogen to an active enzyme.

Table 6.7 lists some of the enzymes, which occur as proenzymes.

Table 6.7. Some of the enzymes that are secreted as proenzymes

Proenzyme	*Activator*	*Enzyme*
Pepsinogen	H^+, pepsin	Pepsin
Trypsinogen	Trypsin, enterokinase	Trypsin
Chymotrypsinogen	Trypsin	Chymotrypsin
Procarboxypeptidase	Trypsin	Carboxypeptidase
Proelastase	Trypsin	Elastase

ISOENZYMES

Isoenzymes (isozymes) are **physically distinct forms of the enzyme,** which have **same specificity** but **differ from each other with respect to their structure, electrophoretic mobility, immunological properties, or source,** e.g. lactate dehydrogenase, creatine phosphokinase, alkaline phosphatase, etc.

LACTATE DEHYDROGENASE

Lactate dehydrogenase (LDH) is a tetramer, i.e. it has four polypeptide subunits. Its each subunit may be one of the two-types, known as the H (heart) type and the M (muscle) type. **LDH** exists, in serum, in **five distinct forms** (isoenzymes), which have different proportions of H and M subunits. LDH_1 has four polypeptide chains of the H type, i.e. as H_4 while LDH_5 has four subunits of the M type (M_4). Other forms of the LDH include LDH_2 (H_3M), LDH_3 (H_2M_2), and LDH_4 (HM_3).

LDH_1 and LDH_2 predominate in the myocardium and erythrocytes, while LDH_4 and LDH_5 predominate in the liver and skeletal muscle. LDH_1 becomes greater than LDH_2 between 12 to 24 hours following myocardial infarction. LDH_5 is diagnostic of secondary congestive liver involvement.

CREATINE PHOSPHOKINASE

Creatine phosphokinase (CPK), also referred to as **creatine kinase (CK), has three isoenzymes**. Each of its **isoenzyme** is a **dimer,** i.e. it is composed of two subunits, which may either be of the M (muscle) type or the B (brain) type. Its three isoenzymes are called as CPK_1 (BB), which is mainly found in the brain; CPK_2 (MB) in the myocardium; and CPK_3 (MM) in skeletal muscle.

CPK_2 is present in very small amount in serum. Its level rises with in 4 hours, reaching maximum with in 1 day, of myocardial infarction.

ALKALINE PHOSPHATASE

Alkaline phosphatase exists in three forms. Different tissues contain a distinct form of the enzyme. Major portion of the enzyme is **derived from liver whose** level **rises in post-hepatic jaundice.**

In **growing children, the enzyme is mainly from bone** and is **related to increased osteoblastic activity.**

During the **last trimester of pregnancy, increase in alkaline phosphatase** is primarily of the placental **origin**. This form of the enzyme is heat-stable; hence placental enzyme is also called as **heat-stable alkaline phosphatase.**

REGULATION OF ENZYME ACTIVITY

Regulation of the reaction velocity of enzyme is essential for the coordination of numerous metabolic processes. Besides changes in substrate concentration, enzyme activity is regulated by modifying the activity of the existing enzyme molecules, e.g. by allosteric effectors and covalent modification, or by altering the rate of its synthesis.

ALLOSTERIC REGULATION

Enzymes having two or more subunits have a **catalytic site,** also called as the regulatory site or the **allosteric site,** which is different from the **substrate-binding site**. These two sites are **located on different subunits of the oligomeric enzymes**. Such enzymes are called as the **allosteric enzymes or the regulatory enzymes**. Allosteric enzymes frequently catalyze the committed step, early in a pathway.

Certain substances called allosteric modulators or effectors, bind reversibly to an enzyme at the allosteric site and regulate activity of these enzymes. For example, HMG CoA reductase is a regulatory enzyme of cholesterol biosynthesis, aspartate transcarbamoylase for pyrimidine synthesis, etc.

An interaction with the effecter molecule brings about conformational changes in the catalytic site of the enzyme. Such an **effecter molecule** may **activate the enzymatic reaction (called allosteric activation)** and is referred to as a **positive effecter or allosteric activator. Binding** of some effecter may result in **the inhibition of the enzymatic reaction (called allosteric inhibition).** Such a molecule is called as a **negative effecter or allosteric inhibitor.**

Due to interaction between the substrate site, the activator site, and the inhibitor site, a characteristic **sigmoid curve** (S-shaped curve) is obtained. The presence of an **allosteric activator (+) shifts** the **curve to right** whereas an allosteric inhibitor (–) **shifts the curve to left** (Fig. 6.13).

Table 6.8 shows some examples of the allosteric modulators.

Table 6.8. Some allosteric modulators

Enzyme	Allosteric activator	Allosteric inhibitor
Hexokinase	ADP	Glucose-6-P, ATP
Isocitrate dehydrogenase	ADP	Glucose-6-P, ATP
Glutamate dehydrogenase	ADP	ATP, NADH
Pyruvate carboxylase	Acetyl CoA	ADP

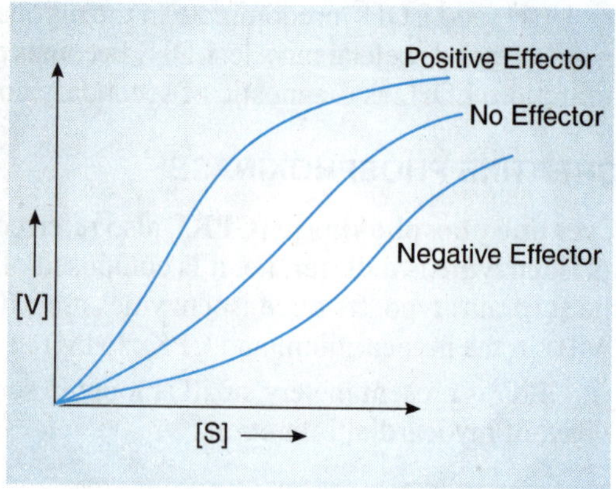

Fig. 6.13. Effect of activator/inhibitor on allosteric enzyme.

REGULATION BY COVALENT MODIFICATIONS

Several enzymes are regulated by covalent modification, most frequently by the addition or removal of a phosphate group that is attached at the serine, threonine, or tyrosine residue of the enzyme. Families of enzymes, called protein kinases that use ATP as a phosphate donor, catalyze phosphorylation of several enzymes. A phosphate group is removed from the phosphorylated enzyme, by the action of phosphoprotein phosphatase. Depending upon the specific enzyme, either the phosphorylated form (such as for glycogen phosphorylase) or the dephosphorylated form (as for glycogen synthase) is more active.

INDUCTION/ REPRESSION OF ENZYME SYNTHESIS

Cells can regulate the amount of the enzyme, usually by altering the rate of enzyme synthesis. Increase (induction) or decrease (repression) of enzyme synthesis leads to the alterations in the total number of the active sites. Enzymes that are needed at only one stage of the development or under selected physiological conditions are regulated in this way. For example, elevated level of insulin, as a result of high blood glucose level, causes an increase in the synthesis of the key enzymes, which are involved in glucose metabolism.

SERUM ENZYMES IN DIAGNOSIS

Measurement of certain enzymes, in serum, is helpful in diagnosis of various diseases. The level of the enzyme increases in serum, when it is released in large amounts due to the damage to the tissue. Some of these enzymes also have a prognostic significance.

Some of the enzymes, which have a diagnostic significance, include transaminases, alkaline phosphatase, etc.

Enzymes of diagnostic significance along with their tissue of origin and clinical applications are listed in Table 6.9.

TRANSAMINASES

Serum levels of aspartate aminotransferase (AST, also called **glutamate oxaloacetate transaminase or GOT)** and **alanine aminotransferase** (ALT, also called **glutamate pyruvate transaminase or GPT)** have clinical significance. In routine, these enzymes are also called as SGOT and SGPT.

In viral hepatitis and other forms of liver disease, serum GOT and GPT levels are raised even before the clinical signs and symptoms of the disease appear. Levels of both the enzymes may reach values up to 100 folds the upper normal limits. Their peak levels are seen between seven and twelve days. Thereafter, their

Table 6.9. Some serum enzymes of diagnostic significance

Enzyme	Principle source	Clinical situation in which altered
Acid phosphatase	Prostate, RBC	Increases in carcinoma of prostate
Alkaline phosphatase	Liver, bone, placenta, kidney	Increases in obstructive jaundice, rickets, Paget's disease, hyperparathyroidism
Aldolase	Skeletal muscle, heart	Increases in muscular dystrophies, acute liver diseases
Amylase	Salivary glands, pancreas, ovaries	Increases in acute pancreatitis, intestinal obstruction, acute parotitis, decreases in acute liver diseases
Ceruloplasmin	Liver	Increases in cirrhosis, decreases in Wilson's disease
Choline esterase	Liver	Increases in nephrotic syndrome, organo-phosphorus poisoning, decreases in acute liver diseases
Creatine phosphokinase	Skeletal muscle, brain, heart	Increases in myocardial infarction, muscular dystrophies
Glutamate oxaloacetate transaminase (GPT)	Liver, skeletal muscle, heart, kidney, RBCs	Increases in myocardial infarction, toxic liver cell necrosis, acute liver diseases, muscle diseases
γ-Glutamyltransferase	Liver, kidney	Alcoholism, hepatobiliary diseases
Lactate dehydrogenase	Heart, liver, skeletal muscle, RBCs, platelets	Increases in acute myocardial infarction, acute hepatitis, muscle disorders
Lipase	Pancreas	Increases in acute pancreatitis, pancreatic carcinoma, decreases in liver diseases, diabetes mellitus
5′-Nucleotidase	Hepatobiliary tract	Increases in liver diseases, obstructive jaundice, hepatic carcinoma
Trypsin	Pancreas	Increases in acute pancreatic diseases

activities gradually decrease and reach towards normal between three to five weeks. Although serum levels of both the enzymes (GPT and GOT) are elevated, GPT is more liver specific.

Five to ten-folds rise also occurs in both the enzymes in-patients with primary or metastatic carcinoma of liver.

After myocardial infarction (MI), increased GOT activity appears in serum, as its concentration is highest in the cardiac muscle. Since GPT concentration is less than GOT in cardiac muscle, there is comparatively lesser rise in GPT. Peak level of GOT is reached after 18 to 24 hours and returns towards normal, by fourth or fifth day.

GOT and occasionally GPT levels are elevated in progressive muscular dystrophy.

CREATINE PHOSPHOKINASE

CPK or CK (creatine kinase) activity is greatly elevated in all types of muscular dystrophies. Usually, only CK_3 is present in serum, in dystrophies and myopathies. However, in a neurogenic muscle disease, such as myasthenia gravis, its activity is normal.

Measurement of the CK_2 in serum is most commonly used for the diagnosis of acute MI. Initial rise occurs with in 4 to 6 hours. Peak levels are observed after approximately 24 hours, which return towards normal with in 48 to 72 hours.

Serum CK activity also increases in-patients with acute cerebro-vascular diseases. This is entirely due to CK_3.

LACTATE DEHYDROGENASE

Rise in LDH starts 12-18 hours after onset of acute MI, with peak after 48 to 72 hours. Its level returns towards normal after 6 to 10 days. Rise in total LDH in MI parallels a rise in **LDH_1**.

A marked elevation in total LDH activity, up to 50 times the upper normal value, may be observed in megaloblastic anemia. Elevation in LDH activity is also observed in liver diseases, renal diseases, and malignancy.

ALKALINE PHOSPHATASE

Estimation of serum alkaline phosphatase (ALP) is of significance in the diagnosis of hepato-biliary diseases, and bone diseases that are associated with increased osteoblastic activity. Amongst the various bone diseases, highest levels are seen in Paget's disease (nearly 10-25 times of the upper normal limit). Only a moderate rise is observed in osteomalacia.

In intrahepatic obstruction of the bile flow, increase in serum ALP is less where the rise is only 2-3 times of the upper normal limit.

γ-GLUTAMYL TRANSPEPTIDASE

γ-Glutamyl transpeptidase, also called **γ-glutamyl transferase (γGT)**, in serum primarily originates from the hepatobiliary system. Its activity is increased in all forms of a liver disease.

Elevated levels are of special significance in detecting alcohol-induced liver disease. Levels are increased not only in-patients with alcoholic cirrhosis but also in majority of people who are heavy drinkers.

AMYLASE

Estimation of amylase in serum and urine is of significance in the diagnosis of the diseases of the pancreas.

In acute pancreatitis, a transient rise (4–6 folds increase) in serum amylase activity occurs with in 2–12 hours of its onset, and the level returns towards normal by third or fourth day.

SOME IMPORTANT QUESTIONS

1. What are enzymes? Classify them. Discuss factors affecting enzyme activity.
2. Define enzyme, coenzyme, and cofactor. Discuss role of vitamins as coenzymes.
3. Define enzyme. What are isoenzymes? Discuss importance of enzymes in clinical diagnosis.
4. What are allosteric enzymes? How their activity is modulated? Give examples.
5. Give brief account of factors affecting enzyme activity.
6. Discuss briefly:
   (i) Various types of enzyme inhibition, giving examples.
   (ii) Apo-enzyme, holo-enzyme, and coenzyme, with examples.
   (iii) Classification of enzymes with examples.
7. Write notes on:
   (i) Diagnostic significance of enzymes.
   (ii) Noncompetitive inhibition of enzyme activity
   (iii) Isoenzymes and their importance
   (iv) Proenzymes

(v) Competitive inhibitors
(vi) Specificity of enzyme action
(vii) Coenzymes
(viii) Classification of enzymes
(ix) Ribozymes
(x) Allosteric regulation
(xi) Covalent modification
(xii) Induction and repression of enzyme activity

CHAPTER

7

Energy Metabolism

Carbohydrates, fats, and **proteins** are called as macronutrients and are the sources of **energy** in a diet. They are also called as the **proximate principles** of food.

Chemical energy, which is stored in these macromolecules, is released in the form of the **high energy phosphate bond** (~P), such as in ATP, creatine phosphate, etc., and in the form of reducing equivalents ($H^+ + e^-$), such as in NADH, $FADH_2$, etc.

In addition to energy, proteins also supply essential amino acids and nitrogen, which are required for the **growth** and **maintenance** of the **tissues.**

Energy stored in the various **foodstuffs is** ultimately **converted to heat hence; energy output** from the food is **measured as heat output** from the body.

CALORIE

Energy content of food is represented in terms of **calories, which is a unit** of **heat.**

A **calorie** is defined as the **amount of heat that is required to raise the temperature of 1g of water by 1°C,** i.e. from 14.5°C to 15.5°C.

International unit of energy is joule.

1 Calorie = 4.18 Joule

A Joule (J) is defined as the amount of heat that is required to move a mass of 1 Kg by 1 meter distance, by a force of 1 Newton.

Since calorie is a very small unit of heat, the amount of heat released by combustion of food is expressed in terms of kilocalories (Kcal or C).

1 Kcal (C) = 1000 calories, or
= 4.18 KJ (approx)

Since daily heat output from the body is replaced by supplying the equivalent amount of calories from the food, **calories requirement** therefore is estimated by measuring **calories output.**

The technique of the measurement of energy expenditure is known as calorimetery.

CALORIMETERY

Energy expenditure of an individual can be determined either **directly** by measuring heat output in a calorimeter, by the process called direct calorimetery, or **indirectly** by estimating oxygen consumption over a fixed period of time, by the process referred as **indirect calorimetery.**

Direct calorimetery

It is a most accurate method though easy in theory but difficult and costly in practice.

For direct calorimetery, a subject is placed in an insulated chamber around which a weighed quantity of the water is circulated, at a known rate and temperature. All the **heat, so produced,** is **directly measured by recording the total amount of heat which is transferred to the circulating water.**

Indirect calorimetery

In indirect calorimetery, **quantity of the heat produced** by the body, as a result of combustion of food, is **calculated from the quantity of the oxygen,** which is **consumed** by an individual.

Technically, it is a simple procedure.

Under normal conditions, **one liter of the O_2 accounts for approximately 4.82 Kcal of energy spent** by the body, as per respiratory quotient (RQ) of a mixed food.

In addition to O_2 utilized and CO_2 produced, the amount of nitrogen excreted during a given period of time can also be measured. Since each g of the urinary nitrogen represents 6.25g of protein, approximate amount of the protein metabolized can also be calculated by this technique.

RESPIRATORY QUOTIENT

Combustion of organic substances, during their oxidation, consumes O_2 and results in liberation of CO_2. **Ratio of the volume of CO_2 expired to the volume of O_2 utilized is known as respiratory quotient (R.Q.).**

$$R.Q. = \frac{\text{Volume of the } CO_2 \text{ expired}}{\text{Volume of the } O_2 \text{ utilized}}$$

R.Q. for the oxidation of carbohydrate is equivalent to **1.0** since on complete oxidation of carbohydrates; **volume of the CO_2 eliminated is equal to volume of the O_2 consumed.** For example, for oxidation of a molecule of glucose, six volumes of CO_2 are expired at the expense of six volumes of O_2.

$$C_6H_{12}O_6 + 6O_2 \longrightarrow 6CO_2 + 6H_2O$$

R.Q. for a carbohydrate therefore is equivalent to:

$$\frac{6CO_2}{6O_2} = 1.0$$

As oxygen content of the lipids is lower than their carbon contents, **lipids** therefore **require more O_2 for their oxidation.** For example, for the oxidation of two molecules of tri-stearin, 114 volumes of CO_2 are liberated while 163 volumes of O_2 are utilized:

$$2C_{57}H_{110}O_6 + 163O_2 \longrightarrow 114CO_2 + 110H_2O$$

R.Q. for the lipids therefore is equal to:

$$\frac{114}{163} = 0.7$$

Oxidation of proteins can not be readily expressed, due to their variable chemical structures. However, **R.Q. value for proteins has been reported to be 0.8.**

As varying proportions of the carbohydrates, fats, and proteins are consumed in the diet, each having its own R.Q., the **R.Q. value for a mixed food is taken as 0.82.**

At this value, every liter of O_2 consumed represents an energy expenditure of 4.82 Kcal.

CALORIFIC VALUE OF FOODS

Different types of foodstuffs release different **amounts of heat,** which is **expressed in terms of the calorific value of the food (Table 7.1).**

Calorific value of the food is defined as the **amount of heat (energy) produced on complete combustion of 1g of the foodstuff, in the presence of O_2.**

Table 7.1. Calorific value of different foodstuffs

Food stuff	*Calorific value (Kcal/g)*	
	In a bomb calorimeter	*In the body*
Carbohydrate	4.1	4.0
Fat	9.4	9.0
Protein	5.4	4.0

From metabolic oxidation of carbohydrate and fat, the heat of combustion in a bomb calorimeter as well as the amount of energy available to the human body is nearly same (Table 7.1).

This is due to the reason that oxidation of the two foodstuffs is complete both outside as well as with in the body. Since actual **calorific values for carbohydrate and fat are** not much different under two conditions, for simplicity these values are taken as **4Kcal/g for carbohydrate and 9 Kcal/g for fat.**

For proteins, the actual heat output, as obtained in a calorimeter, is 5.4 Kcal/g, whereas the value obtained in the body is **4.0 Kcal/g** only. Difference in the two values is due to the reason that proteins are not completely oxidized in the body and that the nitrogenous end products of their catabolism, such as urea, still has some energy though that is not available to the body.

Quantity of the heat produced by the body, as a result of combustion of different foodstuffs, can thus be calculated if quantity of each foodstuff, present in the diet, is known.

ENERGY NEEDS

Energy need of an individual can be calculated by knowing his energy expenditure, which depends upon the basal requirement, SDA, and the requirement for physical activity.

BASAL REQUIREMENT

An individual, even **at complete physical and mental rest,** requires some energy. This requirement of energy is for the activities of the internal organs as well as for the maintenance of body temperature. These processes are called as the basal metabolic processes and energy required for these processes is **referred to as the basal requirement.**

Average basal requirement, per 24 hours, is taken as 1500 Kcal for an adult male and 1300 Kcal for an adult female.

Basal requirement of an individual is determined as the rate of metabolic activities of the body in resting condition and is **expressed as basal metabolic rate.**

BASAL METABOLIC RATE

Basal metabolic rate (BMR) is **defined as the rate of energy utilization in a resting state.**

It is determined experimentally, when the subject is lying down at complete physical and mental rest (with closed eyes but awaken), **wearing light clothing**, at a room temperature of around 20-25°C, and at least 12 hours after the last meal, i.e. in the post-absorptive state.

BMR is determined with the help of indirect calorimetery where oxygen consumption is measured, in a complete resting state, for 6 minutes, and the value per hour is calculated. This value is multiplied with 4.82 (the amount of heat produced per liter of O_2 consumed) and total amount of heat produced, as Kcal/hr, is calculated. This value is divided by surface area, to obtain the value of BMR, which is expressed in terms of Kcal/m^2/hr.

Average BMR for a normal adult male is 40 Kcal/m^2/hr. For a female, this value is 36 Kcal/m^2/hr.

BMR value of an individual is expressed as a percentage of the normal reference value.

BMR value between -15 to +20% of the normal value is considered to be within normal limit.

FACTORS AFFECTING BMR

1. **Age:** Age reflects growth as well as lean muscle mass.

   Infants and children require more energy, for growth. This, in turn, is reflected in terms of the higher basal metabolic rate (BMR).

   Thus BMR is **high in actively growing children** up to around 5 years of age. It again increases at puberty.

   During aging since muscle tissue is gradually replaced with fat and water, adults therefore, have reduced BMR. There is nearly 2% decrease in BMR per decade.
2. **Sex:** Since women have smaller percentage of lean muscle mass than men, women therefore have low BMR.
3. **Climate: BMR is low in temperate** (warm) **climate** than in the cold climate.
4. **Physiological state:** BMR is **increased in severe stress** and after **trauma.**

   It remains **unaltered in the first trimester of pregnancy** but **increases thereafter.** This is due to the additional BMR of the fetus.
5. **Diet: Vegetarians have low BMR. Caffeine, nicotine,** and **alcohol** increase BMR.

   BMR decreases during starvation. It is **also reduced in undernutrition.**
6. **Hormones:** Hormones, such as **thyroxine, sex hormones, growth hormone, epinephrine, and glucocorticoids increase BMR.**

   Thyroxine is most important in this regard. Measurement of BMR is used in assessment of the thyroid functions. BMR is increased up to 75% in hyperthyroidism and reduces up to 50% in hypothyroidism.

Epinephrine also increases BMR.

BMR is also increased in hyperactivity of the **adrenal gland**. In tumor of the adrenal cortex and in Cushing's syndrome, BMR is increased. BMR is reduced in Addison's disease.

BMR is also increased in hyper functioning of the **anterior pituitary.**

7. **Clinical Disorders:** BMR is **increased** during **fever,** in certain **infections,** and **hypermetabolic disorders.**

   During fever, increase in BMR is usually proportional to rise in body temperature. For every 1ºC rise in body temperature above normal, there is nearly 12% increase in BMR.

   Due to enhanced metabolic activity of the cells, BMR is increased in leukemia, polycythemia, anemia, cardiac failure, and hypertension.

NEED ON ACCOUNT OF THE SPECIFIC DYNAMIC ACTION (SDA)

Specific dynamic action (SDA) is defined as the **amount of heat produced, over and above the actual calorific value of the food,** when it is metabolized in the body. This is **also referred to as the thermogenic effect** or **calorigenic action of food.** These terms are used to describe the effect of food in raising metabolic rate, above the value found during fasting.

Dietary protein increases metabolic processes by nearly **30%, fat** by about 12% and **carbohydrate** by about 5%. This extra amount of the calories is actually the amount of heat that body has spent for degradation of food, and which is regained back due to SDA.

Cause of the calorigenic action of food though is uncertain, it may partly account for various activities, which are being performed by the body, such as secretion of juices by the stomach, pancreas, etc.

High value of SDA on feeding a protein rich diet is actually due to requirement of energy for various metabolic activities, such as deamination, urea synthesis, etc. This energy is derived by the oxidation of other metabolites, which are present in the tissues. High SDA for protein is also an important factor in the regulation of body temperature.

Addition of the other foodstuffs to a protein diet lowers its SDA.

The value of SDA for a mixed food is taken as 10% of the basal requirement.

NEED FOR PHYSICAL ACTIVITY

Energy requirement is also determined by the extent as well as type of physical activity, an individual performs.

Several measurements of the energy expenditure, separately for men and women, for various types of activities, have been made, by indirect calorimetery, by several workers. Accordingly –

Those who perform **light type of work are called as the sedentary workers,** e.g. shopkeepers, carpenter, painter, etc.

Moderate category of workers includes those individuals who perform both physical as well as mental activities, e.g. students, farmers doing mechanized farming, soldiers, etc.

Heavy category of workers includes those types of workers who perform more physical work, e.g. plumber, workers working in coal-mining, stone-crushing, rickshaw pulling, etc.

As there are variations in individual efficiency, body weight, and sex, grading of these activities is only the approximations.

Table 7.2 provides some estimates of energy output during various types of activities.

Table 7.2. Approximate calorie requirement for different types of physical activities

Physical activity	*Calorie requirement (Kcal/hr)*
Reading/sitting/standing	35-40
Tailoring/typing/writing	70-75
Household work	100-110
Carpentry/painting	140-150
Light exercise/slow to moderate walk	200-250
Active exercise/Walking downstairs	350-400
Fast walking/running/swimming	450-500
Walking upstairs	1000-1100

Average daily calories requirements for different category of workers are shown in Table 7.3.

On an average, a moderate male worker, e.g. a student, **requires nearly 2800 Kcal/day** while **a female,** performing the same type of work, **needs about 2200 Kcal/day.**

Table 7.3. Average calories requirement for different category of workers

Category of worker	*Requirement (Kcal/day)*			
	Basal	*SDA*	*For physical activity*	*Total (Approx.)*
Males				
Sedentary workers	1500	150	800	2400
Moderate workers	1500	150	1200	2800
Heavy workers	1500	150	2400	4000
Females				
Sedentary workers	1300	130	500	1900
Moderate workers	1300	130	800	2200
Heavy workers	1300	130	1600	3000

SOME IMPORTANT QUESTIONS

1. Define basal metabolic rate. Discuss various factors affecting BMR.
2. Discuss :
   (i) Respiratory quotient.
   (ii) SDA.
   (iii) Calorimetery.

CHAPTER

8

Digestion and Absorption of Macronutrients

DIETARY SOURCES OF ENERGY

Carbohydrates

Carbohydrates are the most efficient and cheapest sources of energy. **Around 40 to 85 per cent of the required calories may be derived from carbohydrates.**

Any excess of the carbohydrates, than what is needed for energy, are converted to glycogen and triacylglycerol and stored in the body. Carbohydrate content of diet thus affects glycogen stores.

Principle sources of carbohydrates include starch **from cereals, pulses, potato, rice, etc.; lactose from milk** and sucrose **from table sugar. Glucose may not form an essential part of diet since all the dietary carbohydrates can be readily converted to glucose in the body.**

Dietary starch and other carbohydrates, which are available **to the body** as a source of energy, are known as available carbohydrates or digestible carbohydrates.

In addition, diet also contains some unavailable carbohydrates or indigestible carbohydrates, called **fibre.**

Fibre

Dietary fiber includes non-starch polysaccharides. They resemble starch but are not digested by the human digestive enzymes, in the gastrointestinal tract. All types of plant foods, such as vegetables, fruits, legumes, and whole grains, contain fiber. Dietary fiber includes cellulose, hemicelluloses, pectin, lignin, gums, and mucilage.

Some of the hemicelluloses, pectin, gum, and mucilage are soluble in water. These are classified as ***soluble fiber***. On the other hand, cellulose and some hemicelluloses and lignin are not soluble in water and are called as ***insoluble fiber.***

Significance of Dietary Fibre

1. High intake of dietary fiber has many health benefits. Diets rich in starch and dietary fiber decrease the risk of obesity, type 2 diabetes, cancer, cardiovascular disease, and gastrointestinal disorders. This is due to the reason that diets rich in complex carbohydrates are usually low in fat and energy. They are also more filling, offer a greater volume of food for fewer calories, and take longer to eat thus, giving a feeling of fullness. Such a diet therefore promotes a healthy body weight and **lowers the risk of obesity**.
2. Higher intake of soluble fiber also delays emptying of stomach and smoothes out blood glucose response. Thus such people have **low incidence of type 2 diabetes.**
3. Diet rich in complex carbohydrates also lowers the risk of certain kinds of cancer. Foods rich in fruits and vegetables contain antioxidants that protect against cell damage and **prevent cancer**.
4. High fiber intake also attracts water and dilutes cancer-causing agents in the gastrointestinal tract. It also speeds up their passage from the body, thereby decreasing their contact in the mucosal cells. This offers a protection against colon cancer.
5. Soluble fiber lowers serum cholesterol by binding bile acids in the GIT and preventing their reabsorption. Thus, diet rich in soluble fiber **lowers the risk for a cardiovascular disease**.
6. Diet rich in insoluble fiber adds to the bulk of the stool and increases its water contents thus, softening the stool and making it easier to pass. When fluid intake is ample, high fiber intake also helps in the **prevention of constipation, hemorrhoids**, and **diverticular disease.**

ENZYMATIC HYDROLYSIS OF DIETARY CARBOHYDRATES

Digestion of carbohydrate begins in the mouth, where salivary amylase hydrolyses starch into smaller polysaccharides and maltose. Chewing stimulates the production of saliva and mixes salivary amylase with the food. Only about 5% of the starch in food is broken down by the time the food is swallowed. When carbohydrate enters the stomach, acidity of the stomach stops the action of salivary amylase by denaturing the enzyme.

As stomach contents enter small intestine, the pancreas secretes pancreatic amylase through the pancreatic duct into the small intestine. Pancreatic amylase continues the digestion of starch, breaking it into maltose. Meanwhile, brush border disaccharidases; break various disaccharides into monosaccharides.

Dietary fiber moves to the large intestine, where bacteria partially ferment these undigested carbohydrates and produce gas and a few short-chain fatty acids. Soluble fiber softens the stool and makes it easier to pass. Insoluble fiber resists bacterial activity and passes unchanged to add bulk to stool.

ABSORPTION OF MONOSACCHARIDES

Different monosaccharides are absorbed into the mucosal cells, lining the small intestine, by two mechanisms. Whereas **fructose is absorbed by facilitated diffusion, the process of active transport absorbs glucose and galactose**. Sodium linked glucose transporter, called SLGT-1, helps in this process.

In the villi, absorbed monosaccharides pass through the intestinal mucosal cells and enter the liver via the portal vein. Within the liver, galactose and fructose are also converted to glucose.

DIETARY LIPIDS

Dietary lipids include triglycerides, cholesterol, and phospholipids. **Fat is a concentrated source of energy** and **provides** comparatively more energy than carbohydrate and proteins. It also reduces bulk of the food.

Amount of fat in the diet may vary from 15 to 45%. According to ICMR, fat should provide about 20% of daily energy requirement. Out of this about 10% of the calorie intake should be in the form of **invisible fat,** such as from milk, cereals, pulses, and legumes. Whereas the remaining 10% of the calories may be added in the form of the **visible fat,** such as from ghee, butter, or oil, etc.

SIGNIFICANCE OF DIETARY LIPIDS

Lipids are important for the body and serve many functions:

1. **Fat** improves palatability of food. **It also produces a feeling of satiety.**
2. **It is also** essential for the absorption of carotenoids and fat-soluble vitamins **(vitamins A, D, E, and K).**
3. Fat from vegetable sources is rich in polyunsaturated fatty acids and thus serves as a source of essential fatty acids, for the body.
4. Phospholipids form an important part of the membrane structure. **They are also essential** for the functioning of the nervous tissue.
5. Cholesterol **is available from foods of animal origin only. It is essential as a** precursor of vitamin D, steroid hormones, **and** bile salts.

Fat included in the diet should preferably be derived from vegetable sources, which are not only low in cost but also superior in quality, as compared to the fat from animal source, due to the presence of polyunsaturated fatty acids (PUFA). Sunflower oil, cottonseed oil, wheat-germ oil, soybean oil, corn oil, etc., are some of the common vegetable sources of fat. These oils have more than 50% of fat, as PUFA.

ESSENTIAL FATTY ACIDS

Three **polyunsaturated fatty acids** have been recognized as essential, in the diet of most animals. These are **linoleic acid, linolenic acid, and arachidonic acid, and are referred to as essential fatty acids.** They are needed for lowering serum cholesterol, maintaining functions and integrity of membrane and synthesis of prostaglandins.

The most common symptom of essential fatty acids deficiency is scaly dermatitis.

Excessive consumption of saturated fat from animal sources, and cholesterol is **associated with hypercholesterolemia** and **atherosclerosis.**

Eggs have the highest concentration of cholesterol. Cholesterol content of the skimmed milk is lower than the whole milk. Pulses do not contain cholesterol. Besides atherosclerosis, **excess cholesterol can also** result in formation of the **biliary stone.** It may also lead to obstructive jaundice and fat indigestion. High fat intake is also associated with cancers of the breast and colon.

Individuals, in prosperous community, who lead a sedentary life and have reached middle age, should limit their fat intake. On the other hand, heavy workers should consume more fat. However, compared to the cost of the carbohydrate, fat has more cost. Thus, it can be said that who require more fat cannot afford it, while those who can afford it, should not consume it.

OBESITY

Obesity is a most common nutritional disorder, due to the **excessive consumption of energy.** Besides overeating, **inadequate exercise** plays an important role in the causation of obesity. **Genetic component** is also important since gene for obesity has been shown to exist.

Striking **features** of the obesity include m**arked elevation in serum free fatty acids, cholesterol,** and **triacylglycerol.** Other findings include high fasting blood glucose and reduced glucose tolerance, as most of the adult-onset diabetics are overweight.

ENZYMATIC HYDROLYSIS OF DIETARY TRIACYLGLYCEROLS AND PHOSPHOLIPIDS

Digestion of triglycerides is initiated in the mouth with chewing and by the action of the lingual lipase. Thereafter, with the action of **gastric lipase**, and churning and contraction by the **stomach**, nearly 30% of the dietary triglycerides get degraded to di-glycerides and free fatty acids, with in 2 to 3 hours. Contents from the stomach pass into the **small intestine**. Presence of the fat in the small intestine stimulates the release of two hormones, i.e. cholecystokinin (CCK) and secretin from the duodenal cells. CCK signals the gallbladder to contract and release bile, down the bile duct and into the duodenum. Bile contains large quantity of bile salts and lecithin. Secretin signals the pancreas to release pancreatic juice, which is rich in pancreatic lipase.

Bile emulsifies fat and breaks fat globules (clumps of triglycerides) into small pieces and keep them suspended in solution. This in turn increases total surface area for the action of **pancreatic lipase**. Pancreatic lipase hydrolyzes all the accessible triglycerides, within minutes into monoglycerides and free fatty acids. Bile salts surround the hydrolyzed products of fat digestion and form water-soluble globules with a fatty core called **micelles.** Micelles transport monoglycerides and free fatty acids through the watery intestinal environment to the brush border of the intestinal mucosal cells for absorption.

Similarly, **phospholipases** hydrolyze phospholipids and release monoglycerides, free fatty acids, phosphate, and a nitrogenous substance.

ABSORPTION OF TRIACYLGLYCEROLS AND PHOSPHOLIPIDS

Most fat absorption takes place in the **duodenum or jejunum** of the small intestine.

Micelles carry monoglycerides and long-chain fatty acids to the surface of the microvilli in the brush border and diffuse into the intestinal cells. The unabsorbed bile salts return to the interior of the small intestine for the transport of more mono-glycerides and fatty acids. Bile salts are absorbed in the ileum and return via the portal vein to the liver where they are again secreted into the bile. This recycling pathway for bile, i.e. from the liver to the intestine and from the intestine to the liver is called **enterohepatic circulation**.

As monoglycerides and fatty acids pass into the intestinal cells, they reform triglycerides. Most of the triglycerides as well as cholesterol and phospholipids join protein carriers and form **chylomicrons.** Chylomicrons make their way to the central lacteal of the villi where they enter the lymph system to be propelled through the thoracic duct and emptied into veins in the neck (Fig. 8.1).

Glycerol and medium and short chain fatty acids are absorbed directly into the blood stream. Dietary fat begins to appear in the blood stream after 1 to 2 hrs of meal, with a peak after 3 to 5 hrs. It is generally cleared by 10 hrs.

Absorption of fat is drastically reduced in the absence of bile salts. As a result of it, bulk of the unabsorbed fat is excreted in the stool. The production of stool with an abnormally high amount of fat is referred as **steatorrhea.** Steatorrhea may follow diseases of malabsorption, such as cystic fibrosis, radiation therapy, or digestive tract surgery. In such conditions triglycerides with medium chain fatty acids are often given in the diet. This is due to the reason that medium chain fatty acids are comparatively more water-soluble than long-chain fatty acids and thus can be emulsified more readily. Breast milk is a rich source of medium and short chain fatty acids.

DIGESTION AND ABSORPTION OF STEROLS

Sterols remain, mostly, unchanged by digestion. Their absorption is also relatively poor. Cholesterol gets esterified prior to its absorption. Dietary fat increases absorption of cholesterol where as plant sterols and dietary fiber decrease cholesterol absorption.

DIETARY PROTEINS

BIOLOGICAL IMPORTANCE OF PROTEINS

Proteins are important for the body and serve many functions:

1. Protein may be used as a source of energy.

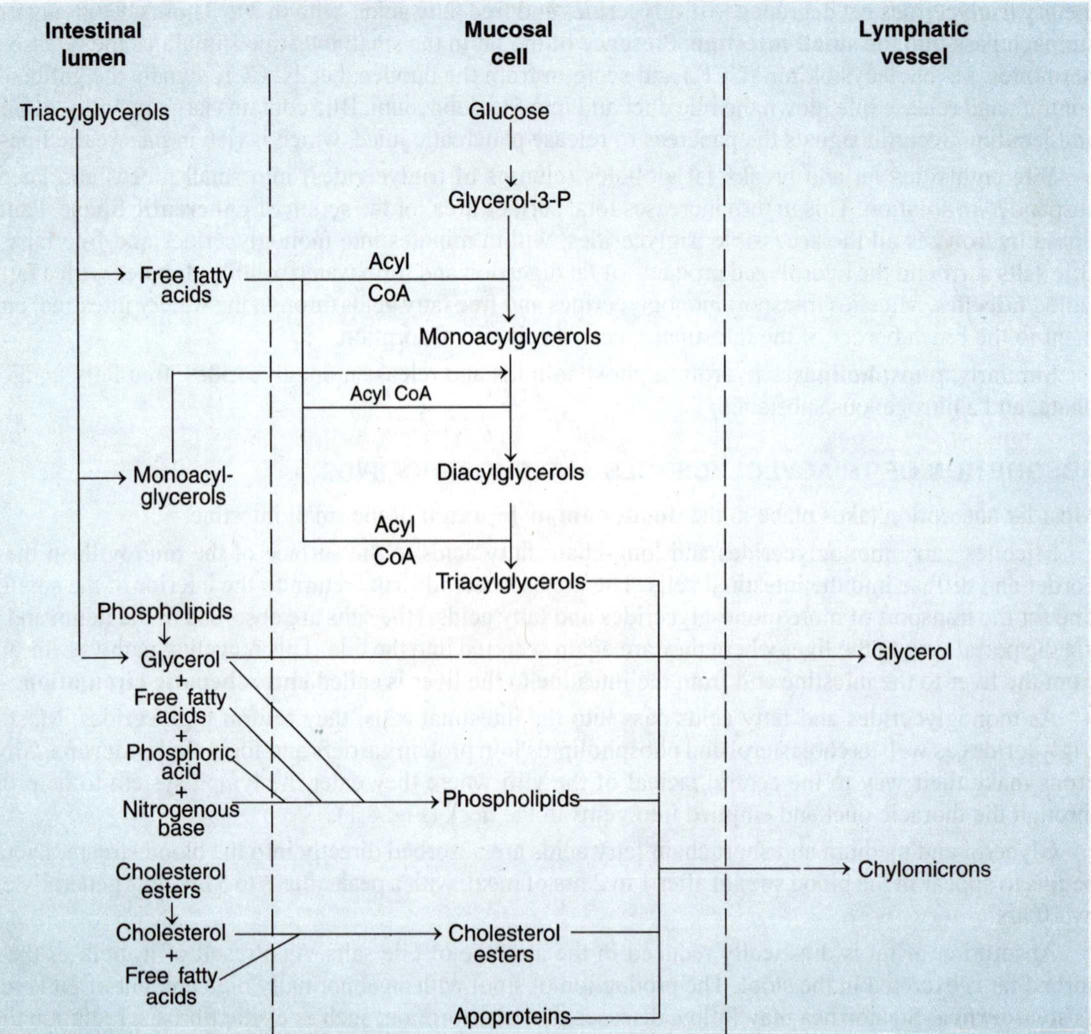

Fig. 8.1. Absorption of lipids in the intestinal mucosa.

2. Proteins are essential **structural components** of the **cell.**
3. Proteins are important for maintaining output of essential **secretions,** such as **digestive enzymes** and peptide/protein **hormones**.
4. These are required for the synthesis of **plasma proteins,** which are essential for maintenance of osmotic balance, transport of substances, and **immunity**.
5. Protein is a source of both essential as well as nonessential **amino acids.**

NITROGEN BALANCE

Comparison of nitrogen intake (dietary protein) to nitrogen excretion (sum of all sources of nitrogen excretion, such as in urine and feces, from the skin and hair, and in body fluids) gives a measure of nitrogen balance and indicates protein status of the body.

When nitrogen intake exceeds nitrogen excretion, body is said to be in a **positive nitrogen balance**. Positive nitrogen balance means body is adding protein, as in the case for growing children, pregnant women, and people recovering from protein deficiency or illness.

When nitrogen excretion exceeds nitrogen intake, body is said to be in **negative nitrogen balance**. This means that body is losing protein, such as during starvation, on weight-loss diets, during fever, severe illness or infection.

When nitrogen intake is equal to nitrogen excretion, the nitrogen balance is zero and body is in **nitrogen equilibrium**, such as in healthy individuals. There is no net gain or loss of the body protein.

ESSENTIAL AMINO ACIDS

Dietary protein is an important source of amino acids, which are required for growth in children and for the maintenance in adults. As growth slows down, need for protein is also decreased.

Isoleucine, leucine, lysine, methionine, phenylalanine, threonine, tryptophan, and valine are called **essential amino acids**. In addition, **histidine and arginine** are also needed during growth. These two amino acids are called **semi essential amino acids.**

Generally, animal proteins, such as egg albumin, milk casein, etc., are rich in essential amino acids.

PROTEIN QUALITY

Both animal and plant foods though contain protein, the quality of protein in the two types of foods differ. Dietary protein, which supplies all the essential amino acids, in the proportions needed by the body, are called **complete proteins** or **high quality proteins**, e.g. protein from meat, poultry, fish, eggs, milk and milk products, and soybeans. On the other hand, proteins that lack adequate amounts of one or more essential amino acids are called **low-quality proteins** or **incomplete proteins**.

Assessment of protein quality

Protein quality of a food may be assessed by several ways, e.g. a**mino acid scoring, protein efficiency ratio, net protein utilization,** etc.

BIOLOGICAL VALUE OF PROTEINS

Biological value is expressed as percentage of the absorbed dietary nitrogen retained by the body for growth and/or maintenance. Since nitrogen retention is a function of absorption, if a protein has an essential amino acid composition similar to our needs, the body will more efficiently retain the particular protein.

Urinary and fecal nitrogen output is measured while the subject is consuming the test protein, and compared with the value on a nitrogen free diet. The final value expresses nitrogen retention as a percentage of the nitrogen absorbed.

$$\text{Biological value} = \frac{\text{Nitrogen retained}}{\text{Nitrogen absorbed}} \times 100$$

Egg protein has a biological value of 100 while biological value of the corn protein is 60.

PROTEIN REQUIREMENT

It is recommended that about 10 to 15% of the total energy requirement, in an adult diet, should come from protein. Recommended daily intake of protein for adult is 0.8g/kg body weight. Accordingly, daily protein recommendation comes out to be 55-60g for an average male and 45-50 g for an average female.

During pregnancy and lactation protein requirement is increased by about 10 to 15g/day. Infants, who are growing rapidly, have the highest protein needs, relative to the body weight. They need about 2.0g of protein / kg body weight.

Protein requirement is increased in severe physical stress, infection, burns, fever, and after surgery.

Dietary intake of carbohydrate and fat are also important in determining protein requirement. As energy content of the diet from carbohydrate is increased, the need for protein decreases. This is referred to as **protein sparing action of carbohydrate**.

Excess of dietary protein is used as a source of energy. The glucogenic amino acids are converted to glucose while ketogenic amino acids are converted to fatty acids and ketone bodies.

Meat, eggs, milk, legumes, grains, and vegetables are good sources of protein. Fruits contain minimal amounts.

COMPLEMENTARY PROTEINS

Proteins in plant foods are low-quality proteins, i.e. they lack one or more essential amino acids. The protein in one plant food generally lacks certain amino acid(s) whereas the protein in another plant food can provide the missing amino acid but lacks some other amino acid, thereby complementing the amino acid pattern when taken together.

Complementary protein may hence be referred to two or more poor quality food proteins whose assortment of amino acids complement for each other's lack of specific essential amino acid, so that the combination provides sufficient amounts of all the essential amino acids. For example, grains, such as wheat, are low in the essential amino acid lysine but high in methionine. On the other hand, legumes, such as beans, are low in methionine but high in lysine. Thus with a combination of wheat with legume, the protein from wheat complements the protein from legume and that the two together provide a complete protein. Protein complementation is important for those people who consume little or no animal protein.

PROTEIN CALORIE MALNUTRITION

Dietary protein deficiency can be harmful for several body systems as protein plays a vital role in many body processes. Normally, it is difficult to separate protein and energy intakes since diets adequate in energy usually are also adequate in protein. Similarly diets, which lack energy also, inhibit the use of dietary protein for protein synthesis in the body. A deficiency of dietary protein and/or energy is called **protein-energy malnutrition (PEM)**. Though PEM can occur at any stage of life, it is most common during the childhood when protein is needed for rapid growth. PEM occurs in all parts of the world but is most common in Southeast Asia, Africa, South and Central America, and Middle East. It occurs most often in population living in poverty, in the elderly people, and in the hospitalized patients with other associated conditions, such as anorexia nervosa, AIDS, cancer, or malabsorption syndromes.

Two common forms of severe PEM include kwashiorkor and marasmus.

Kwashiorkor

Kwashiorkor usually develops when diet is low in protein or the protein is not absorbed easily. The symptoms of kwashiorkor include edema (swelling of body tissues), usually in the feet and legs. The belly becomes bloated from both edema and accumulation of fat in the liver. Other features include stunted weight and height, increased susceptibility to infections, dry and fleshy skin, dry and brittle hair, and changes in the skin color. Kwashiorkor usually develops in children between 18 and 24 months of age, around the time when weaning occurs.

Marasmus

Protein, energy, and nutrients intake are all grossly inadequate, depleting body fat reserves and severely wasting muscle tissue. Growth slows, and children are both short and thin for their age. Their hair is sparse and fall easily. It can also stunt brain development and lead to learning disabilities. Marasmus occurs most often in infants and children 6 to 18 months of age who are fed diluted or improperly mixed formulas.

ENZYMATIC HYDROLYSIS OF DIETARY PROTEINS

Digestion of protein begins **in the stomach** where HCl denatures protein, unfold it, and makes it more accessible to the action of enzymes. Firstly, HCl converts **pepsinogen**, produced by the glands in the stomach lining, to the active enzyme **pepsin**. Pepsin subsequently hydrolyses dietary protein into individual amino acids and peptides of various chain lengths.

From the stomach, amino acids and polypeptides pass into the **small intestine**. In response to the presence of protein, pancreas secretes **trypsinogen and chymotrypsinogen** into the small intestine. These proenzymes are cleaved into their active forms, **trypsin and chymotrypsin,** respectively. Finally, brush border peptidases split the remaining polypeptides into amino acids, dipeptides, and tripeptides. These smaller units are transported across the microvilli membrane into the cell. Inside the cell, many **peptidases** specifically hydrolyze the remaining dipeptides and tripeptides into individual amino acids for their absorption into the bloodstream.

Any part of the protein that is not digested in the small intestine continues through the large intestine and passes out of the body in the feces.

Cystic fibrosis is an inherited disorder due to the deficiencies of pancreatic enzymes that are needed for the digestion of proteins. It results in poor digestion of protein along with widespread dysfunction of the endocrine glands, causing chronic lung disease and abnormally high levels of electrolytes (sodium, potassium, and chloride) in the sweat.

Celiac disease is a defect in the digestion of gluten (a protein found in wheat, rye, oat, and barley). If untreated, it causes flattening of the villi in the intestine, leading to severe malabsorption of nutrients. Symptoms include diarrhea, fatty stool, swollen belly, and extreme fatigue.

ABSORPTION OF AMINO ACIDS

More than 99% of the dietary protein enters the bloodstream as amino acids. Absorption of most of the amino acids takes place in the cells that line the duodenum and jejunum. Absorption of some amino acids takes place by active transport, while others are absorbed via facilitated diffusion. After they are absorbed, most amino acids and few peptides are transported via the portal vein to the liver and released into the circulation.

Active transport is a Na^+-dependent process, which requires ATP, specific transport proteins, and pyridoxal-phosphate. Both, an L-amino acid and Na^+ are attached to a carrier protein that is present on the mucosal surface of the microvillous membrane and form a complex (L-amino acid - carrier protein - Na^+ complex). This complex passes into the inner surface of the membrane and dissociates to liberate amino acid and Na^+. Carrier protein returns to the brush border, while amino acid (through portal blood) enters the liver. Na^+ is actively pumped out of the cell, while ATP is hydrolyzed to release energy, required for this process.

There are several transport proteins for the transport of different amino acids. These include for a group of:

1. Neutral amino acids with a short or polar side chain (Ala, Ser, and Thr);

2. Neutral amino acids with aromatic or hydrophobic side chain (Phe, Tyr, Met, Val, Leu, and Ile);
3. Basic amino acids (Lys, Arg, and Cystine);
4. Acidic amino acids (Asp and Glu); and
5. Imino acids, (Pro and hydroxyproline).

Any part of the dietary protein that is not digested or absorbed in the small intestine enters the large intestine and passes out in the feces.

BALANCED DIET

Balance diet means variety and moderation in choice of food. Balance also means matching the amount of energy (calories) coming into the body via foods, with the amount of energy one expends in daily activities and exercise. No single food possesses unique qualities for health.

A **balanced diet** may therefore be defined as the one, which **contains various groups of foodstuffs,** such as energy-yielding foods, body building foods, and protective foods, in the correct proportions so that an individual is assured of obtaining the minimum requirements of all the nutrients. Their components however, may differ according to age, sex, physical activity, economic status, and the physiological state, viz. pregnancy, lactation, etc.

A balanced diet thus provides quantitatively as well as qualitatively adequate amounts of all the proximate principles of food, for maintaining a good health and physiological efficiency. **In a balanced diet, nearly 65-70% of the calories is derived from carbohydrates, 15-20% from lipids, and 10-15% from proteins.**

Dietary sources of carbohydrate should include both digestible as well as indigestible carbohydrates. **Lipids** should mainly be from the vegetable sources. A balanced diet should be **rich in PUFAs** and **low in cholesterol**. Dietary sources of protein should include **high biological value proteins.**

The diet should have a variety of items from different sources, best possible within one's budget. Green-leafy vegetables, fruits, and milk should also be included to provide the required amounts of vitamins and minerals.

Balanced diets at high cost

Such diets include liberal amounts of costly foods, such as milk, eggs, meat, fish, and fruits, along with moderate quantities of cereals, pulses, nuts, and fats.

Balanced diets at moderate cost

Such diets include moderate amounts of milk, eggs, meat, fish, fruits, and fats with liberal amounts of cereals, pulses, nuts, and green leafy vegetables.

Balanced diets at lower cost

Such diets include small amounts of milk, eggs, meat, fish, and fats with liberal amounts of cereals, pulses, nuts, and green-leafy vegetables.

SOME IMPORTANT QUESTIONS

1. Illustrate dietary sources of carbohydrates. Discuss the process of digestion and absorption of dietary carbohydrates.
2. How are fats digested? Explain the process of absorption of dietary fats.
3. What is a balanced diet? How will you prepare a balanced diet at moderate cost?

4. Write notes on:
   (i) Dietary fibre
   (ii) Enzymatic hydrolysis of dietary carbohydrates
   (iii) Essential fatty acids
   (iv) Obesity
   (v) Significance of dietary lipids
   (vi) Nitrogen balance
   (vii) Essential amino acids
   (viii) Biological value of proteins
   (ix) Complementary proteins
   (x) Protein calorie malnutrition
   (xi) Cystic fibrosis
   (xii) Enzymatic hydrolysis of dietary proteins
   (xiii) Absorption of amino acids
   (xiv) Significance of dietary fibre

CHAPTER 9

Vitamins

Vitamins are the organic constituents of food and are called as the 'protective accessory food factors', as these are essential for the life and well being. Vitamins, in general, can not be synthesized by the body and have to be supplied in the diet though in very small quantities.

Vitamins are classified into two groups as fat-soluble and water soluble vitamins.

WATER SOLUBLE VITAMINS

Water-soluble vitamins include **vitamin B complex** and **vitamin C.**

Typical deficiency symptoms for most of the water-soluble vitamins, particularly those of vitamin B complex, include dermatitis, glossitis, cheilosis, and diarrhea, besides some of the neurological symptoms, such as peripheral neuropathy and malaise.

VITAMIN B COMPLEX

Vitamin B complex includes a group of compounds, most of which are synthesized in the gastrointestinal tract, by the microbial flora.

Certain derivatives of these vitamins also **act as coenzymes**. These vitamins are not stored in the body and thus their toxicity is not generally observed.

Most of these vitamins are heat stable except vitamin B_1, which is heat labile.

Two members of the vitamin B complex group, i.e. folic acid and vitamin B_{12}, are important hemopoietic factors and help in the prevention of anemia.

Various members of the vitamin B complex include **thiamin (B_1), riboflavin (B_2), niacin, pyridoxine (B_6), pantothenic acid, biotin, choline, lipoic acid, folic acid, and cyanocobalamin (B_{12}).**

THIAMIN

Thiamin is a first member of the vitamin B complex, therefore, it is also known as **vitamin B_1**. Due to its role in the prevention of beriberi, **thiamin is also called as the antiberi-beri factor.** Since it has an important role in the nervous system, thiamin is also called as **aneurine**.

Structurally, thiamin consists of a **pyrimidine ring,** which is linked to a **thiazole ring** (Fig. 9.1).

Thiamin occurs in nature as thiaminhydrochloride.

Though thiamin is heat labile, it is quite stable in acidic medium.

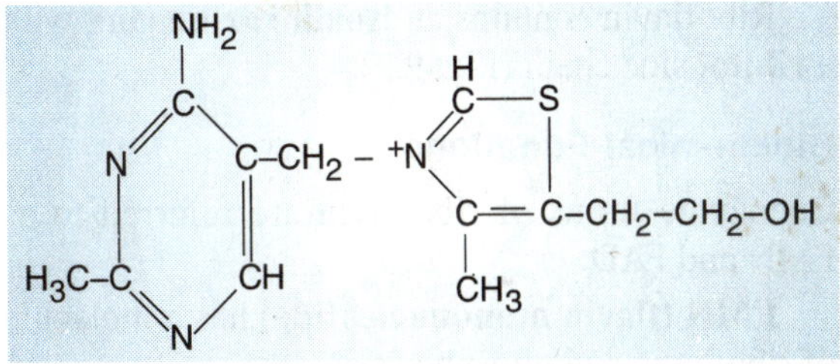

Fig. 9.1. Thiamin (vitamin B_1).

Biochemical Functions

Thiamin pyrophosphate (TPP), i.e. diphosphorylated form of the thiamin, is referred to as the coenzyme of vitamin B_1.

TPP plays an important role in carbohydrate metabolism. It is used as a **coenzyme** in **oxidative decarboxylation of α-keto acids,** e.g.

$$\text{Pyruvate} \xrightarrow{\text{Pyruvate dehydrogenase complex}} \text{Acetyl CoA}$$

$$\alpha\text{-Ketoglutarate} \xrightarrow{\alpha\text{-Ketoglutarate dehydrogenase complex}} \text{Succinyl CoA}$$

TPP also acts as a coenzyme for **transketolase**, an enzyme of the hexose monophosphate shunt.

Deficiency Symptoms

Thiamin deficiency causes **beriberi**. Beriberi is of different types:

1. **Wet beriberi:** It affects cardiovascular system and results in edema and dilated heart.
2. **Dry beriberi:** It normally affects the central nervous system and causes peripheral neuropathy with myelin degeneration, leading to foot-drop, wrist-drop, and sensory changes.
3. **Wernicke's encephalopathy:** It is generally observed in chronic alcoholics, who may develop CNS manifestations, ophthalmoplegia, cerebellar ataxia, and mental impairment.

Thiamin deficiency may also occur in areas where people consume polished-rice or raw-fish as well as in chronic alcoholics.

Deficiency symptoms include nausea, vomiting, weakness, and tenderness of the calf muscles.

Requirements

Average daily requirement is **1.2-1.8 mg/day.**

Daily requirement however, depends upon the carbohydrate intake and has been defined as **0.4-0.5 mg/1000 Kcal**.

Requirement is increased during fever, in hyperthyroidism, alcoholics, and pregnant woman.

Sources

Rich sources of thiamin are **cereal grains, yeast**, liver, kidney, and heart.

RIBOFLAVIN

Riboflavin (B_2) is also called as **lactoflavin,** due to its high content in milk. It is sensitive to light and ultraviolet irradiation. Riboflavin is heat-stable in acidic as well as neutral medium.

Riboflavin contains an **isoalloxazine ring** with a **ribitol** side chain (Fig. 9.2).

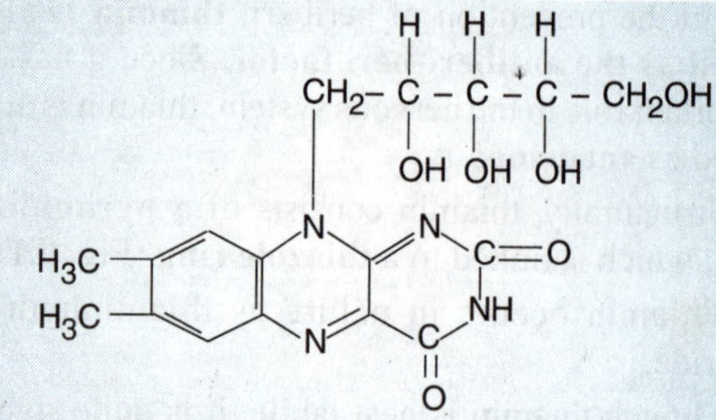

Fig. 9.2. Riboflavin (vitamin B_2).

Biochemical Functions

Coenzyme forms of riboflavin are referred to as FMN and FAD.

FMN (flavin mononucleotide) has a molecule of riboflavin and phosphoric acid.

FAD (flavin adenine dinucleotide) is a dinucleotide of FMN and AMP (Fig. 9.3).

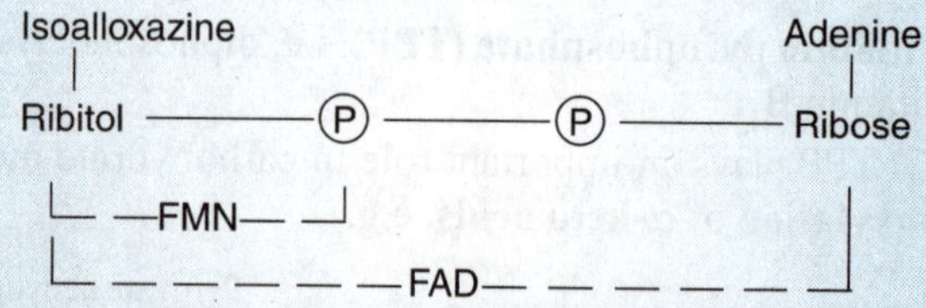

Fig. 9.3. Vitamin B_2 coenzymes.

These two coenzymes form an integral part of the flavoprotein-containing enzymes and participate in oxidation-reduction reactions.

$$\text{FMN} \xrightarrow{+2\text{H}} \text{FMN.H}_2$$

$$\text{FAD} \xrightarrow{+2\text{H}} \text{FAD.H}_2$$

FMN is used as a coenzyme with cytochrome C reductase and **L-amino acid oxidases.**

FAD is used as a coenzyme with **succinate dehydrogenase, glycerol-3-phosphate dehydrogenase, sphingosine reductase, glycine oxidase, xanthine oxidase, D-amino acid oxidases,** and **acyl CoA dehydrogenase**. FAD is important in the metabolism of carbohydrates, lipids, as well as proteins.

Deficiency Symptoms

Deficiency symptoms include **cheilosis** (lesions at the angles of the mouth), **glossitis,** and ocular as well as skin changes, such as localized dermatitis of the face. There also occur functional and organic disorders of the eye, including photophobia, lacrimation, burning, and itching.

Requirements

Its average daily requirement is **1-2 mg/day (0.5-0.6 mg/1000 Kcal).**

Sources

Milk, liver, and kidney are rich sources of vitamin B_2.

NIACIN

Niacin is also known as **pellagra-preventive factor (anti-pellagra factor)** because of its role in the prevention of pellagra.

The vitamin refers to two compounds, which are derivatives of the **pyridine ring** and are referred to as **nicotinic acid** and **nicotinamide** (Fig. 9.4)

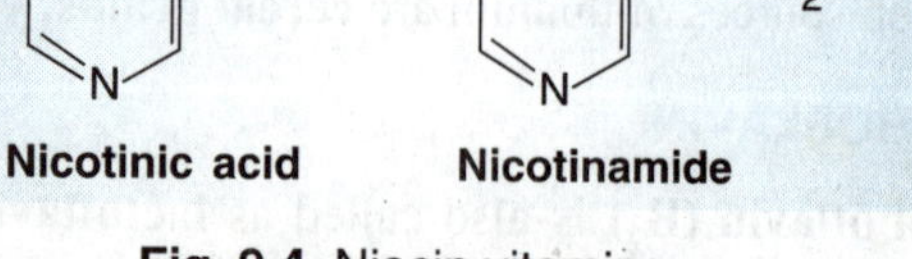

Fig. 9.4. Niacin vitamins.

Biosynthesis

It can be synthesized, by the human beings, from tryptophan.

Sixty mg of tryptophan forms one mg of niacin.

Biochemical Functions

Two coenzyme forms of niacin include NAD (**nicotinamide adenine dinucleotide)** and its phosphorylated from called $NADP^+$ (**nicotinamide adenine dinucleotide phosphate**).

NAD^+ is used as a coenzyme with malate dehydrogenase, which converts malate to oxaloacetate, and lactate dehydrogenase (LDH), which converts lactate to pyruvate.

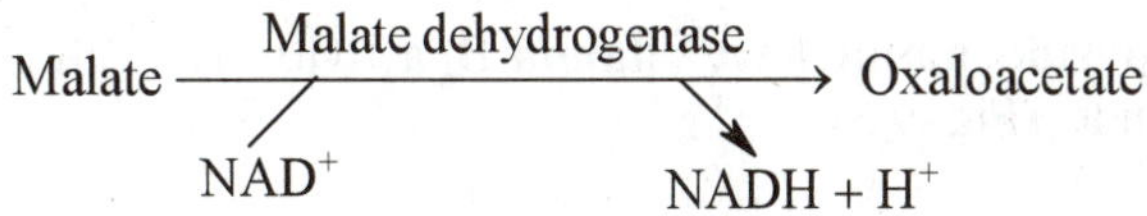

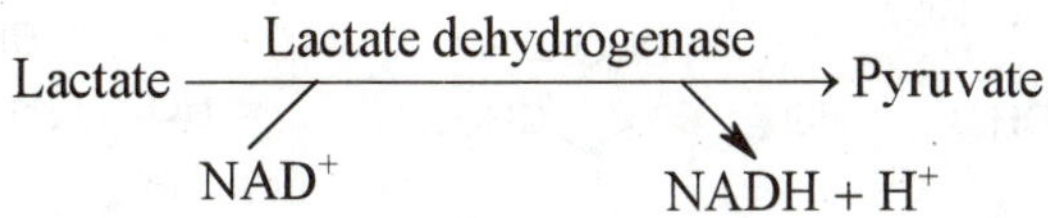

$NADP^+$ is used as a coenzyme with isocitrate dehydrogenase and glucose-6-phosphate dehydrogenase.

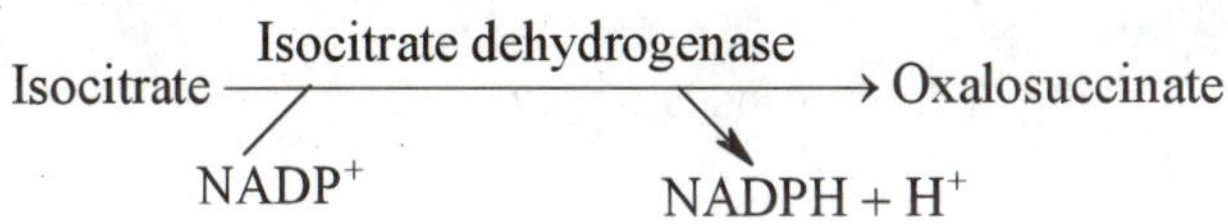

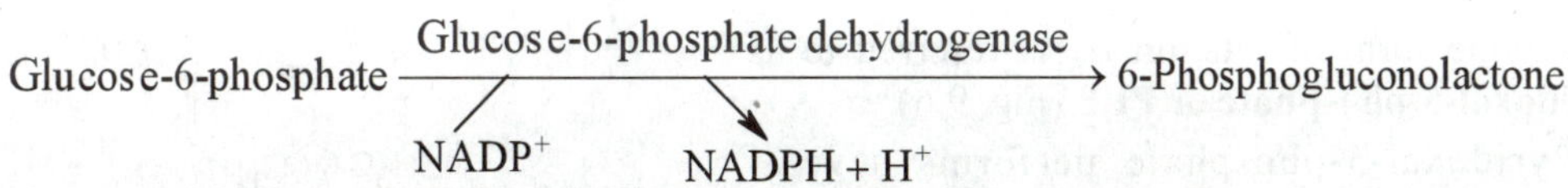

On the other hand, glutamate dehydrogenase can use both **NAD^+ as well as $NADP^+$.**

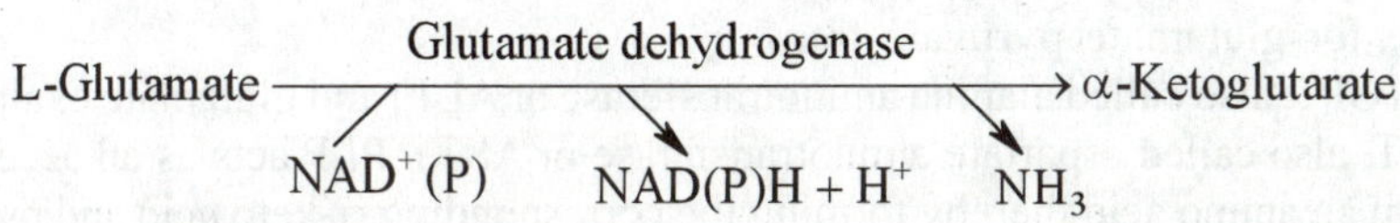

Deficiency Symptoms

Niacin deficiency is common in people whose staple food is **maize or jowar**. Such individuals may develop pellagra-like symptoms since these cereals are **rich in isoleucine** and **deficient in tryptophan.** This amino acid imbalance **affects tryptophan-niacin pathway** and in turn **reduces biosynthesis of niacin.**

Deficiency of niacin leads to a disease, called pellagra. 3D's, i.e. dermatitis, diarrhea, and dementia, characterize it.

Dermatitis results in pain in those parts of the body, which are exposed to sunlight, such as face, neck, hands, and feet. These parts become bronze resembling sunburn and become thickened.

Diarrhea is accompanied with anorexia, abdominal discomforts, and various other symptoms of the gastrointestinal tract.

Dementia is due to the impaired ability of the brain to utilize carbohydrates. Symptoms like depression, confusion, and psychosis are commonly observed.

Prolonged deficiency of niacin may result in **death.**

Requirements

Average daily requirement of niacin is **12-20 mg (5.5-6.5 mg/1000 Kcal).**

Sources

Rice-polish, yeast, liver, poultry, and green vegetables are good sources of niacin.

Milk and milk products though are not common sources of niacin but are important pellagra-preventive factors, due to their high tryptophan content.

PYRIDOXINE

Pyridoxine, pyridoxal, and **pyridoxamine have vitamin B_6** activity. They all contain a pyridine ring and are called **vitamers** of vitamin B_6 (Fig. 9.5).

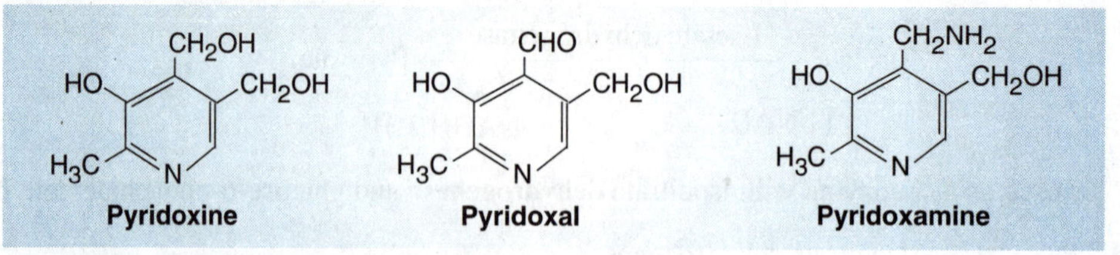

Fig. 9.5. Vitamins B_6.

Biochemical Functions

Coenzyme form of vitamin B_6 is referred to as **pyridoxal-5-phosphate or PLP** (Fig. 9.6).

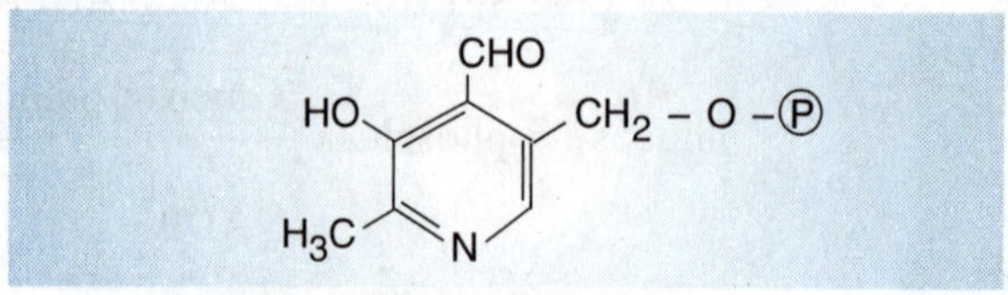

Fig. 9.6. Pyridoxal-5-phosphate.

Pyridoxal-5-phosphate performs several functions:

1. Pyridoxal-5-phosphate is used as a coenzyme for glutamate pyruvate transaminase (GPT, also called alanine aminotransferase or ALT) and glutamate oxaloacetate transaminase (GOT, also called aspartate aminotransferase or AST). PLP acts as an acceptor of the amino group from an amino acid thereby forming the corresponding α-keto acid and pyridoxamine phosphate. Followed by the reversal of the process, pyridoxamine releases its amino group to a α-keto acid and forms the corresponding amino acid (Fig. 9.7).
2. Pyridoxal-5-phosphate is also used with **dehydratases,** and **desulfhydrases** for the metabolism of hydroxyl amino acids and sulphur containing amino acids.
3. Pyridoxal-5-phosphate is used as a coenzyme for **decarboxylases,** e.g. glutamate decarboxylase, which forms γ-aminobutyric acid from glutamic acid; dopa decarboxylase that forms dopamine from dopa; and 5-hydroxytryptophan decarboxylase, which forms serotonin from 5-hydroxytryptophan. Thus, vitamin B_6 regulates neuronal activity.
4. Pyridoxal-5-phosphate is also required by the enzyme kynureninase. Thus, it is important in the conversion of tryptophan to niacin.
5. Pyridoxal-5-phosphate is also required in the **synthesis of heme,** in the formation of δ-aminolevulinic acid, by the enzyme, **δ-aminolevulinic acid synthase.**
6. Pyridoxal-5-phosphate is also essential in glycogen metabolism in the muscle and liver, as it is required as a coenzyme by **phosphorylase.**
7. Pyridoxal-5-phosphate is also essential for **chain elongation of unsaturated fatty acids,** e.g. in the conversion of linoleic acid to arachidonic acid.
8. Vitamin B_6 is also required for the **absorption of amino acids.**

Deficiency Symptoms

Deficiency of vitamin B_6 has been shown to occur in patients with tuberculosis who are taking anti-tubercular drug INH (isonicotinhydrazide) since this drug acts as an antagonist to vitamin B_6 (Fig. 9.8)

Deficiency symptoms include **cheilosis, glossitis,** and **hypochromic anemia.**

In infants, deficiency of B_6 affects central nervous system and results in convulsions, demyelination of the peripheral nerves, and degeneration of axons.

Pyridoxine has also been shown to be helpful in the treatment of nausea and vomiting, during pregnancy, radiation therapy, or muscular dystrophy.

Requirements

Daily requirement is approximately **1-2 mg**.

Sources

Rich sources of vitamin B_6 are **egg, fish, green-leafy vegetables,** and **cereals.**

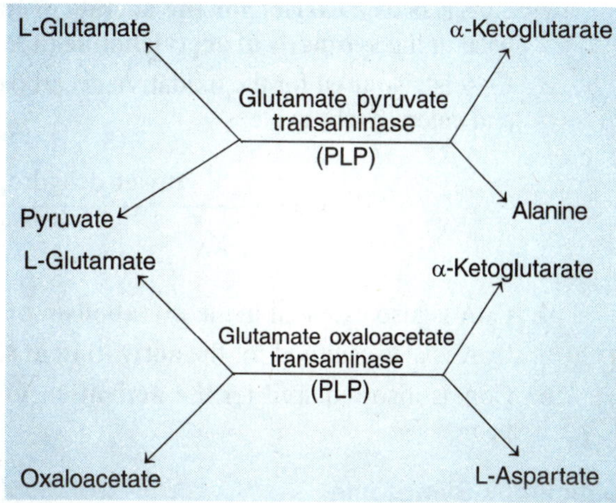

Fig. 9.7. Biochemical role of pyridoxine as a co-enzyme.

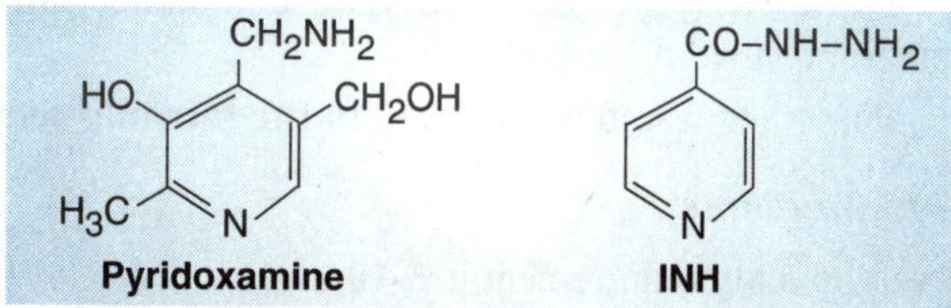

Fig. 9.8. Pyridoxamine and its antagonist INH.

ANTIVITAMINS

Antivitamin is a substance that prevents a vitamin from exerting its typical biologic effects. Most of them have structures like those of vitamins and appear to function as compitive antagonists, e.g. pyridoxine and its antagonist deoxypyridoxine, or pyridoxamine and INH.

PANTOTHENIC ACID

Pantothenic acid is heat stable in the acidic medium. It has a molecule of **pantoic acid** that is linked to **β-alanine** (Fig. 9.9)

Biochemical Functions

Pantothenic acid is an important constituent of **coenzyme** A (Fig. 9.10).

Coenzyme A also contains adenine and a sulfhydryl-group (–SH), which is contributed by β-mercaptoethanolamine.

Due to presence of the –SH group, coenzyme A is also designated as HS-CoA (CoA).

Pantothenic acid as well as coenzyme A performs several functions:

1. Pantothenic acid, as 4-phosphopantotheine, forms prosthetic group of **acyl carrier protein** that participates in **fatty acid synthesis**.

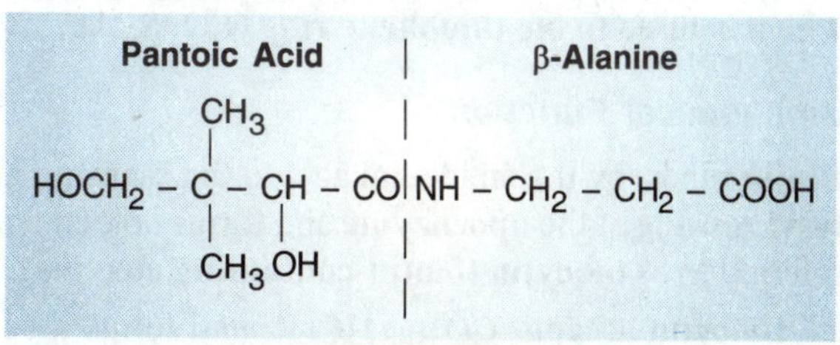

Fig. 9.9. Pantothenic acid.

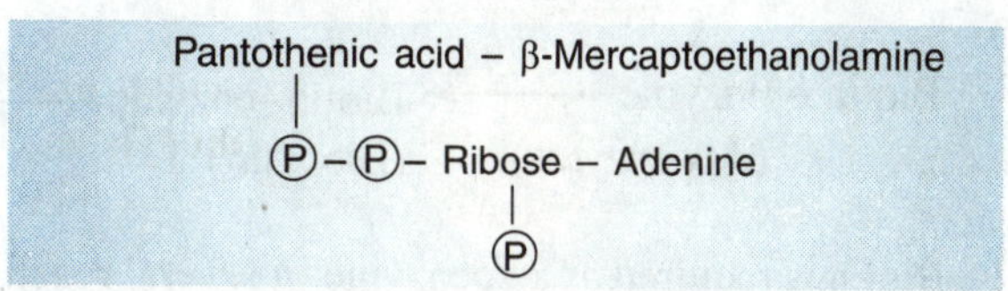

Fig. 9.10. Coenzyme A.

2. CoA acts as a **carrier for the acetate group,** i.e. as **acetyl CoA** also called active acetate, and is used in the **synthesis of acetylcholine** (a transmitter at the nerve synapse), **cholesterol, etc.**
3. CoA is also used for the oxidative decarboxylation of pyruvate, which is converted to acetyl CoA and enters Krebs cycle.

$$\text{Pyruvate} \xrightarrow[\text{CoA} \;\searrow\; CO_2]{\text{Pyruvate dehydrogenase complex}} \text{Acetyl CoA}$$

4. **CoA** is also essential in the **metabolism of branched chain amino acids.**
5. CoA is also required for the **activation of fatty acids** and their oxidation.
6. CoA is also required for the **activation of succinate** and thus is required in the biosynthesis of heme.

Deficiency Symptoms

Pantothenic acid **deficiency,** in human beings, **affects nervous system** as well as **digestive system.** Its deficiency has also been shown to result in adrenal insufficiency.

Deficiency symptoms include headache, fatigue, impaired motor activity, muscle cramps, and gastrointestinal disturbances.

Pantothenic acid is also **used in the burning-feet syndrome** and **healing of the ulcers** and **bedsores.**

Requirements

Average daily requirement is **5-10 mg.**

Sources

Rich sources are **yeast, liver, egg, potato, whole cereals,** and **legumes.**

BIOTIN

Biotin is also called as **anti-egg white injury factor** since it protects animals against toxicity of the raw-egg white.

Structurally, biotin is a **cyclic derivative of urea (ureido ring),** which is fused to the **thiophene ring** (Fig. 9.11).

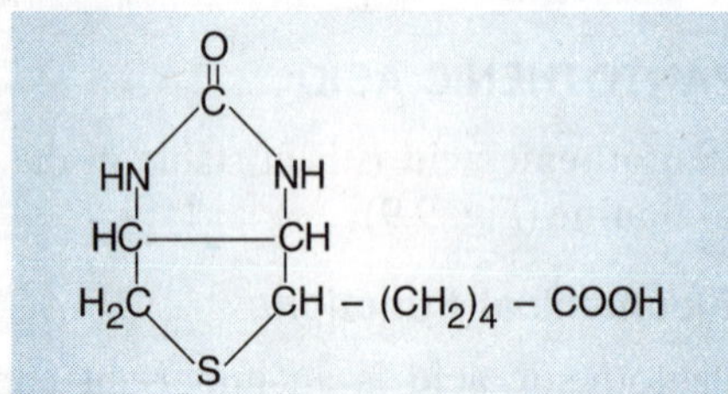

Fig. 9.11. Biotin.

Biochemical Function

Biotin binds, by the amide linkage, to the **ε-amino group of the lysyl residue** of the **apoenzyme** and forms holoenzyme, which is referred to as **biocytin (biotin-containing enzyme).**

Biocytin accepts CO_2 as HCO_3^- and forms a complex, called **active biotin** (carboxybiocytin-enzyme complex).

$$\underset{\text{(Apoenzyme)}}{\text{Biotin + Enzyme}} \longrightarrow \underset{\text{(Biocytin)}}{\text{Biotin–enzyme}} \xrightarrow[\text{ATP} \;\searrow\; \text{ADP + Pi}]{HCO_3^-} \underset{\text{(Active biotin)}}{\text{Carboxybiocytin-enzyme complex}}$$

Biotin is required as a coenzyme in several reactions involving CO_2 **fixation** by the carboxylases, such as:

1. In the carboxylation of **pyruvate, to** form **oxaloacetate,** by the enzyme **pyruvate carboxylase.**
2. In the conversion of propionyl CoA to **succinyl CoA** (via methylmalonyl CoA), by the enzyme **propionyl CoA carboxylase.**
3. In the conversion of **acetyl CoA** to **malonyl CoA** that is used in the formation of long chain fatty acids, by the enzyme acetyl CoA carboxylase.

Deficiency Symptoms

Biotin deficiency is not generally seen, as intestinal flora can synthesize it.

Biotin deficiency has been induced by the ingestion of large amount of raw egg white. Raw egg white contains a heat-labile, biotin-binding protein, called avidin. Avidin binds biotin and prevents its absorption. Heating the egg white can prevent this effect, since heating denatures this protein.

Deficiency of biotin may cause **mild dermatitis, nausea and loss of appetite, muscular pain,** and **anemia.**

Requirement

Daily requirement is **15-30 μg**.

Sources

Rice polishing, whole cereals, milk, yeast, and organ meat, such as liver and kidney are good sources of biotin.

CHOLINE

Choline is **trimethylethanolamine** (Fig. 9.12).

$$HO - CH_2 - CH_2 - N^+ - (CH_3)_3$$

Fig. 9.12. Choline.

Biochemical Functions

Choline performs several biochemical functions in the body:

1. It is converted to betaine, which is used as a **methyl donor for transmethylation reactions.**
2. Choline with acetyl CoA forms **acetylcholine**, a chemical mediator in synaptic transmission.
3. Choline also acts as a lipotropic **factor** and **prevents fatty liver.**

Deficiency Symptoms

Choline deficiency is not generally, observed since it is widely distributed in nature, as a constituent of the phospholipids.

Deficiency symptoms include **fatty liver, hemorrhagic necrosis of the kidney,** and **hemorrhages** into many organs **causing anemia.**

Requirements

Its normal daily requirement is **0.3-1.0 g.**

Sources

Egg yolk, several **animal tissues, cereals,** and **vegetables** are the good sources of choline.

LIPOIC ACID

Lipoic acid contains sulphur and is also called as **thioctic acid**.

Chemically, lipoic acid is a **sulphur containing fatty acid** (Fig. 9.13).

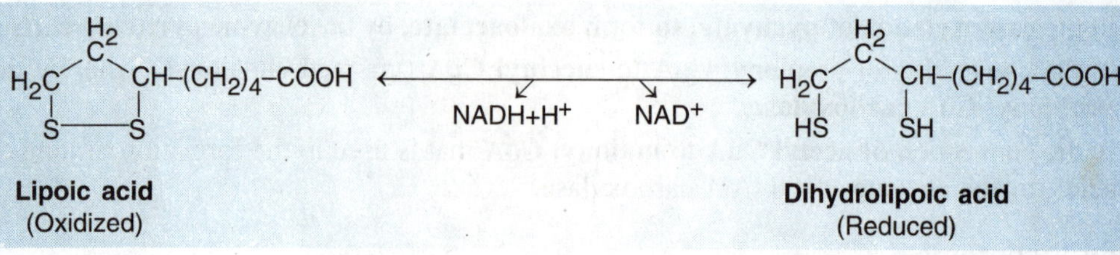

Fig. 9.13. Biochemical role of lipoic acid.

Biochemical functions

Lipoic acid undergoes **reversible oxidation** and **reduction,** and the reduced lipoic acid acts as an acceptor of the activated acyl group (Fig. 9.13).

As a component of the multienzyme complex, reduced lipoic acid mediates the **transfer of electrons** and **activated acyl group,** which is released after decarboxylation and **oxidation of the α-keto acids**. In this way **lipoic acid** is used as a **coenzyme** with several other coenzymes, such as TPP, NAD^+, FAD, and CoA, in the **oxidative decarboxylation of α-keto acids**, e.g. in the conversion of **pyruvate** to **acetyl CoA,** by the **pyruvate dehydrogenase complex,** or **α-ketoglutarate to succinyl CoA,** by the enzyme **α-ketoglutarate dehydrogenase complex.**

Lipoic acid is widely distributed in all natural foods hence; its deficiency symptoms as well as requirements are not well established.

FOLIC ACID

Folic Acid and the related compounds are referred to as **folacin,** since it is derived from the word folium (means leaf).

Folic acid is also called as **pteroylglutamic acid.** It has a **pteridine nucleus**, a molecule of **p-aminobenzoic acid,** and **glutamate, in its structure.**

The number of glutamate molecules may vary from one to seven (Fig. 9.14).

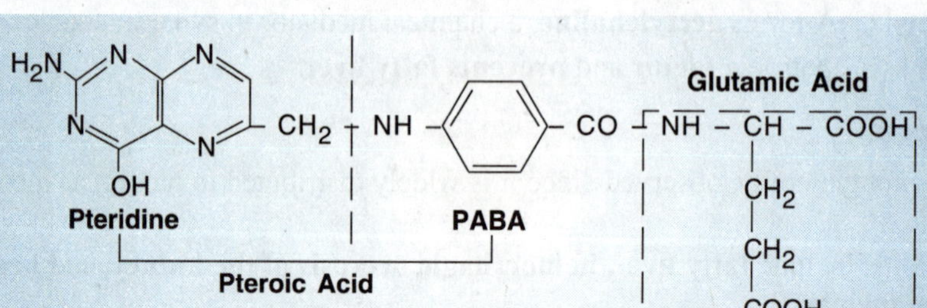

Fig. 9.14. Folic acid.

Biochemical Functions

Coenzyme form of folic acid is called **tetrahydrofolate (FH_4). During its synthesis, folate** is firstly **reduced to dihydrofolate** (FH_2), by the enzyme **folate reductase** and subsequently to **FH_4**, by the enzyme **dihydrofolate reductase** (Fig. 9.15).

Tetrahydrofolate (FH_4) acts as an **acceptor** as well as **donor** of **one-carbon unit** (1-C) in several reactions, such as in the metabolism of amino acids and nucleotides.

Sources of the **one-carbon moiety** may be **histidine** (formimino group), **serine** (hydroxymethyl group), or **choline** and **methionine** (methyl group).

The one-carbon moiety carried by FH_4 may be utilized as carbon numbers 2 and 8 in the biosynthesis of the **purine ring;** in the conversion of **glycine to serine, uracil to thymine, and homocysteine to methionine;** or in the **biosynthesis of choline.**

Some of these reactions also require vitamin B_{12}.

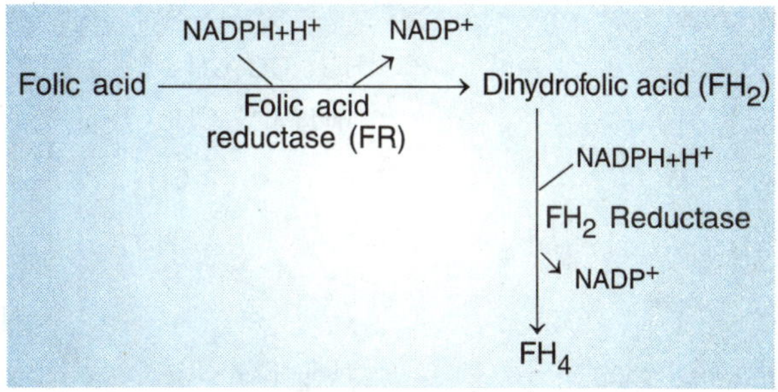

Fig. 9.15. Conversion of folic acid to FH_4.

Deficiency Symptoms

Folic acid deficiency may occur in stress-full conditions, during pregnancy, intestinal malabsorption, such as steatorrhea, and during antibiotic therapy.

Folic acid deficiency may also result in **macrocytic (megaloblastic) anemia, which is** accompanied **by leucopenia.**

Other deficiency symptoms, such as **psychosis** with mental retardation, are due to combined deficiency of folic acid and vitamin B_{12}.

Recently, folic acid deficiency (in early pregnancy) has also been implicated in **neural tube defects**.

Requirement

Average daily requirement for an adult is **150-300 μg**.

Sources

Green-leafy vegetables such as **spinach** and **cabbage, yeast, liver,** and **kidney** are good sources of folic acid.

FOLIC ACID ANTAGONISTS

Certain compounds, which interfere with metabolic functions of folic acid, are called folic acid antagonists. Most potent of these are **aminopterin** and **amethopterin**. They act as **competitive inhibitors** of the enzyme **dihydrofolate reductase,** and are used as **anticancer agents**.

Aminopterin (4-aminofolic acid) inhibits conversion of **folic acid** to **folinic acid** and thus inhibits the **biosynthesis of nucleic acids.** Hence, these drugs are used in the **treatment** of **leukemia,** particularly in children.

Amethopterin (N^{10}-methylfolic acid or methotrexate) **inhibits folic acid reductase** and affects the **conversion of folic acid to FH_4.**

VITAMIN B_{12}

Vitamin B_{12} is also called as the **extrinsic factor of Castle**. Due to the presence of the **cyano** group and the **cobalt** atom, Vitamin B_{12} is also referred to as **cyanocobalamin.**

The central ring structure of the vitamin has a **corrin nucleus**. Cobalt is linked to the cyano group as well as to the nitrogen of the imidazole ring, which is esterified through aminopropanol and propionic acid to ring IV of the corrin nucleus (Fig. 9.16)

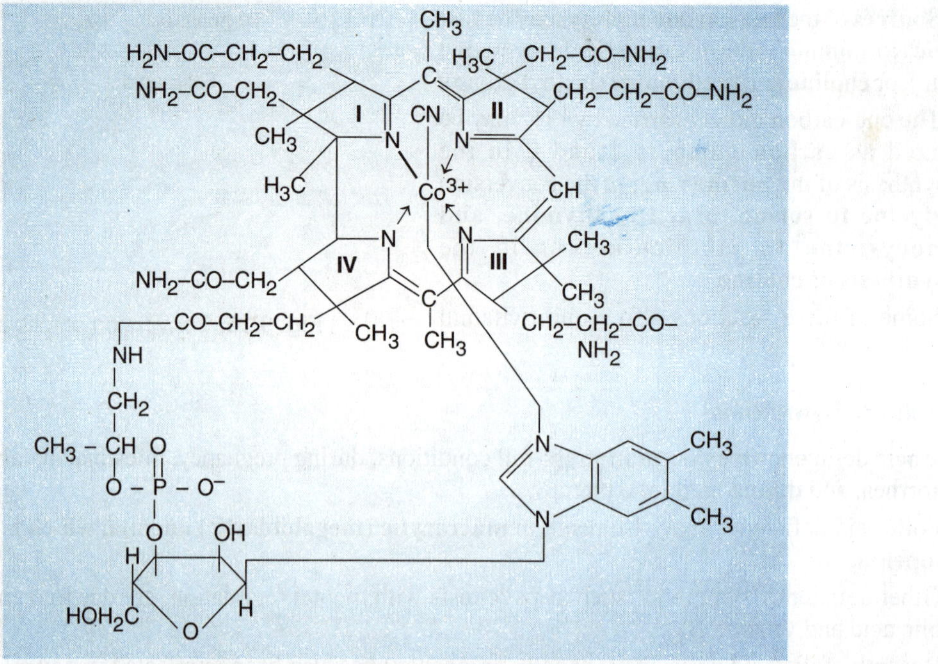

Fig. 9.16. Vitamin B_{12} (cyanocobalamin).

Biochemical Functions

Methylcobalamin and **deoxyadenosylcobalamin** are the **coenzyme forms** of vitamin B_{12}. These are referred to as **cobamides.**

Methylcobalamin is used, as a **coenzyme,** in the **formation of methionine** from **homocysteine.** Vitamin B_{12} thus, maintains methionine stores of the body and spares FH_4 for the biosynthesis of purines and pyrimidines.

Deoxyadenosylcobalamin is important in the metabolism of branched chain fatty acids as well as fatty acids containing odd number of carbon atoms, by converting methylmalonyl CoA to succinyl CoA, by the enzyme **methylmalonyl CoA isomerase.**

Deficiency Symptoms

Vitamin B_{12} deficiency is not generally observed due to its wide spread nature in animal tissues as well as its synthesis by the microbial flora. Deficiency however, can occur in geriatric persons particularly, in those who are strict vegetarians.

Its deficiency may also occur on its prolonged reduced intake, intestinal malabsorption, atrophy of the gastric mucosa, or due to deficiency **of the intrinsic factor,** e.g. in pernicious anemia.

Vitamin B_{12} deficiency can result in **methylmalonic aciduria.** Measurement of the urinary excretion of methylmalonic acid thus, is used to confirm the deficiency of this vitamin.

Requirements

Its average daily requirement is **1-3 μg** only.

Sources

Liver, kidney, egg, fish, and **milk** are good the sources of vitamin B_{12}.

VITAMIN C

Vitamin C is also called as **ascorbic acid, anti-scorbutic factor, or antiscurvy factor.**

Majority of the animals can synthesize vitamin C from glucuronate but men, primates, and guinea pigs can not synthesize it.

Vitamin C is readily absorbed from intestinal tract. Its absorption is reduced during gastrointestinal infections and achlorhydria.

Though it is stored in the liver and adrenals, its highest concentration is found in the adrenal cortex.

Vitamin C is destroyed by heat.

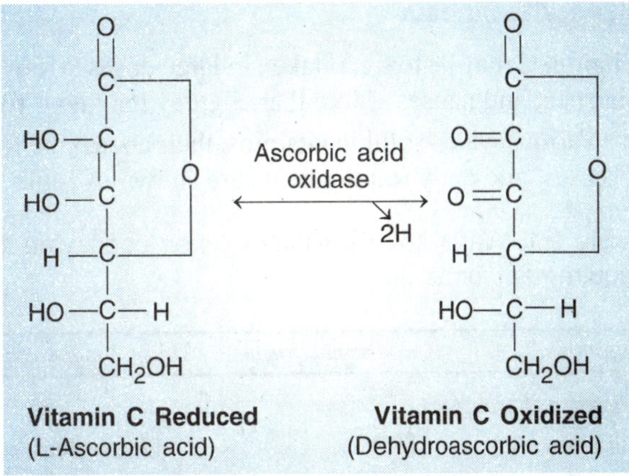

Fig. 9.17. Vitamin C.

Biochemical Functions

Vitamin C has an en-diol group at the second and the third carbon atoms, due to which it is sensitive to oxidizing agents. Oxidation of ascorbic acid converts it to **dehydroascorbic acid** (Fig. 9.17)

Due to its oxidation-reduction properties, ascorbic acid is important for several biological functions in the body:

1. Ascorbic acid is required in the **hydroxylation of amino acids** particularly, the aromatic amino acids.
2. Due to its role in the **hydroxylation of proline** and **lysine (in collagen),** ascorbic acid is required for the **repair of the ground substance.**
3. Vitamin C is essential for the **absorption of iron** from the gastrointestinal tract as well as its **release from the ferritin.**
4. Vitamin C has **stimulating** effect on the **phagocytic activity** of leucocytes. It thus, provides resistance to the body.
5. **Ascorbic acid** is also required for **synthesis of the steroid hormones** in the adrenal cortex. It thus, helps in lowering blood cholesterol level.

Deficiency Symptoms

Prolonged deficiency of vitamin C causes **scurvy,** which is characterized by **multiple hemorrhages.** Early symptoms of the disease include **swollen, spongy, and bleeding gums; loosening of teeth; and joint pain.** In severe cases, there may also be **bleeding from the nose, gastrointestinal tract,** and **genitourinary tract.**

Infants may **lose appetite and body weight** with **painful tenderness of the extremities**, bleeding from **gums** and the **mucous membrane**, and **cessation of osteogenesis** of the long bones.

Because of its role in the absorption, transport, and storage of iron, vitamin C deficiency may also cause **anemia.**

Requirement

Its average daily requirement, for adults, is **40-60 mg.**

Sources

Amla is a **richest source of vitamin C. Citrus fruits, green chillies, guava,** and **tomato** are good sources of vitamin C.

Hypervitaminosis

Vitamin C may be toxic, if taken in large doses. More than 2 g, in a single dose, may result in abdominal pain, diarrhea, and nausea. More than 3 g/day may **lead to urolithiasis,** due to formation of the **oxalate stones.**

Various water-soluble vitamins, their coenzyme forms, major biochemical functions, principal deficiency diseases, and daily requirements are shown in Table 9.1

Table 9.1. Water-soluble vitamins, their coenzyme forms, biochemical role, deficiency diseases and daily requirement for adults

Vitamin	*Coenzyme form*	*Major biochemical role*	*Deficiency diseases*	*Daily requirement*
Vitamin B Complex				
Thiamin (B_1)	TPP	Oxidative decarboxylation	Beriberi	1.2–1.8 mg
Riboflavin (B_2)	FMN, FAD	Oxidation-reduction with flavoproteins	Lesion on the lips, cheilosis	1–2 mg
Niacin	NAD^+, $NADP^+$	Hydrogen acceptor for dehydrogenases	Pellagra	12–20 mg
Pyridoxine (B_6)	Pyridoxal-5-PO_4	Transamination, decarboxylation	Peripheral neuritis	1–2 mg
Pantothenic acid	Coenzyme A	Formation of CoA, component of the acyl carrier protein	Muscle cramps, burning feet	5–10 mg
Biotin	Carboxybiocytin	Cocarboxylase	Anemia, dermatitis	15–30 μg
Folic acid	FH_4	Carrier of one-C moiety	Megaloblastic macrocytic anemia	150–300 μg
Cobalamin (B_{12})	Cobamides	Transmethylation with FH_4	Pernicious anemia	1–3 μg
Vitamin C (Ascorbic Acid)	L-Ascorbate	Hydroxylation	Scurvy	40–60 mg

FAT SOLUBLE VITAMINS

Fat-soluble vitamins are **vitamin A, vitamin D, vitamin E,** and **vitamin K.** They are absorbed in the lumen, in the presence of fat, and are emulsified with bile.

Their **precursors** are called as **provitamins,** which mostly occur in plants.

Due to the fat-soluble nature of these vitamins, they are **stored in the liver** and several other tissues. **Large doses of these vitamins** particularly, for a fairly longer duration, may result in **hypervitaminosis,** leading to various toxic symptoms.

VITAMIN A

Vitamin A is also called as **anti-night blindness factor.** It has a characteristic 6-membered ring known as **β-ionine ring** that is attached to a long **hydrocarbon side chain** (Fig. 9.18)

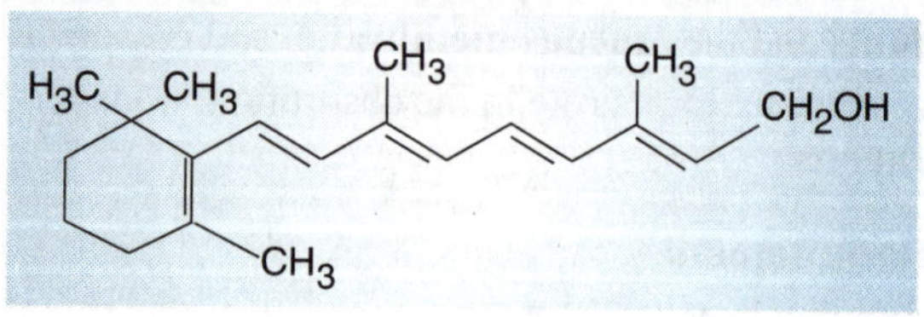

Fig. 9.18. Vitamin A alcohol (retinol).

Vitamin A is an **alcohol** hence; it is also referred to as **retinol**. It may be converted to **aldehyde (retinal**, also called as **retinene**), or **acid (retinoic acid).** Three forms of the vitamin are found in different tissues, in animals.

Precursors of the vitamin A are called carotenoids (provitamin A).

PROVITAMIN A

Carotenoids are called as **provitamin A**. They are **found in plants** and **have** an **additional ionine ring**. Depending upon the presence of the second ionine ring, provitamins are designated as **α, β, or γ-carotenes.**

β-Carotene has **highest vitamin A activity,** as it gives **2 molecules of vitamin A** (retinal). On the other hand, **α- and γ-carotenes** give **one** molecule only. **Provitamins** (carotenoids) are absorbed in the lumen and **converted to retinal in the intestinal epithelium**. Carotenes are splitted at the center of the hydrocarbon chain and give rise to active vitamin A, with in the intestinal wall.

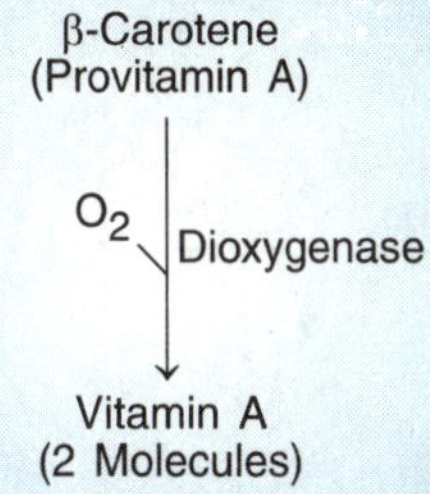

Fig. 9.19. Conversion of β-carotene to vitamin A.

Conversion of β-carotene to retinal requires an enzyme referred to as dioxygenase (Fig 9.19)

β-Carotene is found widely, in plants. Its rich **sources** are **yellow-colored fruits** and **vegetables,** such as **carrot, pumpkin, papaya, and mango.**

Biological Functions

Various biological functions of vitamin A can be performed by retinal as well as retinol (Table 9.2)

Table 9.2. Biological functions of vitamin A
• In vision cycle
• Gluconeogenesis
• Biosynthesis of gluco-corticoids
• Biosynthesis of glycosaminoglycans
• Biosynthesis of cholesterol
• Cell differentiation and growth
• Biosynthesis of membrane glycoproteins
• Immune functions

1. ROLE IN VISUAL PROCESS

Vitamin A aldehyde (retinal) is essential for vision both in rods as well as cones:

In the rods: Rod cells contain a conjugated **transmembrane protein,** called **rhodopsin,** which consists of an apoprotein **opsin** and a nonprotein prosthetic group, called **11-cis- retinal** (11-cis-retinene). It is **essential for vision in the dim light.**

When light falls on retina, **rhodopsin** is **bleached** and generates **all-trans-retinal,** which can not form a complex with opsin. **All-trans-retinal** is **reduced to all-trans-retinol,** by the enzyme all-trans-retinol dehydrogenase (retinene reductase). It is then transported to the liver and **stored there.** In the liver, it is **isomerized** to **11-cis retinol** by an isomerase. After its delivery to the retina, **11-cis-retinol** is **changed to 11-cis-retinal,** which again conjugates **with opsin,** and reforms **rhodopsin, in dark.** This is called **vision cycle** (Fig. 9.20).

In the cones: Similar to the rhodopsin, which is present in the rods for the black and white vision, cones contain 3 different pigments that are sensitive to the three primary colors, i.e. **porphyropsin (for red), iodopsin (for green)** and **cyanopsin (for blue)**. Prosthetic group in these three pigments is the same, i.e. 11-cis-retinal.

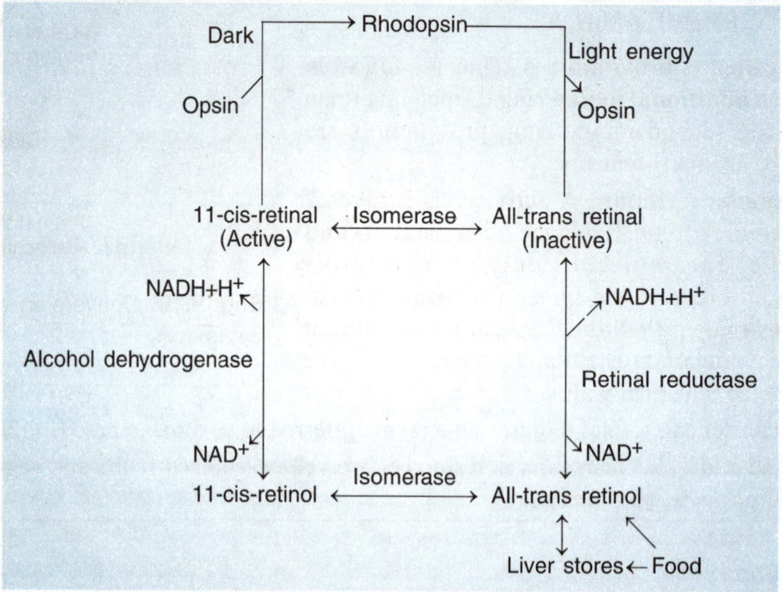

Fig. 9.20. Vision cycle in rod cells.

2. Vitamin A deficiency leads to reduction **in gluconeogenesis**. This is due to decreased **synthesis of the steroid hormones** particularly, synthesis of corticosterone and cortisol.
3. Vitamin A also plays a role in cholesterol biosynthesis.
4. Vitamin A deficiency causes keratinization of mucosal membrane and **decreases synthesis of glycosaminoglycans.**
5. Vitamin A deficiency **impairs spermatogenesis and affects cell growth and differentiation.**
6. Deficiency of vitamin A also **reduces the synthesis** of membrane **glycoproteins.**
7. Vitámin A is also required in maintenance of integrity of the tissues lining eyes, gastrointestinal tract, genitourinary tract, and the respiratory system and ensures **optimal functioning of the immune system.**

Deficiency Symptoms

Vitamin A deficiency is observed, primarily due to its low intake. Its deficiency is aggravated by infections, which reduces its absorption and utilization. Vitamin A deficiency affects many tissues:

1. It is most detrimental for eyes. Deficiency of the vitamin may result in **xerophthalmia,** which is characterized by drying of conjunctiva and cornea, followed by destruction of cornea, leading to blindness.
2. Vitamin A deficiency also affects **osteoblastic activity** and results in **defective resorption of bone,** affecting **growth.**
3. Deficiency of vitamin A also results in **xerosis** and **keratinization of the mucous membrane,** resulting in **dry** and **rough skin.** Keratinization of the mucous membrane increases its susceptibility to infections. Keratinization of the urinary tract may lead to **urolithiasis.**
4. Vitamin A deficiency also results in certain **abnormalities** of the **reproductive** system, such as **degeneration of testes, abortions,** and production of the **malformed-offspring.** Keratinization of the epithelium of the seminiferous tubules may also lead to infertility.

XEROPHTHALMIA

Xerophthalmia occurs when body stores of vitamin A are exhausted and supply fails to meet requirement. Gradual depletion of vitamin A stores results in a condition referred to as xerophthalmia. It may manifest as night blindness, conjunctival xerosis, Bitot's spot, corneal xerosis and ulceration, keratomalacia, and corneal scar.

Night blindness: First symptom of vitamin A deficiency is **night blindness,** i.e. an individual **can not see in dark.** Since retinal is essential for the synthesis of rhodopsin (by the rods) and **vitamin A deficiency interferes with** the **production of rhodopsin,** deficiency of vitamin A thus **impairs rod functions** and results in night blindness.

Night blindness responds to vitamin A therapy, rapidly.

Bitot's spot: Bitot's spot means **accumulation of the foamy-cheesy material on the conjunctiva** often in association with other signs of xerophthalmia, such as conjunctival xerosis. Although the spots may differ in size, location, or shape, they have similar appearance.

Corneal xerosis and ulceration: When **cornea becomes dry**, this condition is referred to as **xerosis**. If the disease is not treated at this stage, it can progress with in hours, to ulcer of the cornea.

Keratomalacia: If the disease is not treated in its early stage, a corneal ulcer can lead to melting or **wasting of cornea**. This is referred to as keratomalacia. It indicates destruction of a part or complete corneal stroma, which in turn results in permanent structural alterations.

Corneal scar: Keratomalacia can lead to **perforation of cornea.** At this stage a corneal scar is formed, which however, remains forever.

Different sites affected by xerophthalmia are shown in Fig. 9.21

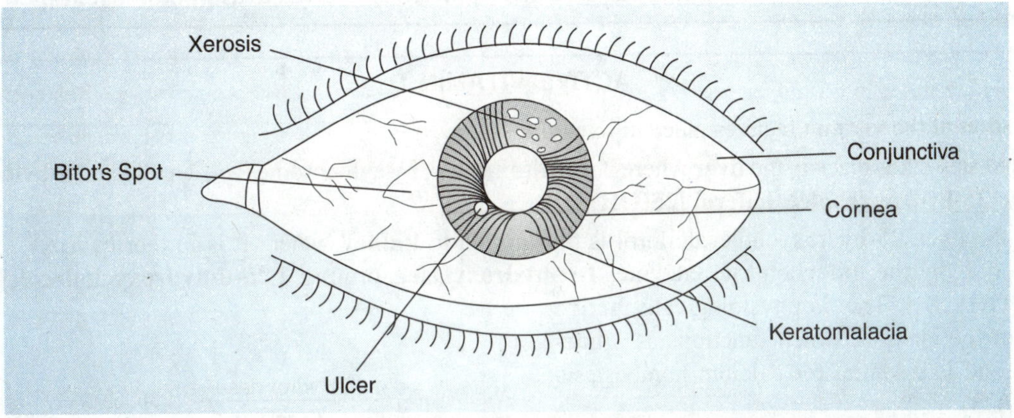

Fig. 9.21. Xerophthalmia.

Requirements

Average daily requirement of **vitamin A,** for an adult, is **2000-3500 IU** (about 750-1000 mg).

Daily requirement of **β-carotene** is **4000-6000 IU** (about 2000 mg).

Sources

Liver oil, fish-liver oil, egg, milk, and milk products are the good sources of **vitamin A.**

On the other hand, **papaya, carrots**, sweet potatoes, and green-leafy vegetables are the good sources of carotene.

Hypervitaminosis

If taken in large quantities, for a longer period, vitamin A is toxic since it is a fat-soluble vitamin and stored in the liver.

Toxicity symptoms include **skin abnormalities,** such as **dry and rough skin, scaly dermatitis**, headache, nausea, vomiting and loss of appetite, **hepatomegaly,** painful joints, and **several bone abnormalities.**

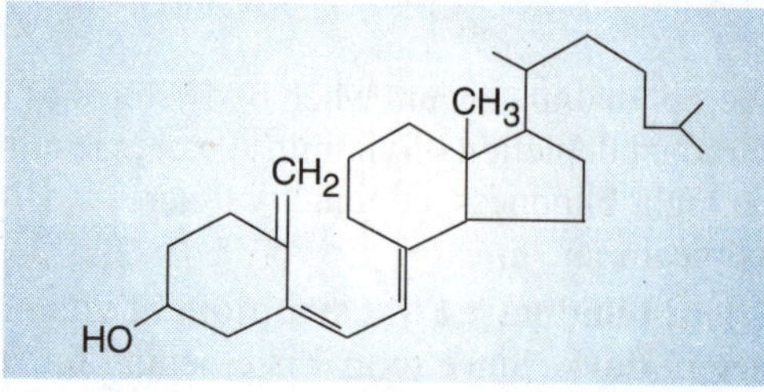

Fig. 9.22. Vitamin D_3 (cholecalciferol).

VITAMIN D

Vitamin D (**calciferol)** is a sterol. It is also called as **anti-rachitic factor** and considered to be a prohormone.

It is present in nature in several forms, two of which are most common. These are referred to as **vitamin** $\mathbf{D_2}$ and $\mathbf{D_3}$.

Vitamin $\mathbf{D_2}$ (ergocalciferol) is of **plant origin**. It is obtained from ergot plant. It can also be synthesized in the laboratory, by irradiating ergosterol.

Vitamin $\mathbf{D_3}$ (cholecalciferol) is of animal origin (Fig. 9.22).

PROVITAMIN D

A derivative of the cholesterol, called 7-dehydrocholesterol, is a **precursor** of **vitamin $\mathbf{D_3}$ in animals.** It is also called as **provitamin D**. It is synthesized in the human beings in the intestinal mucosa and is converted to vitamin D_3 by **UV light in the skin.** This process is referred to as **photobiogenesis.**

ACTIVE VITAMIN D

Activation of the vitamin D takes place in liver and kidney.

The first step takes place in the **liver** where it is hydroxylated, by cytochrome P_{450} dependent **25-hydroxylase,** to **25-hydroxycholecalciferol [25(OH).$\mathbf{D_3}$]**.

From the liver, 25-hydroxycholecalciferol is transported to **kidney**, where it is further hydroxylated at position 1, by the mitochondrial enzyme, **1-α-hydroxylase,** forming **1,25-dihydroxycholecalciferol [1,25$\mathbf{(OH)_2}$.$\mathbf{D_3}$]**. This is physiologically **active** form of the vitamin, which functions as a **hormone** and is essential for calcium homeostasis (Fig. 9.23)

Due to the presence of 3-OH groups, 1, 25$(OH)_2$.D_3 is also called as **calcitriol.**

1-α-Hydroxylase activity is present in renal tubules, bones, and placenta. Parathyroid hormone (PTH), serum phosphorus, and calcitriol regulate it. **Production of 1, 25$\mathbf{(OH)_2}$.$\mathbf{D_3}$** is also **regulated by serum calcium.**

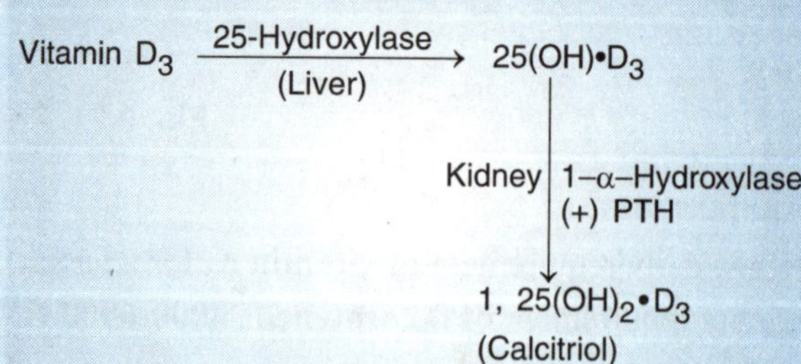

Fig. 9.23. Activation of vitamin D.

Biological Functions

Most important function of active vitamin D is the regulation of serum calcium level.

ROLE IN CALCIUM METABOLISM

Calcitriol induces synthesis of calcium-binding protein, Ca^{2+}-dependent ATPase, and **alkaline phosphatase, which are essential** for the **regulation of serum calcium** and **phosphorus.**

A net result is achieved through its action in the intestine, bone, and kidney:

- **In the intestine,** due to the **stimulation of synthesis** of the **calcium-binding protein,** $1,25(OH)_2.D_3$ increases intestinal absorption of calcium as well as phosphorus.
- **In the bone,** calcitriol **stimulates the synthesis of osteocalcin,** which in turn mobilizes calcium from bone, i. e. it causes **demineralization of bone, and**
- **In the kidney,** active vitamin D **increases tubular reabsorption of calcium** and excretion of phosphorus.

Overall effect of the three processes is to **increase serum calcium** level, towards normal.

Deficiency Symptoms

Deficiency of vitamin D, generally, does not occur, as it can be synthesized in the body. Deficiency however, may occur due to lack of sunshine.

Vitamin D deficiency leads to **rickets** in **children** and **osteomalacia** in **adults.**

Rickets

Rickets is a **disease, which occurs during infancy** and childhood. It is a nutritional disorder due to the deficiency of vitamin D. Besides vitamin D, exposure of the body to sunlight has both, preventive as well as curative effects.

Symptoms, such as **enlarged wrists, ankles,** and poor structural development affecting long bones are frequently seen.

Ends of the long bones become soft and bulky, particularly characteristic of bowed-legs and knock-knees. There may also be extreme stunting of growth (Fig. 9.24).

Deformities may also appear in the bones of the skull, chest, and spine. Teeth may erupt late and are deformed.

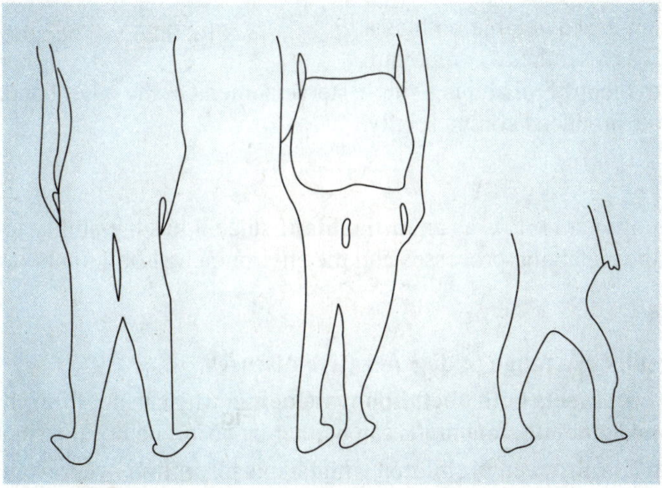

Fig. 9.24. Rickets (bowed legs & knock knees).

Biochemically, a patient with rickets shows **decrease** in **serum calcium** and **phosphorus** along with **increase** in **serum alkaline phosphatase,** and **increased excretion of inorganic phosphate in urine.**

Product of serum calcium and phosphorus, which is normally 40 (10 mg calcium x 4 mg phosphorus), is decreased to below 30 in such children.

Osteomalacia

Deficiency of vitamin D in **adults,** results in a condition called **osteomalacia,** also termed as **adult rickets**. It is commonly observed in females during pregnancy and lactation, or in those who are not exposed to sunlight, may be because of their customs wearing purdah. **Bones** particularly, **of the pelvic region** show characteristic **deformities,** which in turn may complicate parturition.

Requirements

Average daily requirement is **200 IU** (5-10 mg) of cholecalciferol.

Sources

As vitamin D can be synthesized in the body by the action of the ultraviolet light on the skin, hence sunshine is the best source of vitamin D. Besides, rich sources are **milk, butter, egg yolk, fish oil,** and **liver oil.**

Hypervitaminosis

Extremely **large doses** of vitamin D, over a long period, may lead to **hypercalcemia, hyperphosphatemia, anorexia, nausea, vomiting,** and **diarrhea** besides bone pain and **metastatic calcification of the soft tissues,** including kidney, myocardium, pancreas, and uterus.

VITAMIN E

Several compounds belonging to the group tocopherols, such as α, β, γ, and δ tocopherols, exhibit vitamin E activity. Amongst them, α-tocopherol has highest biological activity as well as its widest distribution. It is an alcohol with a **phytol** and **trimethylhydroquinone** (Fig. 9.25).

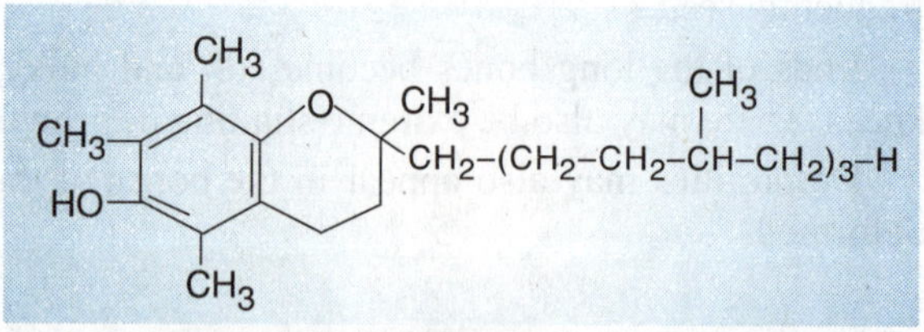

Fig. 9.25. α-Tocopherol (vitamin E).

Commercially, vitamin E is available both as a natural substance as well as a synthetic compound. **Natural** vitamin E is **d-α-tocopherol** and is a single stereoisomer. On the other hand, **synthetic** vitamin E is **dl-α-tocopherol**, which is produced commercially.

Biological Functions

Most important function of vitamin E is as an **antioxidant** since it has the ability to **quench free radicals**, which are generated by the metabolic processes and the environmental pollutants.

Deficiency Symptoms

Vitamin E deficiency **results in** a range of **degenerative diseases.**

Its deficiency is seen **in-patients with abetalipoproteinemia** who can not form chylomicrons and VLDL. As a result of **abetalipoproteinemia,** vitamin E can neither be absorbed nor distributed.

Deficiency of vitamin E is also seen in children with fat malabsorption, where it results in severe progressive **neuropathy** and **retinopathy**.

Hepatic necrosis, muscular dystrophy, defects in vascular system, and certain reproductive defects are also known to exist in various animal species.

Requirements

Daily requirement of vitamin E, for an adult man, is 5-10 mg **(about 15 IU)**.

Requirement of vitamin E however varies, depending upon the level and nature of physical activity, diet, psychological stress, exposure to polluted environment, and intake of polyunsaturated fatty acids. Normally, 0.4 mg vitamin E is required per g of PUFA.

Sources

Tocopherols are present in smaller quantities, **in green-leafy vegetables such as** spinach and lettuce, milk and milk products, and **egg yolk.** Oils, such as **corn oil, cottonseed oil**, and **sunflower oil,** are the rich sources of vitamin E.

VITAMIN K

The name, **vitamin K,** has been derived from the Danish word 'Koagulation' since it has important **role in blood clotting.**

Various compounds related to **2-methyl-1, 4-napthoquinone** have been shown to possess vitamin K activity.

- Its most important form is **vitamin K_1 (phylloquinone),** which occurs naturally, and is found in plants. It has a phytyl- side chain. (Fig. 9.26).
- **Vitamin K_2 (menaquinone or farnequinone)**, which is synthesized by intestinal bacteria. It has a farnesyl- side chain.
- **Vitamin K_3 (menadione),** a synthetic compound, which is water-soluble. It is easily absorbed, on parenteral administration. Vitamin K is available commercially as menadione for therapeutic use.

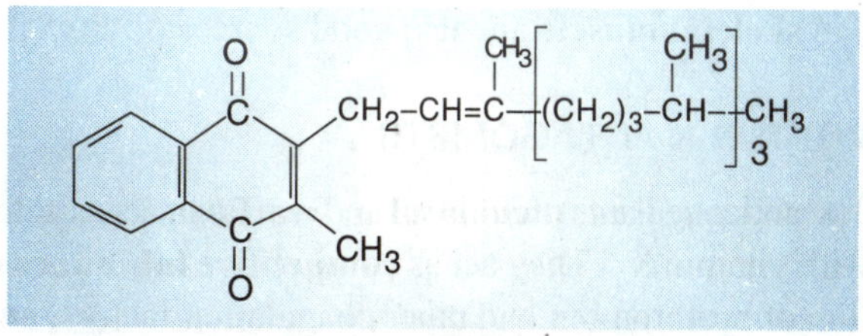

Fig. 9.26. Vitamin K_1.

Biological Functions

Vitamin K is essential for the **maintenance of the normal levels** of various **blood-clotting factors,** such as **prothrombin, factor VII, factor IX,** and **factor X. These proteins** are **synthesized** in the liver **in their inactive forms** and get **converted** to their **biologically active forms** with the help of vitamin K.

ROLE IN GAMMA-CARBOXYLATION

Formation of the clotting factors requires the **vitamin K-dependent carboxylation of glutamic acid residues** (Fig. 9.27).

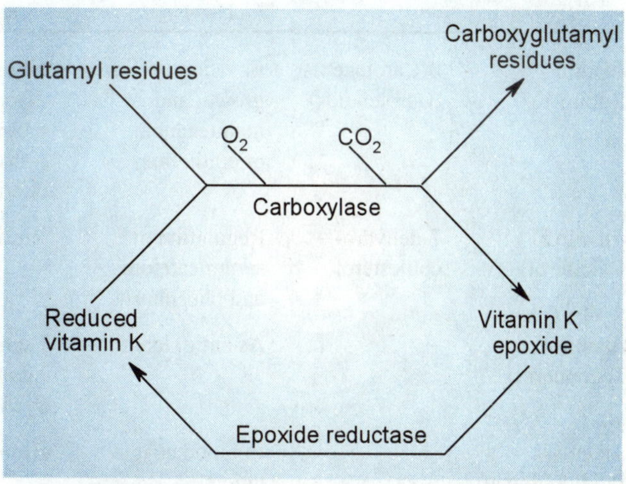

Fig. 9.27. Role of vitamin K in the carboxylation of blood coagulation proteins.

This forms a mature clotting factor that contains γ-carboxyglutamate (Gla) and is capable of subsequent activation.

Deficiency Symptoms

Deficiency of vitamin K is seen in the newborns, due to their sterile intestine, particularly in premature infants who show **reduced** levels of **vitamin K, prothrombin,** and **Christmas factor.**

Common **deficiency symptoms** include **cutaneous** and **intramuscular hemorrhages** with **bluish-red coloration** in different parts of the body.

Requirements

Its requirement is not well established in adults, but it is suggested that **20-100 μg/day** is sufficient to meet its daily needs. It is advised to administer a **single,** prophylactic **dose of 1 mg** of vitamin K_1 to a newborn, on the **first day of life.**

Sources

Green-leafy vegetables, such as spinach, lettuce, and cabbage, are the rich sources of vitamin K. **Fish, liver,** and **skeletal muscle** are also good sources of this vitamin.

VITAMIN K ANTAGONISTS

The anticoagulants **dicumarol** and **warfarin** act as antivitamins for vitamin K, due to their structural similarities with vitamin K_1. They act as **competitive inhibitors for the enzymes, which** are concerned with the activation of prothrombin and other coagulation factors, and require vitamin K for their activation.

Table 9.3 lists various fat soluble vitamins, their biological functions, and daily requirements for adults.

Table 9.3. Fat-soluble vitamins, their biological functions, sources, and daily requirement for adults

Vitamin	*Provitamin*	*Biological functions*	*Deficiency diseases*	*Sources*	*Daily requirement*
Vitamin (Retinol)	β-Carotene (Carotenoids)	In vision cycle, growth and maintenance of epithelium	Night blindness, disorders of mucous mebrane, bone, nerves, and reproduction	Liver oil, fish oil, vegetable oil	2000-3500 IU
Vitamin D (Calciferol)	7-dehydro-cholesterol	Regulation of serum calcium and phosphorus	Rickets, osteomalacia	Fish oil	200 IU
Vitamin E (Tocopherol)	–	As antioxidant	Hemolytic anemia in infants, muscular dystrophy	Plant seed oils	5-10 mg
Vitamin K (Phylloquinone)	–	In blood coagulation	Blood clotting failure	Plant seeds oils	20-100 μg

SOME IMPORTANT QUESTIONS

1. Name fat-soluble vitamins? Mention their dietary sources, biological functions, and associated deficiency disorders.
2. Describe chemistry, biological functions, and deficiency manifestations of Vitamin A.
3. How is vitamin D synthesized in the body? Describe its biochemical role.
4. Describe dietary sources, biological functions, and deficiency manifestations of folic acid and vitamin B_{12}.
5. Given an account of chemistry, dietary sources, biological functions, and deficiency manifestations of vitamin C.
6. Describe the coenzyme form and biochemical role of:
   - (i) Riboflavin
   - (ii) Pantothenic acid
   - (iii) Biotin
   - (iv) Vitamin B_6
   - (v) Thiamin
   - (vi) Niacin
7. Discuss briefly:
   - (i) Role of pyridoxal phosphate in amino acid metabolism
   - (ii) Structure and functions of vitamin D
   - (iii) Role of vitamin A in vision
8. Write notes on:
   - (i) Keratomalacia
   - (ii) Pellagra
   - (iii) Beriberi
   - (iv) Scurvy
   - (v) Cobamide coenzymes
   - (vi) Calcitriol
   - (vii) Role of vitamin D in calcium metabolism
   - (viii) Role of vitamin K in gamma-carboxylation
   - (ix) Pyridoxine
   - (x) Antivitamins
   - (xi) Folic acid antagonists
   - (xii) Provitamin A
   - (xiii) Xerophthalmia
   - (xiv) Provitamin D
   - (xv) Active Vitamin D
   - (xvi) Rickets
   - (xvii) Osteomalacia
   - (xviii) Vitamin K antagonists
   - (xix) Hypervitaminosis

CHAPTER

10

Minerals

The minerals necessary in human nutrition are inorganic elements that are widely distributed in nature. These are classified into two groups as minerals and trace elements. Those that are **required by the body in amounts of more than 100 mg/day** are called **minerals.** These are **calcium, phosphorus, magnesium, etc.**

Elements (micronutrients)**,** which are **required by the body in amounts less than 100 mg/day,** are called **trace elements**. These include **iron, iodine, zinc, fluoride, etc.**

CALCIUM

Amongst the various minerals, **calcium (Ca) is found in the highest concentration** in the body. Nearly all the cells need it. **An adult man** contains nearly **1.0-1.2 kg of calcium**. About 99% of it is present **in skeletal tissue,** i.e. in bones and teeth while the remaining of it is found in the soft tissues, such as muscle and nervous tissue.

Normal serum calcium level is **9-11 mg/100 ml**. It is present in three forms:

1. ***Ionized calcium***: About **45-50%** of total serum calcium is present **in the ionized form, as Ca^{2+} ions.** Ionized calcium is freely exchangeable between the soft tissues, extracellular fluid and blood.
2. ***Protein-bound calcium:*** Nearly **45-50% of total serum calcium is bound to protein**, and
3. ***Calcium salts:*** About **5-10%** of the calcium is present **in the form of calcium salts,** i.e. calcium bound with citrate and/or phosphate.

ABSORPTION OF DIETARY CALCIUM

Calcium is absorbed by all parts of the small intestine, but the most rapid absorption after a meal occurs in the more acidic (< pH 7.0) duodenum. Absorption is slower in the remainder of the small bowl because of the alkaline pH.

Only about 30% of the ingested calcium is absorbed by adults. Calcium is absorbed by two mechanisms, i.e.:

Active transport, which operates predominantly at low luminal concentration is controlled through the action of calcitriol.

The second absorption mechanism, which is ***passive*** in nature, occurs along the entire length of the small intestine.

Numerous factors influence the absorption of calcium within the gut.

Factors Affecting Calcium Absorption

1. Calcium absorption is **impaired in vitamin D deficiency**.
2. **Excess of phosphate reduces** calcium absorption.
3. **Phytic acid** and related substances, which are found in unrefined cereals, **interfere** with calcium absorption.
4. **Excessive amounts of fat, fiber and oxalate,** if present in diet, **reduce** calcium absorption, due to the formation of insoluble salts.
5. **Higher amounts of protein and lactose in the diet and acidic pH promote** calcium absorption.

Excretion

About 50% of the ingested calcium is excreted in the urine each day. Almost an equal amount is also secreted into the intestine and is lost in the feces. A small amount (about 15 mg/day) is also lost through skin.

REGULATION OF SERUM CALCIUM

Maintenance of serum calcium, with in normal limits, **is called calcium homeostasis.**

Ionized calcium (Ca^{2+}) is freely exchangeable between the soft tissues, the extracellular fluid and the blood; hence it is also called as the **diffusible calcium**. The ionized, Ca^{2+}, performs most of the functions of calcium. Parathyroid hormone (PTH), vitamin D, and calcitonin regulate serum Ca^{2+} level (Fig. 10.1).

Parathyroid hormone: PTH plays a key role in the regulation of Ca^{2+}. If Ca^{2+} concentration falls, secretion of PTH is increased. PTH acts directly, on osteoclasts and **increases dissolution of bone minerals**. This process is called as **bone resorption.**

PTH also **increases reabsorption of Ca^{2+} from the kidney.**

The **overall effect** of the above two processes is **to elevate serum Ca^{2+}.**

PTH also **stimulates 1-α-hydroxylase** activity in kidney, **which** in turn **activates vitamin D** and converts it to **1, 25-dihydroxycholecalciferol (calcitriol).**

Active Vitamin D: It **increases serum Ca^{2+}** concentration, by **promoting intestinal absorption of Ca^{2+}, by increasing synthesis of calcium binding protein.**

Calcitonin: It is secreted when serum Ca^{2+} level is increased. Its action is to **lower serum Ca^{2+}** level, by **promoting the deposition of calcium,** by the osteoblasts.

PTH and calcitonin thus **act in opposite directions.**

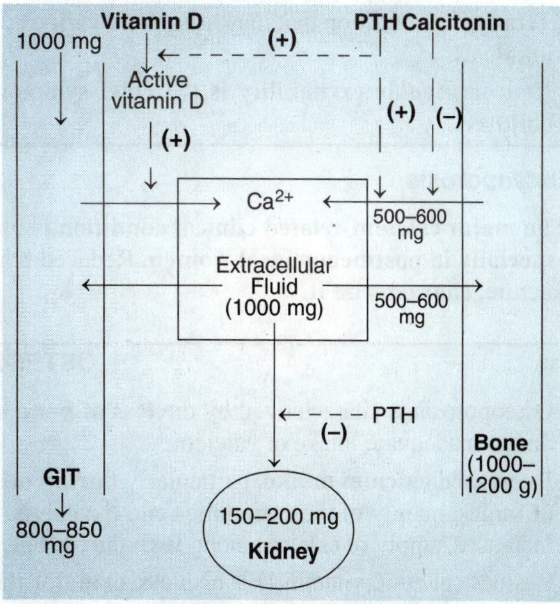

Fig 10.1. Calcium homeostasis.

Biological Functions

Calcium is one of the important elements, which is present in the body. It performs several functions:

1. **Calcification of the growing bones and teeth,** and **maintenance of mature bones** is dependent on adequate dietary intake of calcium and phosphorus.
2. Calcium acts as **activator for several enzymes,** e.g. adenylate cyclase, ATPase, protein kinase, etc.
3. Calcium is essential for the **clotting of blood.**
4. It is also required for the **contraction of muscle.**
5. Calcium is also required to regulate the **permeability of the capillary walls** and **excitability of the nerve fibers.**
6. It is also required for the **secretion of various hormones** and **acts as a second messenger.**
7. Calcium **decreases membrane fluidity.**
8. Ca^{2+} also **regulates citric acid cycle.** It activates pyruvate dehydrogenase phosphatase, which in turn activates pyruvate dehydrogenase complex and produces acetyl CoA. It also activates isocitrate dehydrogenase and α-ketoglutarate dehydrogenase activity.
9. Ca^{2+} also activates phosphorylase kinase, through its binding to calmodulin and **increases rate of glycogen breakdown.**

Deficiency Symptoms

Hypocalcemia may be caused by the deficiency of vitamin D as well as in hypoparathyroidism. Prolonged hypocalcemia may **lead to** faulty calcification of bones, such as in **rickets (in children)** and **osteomalacia (in adults).**

A decrease in calcium in the blood, in relation to phosphorus, results in **tetany,** a condition characterized by abnormal muscle spasm.

> **TETANY**
>
> **Tetany** is a condition that may arise from various causes, such as **hypocalcemia, hypomagnesemia** and **alkalosis.**
>
> **Neuromuscular excitability** is the chief symptom **in adults** while **convulsive seizures are seen in children.**

Osteoporosis

The major calcium-related clinical condition is osteoporosis, **which is an abnormal thinning of bones, especially in postmenopausal women.** Reduced bone mass, increased bone fragility, and a greater risk for fracture, **characterize it.**

> **OSTEOPOROSIS**
>
> Osteoporosis is characterized by the **loss of bone matrix** and **progressive demineralization,** primarily due to inadequate intake of calcium.
>
> **Decreased calcium intake,** particularly **during menopause,** leads to **increased fragility and fractures of bones,** mainly of the extremities and the pelvis. In the postmenopausal women, it can be retarded by increased supply of calcium along with the estrogen therapy.
>
> Besides calcium, vitamin D is also essential, for the absorption and utilization of calcium. Vitamin C is also needed for the formation of bone matrix. Magnesium and phosphorus are also essential since they

also form an essential part of the bone structure. Vitamin K, copper, zinc, manganese and boron are also important in bone formation.

Thus, **an adequate diet, sufficient in all the nutrients along with the regular exercise is important for preventing osteoporosis.**

Requirements

Nearly **800 mg** of calcium is **required daily, by an adult. During pregnancy and lactation,** its **requirement is increased to** about **1.2 g/day.**

Sources

Milk and milk products are the rich sources of calcium. **Egg yolk, dry fruits, legumes, cabbage, cauliflower** and **leafy-vegetables are also good source** of calcium.

Hypercalcemia

Hypercalcemia may be observed due to **increased intake of calcium, increased plasma albumin,** or **increased renal reabsorption of Ca^{2+}.** Hyperactivity of the parathyroid gland (hyperparathyroidism) or hypervitaminosis D may also result in hypercalcemia.

Hypercalcemia may lead to renal stones (calculi). It may also cause loss of appetite, vomiting, constipation, muscle weakness, and sluggish-reflex activities of the central nervous system.

PHOSPHORUS

Phosphorus (P) is widely distributed in most of the tissues. A normal **adult body contains** nearly **600-800 g of phosphorus. About 75% of this is present,** in combination with calcium, **in bones, teeth** and **skeletal tissues.** Blood, muscle, and nerve tissue also contain fairly good amounts of phosphorus.

It is **present** in the body **in two forms** as **inorganic phosphorus** and **organic phosphorus.**

Inorganic phosphorus is essential **for the formation and development of bone and teeth. It** helps in ossification and **gets deposited as calcium phosphate**. It is also **present in the soft tissues and various body fluids as sodium and potassium phosphates.**

Phosphorus containing **organic compounds** includes **phosphate esters of monosaccharides,** such as glucose-6-phosphate, dihydroxyacetone phosphate, phospholipids, **nucleic acids, high-energy compounds** and various **coenzymes like** TPP, $NADP^+$, etc.

ABSORPTION OF DIETARY PHOSPHORUS

Most phosphates are absorbed in the inorganic state. Organically bound phosphate is hydrolyzed in the lumen of the intestine and released as inorganic phosphate, primarily through the action of pancreatic or intestinal phosphatases.

Bioavailability of phosphate depends on the form of the phosphate and the pH. In general, the efficiency of phosphate absorption is 60%-70% in adults, almost twice as high as for calcium.

EXCRETION

The primary route of phosphorus excretion is renal, which also is the primary site of phosphate regulation.

Biological Functions

Phosphorus performs various functions in the body:

1. **Phosphorus** along with calcium **is essential for the mineralization of bone** and **teeth**. It forms **a part of the hydroxyapatite,** which is laid down in bone.
2. Phosphorus also plays an important role **in the maintenance of acid-base balance** thus; it helps in the **regulation of pH of body fluids.**
3. **Phosphorus is also found in phospholipids, which are essential for the transport** and **metabolism of lipids. Phospholipids also form an integral part of the cell membrane.**.
4. **Phosphorus** also forms an important constituent of the nucleic acids in the cell nucleus and thus, is **essential for cell multiplication** and **protein biosynthesis.**
5. **Inorganic phosphorus (Pi) as well as organic esters of phosphoric acid,** such as ADP, **glucose-6-phosphate,** etc., are **necessary for the metabolism of carbohydrates and thus in the production of energy.**
6. As a component of several coenzymes, phosphorus also participates in various enzyme-catalyzed reactions.

Deficiency Symptoms

Deficiency of phosphorus may lead to several neuromuscular, skeletal and renal manifestations.

Low serum phosphorus concentration may be a result of vitamin C deficiency and causes defective bone calcification. Similar to hypocalcemia, **hypophosphatemia** may **lead to rickets in children** and **osteomalacia in adults.**

Requirements

Daily requirement of phosphorus is nearly 50% higher than calcium. It varies from **1.0 to 1.5 g/day.**

Sources

Phosphorus is found in foods containing phosphoproteins, nucleoproteins, phospholipids and glycerophosphates, as well as in the form of inorganic phosphates, chiefly of Ca and Na.

Calcium rich diets, e.g. **milk, cheese, and beans,** are also **rich source** of phosphorus. **Eggs, cereals, fish,** and **meat are** also its **good sources.**

IRON

Total quantity of iron (Fe) **in a normal adult human being is about 4 g.**

Iron may be incorporated in the protoporphyrin ring both in Fe^{2+} or Fe^{3+} form. The **Fe^{2+}-protoporphyrin complex is called as heme** while the **Fe^{3+}-protoporphyrin complex is designated as hematin.**

ABSORPTION, TRANSPORT, STORAGE AND EXCRETION OF IRON

Dietary iron exists in two chemical forms:

Heme iron, which is found in hemoglobin, myoglobin and some enzymes, and

Non-heme iron, which is found predominantly, in plant foods but also in some animal foods, as are non-heme enzymes and ferritin.

Heme iron is absorbed across the brush border (mucosa) of the intestinal absorbing cells (enterocytes) after it is digested from animal sources. After heme enters the cytosol, the **ferrous iron is enzymatically removed from the ferroporphyrin complex**. The **free iron ions combine** immediately **with apoferritin to form ferritin,** similar to free non-heme iron. Ferritin carries bound iron from the brush border to the basolateral membrane of the absorbing cell that involves an active transport mechanism.

The brush border iron transporter called **divalent metal transporter 1** (DMT 1) **transports ferrous iron. Ferric iron** may be **reduced by** a brush border enzyme **ferric reductase**, for its absorption. Several factors affect iron absorption.

The **efficiency of iron absorption** (from gut lumen to blood) by adults with normal hemoglobin values averages **5% to 15% of the iron** (heme and non-heme iron combined) **contained in food.**

Iron (non-heme) is transported, bound to transferrin, from the intestinal absorbing cells to various tissues, to meet their needs.

Between 200-1500 mg of **iron is stored in the body as ferritin and hemosiderin**. Thirty percent of the body's iron store is in the liver, 30% in the bone marrow and the rest is found in the spleen and muscles.

Iron is only lost through bleeding and in very small amounts through defecation, sweat and the normal exfoliation of hair and skin. Unabsorbed iron is lost in the feces. Almost no iron is excreted in the urine. Daily iron loss is **approximately 1 mg**.

HEME AND NON-HEME IRON

Heme containing proteins include **hemoglobin, myoglobin** and **certain enzymes, such as catalase** and **peroxidases.**

Nonheme proteins include **ferritin, transferrin, cytochromes** and **iron-sulphur proteins.**

Ferritin: Ferritin is an iron containing protein, which is involved in the storage of iron.

Protein part of ferritin **is called apoferritin.** Its synthesis is regulated by the concentration of free intracellular iron.

Apoferritin controls absorption of iron, as it has a rapid turn over. **It is converted into ferritin, high concentration of which blocks the absorption of iron in the mucosal cells.** On the other hand, **when more iron is to be absorbed, apoferritin is rapidly synthesized and becomes readily available.** Thus, **ferritin acts** both, **as sink for iron, during its excess intake,** as well as source of iron during its deprivation.

Transferrin: **Transferrin is a nonheme iron protein. It is involved in transport of iron.** It is a serum glycoprotein (β_1-globulin) and is synthesized in the liver.

Protein part of transferrin is designated as apotransferrin. It has affinity for Fe^{3+}.

Hemosiderin: **Excess of iron stimulates the storage capacity of the newly synthesized apoferritin, which may be partially degraded** by the proteolytic enzymes. This in turn results in **release of iron oxide micelles, forming insoluble aggregates, designated as hemosiderin.** These insoluble aggregates are trapped in the secondary lysosomes.

In a normal healthy subject, very little of hemosiderin is detectable. Quantity of the hemosiderin, **as brownish granules in the cells,** increases during iron overload.

Factors affecting Iron Absorption

1. Iron **absorption increases with its intake.**
2. Iron, in the **ferrous form is more effectively absorbed** than in the ferric form.
3. Amino acids, such as **cysteine and reducing substances, e.g. vitamin C, stimulate iron absorption.**
4. Due to the presence of certain complex forming agents, such as oxalates, phosphates, carbonates, phytates and fiber, **iron from the vegetables and cereals is poorly absorbed**.
5. **Iron status of the body** also affects its absorption. Absorption of dietary iron varies inversely with the iron stores of the body.
6. **Hydrochloric acid,** secreted by the gastric mucosa, enhances iron absorption by stimulating digestion of protein, which in turn releases protein-bound iron.

Biological Functions

Iron plays number of roles in the body:

1. As a component of hemoglobin and myoglobin, iron is **required for the transport of O_2 and CO_2**.
2. Several **enzymes contain heme iron, as a part of their prosthetic group,** e.g. **catalase, peroxidase, tryptophan pyrrolase,** etc.
3. As a **component of cytochromes, iron is required for electron transport chain and oxidative phosphorylation.**
4. **As a component of the lysosomal enzyme myeloperoxidase,** iron **is required in phagocytosis.**
5. Iron is also an **essential component of several non-heme proteins,** such as **transferrin, ferritin and iron-sulphur proteins** (ferridoxins).

Deficiency Symptoms

Most common **iron deficiency** disorder is anemia, which is a common feature in children, adolescent girls, and females of the childbearing age, particularly in developing countries.

Children become dull and inactive, have loss of appetite and poor growth. Deficiency of iron in females also **reduces** their **work capacity.**

Iron deficiency is also associated with **reduced immunocompetence.**

ANEMIA

Anemia is **characterized by reduced number of circulating erythrocytes** and/or their **hemoglobin contents**. Anemia may be divided into three types:

1. ***Microcytic anemia*: Erythrocytes** become **small in size** and have **reduced content of hemoglobin.** Their **number may also be reduced** but to a smaller extent.
   It is **caused by the deficiency of iron. Conditions like pregnancy, hookworm infections, and complete or partial gastrectomy, may lead to iron deficiency anemia.**
2. ***Macrocytic anemia*: Size of erythrocytes is increased** while their **number is reduced,** presenting a characteristic blood picture of **pernicious anemia.** It is usually **caused by the deficiency of vitamin B_{12} and/or folic acid.**
3. ***Normocytic anemia*: Size as well as hemoglobin content** of erythrocytes **remains normal but their number is reduced.** It is usually due to **hemorrhages.**

Requirements

Recommended **dietary allowance** for iron is about **10 mg for normal adult males**. For females, the requirement is **18-20 mg/day, particularly during the reproductive stage.** This is on account of the increased iron losses during menstruation and on account of the increasing demand of the body during pregnancy and lactation. **Daily requirement** of iron is increased to **nearly 30 mg/day during pregnancy.**

Sources

Food cooked in **iron cook wares is the best source of iron.**

Animal foods, such as **meat, fish, and egg,** are good **sources of heme iron.**

Green-leafy vegetables, cereals, and legumes (whole grains) **are good sources of the non-heme iron.** Milk is a poor source of iron.

Iron Toxicity

Iron overload may lead to a condition called hemochromatosis (hemosiderosis). It may result in the deposition of the **iron** in **many tissues,** particularly in storage organs, such as liver and spleen, leading to hepatomegaly, pancreatic and cardiac dysfunctions and skin pigmentation.

Hemochromatosis may be a result of failure of regulation of iron absorption, excess dietary intake of iron, alcoholic cirrhosis, chronic pancreatitis, or excessive blood transfusions.

IODINE

About **20-30 mg** of iodine (I^-) is present in an **adult human body.** About **two-third** of it is **present in the thyroid gland as free iodine** as well as in the form of **mono-iodotyrosine, di-iodotyrosine, tri-iodothyronine (T_3), and tetra-iodothyronine or thyroxine (T_4).**

SYNTHESIS OF THYROID HORMONES

Iodine is stored in the thyroid gland where it is used for the synthesis of thyroid hormones. First **iodine** is **activated by peroxidase**. Subsequently, **iodinase catalyzes the iodination of tyrosyl- residues of thyroglobin and sequentially form mono-iodotyrosine (MIT) and di-iodotyrosine (DIT).** Thereafter, **coupling of either a** molecule of **MIT with DIT or two molecules of DIT form tri-iodothyronine** (T_3) or **thyroxine** (tetra-iodothyronine or T_4), respectively (Fig. 10.2).

$$2I^- \xrightarrow{\text{Peroxidase}} I_2$$

$$\text{Tyrosine} \xrightarrow{\text{Iodinase}} \text{MIT} \longrightarrow \text{DIT}$$

$$\text{MIT} + \text{DIT} \xrightarrow{\text{Coupling enzyme}} T_3$$

$$\text{DIT} + \text{DIT} \longrightarrow T_4$$

Fig. 10.2. Synthesis of thyroid hormones.

Thyroid hormone is degraded in the target cells and in the liver, and the **iodine is highly conserved under normal conditions.**

Biological Functions

Important function of iodine is the **synthesis of iodine-containing hormones,** which are physiologically active substances, formed **by thyroid gland.**

These hormones in turn regulate basal metabolic rate in adults, and growth and development in children.

Deficiency Symptoms

Lack of iodine leads to a condition called endemic goiter. Most characteristic symptom of which is enlargement **of the thyroid gland.**

Endemic goiter: **Dietary iodine deficiency causes** depletion of thyroid stores and **reduces the output of** thyroid stimulating hormone **(TSH) from the pituitary.** This in turn **results in hyperplasia of the thyroid gland,** which traps and processes available iodine, more efficiently. The gland returns to its normal size, after sufficient amount of dietary iodine is available. This is called as **simple goiter** and is endemic in many areas.

Cretinism: **Cretinism is** a condition of **hypothyroidism in infants and children. A cretin child is dwarf in size with thick tongue and skin, and is mentally retarded and sexually underdeveloped.**

Myxedema: **Severe hypothyroidism in adults** leads to a condition **called myxedema.**

Due to the deposition of the mucous-like viscous material (myxomatous material) in the subcutaneous layer of face and hands, **skin of these individuals becomes thick and puffy. Body weight is increased** due to retention of water and NaCl. **There is also mental dullness and hypersensitivity to cold.**

Requirement

Daily requirement of iodine is about **50-100 µg.**

Sources

Iodine requirement is mostly fulfilled from **drinking water.** Adequate supply of iodine can also be met from **iodized salt.**

Seafoods, fruits, vegetables, cereals, and **meat are good sources of** iodine.

Iodine Toxicity

Iodine toxicity may result in **thyrotoxicosis.**

FLUORIDE

Fluoride (F) is present in **traces in several tissues,** mainly in bone, teeth, thyroid gland, and skin.

Biological Functions

1. **Fluoride promotes normal bone development, increases retention of calcium and phosphorous** and **prevents osteoporosis during aging.**
2. Its incorporation into the hydroxyapatite **helps in the maintenance and hardening of dental enamel and makes it resistant to acid.**

Deficiency Symptoms

Deficiency of fluoride promotes development **of dental caries in children** and **osteoporosis in adults** (particularly in the postmenopausal women).

Requirement

Average daily requirement for fluoride is **2-3 mg.**

Sources

Drinking water is an important source of fluoride **in human diet.**

Tea is also a good source of fluoride.

Fluoride Toxicity

Excess of fluoride causes several health problems including **dental and skeletal fluorosis.**

Dental Fluorosis: Fluorosis occurs mainly in children who are exposed to excess fluoride intake before the completion of mineralization of tooth enamel.

Skeletal Fluorosis: Clinical features of skeletal fluorosis include **pain, inflammation, and restricted movements of joints, and stiffness of spine.**

Genu Valgum: Individuals with **Genu Valgum (Knock-knee syndrome)** exhibit **extensive osteoporosis of the bones of the limbs, besides features of dental and skeletal fluorosis.**

COPPER

Adult human body contains nearly 100-150 mg of copper (Cu), out of which 50% is found in muscle and 25% in bone.

Some of the copper in plasma is loosely bound to albumin. It is called direct reacting copper. Most of it is bound to a specific copper-binding protein, called **ceruloplasmin.**

CERULOPLASMIN

Ceruloplasmin, also called as ferroxidase I, is a copper containing α_2-globulin, present in plasma. It is **synthesized in liver, in the form of apoprotein, called apoceruloplasmin.** After nearly 6-8 atoms of copper are incorporated in a molecule **of the apoprotein,** it **is converted into ceruloplasmin.**

Ceruloplasmin helps in the conversion of Fe^{2+} to Fe^{3+} form of iron, for its incorporation into transferrin and ferritin. Copper thus, **helps in the transport of iron, to the extrahepatic tissues.**

Biological Functions

1. Copper is a **component of many enzymes,** particularly those, which require vitamin C, **such as cytochrome oxidase, ferroxidase (ceruloplasmin), tyrosinase, ascorbic acid oxidase, superoxide dismutase,** etc.
2. It is also an important **constituent of several proteins,** such as **erythrocuprein, cerebrocuprein,** and **hepatocuprein,** which are present in bone marrow, brain and liver, respectively.
3. Copper also **helps in the formation of bone and the elastin fibers.**
4. It is also **required for the maintenance of myelin sheath, in nerve fibers.**
5. Copper, as a **constituent of δ-aminolevulinate synthase and ferroxidase I, also helps in the metabolism of iron** and **biosynthesis of hemoglobin.**

After its absorption, **copper** is stored in liver and is **excreted via bile**. Very little of it is excreted in urine.

Deficiency Symptoms

Symptoms of copper deficiency include **hypercholesterolemia, demineralization of bone, leukopenia, demyelination of the neural tissue, and alopecia** (loss of hair).

Copper deficiency may also lead to **microcytic normochromic anemia, which can not be cured by iron supplementation alone,** since copper is essential for the intestinal absorption and metabolism of iron.

Copper deficiency has also been found to be associated with a condition, called **Menke's disease**.

MENKE'S DISEASE

Menke's disease **also called as Kinky-hair syndrome, due to the failure to keratinize hair. Hairs become kinky and steel gray.**

It is an X-linked hereditary disease, **due to failure of copper absorption and transport.** This in turn leads to low concentration of copper in plasma and liver. Skeletal malformation, mental retardation, defective thermoregulation, and immunological deficiency characterize it.

Most of these abnormalities are **due to the deficiency of various copper-containing oxidases,** such as tyrosinase, lysyl-oxidase, etc.

Requirement

A normal adult requires nearly **2-3 mg** of copper **per day.**

Sources

Nuts, leafy vegetables, dried legumes, egg-yolk, fish, and liver-meat are the good sources of copper. Milk is its poor source.

Copper Toxicity

Copper toxicity may manifest as diarrhea, blue-green discoloration of saliva, hemolysis, proteinuria, and renal failure.

It may also lead to the deposition of copper in liver and brain. This condition is called **Wilson disease.**

> **WILSON DISEASE**
>
> **Wilson disease, also called hepatolenticular degeneration,** is an autosomal recessive inherited disorder. It is **due to defect in incorporation of Cu^{2+} into apoceruloplasmin.** As a result of which, **excess of copper gets accumulated** in various tissues, mainly the **liver** and the **basal nuclei of the brain.** This in turn also results in **increased excretion of copper, causing renal tubular damage with hemoglobinuria and generalized aminoaciduria.**

ZINC

Total body content of zinc (Zn), in an adult man, is **about 2.0 g.**

Choroid of eye, liver, prostate gland and **prostate fluid contain high concentrations of zinc.**

Biological Functions

1. **Zinc is a component of several enzymes,** such as **carbonic anhydrase, lactate dehydrogenase, alcohol dehydrogenase, alkaline phosphatase, DNA and RNA polymerases,** and **retinene-retinal reductase,** etc.
2. It is also **an important constituent of insulin.** Zinc forms a complex with insulin and **helps in its storage and release from β-cells of the pancreas.**
3. Zinc is also **necessary for maintaining the plasma concentration of vitamin A,** by stimulating its release from liver into blood.
4. As a component of **gustin** (a salivary polypeptide **necessary for the normal development of the taste buds),** zinc is also **important in taste sensation.**
5. Zinc has also been shown to be **essential for normal growth and reproduction in animals.**

Deficiency Symptoms

Severe zinc deficiency is seen primarily, **in alcoholics, or in-patients with chronic renal disease, severe malabsorption, and protein-energy malnutrition.**

1. Its deficiency may result in **poor wound healing, loss of appetite, poor growth, and alopecia** (loss of hair).
2. Zinc deficiency in children, may result in the **impairment of sexual development.**
3. Its deficiency may also **impair brain functions, DNA synthesis, and carbohydrate metabolism.**
4. **Zinc deficiency may also cause fetal abnormalities during pregnancy,** besides hypogonadism, dwarfism (stunted growth), and gross skin lesion with severe acrodermatitis.
5. Zinc deficiency has also been shown to affect spermatogenesis, parturition, and lactation, in experimental animals.

Requirement

Daily requirement of zinc is about **10-15 mg.**

Sources

Good dietary sources are **meat, seafoods, egg, legumes, and milk.**

Colostrums are a very rich source of zinc.

Zinc Toxicity

When consumed in **excess,** zinc **produces** toxic effects, such as **acute gastrointestinal irritation, gastric ulcer, nausea, and vomiting.**

Zinc also interferes with the utilization and functions of copper.

MAGNESIUM

Adult human body contains nearly **20-25 g of magnesium** (Mg).

About 75% of it is combined with calcium and phosphorous, and is present in **bones. Remaining** of it is present in **soft tissues,** such as muscle and nervous tissue, **and in body fluids.**

In blood, most of the magnesium is intracellular.

Biological Functions

1. Magnesium is a **component of the bone structure.**
2. It also plays an important **role in nerve impulse transmission.**
3. **Magnesium ions, (Mg^{2+}), acts as activator for several enzymes particularly, those requiring ATP,** such as glucokinase, hexokinase, acyl CoA synthetase, alkaline phosphatase, DNA and RNA polymerases, etc.
4. Magnesium is also **involved in the formation of cAMP,** and thus mediates the effects of numerous hormones.
5. Mg^{2+} also **participates in electron transfer** and stabilizes the arrangement of the redox centers, in cytochrome C oxidase.
6. Mg^{2+} **also helps in the contraction of the cardiac and smooth muscles.**

Deficiency Symptoms

Magnesium **deficiency is** often **observed in alcoholics, in-patients taking certain types of diuretics, and in metabolic acidosis.** Magnesium deficiency may also be observed in **uremics** and in children suffering from **kwashiorkor.**

Low serum magnesium levels are also observed in pregnancy (particularly during toxemia of pregnancy), rickets, diarrhea and vomiting.

Deficiency symptoms include tremors, depression, hyperirritability, cardiac arrhythmia, muscular weakness, and **convulsions.**

Low levels of serum magnesium **may also result in tetany.**

Requirement

Average **daily requirement is 250-300 mg.**

Sources

Whole grains, **cereals, potato,** and **seafoods are good sources** of magnesium. Beverages, such as **coffee, tea** and **cocoa, are** also rich in **magnesium.**

Magnesium Toxicity

Toxicity may be observed due to increased use of magnesium containing laxatives and antacids. Chief **symptoms include drowsiness, lethargy,** and **weakness.**

MANGANESE

Total Body manganese (Mn) **content** in an adult man is about **10-12 mg.**

It is mainly concentrated in bone, liver, and kidney.

Biological Functions

1. **Manganese is a cofactor for several enzymes,** such as **hydrolases, decarboxylases, phosphorylases,** and **phosphotransferases.**
2. It is essential for the **synthesis of glycoproteins and proteoglycans, in the cartilage.**
3. Manganese also **stimulates the biosynthesis of cholesterol and long chain fatty acids.**
4. **It also prevents lipid peroxidation,** and **exhibits lipotropic effects.**

Deficiency Symptoms

Manganese **deficiency leads to bone deformities, poor growth, and ataxia,** in several animal species. Its deficiency has also been shown to **decrease synthesis of oligosaccharides, glycoproteins, and proteoglycans.**

Requirement

Daily requirement of manganese is about **2-5 mg.**

Sources

Nuts, whole grains cereals, legumes, and **leafy-vegetables** are the good sources of manganese.

Tea is also a rich source of manganese.

Manganese Toxicity

Manganese **toxicity** can occur in manganese-ore mine workers, in whom its excessive inhalation **produces severe psychotic symptoms and Parkinsonism.**

CHROMIUM

Total Body chromium **(Cr) content** of adult men varies between **5-10 mg.**

Chromium exists in several forms but it is the trivalent form of chromium **(Cr^{3+}), which is biologically** active. It is found in an **organic compound** termed **glucose tolerance factor,** which potentiates the effects of insulin, may be by facilitating its binding to the cell receptor sites. Chromium is thus, **important in the removal of the ingested glucose.**

Biological Functions

1. **Chromium,** as a component of glucose tolerance factor, **is important in the regulation of blood glucose since it potentiates insulin secretion.**
2. It is also **important in the metabolism of lipoproteins,** and maintains normal level of blood cholesterol.

Deficiency Symptoms

Chromium deficiency can impair glucose tolerance.

Requirement

Daily requirement of chromium is about 50-100 μg.

Sources

Brewer yeast, mushrooms, black pepper, liver meat, whole grains cereals, nuts, and **cheese are the good sources of chromium.**

Chromium Toxicity

Chromium toxicity may be observed in workers who are exposed to chromium dust. Excess of chromium may **induce lung cancer.**

SELENIUM

Selenium (Se) is present in higher amounts in renal cortex, pancreas, pituitary, and liver.

Biological Functions

1. Selenium is **an essential component of selenoproteins** (selenium-containing proteins), which **have selenocysteine (SeC) residues.** In mammals, an essential selenoprotein is **glutathione peroxidase,** which **protects the cells against the damage caused by H_2O_2.**
2. Selenium **acts as a synergic antioxidant with vitamin E** and protects cells against free radicals. Both selenium and vitamin E are therefore, necessary for efficient scavenging of peroxides, by peroxidases.

Deficiency Symptoms

Selenium **deficiency may lead to liver necrosis, muscular dystrophy, cardiomyopathy, and dilatation of heart.**

Requirement

Daily intake of selenium is **about 50-100 μg.**

Sources

Plant foods, cereals, fish, and meat are the rich sources of selenium.

Selenium Toxicity

Selenium toxicity has been observed in persons working in the paint, glass, and ceramic industry. They suffer from **difficulty in breathing.**

High selenium intake may also induce weight loss, hair loss, dermatitis, diarrhea, and emotional disturbances (irritability).

COBALT

An adult human **body contains** about **2-3 mg of cobalt** (Co).

It is mainly present in **liver and kidney.**

Biological Functions

1. Cobalt is **an important constituent of vitamin B_{12} (cobalamin).**
2. It also **acts as a cofactor for enzymes,** such as **glycylglycine dipeptidase.**
3. Cobalt **stimulates the production of erythropoietin,** and thus promotes erythropoiesis.

Deficiency Symptoms

Cobalt deficiency may cause pernicious anemia, which is due to the deficiency of vitamin B_{12}.

Requirement

Its daily requirement is about **1-2 μg/day.**

Sources

Foods from animal origin are the good sources of cobalt. **Liver meat** is its rich source.

Cobalt Toxicity

High doses of cobalt **may produce polycythemia, hypothyroidism, cardiomyopathy, and heart failure.**

MOLYBDENUM

An adult human **body contains** nearly **5 mg** of molybdenum (Mo). It is present in large amounts in **liver and kidney.**

Biological Functions

Molybdenum is an integral part of several flavoprotein-containing oxidases, e.g. **xanthine oxidase, aldehyde oxidase, sulfite oxidase,** etc. It thus helps in the transport of electrons.

Deficiency Symptoms

Molybdenum deficiency may result in the deficiency of the molybdenum-containing enzymes, which in turn **may lead to reduced food consumption and cause mental retardation.**

Decreased xanthine oxidase activity may also increase the excretion of xanthine and reduce the excretion of uric acid.

Requirement

Daily requirement of molybdenum is about 100-200 μg.

Sources

Pulses, cereals, green-leafy vegetables, and meat are the good sources of molybdenum.

Toxicity

Molybdenum toxicity may cause weight loss, anorexia, anemia, severe diarrhea, and skeletal deformities.

Very high amount of molybdenum may also inhibit the absorption and utilization of copper.

Important biological functions, sources, daily requirement, deficiency disorders, and toxicity symptoms of various minerals are shown in Table 10.1.

Table 10.1. Minerals and trace elements, their important biological functions, sources, daily requirements, deficiency disorders and toxicity symptoms

Mineral/trace element	*Biological functions*	*Sources*	*Daily requirement*	*Deficiency disorders*	*Toxicity*
Calcium (Ca)	Calcification of teeth and bone, blood clotting, and cofactor for enzymes, such as adenylate cyclase, glycogen synthase, etc.	Milk and milk products, legumes, and dry fruits	800-1200mg	Tetany, osteoporosis	Renal stones
Phosphorus (P)	Calcification of teeth and bone, component of	Milk and milk products,	1.0-1.5 g	Neuromuscular, skeletal, and	–

(Contd.)

Mineral/trace element	*Biological functions*	*Sources*	*Daily requirement*	*Deficiency disorders*	*Toxicity*
	nucleic acids, regulation of blood pH, and activator for enzymes involved in phosphorylation/ dephosphorylation	eggs, meat, legumes, and cereals		renal manifestations	
Iron (Fe)	Component of heme and nonheme proteins, e.g. hemoglobin, catalase, cytochromes, etc.	Meat, green-leafy vegetables	10-20 mg	Anemia	Hemosiderosis
Copper (Cu)	Component of many enzymes, such as cytochrome oxidase, ceruloplasmin, tyrosinase, etc., also helps in iron metabolism	Meat, egg, and legumes	2-3 mg	Menke's disease, anemia, neutropenia	Wilson disease
Zinc (Zn)	Cofactor for various enzymes, such as carbonic anhydrase, DNA and RNA polymerases, alkaline phosphatase; also has role in insulin secretion and taste development	Meat, seafoods, and legumes	10-15 mg	Poor wound healing, growth retardation	Gastrointestinal irritation
Iodine (I_2)	Synthesis of thyroid hormones	Iodized salt, seafoods	50-100 μg	Endemic goiter, myxedema, cretinism	Thyrotoxicosis
Fluoride (F)	Promotes normal bone and teeth development	Drinking water and tea	2-3 mg	Dental caries	Fluorosis
Magnesium (Mg)	Component of the bone structure, in nerve impulse transmission, also acts as cofactor for various ATP-dependent enzymes	Cereals, seafoods, coffee, and tea	250-300 mg	Depression, muscle weakness, and tetany	Drowsiness and lethargy
Manganese (Mn)	Cofactor for various enzymes, such as hydrolases, decarboxylases, transferases, etc.	Nuts, whole grains, and tea	2-5 mg	Bone deformities	Psychotic symptoms
Chromium (Cr)	Regulation of blood glucose	Mushrooms, nuts, and black pepper	50-100 μg	Glucose intolerance	Lung cancer
Selenium (Se)	Component of selenoproteins, such as glutathione peroxidase	Cereals, fish, and meat	50-100 μg	Liver necrosis	Hair loss
Cobalt (Ca)	Component of vitamin B_{12}	Liver meat	1-2 μg	Pernicious anemia	Polycythemia, hypothyroidism
Molybdenum (Mo)	Component of flavoprotein containing oxidases, such as xanthine oxidase	Pulses and cereals	100-200 μg	Affects growth, causes mental retardation	Anorexia and diarrhea

SOME IMPORTANT QUESTIONS

1. Describe dietary sources, daily requirement, and biological functions of calcium.
2. Describe role of parathyroid hormone, vitamin D, and calcitonin in calcium metabolism.
3. Name iron containing proteins that are found in the body and explain their functions. Describe the disorders related to iron metabolism.
4. Describe:
   (i) Calcium homeostasis
   (ii) Fluoride as a nutrient
   (iii) Role of copper in iron metabolism
   (iv) Significance of zinc for the body
   (v) Factors affecting absorption of iron
   (vi) Biological functions of phosphorus
   (vii) Biological functions of chromium
5. Write notes on:
   (i) Copper
   (ii) Biological functions of selenium
   (iii) Wilson disease
   (iv) Biological functions of calcium
   (v) Tetany
   (vi) Ferritin
   (vii) Transferrin
   (viii) Hemosiderin
   (ix) Anemia
   (x) Ceruloplasmin
   (xi) Hemosiderosis
   (xii) Menke's disease
   (xiii) Kinky-hair syndrome
   (xiv) Glucose tolerance factor
6. Discuss:
   (i) Biological functions of magnesium
   (ii) Hepatolenticular degeneration
   (iii) Endemic goiter
   (iv) Biological functions of manganese
   (v) Biological functions of cobalt
   (vi) Factors affecting absorption of calcium

CHAPTER 11

Electron Transport Chain

REDUCING EQUIVALENTS

Ability of the body to derive comparatively, more energy from lipids than carbohydrate or proteins is related to the oxidative state of the carbons in these molecules. The carbons in the lipid are more reduced (or less oxidized) than the carbohydrate or protein, which are comparatively more oxidized (or less reduced). Hence, during the sequential breakdown of lipids, more reducing equivalents are generated than from the carbohydrate or protein (Fig. 11.1).

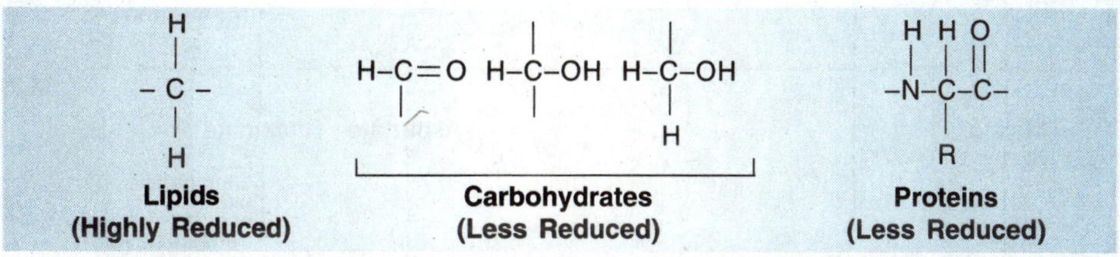

Fig. 11.1. State of different carbon atoms in a nutrient molecule.

A **reducing equivalent** is defined as a **proton plus electron ($H^+ + e^-$).** They are generated in the cytoplasm and are accepted by NAD^+ or FAD, which are converted to their reduced state as NADH or $FADH_2$, respectively. These reducing equivalents **are utilized for ATP synthesis** in the mitochondria, by a system of electron carriers, in or association with the inner mitochondrial membrane. This system of electron carriers, in the presence of O_2, converts these reducing equivalents into the utilizable energy, by the process called **electron transport chain.**

TRANSPORT OF REDUCING EQUIVALENTS INTO MITOCHONDRIA

Reducing equivalents however, can not cross the inner mitochondrial membrane, where they are utilized, because the inner mitochondrial membrane is impermeable to the reducing equivalents. For the transport of reducing equivalents from the cytoplasm to the mitochondria, there are two shuttle systems, called as **malate-aspartate shuttle** and **glycerol phosphate shuttle**.

Malate aspartate shuttle

In the malate-aspartate shuttle, oxaloacetate, which is present in the cytoplasm, is converted to either aspartate, through the action of aspartate aminotransferase or malate, by malate dehydrogenase.

With the use of the **reducing equivalents** from **NADH**, oxaloacetate is reduced **by malate dehydrogenase** to malate, and gets **transported into mitochondria**. After its reoxidation in the matrix, by the same enzyme, malate releases these reducing equivalents and is reoxidized to oxaloacetate. Since oxaloacetate is impermeable through the mitochondrial membrane, it is first converted to aspartate, by glutamate oxaloacetate transaminase. This enzyme converts oxaloacetate to aspartate, and glutamate to α-ketoglutarate. Both, aspartate and α-ketoglutarate are transported across the mitochondrial membrane and return to the cytoplasm where aspartate is reconverted to oxaloacetate.

As both, aspartate as well as malate are freely permeable through the inner mitochondrial membrane, the reducing equivalents, which were accepted by NAD^+ and originated in the cytoplasm, are transported into the mitochondria for their entry into the electron transport chain (Fig. 11.2).

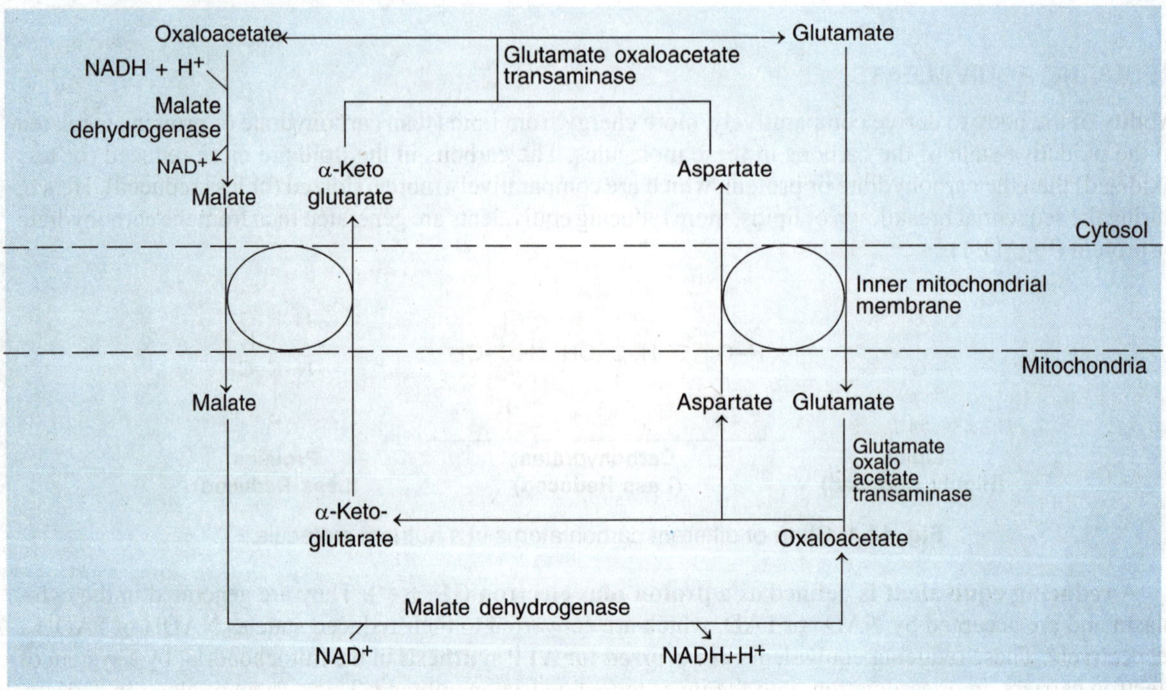

Fig. 11.2. Malate-Aspartate shuttle.

Glycerol phosphate shuttle

Electrons, through the glycerol phosphate shuttle, are **transported to the mitochondrial electron-transport chain, via FAD.**

In the first step, 3-phosphoglycerol dehydrogenase, with the help of dihydroxyacetone phosphate, catalyzes the oxidation of NADH to NAD^+, which reenters glycolysis.

In the next step, electrons, from 3-phosphoglycerol (glycerolphosphate), are transferred to a flavoprotein

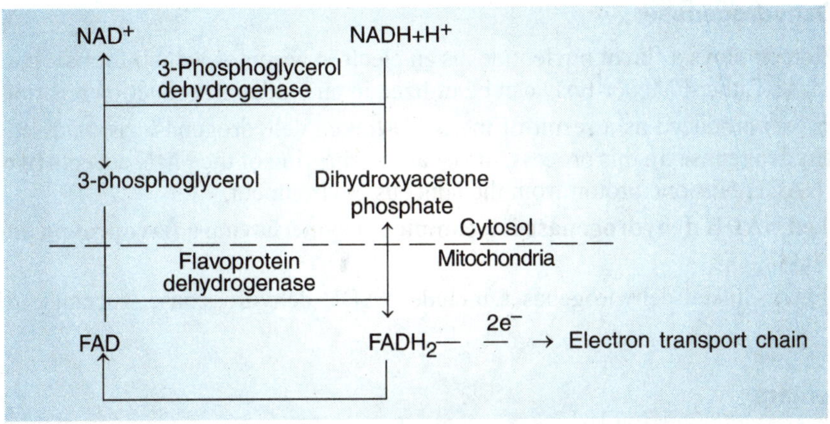

Fig. 11.3. Glycerolphosphate shuttle.

dehydrogenase. Oxidation of 3-phosphoglycerol in turn causes the reduction of FAD to $FADH_2$. Since flavoprotein dehydrogenase is situated on the outer surface of the inner mitochondrial membrane, it supplies electrons directly to the electron-transport chain and results in reoxidation of $FADH_2$ to FAD, within mitochondria. The overall process thus, results in transport of reducing equivalents from the cytoplasm directly into the mitochondrial electron transport chain (Fig. 11.3).

ELECTRON TRANSPORT CHAIN

Electrons, which are transferred from cytoplasm to the mitochondria, participate in sequential oxidation/ reduction of the various redox centers that are present in the four enzyme complexes with in the mitochondria. This sequence of electron carriers is called electron transport chain or mitochondrial respiratory chain.

COMPONENTS OF THE CHAIN

The electron transport chain has various components, which include NAD^+-linked dehydrogenase, flavin-linked dehydrogenase, iron-sulphur proteins, coenzyme Q and various cytochromes.

NAD^+-Linked Dehydrogenase

Initial step in the mitochondrial electron transport chain consists of the generation of reducing equivalents in several processes, such as citric acid cycle, β-oxidation of fatty acids, etc.

NAD^+-linked dehydrogenase reaction **reduces NAD^+ to NADH and** in turn converts a reduced member of the oxidation-reduction reaction to the oxidized form, such as the oxidation of malate to oxaloacetate:

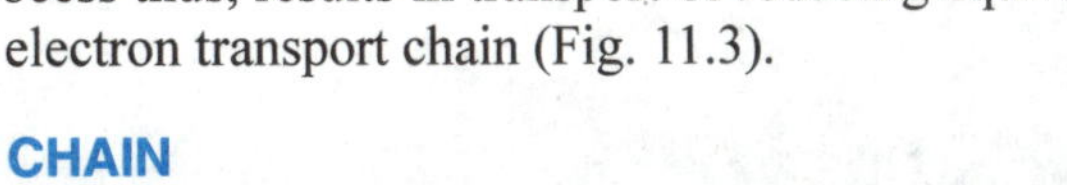

In the dehydrogenation of a metabolite, **two electrons** and **two protons are removed**, out of which both the electrons and one of the protons are transferred to NAD^+. Since only one of the protons (as an anhydride ion, i.e. H^-, one hydrogen atom containing an additional electron), is accepted by NAD^+, the second proton (H^+) therefore, is released free into the aqueous environment.

Some of the NAD-linked dehydrogenases include malate dehydrogenase, lactate dehydrogenase, etc.

NADPH is not a substrate for the mitochondrial respiratory chain as it is used in reductive biosynthesis, such as in the biosynthesis of fatty acids and cholesterol, etc.

Flavin-Linked Dehydrogenase

This type of reaction employs a flavin nucleotide, as an electron acceptor, which forms a part of the flavin-linked dehydrogenase. Either FMN or FAD can be utilized in an oxidation-reduction reaction.

NADH, which was produced as a result of the NAD-linked dehydrogenase, is oxidized by the **FMN-linked NADH dehydrogenase**. In this process, the isoailoxazine ring of the FMN accepts **two electrons** and one **proton** from NADH plus one proton from the aqueous environment.

The FMN-**linked NADH dehydrogenase is a complex** enzyme, having a **flavoprotein and at least four iron-sulphur centers.**

Some of the Flavin-linked dehydrogenases include NADH dehydrogenase, succinate dehydrogenase, etc.

Iron-Sulphur Centers

Iron-sulphur centers, also called as the iron-sulphur clusters, form prosthetic group of iron-sulphur protein, a nonheme iron protein. Iron component of the iron-sulphur center is bound to the cysteine residue of the protein as well as to the acid-labile sulphur.

Iron-sulphur clusters undergo **one-electron oxidation** and **reduction,** and during transfer of the reducing equivalents, iron is converted from Fe^{3+} to Fe^{2+}, on and off the flavin moiety.

Iron-sulphur centers function in the **transfer of electrons from $FMNH_2$ to coenzyme Q** and **from cytochrome b to cytochrome c_1.**

Coenzyme Q

The acceptor of the electrons and protons from NADH dehydrogenase is **coenzyme Q** (CoQ) also called **ubiquinone.** It is neither a protein nor nucleotide, but a lipophilic electron carrier.

It serves as a **mobile electron transporter** within the mitochondrial membrane, which operates **between the flavin-linked dehydrogenase** and cytochrome b. With the addition of two reducing equivalents ($2H^+ + 2e^-$), CoQ is reduced to $CoQ.H_2$. Hydrogen atoms, which have been collected by CoQ, are released into the mitochondrial matrix and ultimately form water, with the molecular oxygen.

Cytochromes

Cytochromes are a class of proteins, called **hemoproteins,** which are characterized by the presence of an iron-containing heme, which is bound to a protein. Unlike the heme group found in hemoglobin or myoglobin, where heme iron remains in the Fe^{2+} State, iron in the heme of the cytochrome is reduced (Fe^{2+}) and oxidized (Fe^{3+}), alternatively.

Various cytochromes of the mammalian mitochondria are designated as cytochrome a, b, c, etc. They carry electrons from CoQ to molecular oxygen, sequentially and thus act as transelectronases.

Each cytochrome accepts a pair of electrons from its predecessor, converting Fe^{3+} into Fe^{2+}. Transfer of electrons from one cytochrome to another, and eventually to cytochrome oxidase, accomplishes regeneration of Fe^{3+}. No hydrogen transfer takes place with in this segment of the electron transport chain.

Cytochrome oxidase (cytochrome $a.a_3$) is a terminal unit of the electron transport chain. This component functions in the transport of electrons, by the reversible oxidation and reduction of its iron, whereas the a_3 component is capable of reacting with oxygen. Copper ions are also involved in the transfer of electrons from cytochrome a to a_3.

Cytochrome oxidase thus finally, transfers its electrons to oxygen, which in its negatively charged state combines with hydrogen ions that were released from $CoQ.H_2$ to form water.

SEQUENTIAL ARRANGEMENT OF VARIOUS COMPONENTS

Various components of the electron transport chain are arranged in the inner mitochondrial membrane and participate in a sequential manner, as follows:

Reducing equivalents are fed into the respiratory chain at the level of NAD or CoQ, from either NAD-linked dehydrogenase or flavin-linked dehydrogenase, and are transferred through the chain of cytochromes to molecular oxygen.

First three components of the electrons transport chain, i.e. NAD-linked dehydrogenase, flavin-linked dehydrogenase, and CoQ, are involved in the transfer of both, hydrogen and electrons.

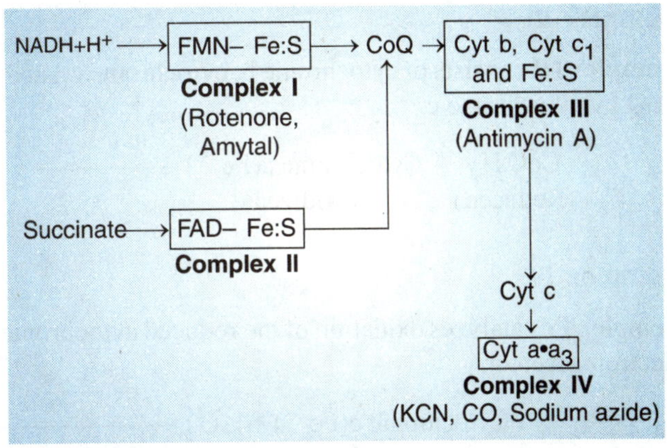

Fig. 11.4. Four complexes containing various components of the electron transport chain (inhibitors are shown in parenthesis).

Electron transfer reactions from NADH through CoQ involves the transport of two e^- whereas reactions between CoQ and O_2 involving various cytochromes, are one e^- transfer reactions.

Various components of the electron transport chain are located asymmetrically, in four complexes (Fig. 11.4).

These **four complexes** contain redox centers, with progressively greater affinity for electrons, i.e. with the increasing standard redox potentials.

Electrons travel through this chain, from lower to higher standard redox potentials, and are carried from complex II, to complex III by CoQ and from complex III to IV by cytochrome c.

Complex I

Initial reaction is catalyzed by NADH dehydrogenase complex [NADH dehydrogenase (FMN-Fe:S protein)], which is also designated as **Complex I.** It accepts protons and electrons from NADH+H^+ and transfers them to CoQ. Complex I thus, catalyze oxidation of NADH by the reduction of CoQ.

This is a largest protein complex found in the inner mitochondrial membrane. Complex I contains one molecule of FMN and 6-7 iron sulphur centers.

FMN and CoQ can transfer either one or two electrons at a time and provide electrons conduit between the two-electron donor (NADH) and the one-electron acceptor (cytochrome c).

As electrons are transferred between the redox centers of complex I, four protons are translocated from matrix to the inter-membrane space.

$$\text{NADH} + \text{H}^+ + \underset{\text{(Oxidized)}}{\text{CoQ}} \longrightarrow \text{NAD}^+ + \underset{\text{(Reduced)}}{\text{CoQ.H}_2}$$

Complex II

Complex II consists of succinate dehydrogenase-flavoprotein component [succinate dehydrogenase (FAD-Fe:S.protein)] which accepts reducing equivalents from succinate and reduces FAD to $FADH_2$.

$$\text{FADH}_2 + \underset{\text{(Oxidized)}}{\text{CoQ}} \longrightarrow \text{FAD} + \underset{\text{(Reduced)}}{\text{CoQ.H}_2}$$

CoQ thus, is a mobile component and facilitates transfer of electrons from both the complexes, i.e. from complex I as well as complex II, to complex III.

Complex III

Complex III consists of cytochrome b, cytochrome c_1, and Fe:S protein. It catalyzes oxidation of the reduced CoQ by cytochrome c.

$$\underset{\text{(Reduced)}}{CoQ.H_2} + \underset{\text{(Oxidized)}}{\text{Cytochrome } c(Fe^{3+})} \longrightarrow \underset{\text{(Oxidized)}}{CoQ} + \underset{\text{(Reduced)}}{\text{Cytochrome } c(Fe^{2+})}$$

Complex IV

Complex IV catalyzes oxidation of the reduced cytochrome c by molecular oxygen (1/2 O_2). It is the terminal electron acceptor.

$$\underset{\text{(Reduced)}}{\text{Cytochrome } c(Fe^{2+}) + \tfrac{1}{2}O_2} \longrightarrow \underset{\text{(Oxidized)}}{\text{Cytochrome } c(Fe^{3+}) + H_2O}$$

INHIBITORS OF ELECTRON TRANSPORT CHAIN

Inhibition of electron transport chain is assessed by the effect of some inhibitory compound on the consumption of O_2.

A variety of compounds inhibit electron transport chain specifically, at different points. These include **rotenone (a plant toxin), amytal, barbiturates, actinomycin A (an antibiotic), cyanide, azide, and carbon monoxide (CO).**

Rotenone and **amytal** inhibit oxygen consumption between NADH dehydrogenase and CoQ (complex I). They however, do not affect addition of succinate. Respiratory chain, in the presence of these inhibitors, does not oxidize reducing equivalents that are derived from NAD-linked dehydrogenase whereas those derived from flavin-linked dehydrogenase are freely oxidized (Fig. 11.4).

Inhibition of the mitochondrial electron transport chain results in impairment in energy generating function and may cause cell death.

OXIDATIVE PHOSPHORYLATION

The process of formation of ATP, from ADP and Pi, is termed as **phosphorylation.**

When phosphorylation is coupled with biological oxidation, this process is called as **oxidative phosphorylation.**

Oxidative phosphorylation thus, is a descriptive blend of the two processes, which are operating simultaneously, i.e. **the oxidation of a metabolite by oxygen via electron transport chain coupled with the phosphorylation of ADP and Pi.**

During the transfer of electrons from NADH-NAD^+ redox couple (E_o' = -0.32 volt) to molecular oxygen (E_o' = +0.82 volt), oxidation-reduction potential is decreased by 1.14 volts. Within this sequential process, there are three different sites, with a decrease of at least 0.3-volt at each site, which is required for the phosphorylation of ADP. This, in turn, suggests that each molecule of NADH reoxidized to NAD^+ by oxygen, via electron transport chain, generates 3 ATP.

Number of ATP produced by oxidative phosphorylation is less if a dehydrogenase reaction uses FAD rather than NAD^+ as a co-substrate. This is because CoQ accepts hydrogen, directly from $FADH_2$, bypassing the NAD^+-FMN phosphorylation site. FAD utilizing reactions therefore generate only 2 ATP.

P/O RATIO

P/O ratio is the ratio of the number of moles of ATP generated to the number of moles of oxygen reduced in the electron transport chain. It is used to express efficiency of oxidative phosphorylation of the system. There are 3 sites of generation of ATP in the electron transport chain, i.e. one molecule of ATP is produced between NAD and flavoprotein. The second phosphorylating site exists between cytochrome b and cytochrome c_1 while the third molecule of ATP is generated between cytochrome c and cytochrome oxidase (cytochrome $a.a_3$)

Thus, P/O ratio is 3 if reducing equivalents enter the electron transport chain through NAD. On the other hand, P/O ratio is 2 for FAD requiring reactions.

MECHANISM OF OXIDATIVE PHOSPHORYLATION

Most acceptable mechanism for coupling the synthesis of ATP to the electron transport chain is called **chemi-osmotic process.**

According to this theory, protons are transported across the mitochondrial membrane, into the spaces between the inner and the outer membrane. This in turn creates H^+ gradient across the membrane and each pair of electrons (originating in NADH), results in the outward flow of six protons.

In the first step, two electrons and a proton from NADH, in addition to one proton from the aqueous matrix, are added to FMN (of the NADH dehydrogenase) thereby reducing the prosthetic group (FMN to $FMNH_2$). Two electrons from $FMNH_2$ are then accepted by the iron-sulphur centers, which cycle these electrons back across the membrane, to the interior. Simultaneously, $2H^+$ are released into the inter-membrane space. Two electrons from Fe:S centers are then transferred to CoQ, accompanied by $2H^+$, which are derived from the aqueous matrix. Reduced CoQ then translocates $2H^+$ to the exterior. Thus, two electrons are donated to cytochrome b and protons are released into the medium. Electrons from cytochrome b are returned to the inner surface, where together with $2H^+$ from the matrix, they again join CoQ. Once third pair of the H^+ has been released, electrons are donated to cytochrome c_1 and then to cytochrome c on the outer membrane surface. These electrons are finally accepted by cytochrome a, and cross the membrane.

On the matrix side, electrons are transferred by cytochrome a_3 to an atom of oxygen and with the acquisition of two protons; a molecule of water is formed.

This cyclic process involves flow of electric current in the membrane and establishes a gradient of H^+, as a result of which pH is reduced, outside the matrix. Once the gradient is established, the H^+ flow spontaneously, back across the membrane, in a downhill fashion.

Protons transverse the membrane at the site, which is designated as F_0 protein of the F_1-F_0 complex. Two protons enter F_0 protein, which provides ion channel through the lipid bilayer into the headpiece, i.e. F_1. Near the proton channel, F_1 has binding sites for inorganic phosphate. The energy of proton gradient and also the membrane potential promotes a reaction of two protons with oxygen of the phosphate. As a result of this, water is eliminated and the highly reactive Pi joins ADP, to form ATP (Fig. 11.5).

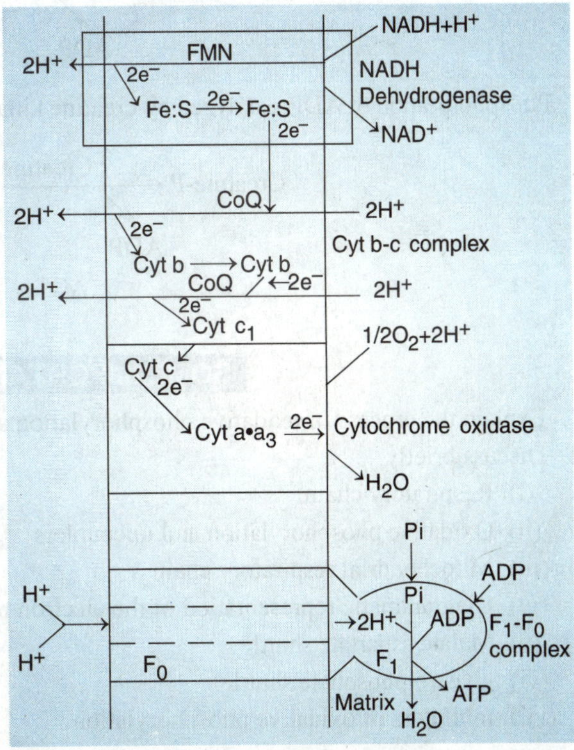

Fig. 11.5. Mechanism of oxidative phosphorylation.

INHIBITORS/UNCOUPLERS OF OXIDATIVE PHOSPHORYLATION

Uncouplers and inhibitors of the electron transport with the process of oxidative phosphorylation inhibit ATP synthesis.

Oligomycin is an **inhibitor of oxidative phosphorylation**. It suppresses the consumption of oxygen and affects the process of phosphorylation.

On the other hand, **2,4-dinitrophenol** is an **uncoupler,** as it uncouples the process of electron transport chain to the process of oxidative phosphorylation. It thus, results in the accumulation of ADP. Energy, which is normally conserved as ATP, is lost as heat. In this situation, though electron transport may continue but it is without the generation of ATP.

SUBSTRATE-LEVEL PHOSPHORYLATION

ATP is also synthesized in the cytosol, in some of the step of a metabolic pathway.

This process transfers a phosphate group from a high-energy phosphate donor to ADP, and is called **substrate-level phosphorylation,** e.g. the reactions of the glycolysis, which are catalyzed by phosphoglycerokinase and pyruvate kinase.

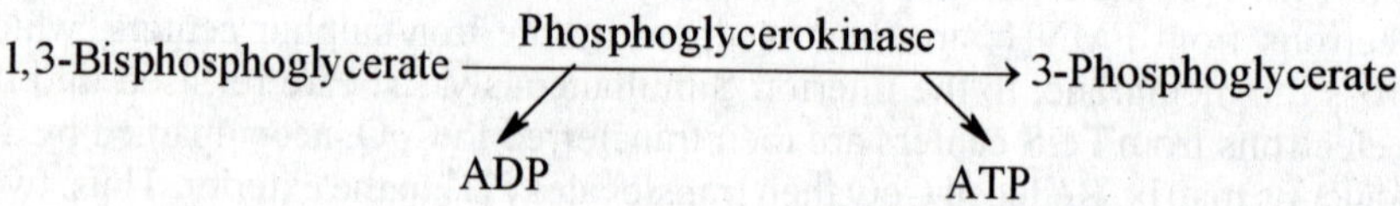

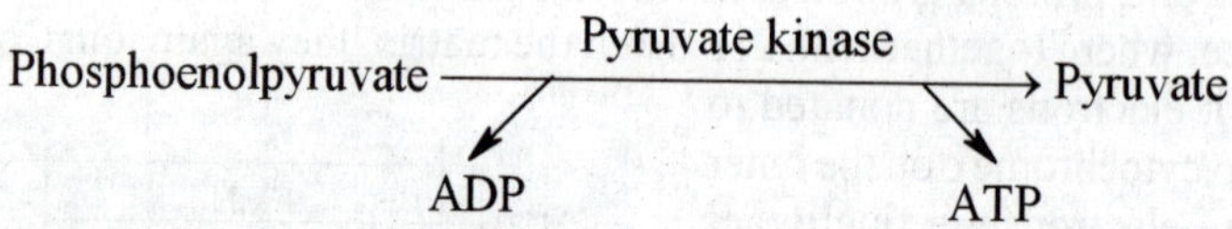

Phosphorylation of ADP, catalyzed by creatine kinase is an important mode of ATP formation in muscle.

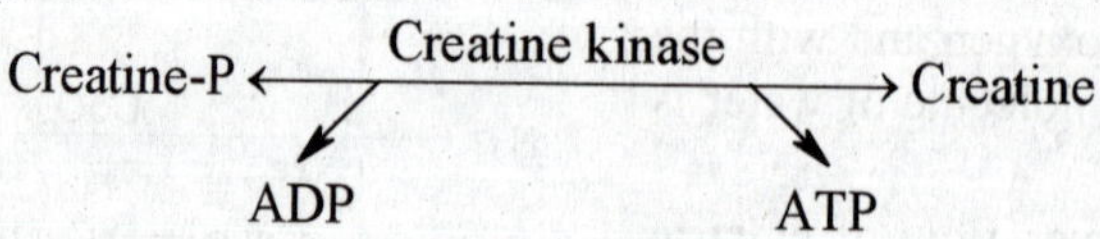

$\Delta G^o = -3Kcal$

SOME IMPORTANT QUESTIONS

1. Explain the process of oxidative phosphorylation and its inhibitors.
2. Discuss briefly:
   (i) Respiratory chain
   (ii) Oxidative phosphorylation and uncouplers
   (iii) Mitochondrial respiratory chain
   (iv) Diagrammatic representation of the electron transport chain
   (v) Malate aspartate shuttle
   (vi) glycerolphosphate shuttle
   (vii) Inhibitors of oxidative phosphorylation

3. Write notes on :
   (i) Respiratory chain
   (ii) Oxidative phosphorylation
   (iii) Substrate level phosphorylation
   (iv) Reducing equivalents
   (v) Iron-sulphur centers
   (vi) Cytochromes
   (vii) P/O ratio

CHAPTER

12

Metabolism of Carbohydrates

METABOLISM OF GLUCOSE

Glucose is the major **monosaccharide,** which enters the **liver**. Thereafter, it is both, converted to glycogen and **stored in the liver and muscle** as well as is **oxidized** in the liver to **produce energy** (Fig. 12.1).

Various metabolic **pathways**, which **utilize glucose, include glycolysis, glycogenesis and pentose phosphate pathway.**

On the other hand, **gluconeogenesis** and **glycogenolysis** are the **pathways,** which generate **glucose.**

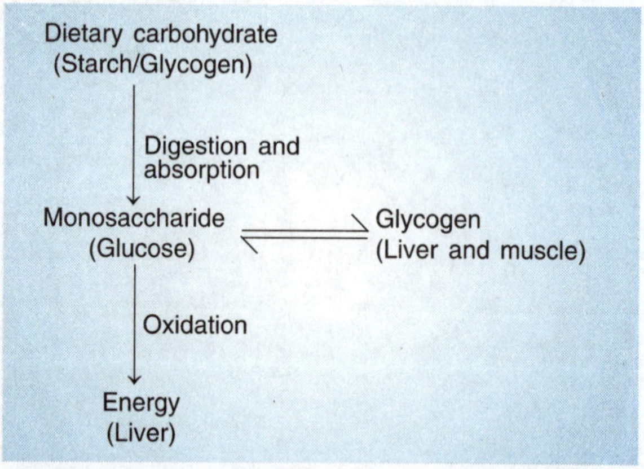

Fig. 12.1. Metabolic fates of glucose.

GLYCOLYSIS

Glycolysis is also called as the **Embden-Meyerhof Parnas pathway** or **the Embden-Meyerhof Pathway.** It is a process of **catabolism** of **glucose** either in the presence of oxygen, such as in the liver (aerobic glycolysis), or lack of oxygen, such as in skeletal muscle (anaerobic glycolysis).

Glycolytic enzymes are present in the extra-mitochondrial compartment of the cell. Although aerobic glycolysis occurs in most of the tissues like liver, kidney and erythrocytes, anaerobic glycolysis occurs only in muscle (Fig. 12.2).

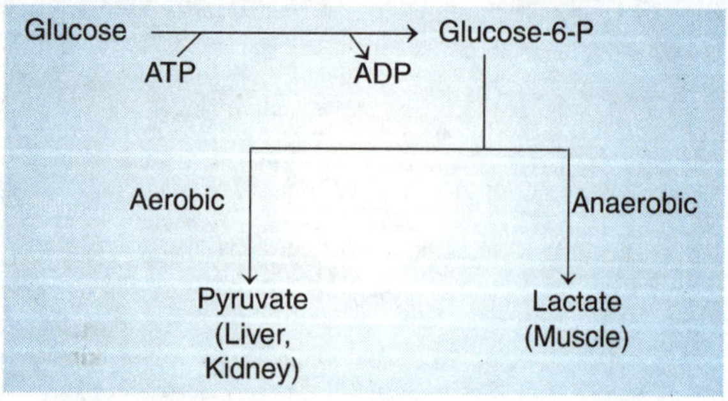

Fig. 12.2. Aerobic and anaerobic glycolysis.

Various reactions of the glycolytic pathway are shown in Fig. 12.3

1. **Activation of Glucose : Glucose** is activated, irreversibly, to **glucose-6-phosphate** by **glucokinase** or **hexokinase**, in the presence of ATP and Mg^{2+} (Fig. 12.4)

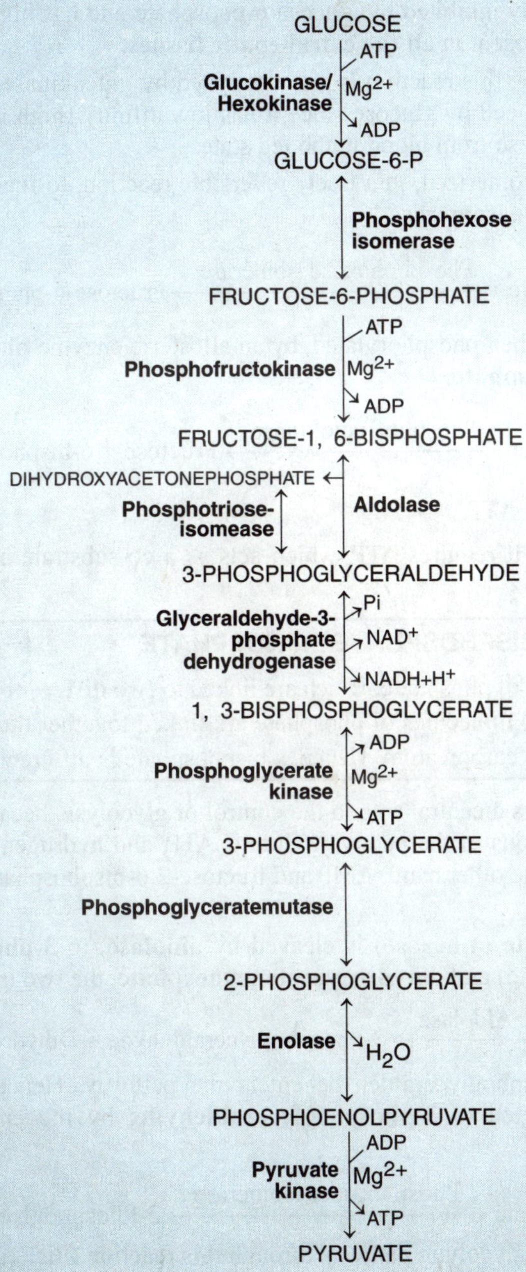

Fig. 12.3. Reactions of the glycolysis.

$$\text{Glucose} \xrightarrow[\text{ATP} \quad \text{Mg}^{2+} \quad \text{ADP}]{\text{Hexokinase/Glucokinase}} \text{Glucose-6-phosphate}$$

Fig. 12.4. Activation of glucose.

Hexokinase is allosterically inhibited by glucose-6-phosphate and has high affinity (low K_m) for glucose. This enzyme is present in **all the extrahepatic tissues.**

In the liver, in the fed state, this reaction is also catalyzed by glucokinase, which is an inducible enzyme. Its activity is induced by glucose since it has low affinity (high K_m) for glucose and its function is to remove glucose from blood in the fed state.

2. **Glucose-6-phosphate** is isomerized, in a freely reversible reaction, to **fructose-6-phosphate,** by the enzyme **phosphohexose isomerase.**

$$\text{Glucose-6-phosphate} \xleftrightarrow{\text{Phosphohexose isomerase}} \text{Fructose-6-phosphate}$$

3. **Fructose-6-phosphate** is then phosphorylated, by an allosteric enzyme **phosphofructokinase**, to form **fructose-1, 6-bisphosphate.**

$$\text{Fructose-6-phosphate} \xrightarrow[\text{ATP} \quad \text{Mg}^{2+} \quad \text{ADP}]{\text{Phosphofructokinase}} \text{Fructose-1,6-bisphosphate}$$

This is an irreversible reaction. It requires ATP, which acts as a co-substrate as well as an allosteric inhibitor of the enzyme.

> **BISPHOSPHATE/BIPHOSPHATE**
>
> A **bisphosphate** has two molecules of phosphate, which are linked to **two different carbon atoms,** while in a biphosphate (diphosphate) two molecules of phosphate are linked together through each other by a phosphodiester linkage to the same carbon atom. Hence, a bisphosphate is different from a biphosphate.

Phosphofructokinase plays a central role in the control of glycolysis because it catalyzes one of the rate determining reactions of the pathway. Citrate, ATP, and hydrogen ions (low pH) inhibit phosphofructokinase. On the other hand, AMP and fructose-2,6-bisphosphate are activators of this enzyme

4. **Fructose-1, 6-bisphosphate** (a hexose) is cleaved by **aldolase,** to **3-phosphoglyceraldehyde** (glyceraldehyde-3-phosphate) and **dihydroxyacetonephosphate**, the two trioses.

$$\text{Fructose-1, 6-biphosphate} \xleftrightarrow{\text{Aldolase}} \text{3-Phosphoglyceraldehyde + Dihydroxyacetone phosphate}$$

5. Subsequently, only 3-phosphoglyceraldehyde enters the pathway. Hence, **dihydroxyacetone-phosphate** is also converted to **3-phosphoglyceraldehyde,** by the enzyme **phosphotriose isomerase.**

$$\text{Dihydroxyacetonephosphate} \xleftrightarrow{\text{Phosphotriose isomerase}} \text{3-Phosphoglyceraldehyde}$$

Glycerol can also enter the glycolytic pathway through this reaction (Fig. 12.19).

6. In the presence of NAD^+ and inorganic phosphate (Pi), **glyceraldehyde-3-phosphate dehydrogenase** oxidizes 3-phosphoglyceraldehyde to **1, 3-bisphosphoglycerate**.

3-Phosphoglyceraldehyde ⟷ 1,3-Bisphosphoglycerate (Glyceraldehyde–3–phosphate dehydrogenase; with Pi, NAD^+ → $NADH + H^+$)

7. In the next step, **1, 3-bisphosphoglycerate** is converted to **3-phosphoglycerate**. This reaction is catalyzed by the enzyme **phosphoglycerate kinase**.

1,3-Bisphosphoglycerate ⟷ 3-Phosphoglycerate (Phosphoglycerate kinase; ADP → ATP, Mg^{2+})

In this reaction, there is production of ATP. It is called **substrate level production of ATP** (i.e. substrate level phosphorylation).

Arsenic acid inhibits phosphorylation at this step and thus, ATP production.

RAPAPORT-LUEBERING CYCLE

In erythrocytes, conversion of 1, 3-bisphosphoglycerate to 3-phosphoglycerate, by phosphoglycerate kinase, is bye-passed. Instead, 1, 3-bisphosphoglycerate is converted to 2, 3-bisphosphoglycerate (2, 3-BPG), which is subsequently converted to 3-phosphoglycerate. This results in loss of high-energy phosphate bond and there is no production of ATP. This is called Rapaport-Luebering cycle (Fig. 12.5)

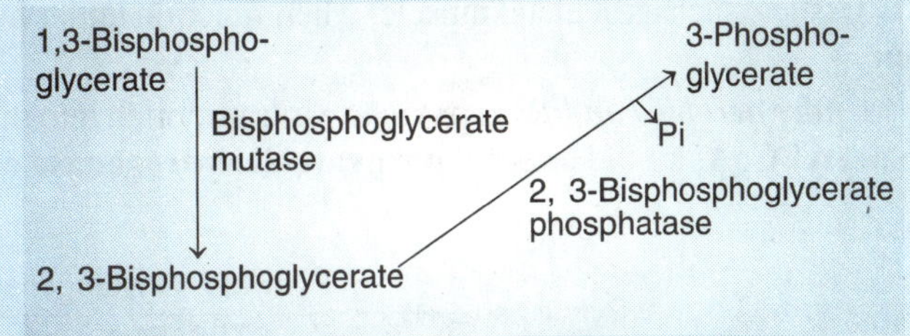

Fig. 12.5. Rapaport-Luebering cycle.

8. Thereafter, **3-phosphoglycerate** is converted to **2-phosphoglycerate,** by the enzyme phosphoglycerate mutase.

3-Phosphoglycerate ⟷ 2-Phosphoglycerate (Phosphoglycerate mutase; 2,3–BPG)

2,3-Bisphosphoglycerate (2,3-BPG) acts as coenzyme for this reaction.

9. **Enolase** converts **2-phosphoglycerate** to a high-energy compound, called **phosphoenolpyruvate.**

2-Phosphoglycerate ⟷ Phosphoenolpyruvate (Enolase; Mg^{2+} or Mn^{2+}; → H_2O)

Enolase requires Mg^{2+} or Mn^{2+} for its activity but is inhibited by fluoride. Since **fluoride** inhibits this reaction, therefore, fluoride is added to the blood, as a preservative, which is collected for glucose estimation.

10. Subsequently, **phosphoenolpyruvate** is converted to **pyruvate,** irreversibly. This reaction is catalyzed by the enzyme pyruvate kinase. It also phosphorylates ADP to ATP.

Phosphoenolpyruvate → Pyruvate (Pyruvate kinase; ADP → ATP, Mg^{2+})

Deficiency of pyruvate kinase leads to hemolytic anemia.

Regulation of glycolysis

There are three irreversible steps, which are catalyzed by hexokinase, phosphofructokinase, and pyruvate kinase. These are the sites of the regulation of glycolysis.

Insulin stimulates these enzymes and increases utilization of glucose by glycolysis. On the other hand, **glucagon inhibits** this process.

PYRUVATE OXIDATION

Under anaerobic conditions **pyruvate** is reduced to **lactate**. This reaction is catalyzed by the enzyme **lactate dehydrogenase**, which requires NADH + H^+.

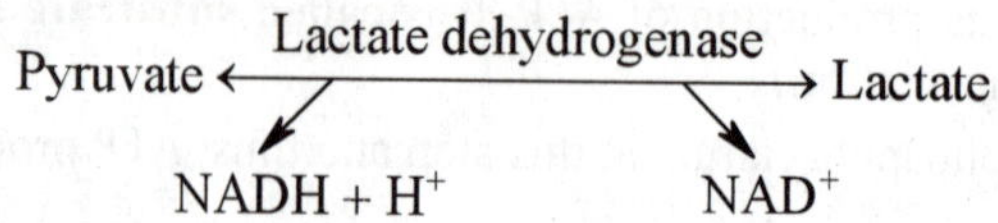

Tissues, such as skeletal muscle, when function under hypoxic conditions, produce large amount of lactic acid.

Under aerobic conditions **pyruvate** is transported into mitochondria where it is oxidatively decarboxylated to **acetyl CoA**, by the enzyme **pyruvate dehydrogenase complex** (Fig. 12.6).

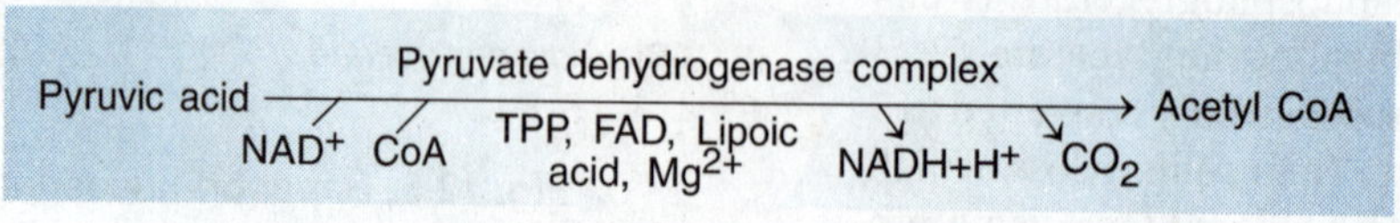

Fig. 12.6. Fate of pyruvate under aerobic conditions.

Pyruvate dehydrogenase complex requires five coenzymes, i.e. **TPP, CoA, NAD$^+$, FAD,** and **lipoic acid**. Insulin stimulates its activity whereas it is inhibited by acetyl CoA, NADH, and increased ATP/ADP ratio.

This enzyme is also inhibited by arsenate and mercuric ions, as well as by dietary deficiency of thiamin. Inhibition of the enzyme results in accumulation of pyruvate and lactate, resulting in **lactic acidosis.** This in turn may manifest several neurological disturbances.

ENERGY PRODUCTION DURING GLYCOLYSIS

Number of ATP produced during glycolysis varies, depending upon the conditions of the reaction.

Under Anaerobic Conditions

Since each of the energy-yielding steps, i.e. conversion of 1,3-bisphophoglycerate to 3-phosphoglycerate and phosphoenolpyruvate to pyruvate, produce one ATP, **total** 2 ATP are produced per molecule of triose or **4** molecules of **ATP per** molecule of **hexose** (Fig. 12.7).

As 2 ATP are used in the initial two reactions of the process, i.e. conversion of glucose to glucose 6-phosphate and fructose-6-phosphate to fructose-1,6-bisphosphate, **net energy yield** per molecule of glucose is **2 ATP**.

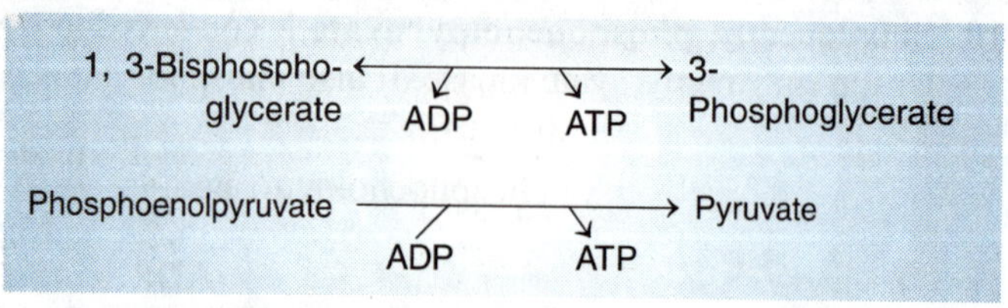

Fig. 12.7. Energy-yielding steps in glycolysis.

Under Aerobic Conditions

Under aerobic conditions, NADH, produced during the conversion of 3-phosphoglycerte to 1,3-bisphosphoglycerate, enters electron transport chain and releases 3 ATP. Thus, additionally, 6 ATP are produced per molecule of glucose. Total yield under aerobic conditions therefore, is 10 ATP while the **net yield** is **8 ATP**.

CITRIC ACID CYCLE

Citric acid cycle is also called as the **tricarboxylic acid cycle** or the **Krebs cycle.** It is a process of **oxidation of acetyl CoA** (active acetate) to **CO_2** and **H_2O**.

During the course of the oxidation of acetyl CoA, reducing equivalents are produced, which enter respiratory chain and generate large amount of ATP.

Reactions of the Krebs cycle are shown in Fig. 12.8.

1. In the first step, **acetyl CoA** (formed from pyruvate under aerobic conditions) combines with **oxaloacetate** and forms citric acid (a tricarboxylic acid).

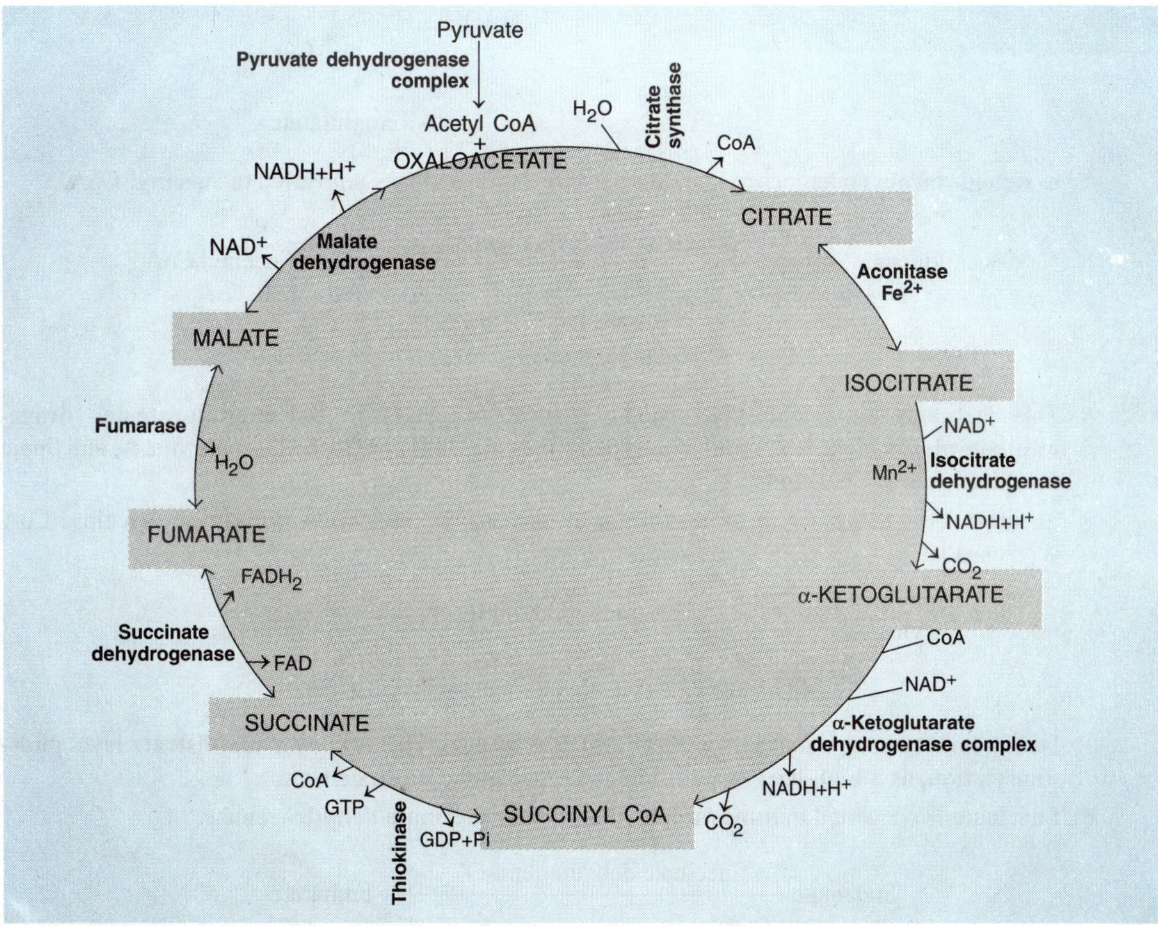

Fig. 12.8. Tricarboxylic acid cycle.

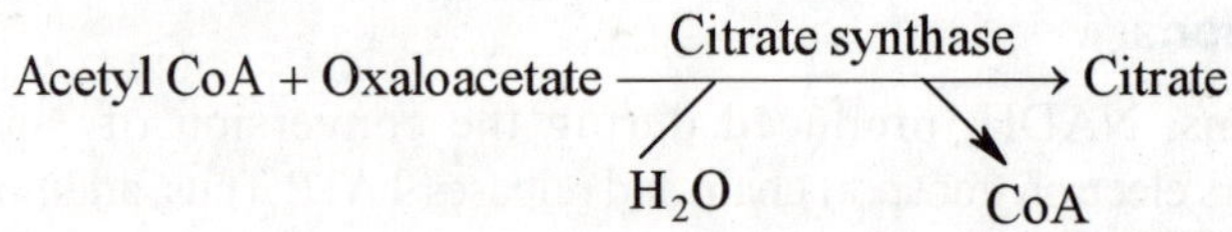

This reaction is catalyzed by the enzyme **citrate synthase,** also called as the **condensing enzyme.**

2. **Citrate** is then rearranged to **cis-aconitate**, which is subsequently changed to isocitrate. Both of these steps are catalyzed by **aconitase**.

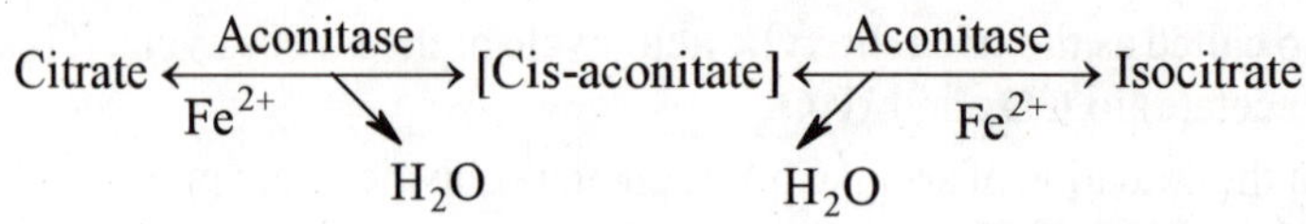

3. In the presence of **isocitrate dehydrogenase, isocitrate** is converted to oxalosuccinate, which is subsequently decarboxylated to **α-ketoglutarate**.

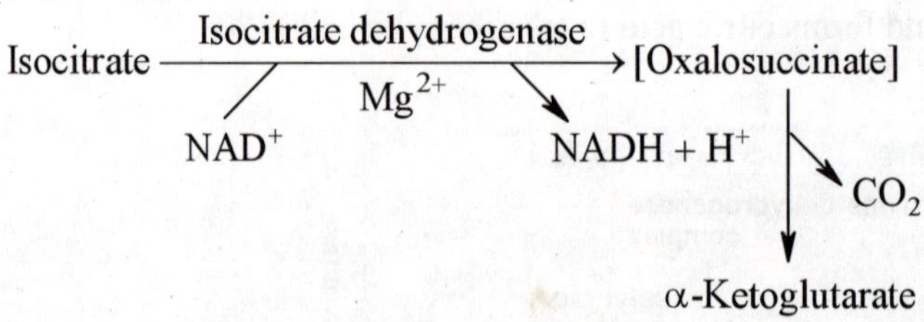

4. **α-Ketoglutarate** undergoes oxidative decarboxylation and gets converted to **succinyl CoA.**

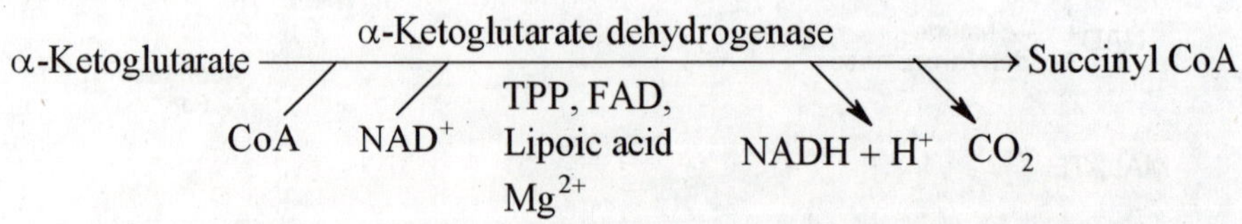

This reaction is similar to the conversion of pyruvate to acetyl CoA. **α-Ketoglutarate dehydrogenase complex,** which also requires five coenzymes, i.e. TPP, NAD^+, FAD, coenzyme A, and lipoic acid, catalyzes this reaction.

5. **Succinyl CoA** is converted to **succinate,** by the enzyme **succinate thiokinase** (succinyl CoA synthetase).

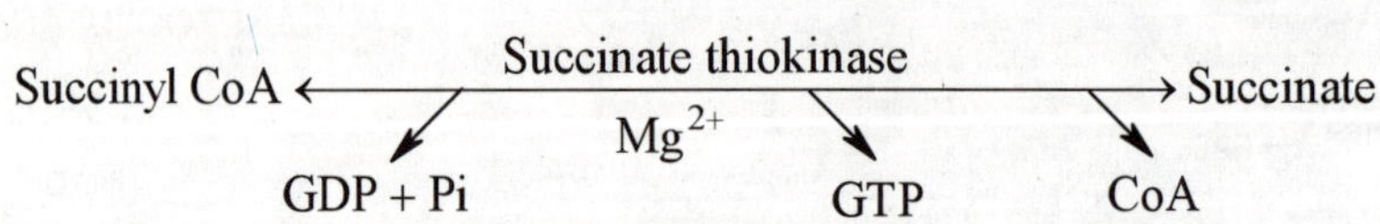

During this reaction, a molecule of GTP (ATP) is formed. This is known as **substrate level phosphorylation, as a high-energy** molecule is formed at the substrate level.

6. **Succinate** is converted to **fumarate,** by the enzyme **succinate dehydrogenase.**

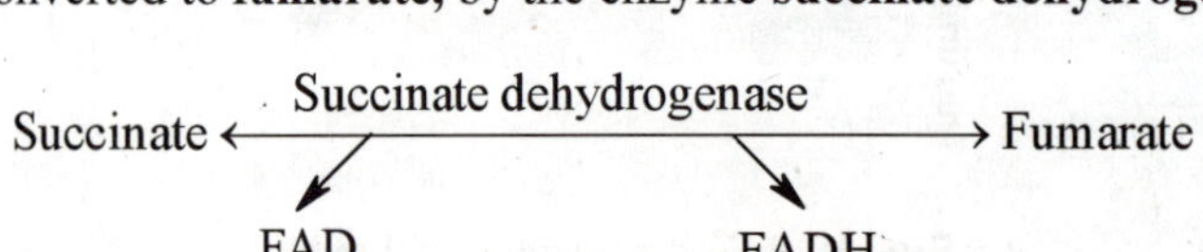

Due to structural similarities between malonate and succinate, **malonate inhibits** succinate dehydrogenase, **competitively.**

7. With the addition of a molecule of water, by the enzyme **fumarase** (fumarate hydratase), **fumarate** is converted to **L-malate**.

$$\text{Fumarate} \xleftrightarrow[\text{H}_2\text{O}]{\text{Fumarase}} \text{L – Malate}$$

8. Finally, **malate dehydrogenase,** in the presence of NAD^+, converts **malate** to **oxaloacetate.**

$$\text{L – Malate} \xleftrightarrow[\text{NAD}^+ \quad\quad \text{NADH + H}^+]{\text{Malate dehydrogenase}} \text{Oxaloacetate}$$

ENERGY PRODUCTION DURING CITRIC ACID CYCLE

As a result of oxidation of one molecule of acetyl CoA in the Krebs cycle, three molecules of NAD^+ and one molecule of FAD are reduced.

Reducing equivalents from NADH + H^+ enter respiratory chain and result in the production of three molecules of ATP. Similarly, $FADH_2$ yields 2 ATP. Besides, there is also substrate level production of GTP.

Thus, **total ATP yield**, per molecule of acetyl CoA, is **12 ATP** (Table 12.1).

Table 12.1. Energy production from citric acid cycle

Reaction	*Reducing equivalents produced as*	*Number of ATP produced*
Isocitrate ⟶ α-Ketoglutarate	NADH + H^+	3
α-Ketoglutarate ⟶ Succinyl CoA	NADH + H^+	3
Succinyl CoA ⟶ Succinate	—	1
Succinate ⟶ Fumarate	$FADH_2$	2
Malate ⟶ Oxaloacetate	NADH + H^+	3
	Total	**12**

As mentioned above, conversion of pyruvate to acetyl CoA also generates NADH + H^+ and gives 3 ATP. Thus, total number of ATP produced, from oxidation of pyruvate, is 15.

Since 2 molecules of pyruvate are formed from one molecule of glucose, therefore, in addition to energy yield during aerobic glycolysis (8 ATP) a molecule of glucose produces 30 ATP via the Krebs cycle. Thus, a total of 38 ATP are obtained when a molecule of glucose is completely oxidized to CO_2 and H_2O under aerobic conditions, i.e. via glycolysis and Krebs cycle.

ROLE OF VITAMINS IN KREBS CYCLE

Five vitamins of the B complex group, i.e. **vitamin B_1** (as thiamine pyrophosphate or TPP), **vitamin B_2** (as FAD), **niacin** (as NAD), **lipoic acid,** and **pantothenic acid** (a constituent of the coenzyme A), play important role in citric acid cycle.

BIOLOGICAL SIGNIFICANCE OF KREBS CYCLE

Citric acid cycle has a **dual role**, i.e. it is important in oxidation as well as synthetic processes. It is thus **amphibolic** in nature.

It is **catabolic** for the oxidation of carbohydrates, lipids, and proteins, as they are completely oxidized to CO_2 and H_2O, and release energy.

It is also important in the **anabolic** reactions, as various intermediates of the cycle can be used for the biosynthesis of the nonessential amino acids. Various intermediates of the cycle are also potentially glucogenic and thus, can give rise to glucose in liver and kidney (Fig 12.9).

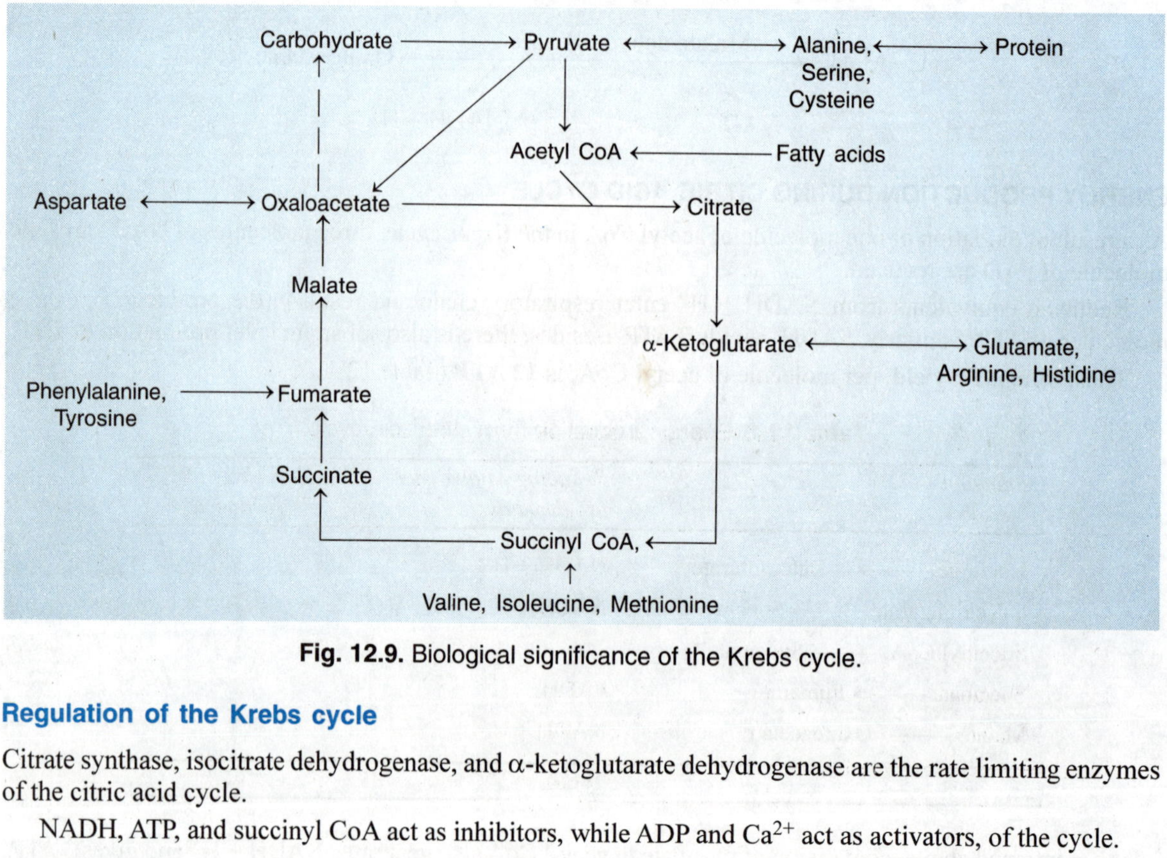

Fig. 12.9. Biological significance of the Krebs cycle.

Regulation of the Krebs cycle

Citrate synthase, isocitrate dehydrogenase, and α-ketoglutarate dehydrogenase are the rate limiting enzymes of the citric acid cycle.

NADH, ATP, and succinyl CoA act as inhibitors, while ADP and Ca^{2+} act as activators, of the cycle.

GLYCOGENESIS

Glycogenesis (glycogen synthesis) is the process of the **conversion of glucose to glycogen**. Although, it is operative in several tissues, liver and muscle are the main organs for the synthesis of glycogen. Glycogenesis is stimulated by insulin.

Various reactions of glycogenesis are shown in Fig. 12.10.

1. **Glucose** is first activated (phosphorylated) to **glucose-6-phosphate.**

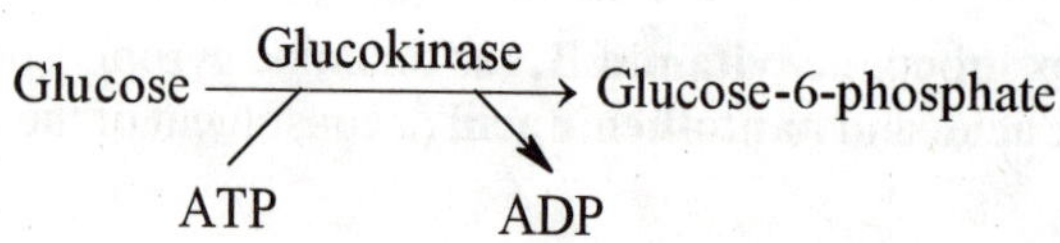

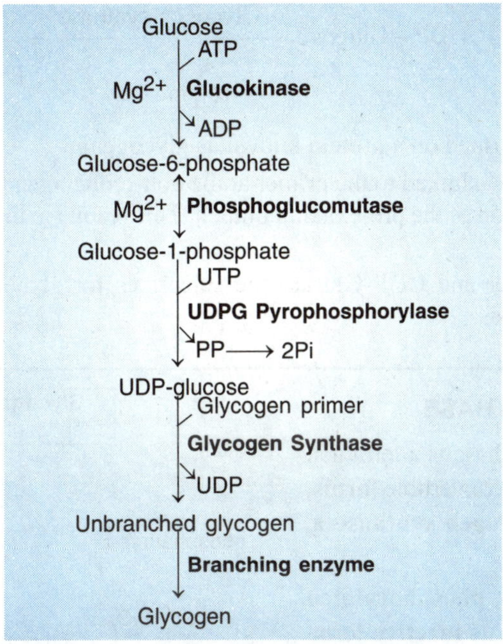

Fig. 12.10. Glycogenesis.

In the liver, **glucokinase** converts most of the glucose into glucose-6-phosphate, in the fed state. This is an inducible enzyme and has greater specificity for its substrate.

In the muscle and other tissues, this reaction is catalyzed by **hexokinase.**

2. **Glucose-6-phosphate** is epimerised to form **glucose-1-phosphate**, by the enzyme **phosphogluco-mutase.**

$$\text{Glucose-6-phosphate} \xleftrightarrow{\text{Phosphoglucomutase}} \text{Glucose-1-phosphate}$$

3. **Glucose-1-phosphate** reacts with UTP and gets converted to **uridinediphosphate glucose** (UDP-Glu). The reaction is catalyzed by **UDPG pyrophosphorylase** (glucose-1-phosphate uridyltransferase).

   Pyrophosphate, so released during this process, is immediately hydrolyzed to two molecules of **inorganic phosphate,** by **pyrophosphatase** (Fig. 12.11).

4. From **UDP-Glu**, glucose is transferred to the **glycogen primer** (i.e. the preformed oligosaccharide). This reaction is catalyzed by the enzyme **glycogen synthase**.

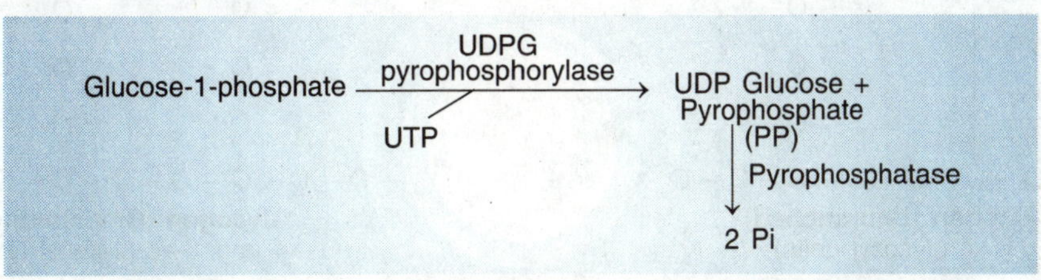

Fig. 12.11. Conversion of glucose-1-phosphate to UDP glucose.

$$\underset{\text{Glycogen primer}}{(\text{Glucose})_n} + \text{UDP} - \text{Glucose} \xrightarrow[\searrow \text{UDP}]{\text{Glycogen synthase}} \underset{\text{Unbranched glycogen}}{(\text{Glucose})_{n+1}}$$

Glycogen primer is formed on a protein known as glycogenin.

The incoming glucose is linked to the primer at the non-reducing end, by 1, 4-α-glycosidic linkage and results in elongation of the pre-existing branch. This results in the formation of an **unbranched glycogen**.

Both, glycogen primer and UDP-Glu are the substrates for glycogen synthase, which is a key enzyme of glycogenesis.

GLYCOGEN SYNTHASE

Human muscle glycogen synthase is a tetramer. It has **two**, enzymatically, interconvertible **forms**, which are referred to as **glycogen synthase a,** and **glycogen synthase b.**

Glycogen synthase b is the **phosphorylated** form of the enzyme, which is its **inactive** form. On the other hand, **glycogen synthase a** is the **dephosphorylated** enzyme that is biologically **active** (Fig. 12.12).

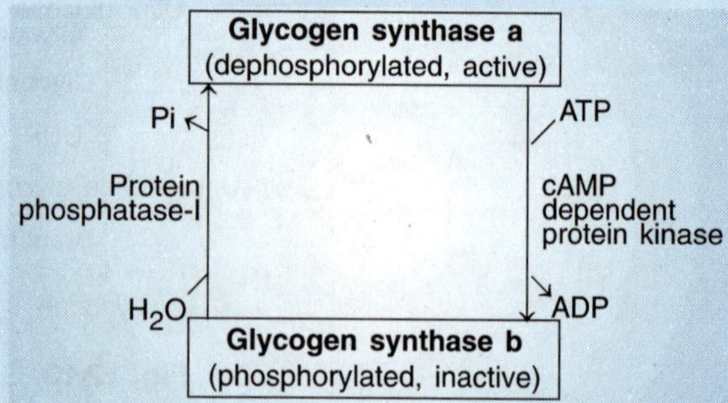

Fig. 12.12. Activation and inactivation of glycogen synthase.

5. Once the straight chain containing nearly11 glucose residues is formed, **branching enzyme** removes a block of 7-8 glycosyl-residues from the growing chain and transfers it to the neighboring chain (Fig. 12.13).

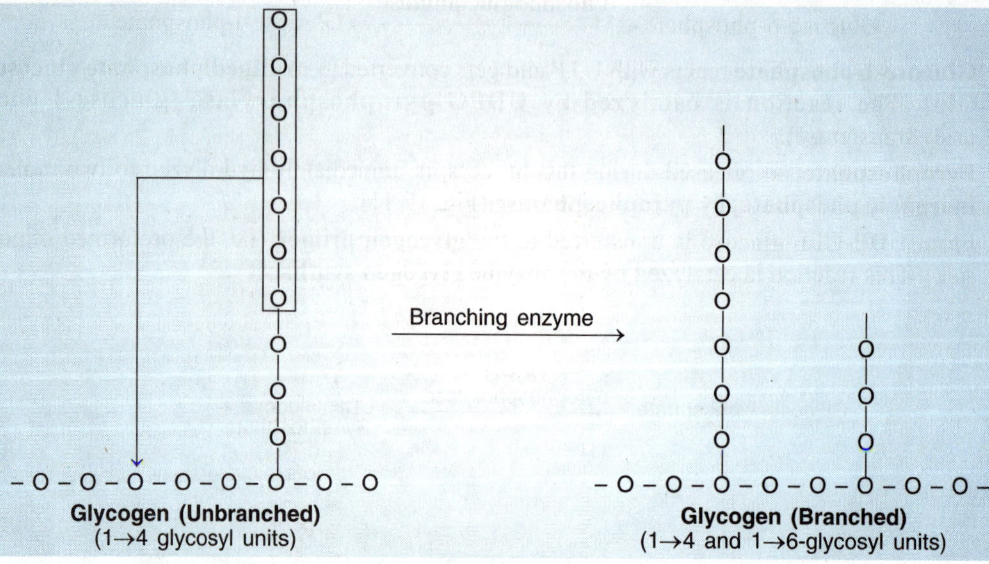

Fig. 12.13. Branching of glycogen.

This branch point again grows with the addition of the glucose molecules at the 1→4 linkage. This in turn results in the formation of a highly branched glycogen structure.

GLYCOGENOLYSIS

Glycogenolysis is the process of the breakdown of **glycogen** to either **glucose-6-phosphate** in muscle or **free glucose** in **liver** and kidney (Fig 12.14).

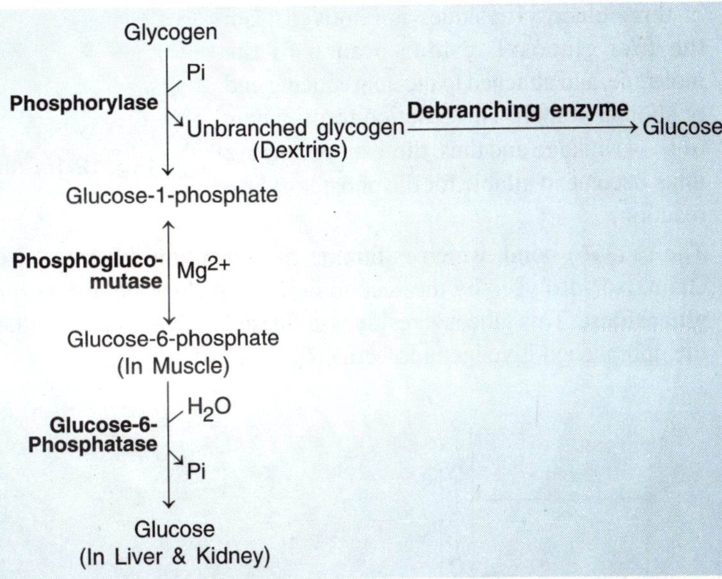

Fig. 12.14. Glycogenolysis.

1. In the first step, glucose molecules are sequentially removed from **glycogen** as **glucose-1-phosphate**. This reaction is catalyzed by the enzyme **phosphorylase**. It is the rate-limiting step of this pathway.

$$\underset{\textbf{Glycogen}}{(\text{Glucose})_n} \xrightarrow[\text{Pi}]{} (\text{Glucose})_{n-1} + \text{Glucose}-1-\text{phosphate}$$

   Phosphorylase hydrolyzes the α-1,4-glycosidic bonds and removes glucose units, as glucose-1-phosphate, until nearly four glucose residues are left. After the action of phosphorylase, **glycogen** is partially hydrolyzed, leaving **limit dextrin**.

PHOSPHORYLASE

Phosphorylase is a dimmer and has two identical subunits. Allosteric interaction as well as covalent modification (phosphorylation and dephosphorylation) regulates it.

Phosphorylated form of this enzyme is called **phosphorylase a**, which is its **active** form. The **dephosphorylated** form of the enzyme is called **phosphorylase b**. It is **inactive** form of the enzyme.

Two forms of the enzyme are interconvertible by **phosphorylase kinase** and **phosphoprotein phosphatase** (Fig. 12.15).

2. Limit dextrin is further hydrolyzed by the debranching enzyme to glucose-1-phosphate and free glucose.

   Debranching enzyme is a bifunctional enzyme. Its first unit has **glycosyltransferase,** i.e. 1→4 α D-glucantransferase [α-(1→4) transglycosylase], **activity** in which a strand of three glucosyl residues is removed from the four glucosyl residue branch of the molecule, and attached to the nonreducing end of another branch. This reaction forms a new α(1→4) linkage and thus, three more glucose units become available for the phosphorylase reaction.

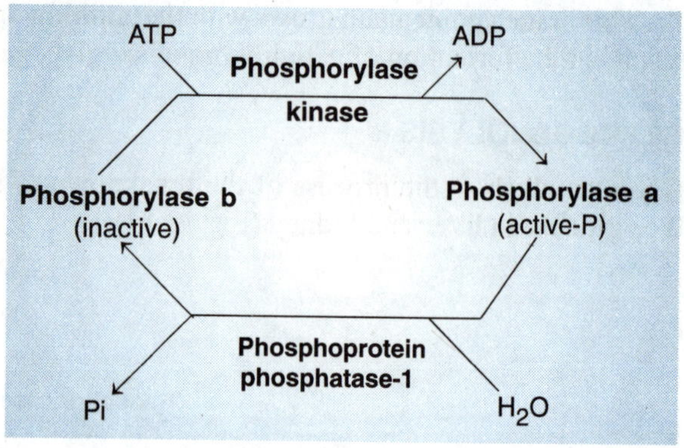

Fig. 12.15. Activation/inactivation of phosphorylase.

The α(1→6) bond, which is linking the remaining glucosyl residue on the branch point to the main chain, is hydrolyzed by the second unit of the debranching enzyme that is referred to as **amylo-α-1,6-glucosidase**. This glucosyl residue is released as free glucose, rather than as glucose-1-phosphate, leaving the unbranched glycogen molecule (Fig. 12.16).

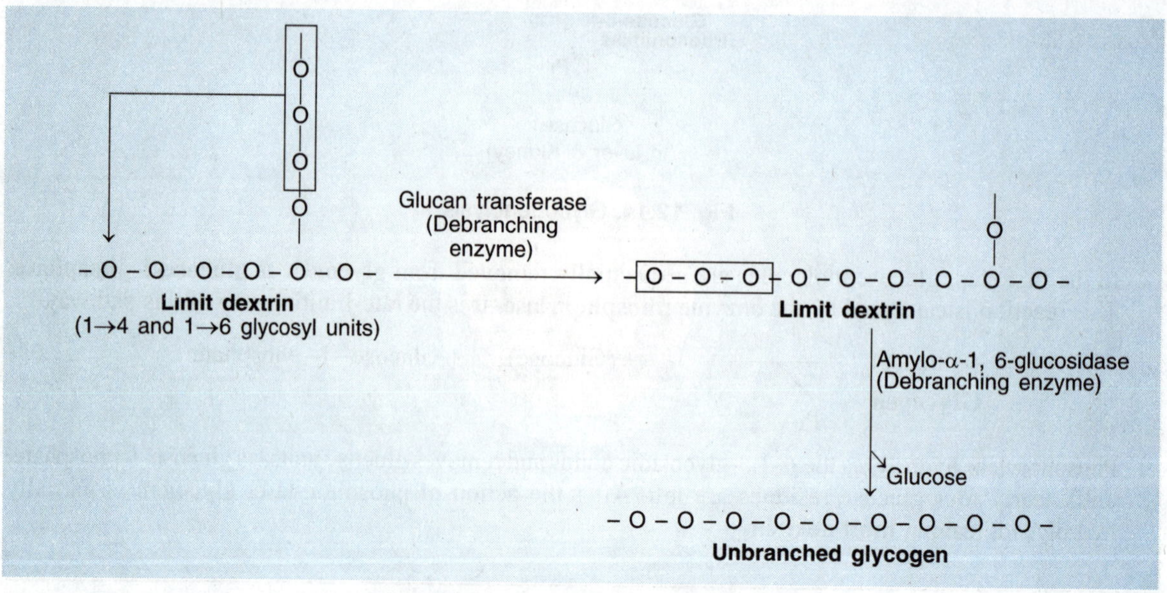

Fig. 12.16. Debranching of glycogen.

Cooperative and repetitive actions of phosphorylase and debranching enzyme result in complete hydrolysis of glycogen.

During glycogenolysis, glucose-1-phosphate and glucose are liberated in the ratio of approximately 10:1.

3. **Glucose-1-phosphate**, produced as a result of the action of phosphorylase, is converted to **glucose-6-phosphate** by the enzyme **phosphoglucomutase**.

$$\text{Glucose-1-phosphate} \xleftrightarrow[\text{Mg}^{2+}]{\text{Phosphoglucomutase}} \text{Glucose-6-phosphate}$$

In the muscle, glucose-6-phosphate is the end product of glycogen breakdown and is used in the glycolytic pathway to liberate energy that is required during exercise. Thus, glycogenolysis is followed by glycolysis, due to the absence of the enzyme glucose-6-phosphatase in the muscle.

4. In liver and kidney, glucose-6-phosphate is further hydrolyzed to **glucose.** This reaction is catalysed by **glucose-6-phosphatase.**

$$\text{Glucose-6-phosphate} + H_2O \xleftrightarrow[\text{Liver and kidney}]{\text{Glucose–6–phosphatase}} \text{Glucose} + \text{Pi}$$

Glycogen, which is stored **in the liver,** is thus converted to free glucose and is used to **maintain blood glucose level** in a hypoglycemic state. On the other hand, glycogen that is stored **in the muscle** is used to **provide energy during exercise.**

GLYCOGEN STORAGE DISEASES

This is a group of inherited disorders that are associated with glycogen metabolism, where an abnormal type or quantity of the glycogen is deposited in different tissues.

According to the deficiency of the enzyme involved, there are several types of glycogen storage diseases (Table 12.2).

Table 12.2. Glycogen storage diseases

Type	*Glycogen storage disease*	*Deficient enzyme*	*Features*
I	Von Gierke's disease	Glucose-6-phosphatase	Liver, renal, and intestinal epithelial cells are loaded with glycogen. There also occurs hypoglycemia, lactic acidosis, ketosis, hyperlipemia, and hyperuricemia
II	Pompe's disease	Lysosomal acid maltase	Accumulation of glycogen in the lysosomes. It is fatal and may result in heart failure
III	Limit dextrinosis/ Forbe's disease or Cori's disease	Debranching enzyme	Accumulation of the branched polysaccharide in liver, muscle, heart, and leucocytes.
IV	Amylopectinosis or Anderson's disease	Branching enzyme	Accumulation of the polysaccharide having few branch points. Death may occur due to liver or cardiac failure with in first year of life.
V	McArdle's syndrome	Muscle phosphorylase	Muscle has abnormally high glycogen content. There is diminished exercise tolerance with little or no lactate in blood after exercise
VI	Her's disease	Liver phosphorylase	High glycogen content in liver. There is also a tendency towards hypoglycemia
VII	Tarui's disease	Phosphofructokinase	As in type V, but there is also a possibility of hemolytic anemia
VIII	–	Liver phosphorylase kinase	As in type VI

GLUCONEOGENESIS

Gluconeogenesis (neoglucogenesis) is the process of the **formation of glucose** from various **non-carbohydrate sources,** such as the glucogenic amino acids, lactate, glycerol, or propionate. Gluconeogenesis takes place in the fasting state or on a low carbohydrate diet, particularly in the liver and some other tissues, which are solely dependent on glucose for their energy demand. It does not take place in muscle.

Gluconeogenesis thus, enables maintenance of blood glucose when all the dietary glucose has been absorbed and oxidized. This process is essential since blood glucose level has to be maintained to support metabolism of the tissues that use glucose as the primary substrate, such as the brain, red blood cells, and lens.

LACTATE METABOLISM

Lactate is produced during the process of anaerobic glycolysis. For its conversion to glucose, firstly, **lactate** is oxidized to **pyruvate**. This reaction is catalyzed by the enzyme **lactate dehydrogenase**, which requires NAD^+.

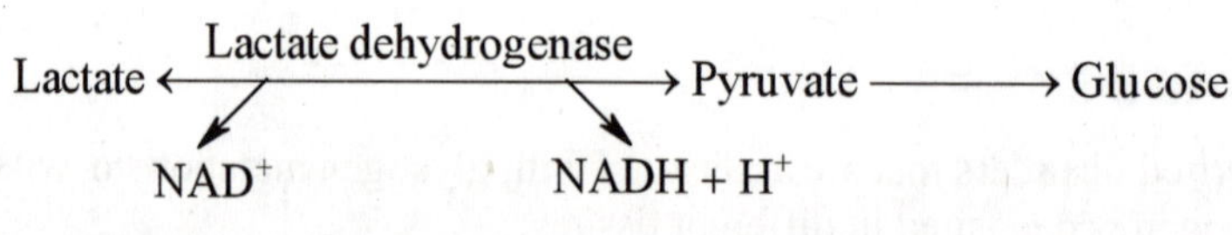

The direction of LDH reaction depends on the relative intracellular concentrations of pyruvate and lactate, and on the ratio of $NADH/NAD^+$ in the cell. The formation of lactate is the major fate of pyruvate in several tissues, such as red blood cells, lens, and cornea of the eye, etc.

In exercising skeletal muscle – NADH production exceeds the oxidative capacity of the respiratory chain. This results in elevated $NADH/NAD^+$ ratio, which in turn favors reduction of pyruvate to lactate. Thus, during intense exercise, lactate accumulates in muscles causing a drop in the intracellular pH, potentially resulting in cramps. Eventually, lactate diffuses into the blood stream and can be used by the liver to make glucose.

In the liver and heart - the ratio of $NADH/NAD^+$ is lower than the exercising muscle. These tissues oxidize lactate to pyruvate.

Subsequently, pyruvate is converted to glucose by the **reversal of the glycolytic reactions**. It is actually, the reversal of the three irreversible reactions of the glycolytic pathway (Fig.12.17).

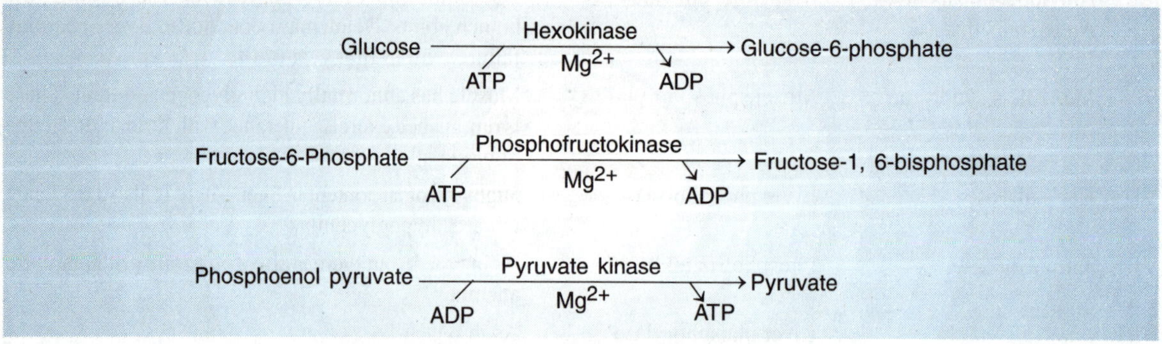

Fig. 12.17. Irreversible steps in glycolysis.

LACTIC ACIDOSIS

Elevated concentration of lactate in the blood is termed as lactic acidosis. Lactic acidosis occurs when there is reduced supply of oxygen, such as in myocardial infarction, pulmonary embolism, or during shock. Supply of inadequate amount of oxygen to the tissues results in inadequate oxidative phosphorylation and decreases ATP synthesis. To survive, the cells use anaerobic glycolysis for the generation of ATP and produce lactic acid as the end product. The excess oxygen required to recover from a period when the availability of oxygen has been inadequate is termed as **oxygen debt**. It is often related to patient's morbidity or mortality. In clinical situations, such as to know the presence and severity of shock, measuring the blood levels of lactic acid provides help for rapid and early detection of oxygen debt in these patients.

REVERSAL OF GLYCOLYSIS

Conversion of pyruvate to phosphoenolpyruvate

For the reversal of the pyruvate to phosphoenolpyruvate, **pyruvate** is first converted to **oxaloacetate** by the enzyme **pyruvate carboxylase,** in mitochondria.

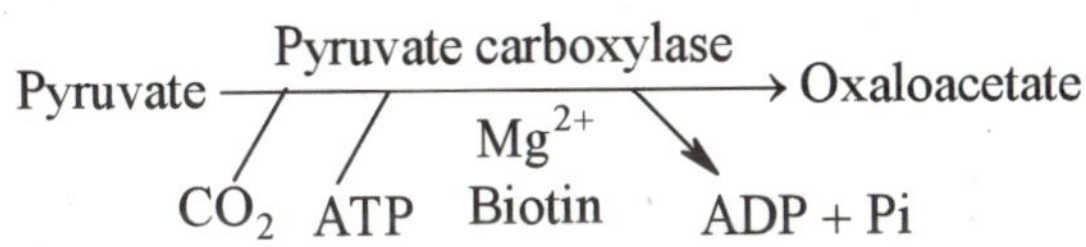

Thereafter, malate dehydrogenase converts oxaloacetate to malate, which is freely transported across the mitochondrial membrane. Malate thus, comes out from the mitochondria to the cytosol where it is reconverted back to oxaloacetate by the same enzyme. This also reduces NAD^+ to $NADH+H^+$. This enzyme thus, not only transports oxaloacetate (via malate) but also reducing equivalents from mitochondria into cytosol. Reactions of gluconeogenesis thus occur in the cytosol as well as mitochondria.

In the cytosol, **oxaloacetate** is converted to **phosphoenolpyruvate**, by the enzyme **phosphoenolpyruvate carboxykinase** (PEP-carboxykinase).

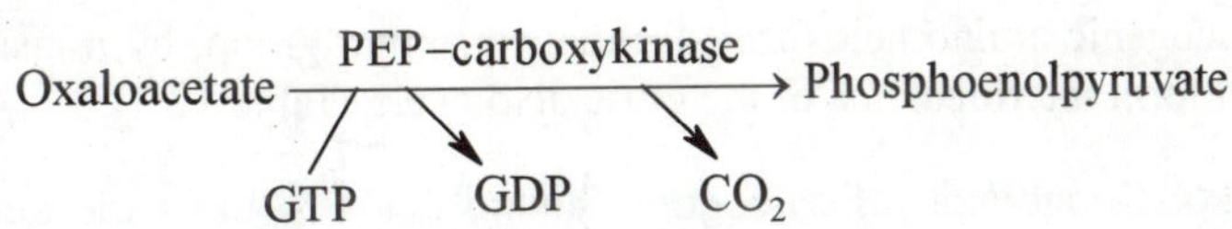

Conversion of fructose-1,6-bisphosphate to fructose-6-phosphate

Fructose-1,6-bisphosphate is converted to fructose-6-phosphate, by the enzyme **fructose-1,6-bisphosphatase.**

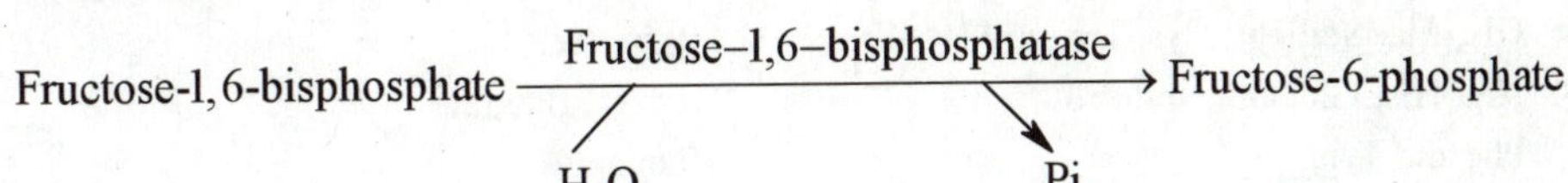

Conversion of glucose-6-phosphate to glucose

Glucose-6-phosphate is converted to glucose by the enzyme **glucose-6-phosphatase.** This enzyme is not found in the muscle and adipose tissue.

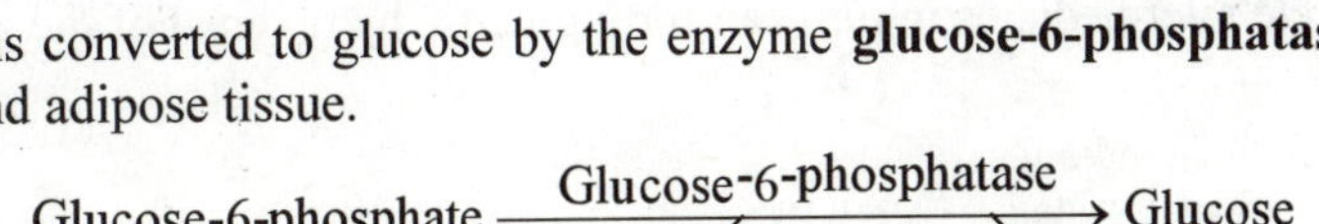

In the muscle, end product of glycogen breakdown, during glycolysis, is glucose-6-phosphate and not free glucose. This is due to absence of the enzyme glucose-6-phosphatase. This, glucose-6-phosphate, is used for energy production, particularly during exercise via anaerobic glycolysis, and results in the production of lactate. Lactic acid is transported to the liver and reforms glucose by the process of gluconeogenesis and becomes available for the muscle and other tissues. This is called **Cori cycle**.

CORI CYCLE

Process of the transport of **lactate** from the **muscle** to the liver, for its conversion into **glucose**, which again goes to the muscle and reforms glycogen, for its re-utilization during exercise is called lactic acid cycle or **Cori cycle.** It results in the net exchange of glycogen via glucose-6-phosphate, and lactate in the two tissues, i.e. the muscle and the liver (Fig. 12.18).

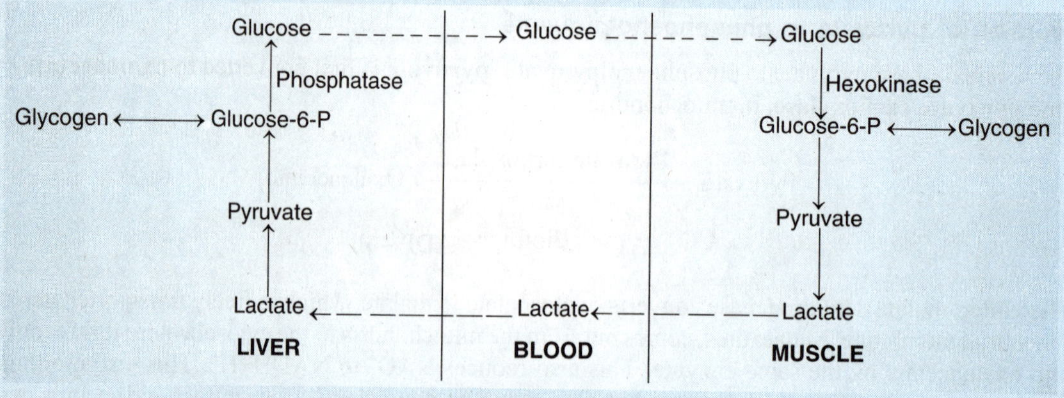

Fig. 12.18. Cori cycle.

SYNTHESIS OF GLUCOSE FROM GLUCOGENIC AMINO ACIDS

In the liver, various glucogenic amino acids transfer their α-amino group, by transamination, and release carbon skeletons, which form intermediates of the citric acid cycle (Table 12.3).

Table 12.3. Conversion of glucogenic amino acids to the citric acid cycle intermediates

Amino Acid	*Citric acid cycle intermediate formed*
Gly, Ala, Ser, Thr, Cys, Trp, and HO-Pro	Pyruvate
Arg, His, Glu, Gln, and Pro	α-Ketoglutarate
Phe and Tyr	Fumarate
Val, Ile, and Met	Succinyl CoA

These citric acid cycle intermediates in turn can form glucose by reversal of the glycolytic reactions via pyruvate (Fig. 12.9).

SYNTHESIS OF GLUCOSE FROM GLYCEROL

Glycerol is produced as a result of lipolysis in the adipose tissue. **Glycerol kinase** converts it to α-

glycerolphosphate in the liver, which is later reduced by a dehydrogenase to **dihydroxyacetone phosphate** and can enter glycolysis at this point (Fig. 12.19).

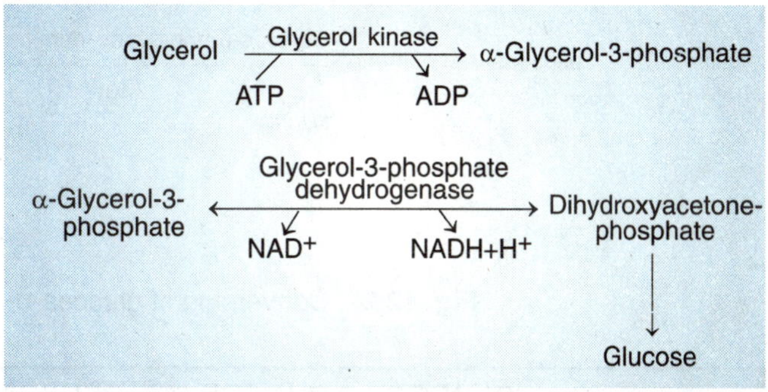

Fig. 12.19. Conversion of glycerol to glucose.

SYNTHESIS OF GLUCOSE FROM PROPIONATE

Oxidation of fatty acids containing odd number of carbon atoms, in addition to acetyl CoA also produces a molecule of **propionyl CoA,** particularly in ruminants. In human beings, propionyl CoA is obtained from Ile, Val and Thr. It is converted to **D-methylmalonyl CoA** by **propionyl CoA carboxylase**. D-Methylmalonyl CoA is then converted to **L-methylmalonyl CoA** and finally, by an isomerase to **succinyl CoA,** which is an intermediate of the citric acid cycle. Succinyl CoA in turn can be converted to glucose via pyruvate (Fig. 12.20).

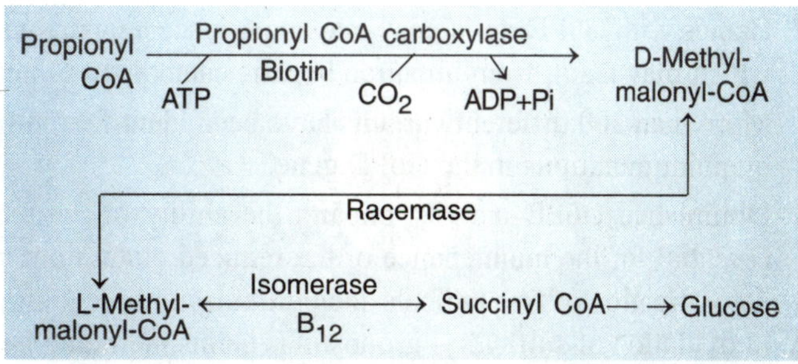

Fig. 12.20. Conversion of propionyl CoA to glucose.

PENTOSE PHOSPHATE PATHWAY

Pentose phosphate pathway, also called hexose monophosphate shunt (HMP shunt) is the second major pathway for the metabolism of glucose. Enzymes for this pathway are localized in the cytosol, while reducing equivalents are accepted by the $NADP^+$, instead of NAD^+. This pathway is operative in many tissues, such as liver, erythrocytes, lactating mammary glands, testes, and adipose tissue. Rate of the HMP shunt reactions is increased by insulin.

In the overall process, six molecules of glucose are utilized to give six molecules of CO_2 and six molecules of pentoses. The pentoses are subsequently, rearranged to give four molecules of fructose-6-phosphate and two molecules of glyceraldehyde-3-phosphate. Two trioses can also form a hexose by the reversal of glycolysis thus, regenerating five molecules of hexoses (Fig. 12.21).

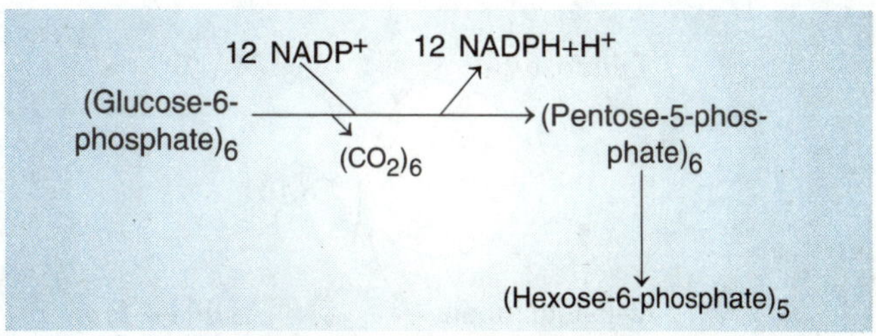

Fig. 12.21. HMP shunt—an overall view.

1. Firstly, **glucose** is activated to **glucose-6-phosphate**, by the enzyme **hexokinase.**
2. Thereafter, **glucose-6-phosphate** is changed to **6-phosphogluconolactone** and subsequently, to **6-phosphogluconate**, by the enzyme **glucose-6-phosphate dehydrogenase.** This enzyme is induced by insulin.

   During this process $NADP^+$ is reduced to $NADPH+H^+$ (Fig. 12.22).

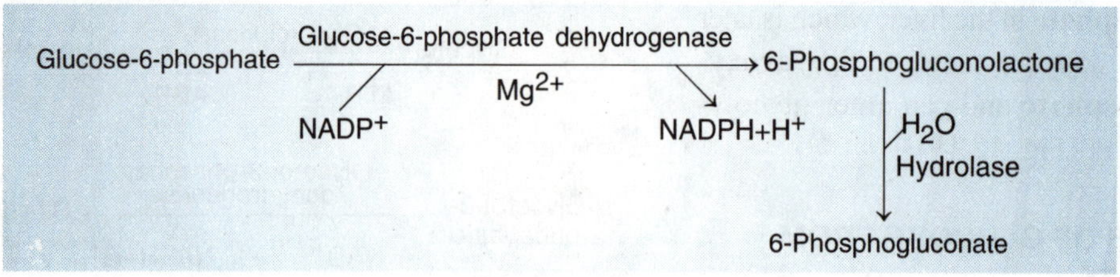

Fig. 12.22. Conversion of glucose-6-P to 6-phosphogluconate

GLUCOSE-6-PHOSPHATE DEHYDROGENASE DEFICIENCY

Glucose-6-phosphate dehydrogenase (G6PD) deficiency is an X-linked inherited disease, characterized by hemolytic anemia, caused by the inability to detoxify oxidizing agents. This deficiency has the highest prevalence in the Middle East, tropical Africa and Asia, and parts of Mediterranean. The life span of many individuals with G6PD deficiency is somewhat shortened as a result of complications arising from chronic hemolysis. Commonly used drugs that produce hemolytic anemia in patients with G6PD deficiency are antibiotics (sulfa-methoxazole and chloramphenicol), anti-malarials (primaquine) and antipyretics (acetanilide).

Babies with G6PD deficiency may experience neonatal jaundice, appearing one to four days after birth, which may result from impaired hepatic catabolism of heme or increased production of bilirubin.

More than 300 different variants have been identified in G6PD gene, and almost all variants are caused by point mutations in the G6PD gene.

Diminished G6PD activity impairs the ability of the red blood cells to form the NADPH, which is essential for the maintenance of the reduced glutathione pool. This results in a decrease in the cellular detoxification of free radicals and peroxides formed within the cell. Reduced level of glutathione results in oxidation of sulfhydryl groups in proteins including hemoglobin and leads to the formation of denatured proteins that form insoluble masses, called Heinz bodies, which gets attached to the red cell membrane.

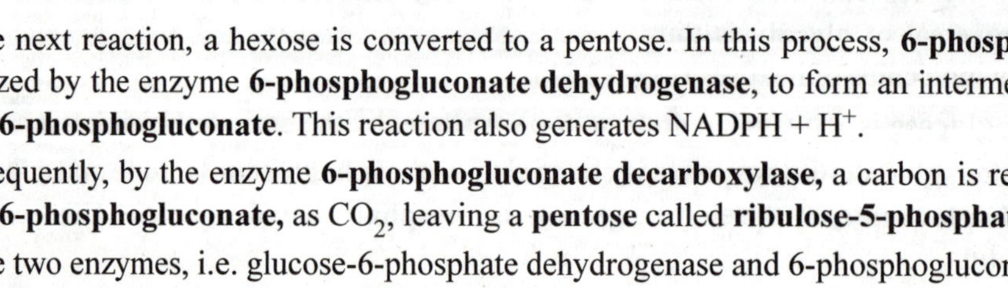

3. In the next reaction, a hexose is converted to a pentose. In this process, **6-phosphogluconate** is oxidized by the enzyme **6-phosphogluconate dehydrogenase**, to form an intermediate, called **3-keto-6-phosphogluconate**. This reaction also generates NADPH + H^+.

   Subsequently, by the enzyme **6-phosphogluconate decarboxylase,** a carbon is removed from **3-keto-6-phosphogluconate,** as CO_2, leaving a **pentose** called **ribulose-5-phosphate** (Fig. 12.23).

   These two enzymes, i.e. glucose-6-phosphate dehydrogenase and 6-phosphogluconate dehydrogenase, are the regulatory enzymes of this shunt.

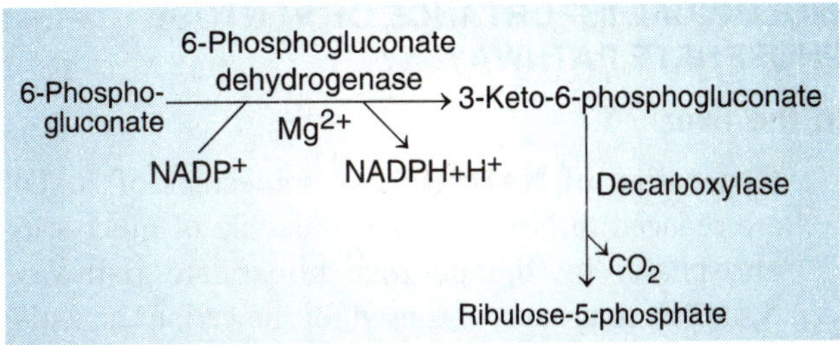

Fig. 12.23. Conversion of a hexose to a pentose.

4. In the second stage of the shunt, ribulose-5-phosphate changes to other pentoses.

   Ribulose-5-phosphate is changed to **ribose-5-phosphate,** by the enzyme **ribose-5-phosphate keto-isomerase,** and to **xylulose-5-phosphate** by the enzyme **ribulose-5-phosphate epimerase** (Fig. 12.24).

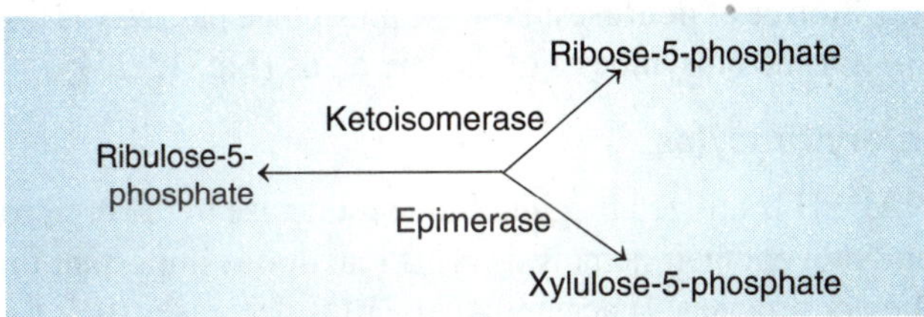

Fig. 12.24. Interconversion of pentoses.

5. In the next reaction, carbon skeletons of the two pentoses are rearranged, as follows:

   A **transketolase** transfers a ketol-group (the first 2 carbon atoms) from **xylulose-5-phosphate** to **ribose-5-phosphate**, forming **sedoheptulose-7-phosphate** and **glyceraldehyde-3-phosphate.** Transketolase requires TPP as a coenzyme.

   Subsequently, an aldol- group (3 carbons moiety) is transferred by the enzyme **transaldolase,** from **sedoheptulose-7-phosphate** to **glyceraldehyde-3-phosphate**, forming **fructose-6-phosphate** and **erythrose-4-phosphate** (Fig. 12.25).

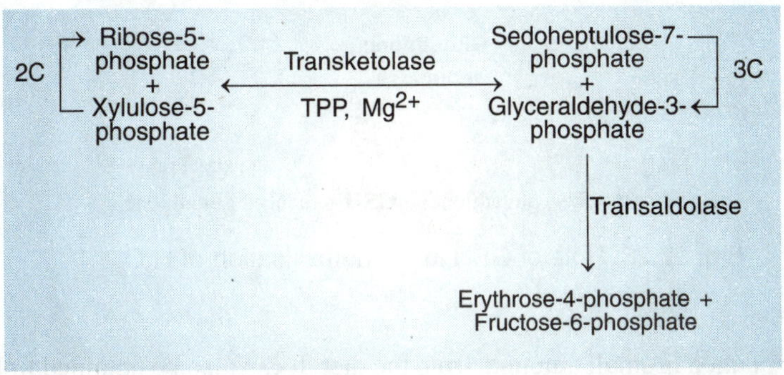

Fig. 12.25. Rearrangement of various carbons of pentoses.

6. **Transketolase** also transfers a ketol group (2 carbons moiety) from **xylulose-5-phosphate** to **erythrose-4-phosphate**, forming **fructose-6-phosphate** and **glyceraldehyde-3-phosphate** (Fig. 12.26).

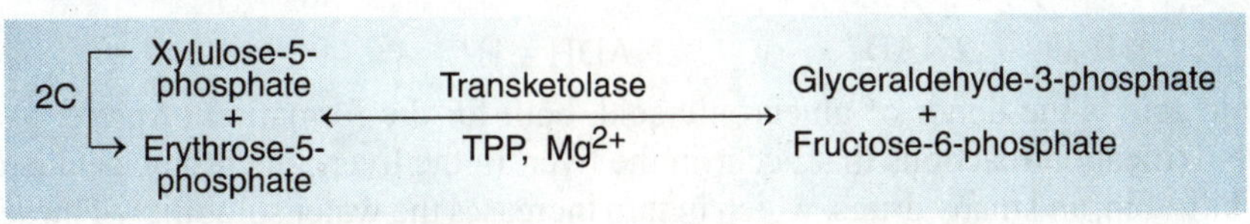

Fig. 12.26. Conversion of pentoses to a hexose and a triose.

BIOLOGICAL IMPORTANCE OF PENTOSE PHOSPHATE PATHWAY

In the liver

1. **Generation of NADPH:** Two molecules of NADP are reduced to NADPH, per molecule of glucose-6-phosphate, by the pentose phosphate pathway. **NADPH,** so produced, is used for the various anabolic reactions, such as synthesis of fatty acids and cholesterol.
2. **Source of pentoses:** Pentose phosphate pathway is also important source of **pentoses,** which are required for the biosynthesis of nucleic acids (Fig. 12.27).

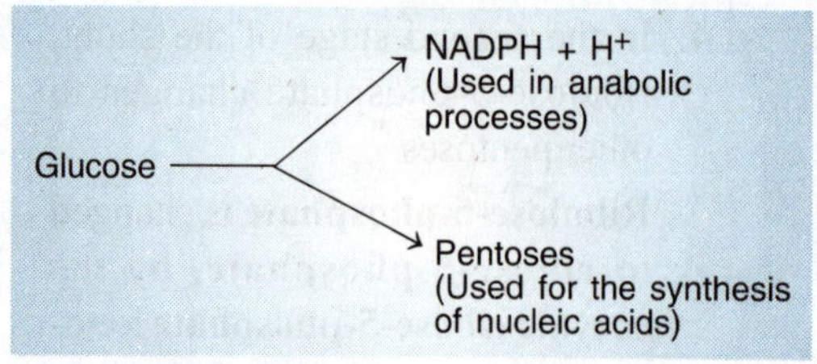

Fig. 12.27. Biological significance of HMP shunt in the liver.

In erythrocytes

NADPH is utilized by glutathione reductase in the erythrocytes, to maintain the reduced state of glutathione and prevent their hemolysis. This reaction is important for the detoxification of H_2O_2, which is produced in the erythrocytes. If accumulated, H_2O_2 decreases their life span and causes hemolysis (Fig. 12.28).

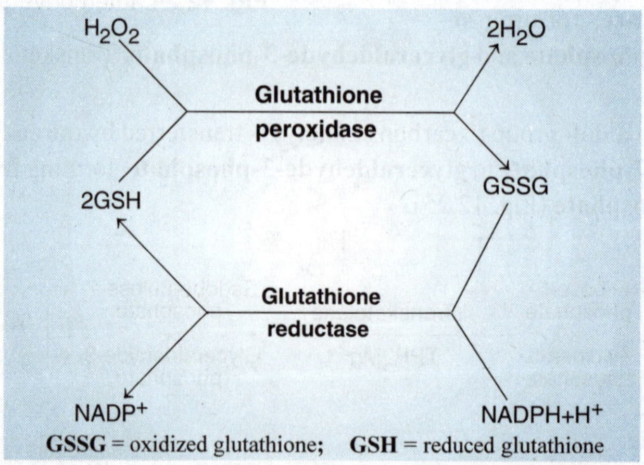

Fig. 12.28. Role of GSH in the detoxification of H_2O_2.

GLUCURONIC ACID

Glucuronic acid can be obtained in small amounts from the diet. It can also be obtained from the intracellular lysosomal degradation of glycosaminoglycans (proteoglycans) or via the **uronic acid pathway.**

The active form of glucuronic acid is UDP-glucuronic acid, which is produced by oxidation of UDP-glucose, by UDP-glucose dehydrogenase.

$$\text{UDP} + H_2O + 2NAD^+ \xrightarrow{\text{UDP-Glucose dehydrogenase}} \text{UDP-Glucuronic acid} + 2NADH + H^+$$

UDP-Glucuronic acid is the donor of glucuronic acid, both for the formation of proteoglycans and for conjugation and detoxification reactions that occur in the liver. In the liver, glucuronic acid is conjugated to steroid hormones, bilirubin, and many drugs, which in turn increases the water solubility of these hydrophobic compounds, facilitating their excretion in urine.

REGULATION OF BLOOD GLUCOSE

Blood glucose level is maintained with in the **normal** physiological **range** of **60-90 mg per 100 ml,** in the fasting (post-absorptive) state by various **hormones** and also by the **kidney.**

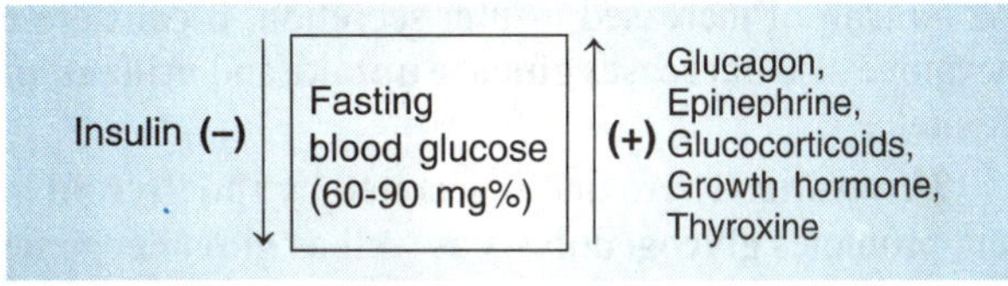

Fig. 12.29. Regulation of blood glucose by hormones.

BY HORMONES

Several hormones regulate blood glucose concentration. While insulin lowers blood glucose, various other hormones increase blood glucose level (Fig. 12.29)

Hormone which has Hypoglycemic Action

Insulin is the only hormone, which has hypoglycemic action. It is released into the blood stream, under the direct influence of hyperglycemia. It is a polypeptide containing 2 chains and produced by **β-cells of the islets of Langerhans** of the pancreas.

Insulin **lowers blood glucose** concentration, by increasing uptake of glucose by the extrahepatic tissues. Insulin also **promotes glycolysis** and **glycogenesis**, both in the liver and the muscle. At the same time, insulin also **suppresses glycogenolysis** in the liver and the kidney. Besides, insulin also suppresses **gluconeogenesis.**

Insulin also **stimulates synthesis of various enzymes**, such as glucose-6-phosphate dehydrogenase, 6-phosphogluconate dehydrogenase, ATP-citrate lyase, etc. Insulin also **represses synthesis** of pyruvate carboxylase; PEP-carboxykinase, and fructose-1,6-bisphosphatase.

Insulin also **promotes transport of amino acids** across the cell membrane and thus **stimulates protein synthesis.**

Insulin also **inhibits ketogenesis** and **promotes lipogenesis.**

Hormones which have Hyperglycemic Action

Several hormones have hyperglycemic action. These are called diabetogenic hormones and include **glucagon, epinephrine, gluco-corticoids, growth hormone,** and **thyroxine.**

Glucagon: Glucagon is produced by **α-cells** of the **islets of langerhans** of pancreas. Its synthesis is stimulated under the influence of hypoglycemia. It acts only in the liver and **promotes glycogenolysis.** It also promotes **gluconeogenesis** from amino acids and lactate.

Epinephrine: Epinephrine, also called **adrenaline**, is secreted by **adrenal medulla**. It is a hormone in the first line of defense against hypoglycemia. It is a derivative of tyrosine.

Epinephrine **promotes glycogenolysis**, both in the liver and muscle. Epinephrine also promotes **gluconeogensis** in the liver. It **also inhibits release of insulin** from the pancreas, and decreases transport and utilization of glucose in different tissues. At the same time, epinephrine also **stimulates secretion of glucagon.**

Gluco-corticoids: Gluco-corticoids are steroids secreted by **adrenal cortex.** They are antagonists to insulin.

Cortisol is a major gluco-corticoid present in blood. It **stimulates protein catabolism** in the **muscle** and **promotes gluconeogenesis** in the **liver**. It also **stimulates lipolysis** and **inhibits glucose oxidation,** by the liver. Cortisol also facilitates actions of other hyperglycemic hormones (permissive effects), such as glucagon, epinephrine, and growth hormone, which further inhibit uptake and utilization of glucose by the peripheral tissues.

Growth Hormone: Anterior pituitary secretes growth hormone. Its secretion is stimulated under the influence of hypoglycemia. Prolonged administration of the growth hormone **stimulates secretion of insulin.**

As a result of increased insulin secretion, β-cells are exhausted, producing diabetes like situation. Growth hormone also **decreases glucose uptake** and **utilization by muscle.** It also **promotes lipolysis in the adipose tissue.**

Thyroxine: Thyroxine is secreted by **the thyroid gland.** It **stimulates intestinal absorption of glucose** and promotes **glycogenolysis** as well as **gluconeogenesis** in the liver. Thyroxine also causes **destruction of insulin.** Hyperthyroidism is generally associated with hyperglycemia and mild diabetes.

BY KIDNEY

Kidney also regulates blood **glucose** concentration, which is continuously **filtered by the glomeruli** and is completely **reabsorbed by the renal tubules.** However, when blood glucose concentration exceeds 180 mg/dl (renal threshold value), tubules fail to reabsorb all of the filtered glucose, some of which starts appearing in the urine.

DIABETES MELLITUS

Diabetes mellitus is characterized by persistent **hyperglycemia** with or without glycosuria **(glucosuria).** This is the commonest endocrine disease caused by the **deficiency in secretion** or **action of insulin**. Besides insulin, several diabetogenic hormones influence metabolism of glucose.

Diabetic mellitus is defined as a state of **chronic hyperglycemia**, which may be a result of genetic and/or environmental factors. It is a multifactorial disease. There are two major clinical classes of diabetes mellitus, which are referred to as:

- Insulin dependent diabetes mellitus, and
- Noninsulin dependent diabetes mellitus

INSULIN DEPENDENT DIABETES MELLITUS

Insulin dependent diabetes mellitus (IDDM), or **type I diabetes** is also called as **juvenile-onset diabetes** because it usually appears in the childhood or in **younger age group** (commonly less than 40 years of age). There is absolute deficiency of insulin, due to a gradual **depletion of β-cells** of the pancreas, which may get destroyed by an autoimmune process.

IDDM is characterized by **hyperglycemia, hyperlipoproteinemia** (raised chylomicron and VLDL), and **severe ketoacidosis.** This in turn suggests that besides defects in carbohydrate metabolism, there are abnormalities in fat and protein metabolism also, in such patients.

Hyperglycemia in IDDM is a result of **inability** of the insulin-dependent tissues, **to take up glucose** as well as due to **accelerated hepatic gluconeogenesis** from amino acids (derived from muscle protein).

Increased lipolysis (in the **adipose tissue)** and **accelerated fatty acid oxidation** (in the **liver**) result in **ketoacidosis.**

Insulin deficiency also **reduces lipoprotein lipase** activity, thereby resulting in **hyperchylomicronemia.**

Patients with IDDM can usually be recognized by abrupt appearance of **polyuria** (frequent urination), **polydypsia** (excessive thirst), and **polyphagia** (excessive hunger), often triggered by the stress or some illness. These symptoms are usually accompanied with fatigue, weight loss, and weakness.

Its diagnosis is confirmed by the **high fasting blood glucose,** commonly accompanied with **ketoacidosis**. Insulin injection, though does not cure the disease, but promotes glucose uptake by the tissues and inhibits gluconeogenesis, lipolysis, and proteolysis.

Life span of the patient is reduced, as a result of the degenerative complications, such as kidney malfunction, nerve impairment, and cardiovascular disease.

Hyperglycemia also leads to blindness through retinal degeneration, and glycosylation of the lens proteins, which in turn causes cataract.

NON-INSULIN DEPENDENT DIABETES MELLITUS

Majority of the diabetic patients (over 80%) suffer from noninsulin dependent diabetes mellitus (NIDDM) or **type II diabetes**. It is also called as the **maturity-onset-diabetes** since it usually occurs in the middle age group (usually more than 40 years of age), who are generally obese. Occurrence of the disease is almost completely determined by the genetic factors. NIDDM develops gradually, without obvious symptoms. Metabolic alterations are milder than in IDDM.

NIDDM is characterized by **hyperglycemia,** often with **hypertriglyceridemia**. Inspite of high level of insulin, glucose levels are poorly controlled because of the lack of normal response to insulin. **Insulin resistance** in these patients may be due to increased expression of the tumor necrosis factor-α, in the adipocytes of obese individuals. Hyperglycemia is mainly, a result of the **poor peripheral utilization of glucose**, especially in muscle.

Ketoacidosis does not develop because adipocytes remain sensitive to the effect of insulin.

Rapid de novo synthesis of fatty acids and VLDL lead to **hypertriglyceridemia** without hyperchylomicronemia.

Blood glucose concentration is much higher than normal, particularly after a meal.

Weight reduction and dietary modifications often correct hyperglycemia of type II diabetes. **Hypoglycemic agents,** such as **sulphonylureas**, may be required to achieve a satisfactory fall in blood glucose level.

Salient features of two types of diabetes mellitus are shown in Table 12.4.

Table 12.4. Salient features of two types of diabetes mellitus

	IDDM	*NIDDM*
Type of Diabetes	Juvenile onset (Type I)	Maturity onset (Type II)
Prevalence	About 20%	About 80%
Age of onset	<40 years	> 40 years
Body habitués	Normal to wasted (weight loss)	Obese
Plasma insulin	Low (due to β-cell destruction)	Normal to high (insulin resistance)
Plasma glucagon	High (suppressible)	High (resistant)
Acute complications	Ketoacidosis	Hyperosmolar coma (ketoacidosis is rare)
Insulin therapy	Responsive	Resistant
Oral hypoglycemic agents	Unresponsive	Responsive

For any form of diabetes, metabolic derangement is due to elevated glucagon/insulin ratio. In addition, there may be weight loss in IDDM.

Metabolic complications of the uncontrolled diabetes include ketoacidosis and coma in IDDM, hyperosmolar non-ketotic coma in NIDDM, or hypoglycemia due to insulin overdose.

Long-term complications of the disease include acute myocardial infarction (diabetic patients often present with painless acute myocardial infarction, i.e. silent MI), due to accelerated atherosclerosis and coronary heart disease, nephropathy, retinopathy, neuropathy, infections, and delayed wound healing.

METABOLIC SYNDROME

Obesity and insulin resistance resulting in either glucose intolerance or diabetes may coexist with dyslipidemia and increased arterial blood pressure. Such combination is referred to as metabolic syndrome and is associated with an increased risk of cardiovascular disease.

GLYCEMIC STATUS

Measurement of plasma glucose though is a good index of diabetes mellitus, however, it changes quickly, and therefore in the monitoring of diabetic patients, it is advised to measure glucose-modified hemoglobin, called glycated-hemoglobin (HbA_{1c}). Native hemoglobin (HbA) gets converted to a glycated form, which increases in proportion to the mean blood glucose concentration, during hyperglycemia. Glycation of proteins may contribute to the medical complications and diabetes, e.g. coronary heart disease, retinopathy, nephropathy, cataract, and neuropathy. Because the formation of HbA_{1c}, at physiologic pH is irreversible, glycation leaves a record of glycemia throughout the rest of the life of erythrocytes. The HbA_{1c} concentration in blood thus reflects the time-average plasma glucose level over the 3-6 weeks preceding the measurement. The normal concentration of HbA_{1c} is 4-6% of total HbA. The concentration of HbA1c increases in uncontrolled diabetes. Higher levels suggest poor control.

SOME IMPORTANT QUESTIONS

1. Outline reactions of the citric acid cycle. Give energetic of the cycle and explain the amphibolic role of this cycle.
2. Outline pentose phosphate pathway reactions. Discuss significance of the pathway in different tissues.
3. Give outline of glycolysis. What are its regulatory steps? What is the energy yield of this pathway?
4. Define glycogenolysis. Outline reactions of this pathway.
5. What is glycogenesis? Give reactions of glycogenesis.
6. Explain :
   (i) Why aerobic glycolysis releases more energy than anaerobic glycolysis?
   (ii) How glycolysis can be reversed?
   (iii) Citric acid cycle and its energetics
7. Discuss briefly:
   (i) Regulation of blood glucose
   (ii) Glycogenolysis
8. Write notes on:
   (i) Diabetes mellitus
   (ii) Glycogenesis
   (iii) Gluconeogenesis
   (iv) Glycogen storage diseases
   (v) Energetics of the citric acid cycle
   (vi) Oxidation of pyruvate to acetyl CoA
   (vii) Von Gierke's disease
   (viii) Lactate metabolism
   (ix) Lactic acidosis
   (x) Glucose-6-phosphate dehydrogenase deficiency
   (xi) Glycemic status

CHAPTER 13

Metabolism of Lipids

The hydrolysed products of lipids absorbed by enterocytes migrate to the endoplasmic reticulum where resynthesis of complex lipids takes place. The fatty acids are stored in the liver and the adipose tissue as triacylglycerols.

METABOLISM OF FATTY ACIDS

Major pathway for the catabolism of fatty acids is a mitochondrial pathway called **β-oxidation,** which was proposed by **Knoop.**

β-OXIDATION OF FATTY ACIDS

Major pathway for catabolism of the saturated fatty acids is a mitochondrial pathway called **β-oxidation,** which was proposed by **Knoop.** In this process, **oxidation** of fatty acids **occurs at the β-carbon atom** (carbon-3) and two-carbon fragments are successively removed from the carboxyl end of fatty acyl CoA. This in turn results in the **elimination of two terminal carbon atoms as acetyl CoA,** thereby leaving fattyacyl CoA that has two carbons less than the original fatty acid (Fig. 13.1)

Activation of A Fatty Acid

A long chain fatty acid (fatty acid containing >12 carbons) enters a cell where it is converted to its CoA derivative, by the enzyme long-chain fatty acyl CoA synthetase (thiokinase) in the cytosol.

$$\text{Fatty acid} + \text{CoA} + \text{ATP} \xrightarrow[\text{Mg}^{2+}]{\text{Acyl CoA synthetase}} \text{Fattyacyl CoA} + \text{AMP} + \text{PP}$$

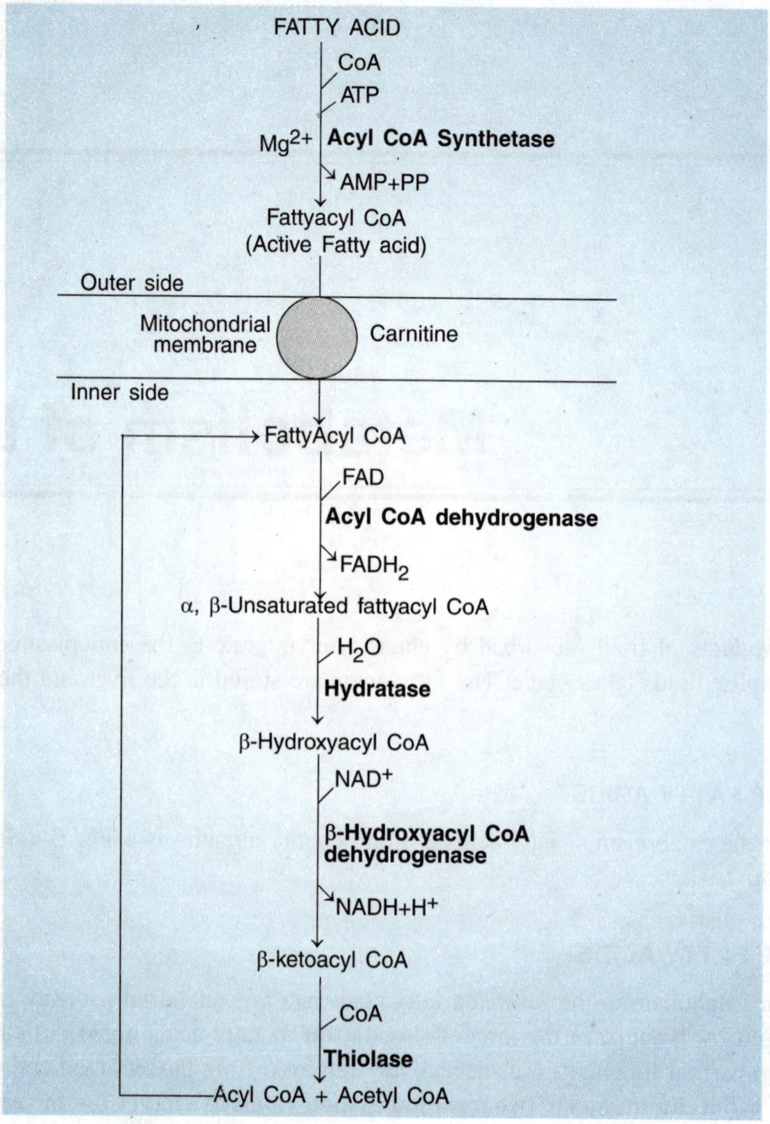

Fig. 13.1. The process of β-oxidation of a fatty acid.

Transport across the Inner Mitochondrial Membrane

The process of **β-oxidation** occurs in the mitochondrial matrix thus, fatty acid must be transported across the mitochondrial membrane. Short chain fatty acids can cross the inner mitochondrial membrane and are activated to their CoA derivatives with in the mitochondria. However, it is impermeable to a long chain fatty acid. A long chain fatty acid is transported from cytosol to the mitochondrial matrix with the help of a specialized carrier called **carnitine.** This process is called carnitine shuttle (Fig. 13.2).

In this process, an acyl group is first transferred from the cytosolic CoA to carnitine, by the enzyme carnitine palmitoyl transferase-I (CPT-I). This enzyme is associated with the outer mitochondrial membrane, and is also referred as carnitine acyl transferase-I (CAT-I). This reaction forms acylcarnitine and regenerates

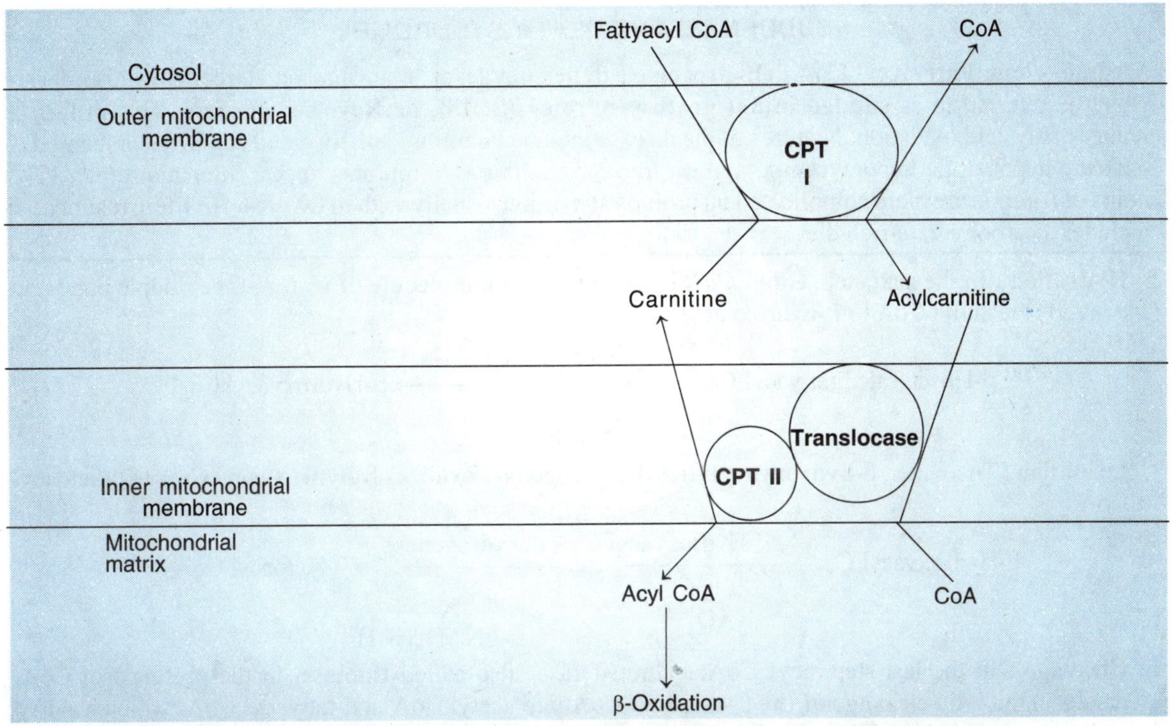

Fig. 13.2. Transfer of a fatty acid from the cytosol through the inner mitochondrial membrane.

free CoA. Thereafter, acyl carnitine is transported into the mitochondrial matrix, in exchange for free carnitine, by a protein called carnitine acyltranslocase. Finally, CPT-II (CAT-II), which is present in the inner mitochondrial membrane, catalyzes transfer of the acyl group, from carnitine to CoA, into the mitochondrial matrix and regenerates carnitine.

Malonyl CoA inhibits CPT-I.

Carnitine is obtained from dietary meat. A small amount of it can also be synthesized in the liver and kidney, from lysine and methionine. Carnitine deficiency can be observed in the patients with a liver disease, malnutrition, or in strict vegetarians. Congenital deficiency of CPT-I or CPT-II is also observed. Such a deficiency can result in the decreased ability to use long-chain fatty acids, by the tissues.

Process of β-oxidation

The process of β-oxidation consists of four reactions, which result in shortening of the fatty acid chain by two carbons. It includes:

1. **Oxidation**- After activation of the fatty acid, such as palmitic acid, and its entry into the mitochondrial matrix, flavoprotein containing **acyl CoA dehydrogenase removes two hydrogens** from the α- and β-positions of the fatty acyl CoA and **produces $FADH_2$.** The fatty acyl CoA is changed to α, β-unsaturated fatty acyl CoA (enoyl CoA).

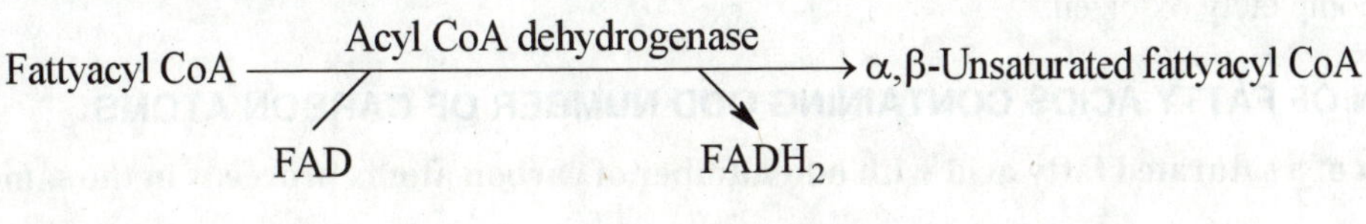

SUDDEN INFANT DEATH SYNDROME

Medium-chain Fatty Acyl CoA dehydrogenase deficiency leads to an autosomal, recessive disorder, which is referred to as **sudden infant death syndrome (SIDS), or Reye's syndrome**. This in turn reduces fatty acid oxidation. Features of the disease include vomiting, lethargy, and coma, accompanied with the hypoketotic hypoglycemia, and dicarboxylic aciduria. Symptoms appear after more than 12 hours of fast, and are more complicated on prolong starvation, usually with in two years of life. Treatment includes a carbohydrate-rich diet.

2. **Hydration :** In the next step, **enoyl CoA hydratase adds a molecule of water** at the double bond and converts the enoyl CoA to β-hydroxyacyl CoA.

$$\alpha,\beta\text{-Unsaturated fattyacyl CoA} \xrightarrow[H_2O]{\text{Enoyl CoA hydratase}} \beta\text{-Hydroxyacyl CoA}$$

3. **Oxidation :** Thereafter, **β-hydroxyacyl CoA dehydrogenase oxidizes β-hydroxyacyl CoA** to β-ketoacyl CoA.

$$\beta\text{-Hydroxyacyl CoA} \xrightarrow[NAD^+ \quad\quad NADH + H^+]{\beta\text{-Hydroxyacyl CoA dehydrogenase}} \beta\text{-Ketoacyl CoA}$$

4. **Cleavage :** In the last step, acyl CoA:acyltransferase, also called **thiolase,** in the presence of CoA, results in thiolytic **cleavage of the β-ketoacyl CoA** into acetyl CoA and fattyacyl CoA, which has two carbons less than the original fattyacyl CoA.

$$\underset{\text{(n carbon)}}{\beta\text{-Ketoacyl CoA}} \xrightarrow[\text{CoA}]{\text{Thiolase}} \text{Acetyl CoA} + \underset{\text{(n-2 carbon)}}{\text{Fattyacyl CoA}}$$

These four steps are repeated, i.e. the fattyacyl CoA again undergoes similar set of reactions starting with acyl CoA dehydrogenase. Each cycle produces acetyl CoA, $FADH_2$, and NADH. Thus, the fatty acid is sequentially degraded to acetyl CoA.

Energy production from β-oxidation

When a molecule of **palmitic acid ($C_{15}H_{31}COOH$)** undergoes β-oxidation, it **releases 8 molecules of acetyl CoA** in seven rounds. In each round, one molecule each of $FADH_2$ and $NADH + H^+$ are produced, which in turn generate 2 and 3 ATP, respectively.

Thus, a total of 35 ATP are produced during this process. In addition, each molecule of acetyl CoA, when oxidized via the citric acid cycle produces 12 ATP (Table 12.1). Therefore, additionally, 96 ATP are produced from 8 molecules of acetyl CoA. Hence, a total of **131 ATP** are produced from one molecule of palmitic acid.

As two high energy phosphate bonds are hydrolyzed from one molecule of ATP, which is changed to AMP, thus 2 ATP are used during activation of the fatty acid.

Therefore, there is a **net yield of 129 ATP,** when one molecule of palmitic acid (fatty acid with 16 carbons) is completely oxidized.

OXIDATION OF FATTY ACIDS CONTAINING ODD NUMBER OF CARBON ATOMS

β-Oxidation of a saturated fatty acid with odd number of carbon atoms proceeds in the same way as a

saturated fatty acid with even number of carbons, until final three carbons are reached. Thus, in addition to acetyl CoA, it also produces a molecule of propionyl CoA (containing 3 carbons), which is used as follows :

(i) Firstly, propionyl CoA is carboxylated by the enzyme propionyl CoA carboxylase, to D-methylmalonyl CoA. This enzyme requires biotin (Fig. 13.3).

(ii) D-Methylmalonyl CoA is then converted to L-methylmalonyl CoA, by the enzyme methylmalonyl CoA racemase.

(iii) Finally, L-methylmalonyl CoA is converted to succinyl CoA by the enzyme methylmalonyl CoA mutase. This enzyme requires deoxyadenosylcobalamin (coenzyme form of vitamin B_{12}).

METHYLMALONIC ACIDEMIA AND METHYLMALONIC ACIDURIA

In the patients with vitamin B_{12} deficiency, methylmalonate levels are increased in the blood (methylmalonic acidemia) and it is also excreted in the urine (methylmalonic aciduria). In this condition, either the enzyme, mutase, is deficient or the patient is unable to convert vitamin B_{12} to its coenzyme form. This in turn also results in metabolic acidosis and mental retardation.

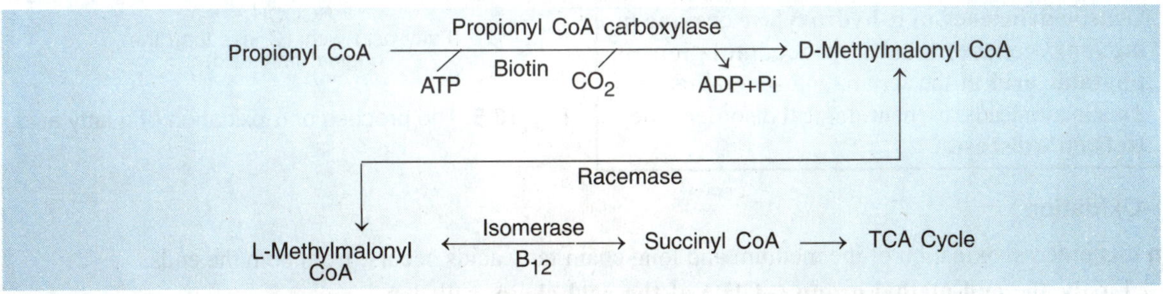

Fig. 13.3. Conversion of propionyl CoA to succinyl CoA.

OXIDATION OF UNSATURATED FATTY ACIDS

Unsaturated fatty acids are also activated, transported across the inner mitochondrial membrane, and **undergo β-oxidation,** by the process similar to that of a saturated fatty acid. However, since the double bonds of the naturally occurring unsaturated fatty acids are found in cis-configuration (compared to those produced during β-oxidation, which have trans-configuration) hence, **three additional enzymes are required** for their oxidation. These include:

1. **Enoyl CoA isomerase,**
2. **Dienoyl CoA reductase, and**
3. **3,2-Enoyl CoA isomerase**

In addition to the other enzymes of β-oxidation, these three enzymes are required for the oxidation of the unsaturated fatty acids (Fig. 13.4).

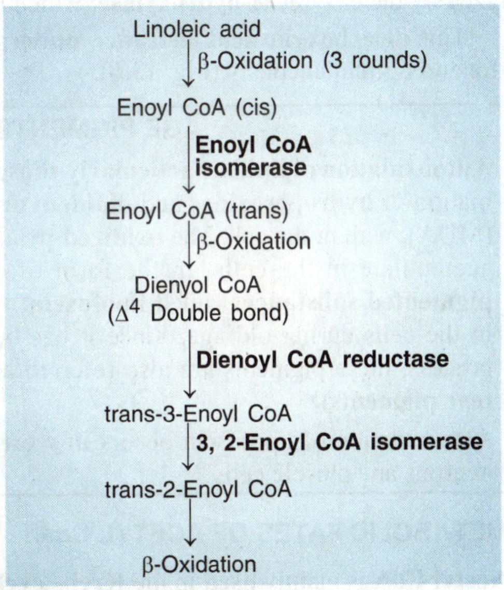

Fig. 13.4. Oxidation of an unsaturated fatty acid.

ALTERNATIVE PATHWAYS FOR FATTY ACID OXIDATION

α-Oxidation

Fatty acids are also oxidized by another process, called α-oxidation, in microsomes, in the liver and brain.

During α-oxidation, a fatty acid is metabolized by α-hydroxylation, followed by dehydrogenation, and decarboxylation (Fig. 13.5).

In this process, there is **sequential removal of a carbon atom, from the carboxyl end** of the fatty acid as CO_2. This process neither produces CoA intermediates nor generates ATP.

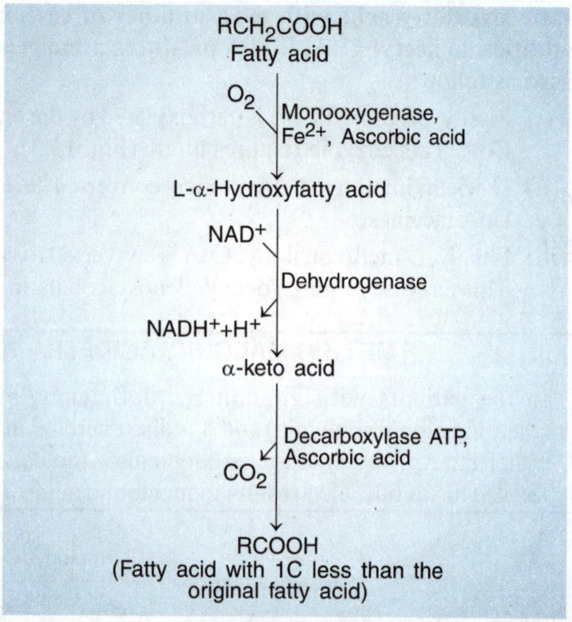

Fig. 13.5. The process of α-oxidation of a fatty acid.

REFSUM DISEASE

Genetic **deficiency of α-hydroxylase enzyme** (a monooxygenase) results in accumulation of **phytanic acid** in the serum, and several tissues. This in turn leads to a neurological disorder called **Refsum's disease.**

ω-Oxidation

In this process, oxidation of the medium and long chain fatty acids occurs, from both the ends.

Firstly, the **end-methyl group ($-CH_3$) of the acyl chain,** called ω-carbon, **is oxidized** and forms a dicarboxylic acid. This reaction is catalyzed by the enzyme **ω-hydroxylase,** which requires cytochrome P_{450}.

This **dicarboxylic acid** thereafter, **undergoes β-oxidation from both the ends**, simultaneously (Fig. 13.6).

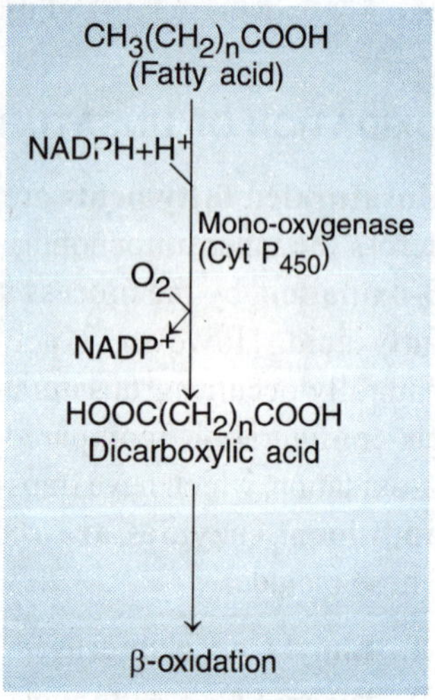

Fig. 13.6. The process of ω-oxidation of a fatty acid.

AGE PIGMENTS

Autooxidation of lipids, particularly those of PUFA, results in the formation of **hydroperoxides** and **dialdehydes,** such as malondialdehyde (MDA), with in the cell. The **oxidized products of lipids and proteins** accumulate in the cells, in the form of chemically **heterogeneous pigmented substances** called **lipofuscin.** Lipofuscin also accumulates in the cells during old age. Since it has been implicated in the aging process, these pigments are also referred as **age-pigments (wear and tear pigments).**

Accumulation of lipofuscin occurs in most of the cells particularly, in neurons and muscle cells.

METABOLIC FATES OF ACETYL CoA

Acetyl CoA is mainly **used** in the **Krebs cycle.**

Besides **Krebs cycle,** acetyl CoA can also be used for the **synthesis of fatty acids** and **cholesterol.** A small quantity of it is also converted to **ketone bodies** in the liver (Fig. 13.7).

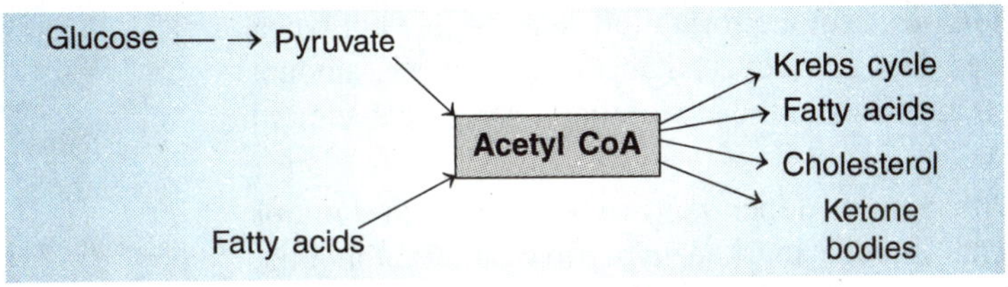

Fig. 13.7. Metabolic fates of acetyl CoA.

KETONE BODIES

Acetoacetate, β-hydroxybutyrate, and **acetone** are collectively referred as **ketone bodies** (acetone bodies).

FORMATION OF KETONE BODIES

The process of the **formation of ketone bodies** is called **ketogenesis.**

In a normal man, concentration of the ketone bodies is usually less than 3 mg/100 ml of blood. In certain conditions, such as during prolonged starvation or impaired glucose oxidation like diabetes mellitus, when fat becomes the source of energy and lipolysis is accelerated, there is increased production of acetyl CoA. This in turn can not be fully utilized through Krebs cycle (due to lack of oxaloacetate) and is converted to ketone bodies.

Clinical condition resulting from the **increased synthesis of ketone bodies** is called **ketosis.** They are diffused into the **blood. Increased** concentration of ketone bodies in the blood is called ketonemia. This in turn also results in their increased excretion in the urine, which is referred to as **ketonuria.**

Formation of ketone bodies occurs in the mitochondria, in the liver since liver has a highly active system for the production of acetoacetate, which is the principal ketone body.

Firstly, **2 molecules of acetyl CoA condense** and **form acetoacetyl CoA,** which further **reacts with one more molecule of acetyl CoA** and **forms HMG CoA.** Thereafter, **HMG CoA lyase splits HMG CoA to acetyl CoA** and **acetoacetate** (Fig. 13.8).

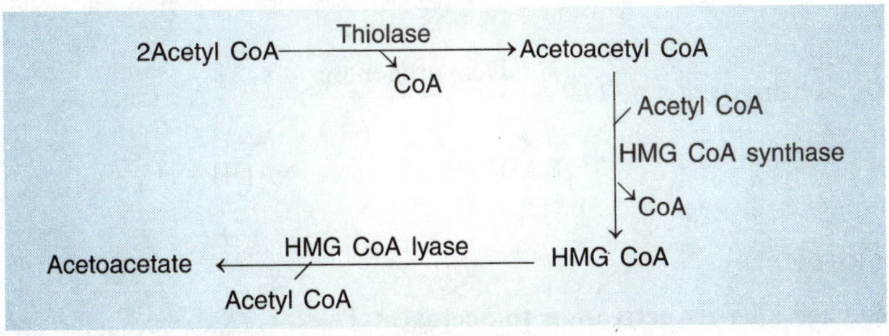

Fig. 13.8. Formation of acetoacetate.

Acetoacetate is the parent ketone body that is first synthesized. In the mitochondria, a part of it **is reduced by NADH-dependent β-hydroxybutyrate dehydrogenase, to β-hydroxybutyrate**. Some of the **acetoacetate** is also **spontaneously decarboxylated,** by a non-enzymatic reaction, **to acetone** (Fig. 13.9).

Both, acetoacetate and β-hydroxybutyrate are the strong acids. Slowly they deplete the alkali reserve of the body and cause **metabolic acidosis**. Hence, this condition is also called as **ketoacidosis.**

Ketosis occurs **in severe diabetes, starvation,** or **on high-fat low-carbohydrate diet.**

Under normal conditions, acetone formation is negligible but when acetoacetate accumulates, such as in severe diabetic ketoacidosis, amount of acetone in the blood increases to the extent that it can be detected in breath of the patient.

In the patients with insulin-dependent diabetes mellitus, major metabolic derangements include marked hyperglycemia, ketonemia, and ketonuria. It may also be associated with water and electrolyte imbalance.

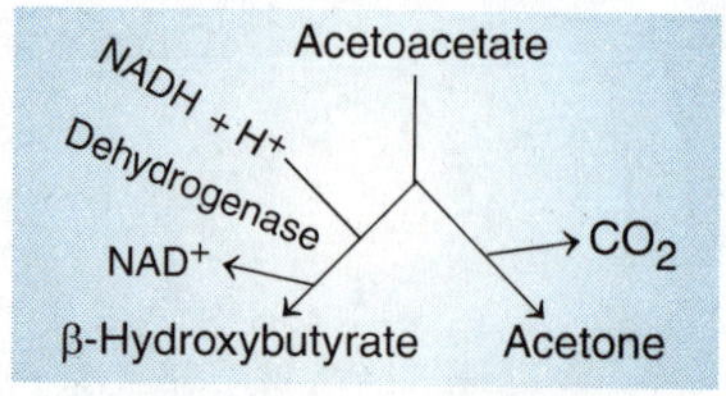

Fig. 13.9. Conversion of acetoacetate to other ketone bodies.

> **DIABETIC KETOACIDOSIS**
>
> **Diabetic ketoacidosis** is a common feature observed **in patients with insulin dependent diabetes mellitus.** This is due to the severe deficiency of insulin with excess of glucagon and other hyperglycemic hormones, such as epinephrine, cortisol, and growth hormone.
>
> Plasma free fatty acid concentration is increased. This in turn leads to increased production of ketone bodies by the liver.
>
> There is also **marked hyperglycemia, ketonemia, ketonuria,** and **water and electrolyte imbalance.** Various features of the disease can be corrected by insulin administration.

UTILIZATION OF KETONE BODIES

Acetoacetate and β-hydroxybutyrate, which are produced by the liver, can be used as a source of energy in the peripheral tissues, such as kidney and muscle. Although, glucose is the major fuel for brain in the well-nourished state, but during starvation even brain starts utilizing ketone bodies.

The process of the **oxidation of ketone bodies** is called **ketolysis.**

Oxidation of β-Hydroxybutyrate

A mitochondrial enzyme, **β-hydroxybutyrate dehydrogenase, oxidizes β-hydroxybutyrate to acetoacetate.**

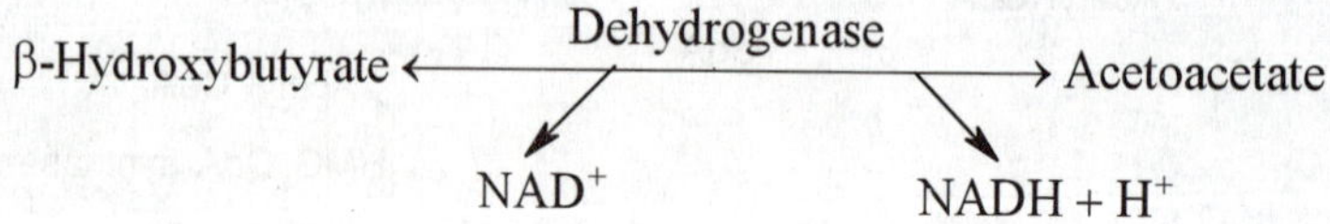

Oxidation of Acetoacetate

Acetoacetate is oxidized after its **activation to acetoacetyl CoA.** Since liver does not contain this enzyme, ketone bodies can not be oxidized in the liver.

Acetoacetate reacts **with succinyl CoA,** in the presence of the enzyme **transacylase** (acetoacetate-succinyl CoA transferase, **also called thiophorase)**, and is converted to **acetoacetyl CoA** (Fig. 13.10).

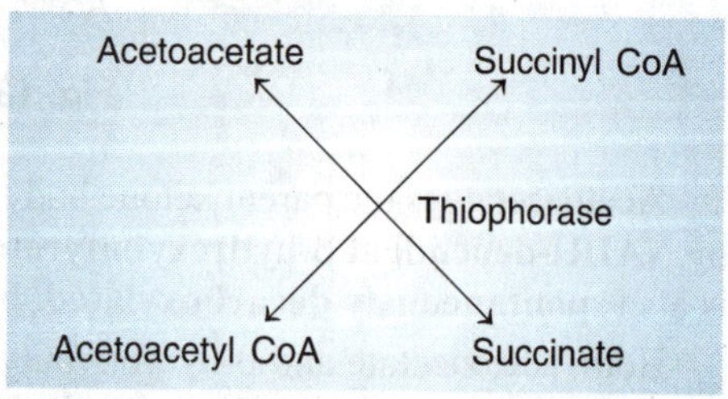

Fig. 13.10. Activation of acetoacetate by thiophorase.

Thereafter, **acetoacetyl CoA is hydrolyzed to two molecules of acetyl CoA, by the enzyme thiolase** (β-ketothiolase).

$$\text{Acetoacetyl CoA} \xrightarrow[\text{CoA}]{\text{Acetoacetyl CoA thiolase}} 2\ \text{Acetyl CoA}$$

Acetone is oxidized very slowly. The lungs mainly remove it.

FATTY ACID SYNTHESIS

Mammals can synthesize a major portion of the saturated as well as monounsaturated fatty acids. First, a saturated, straight chain, 16 carbon containing fatty acid, i.e. palmitic acid, is synthesized, which is subsequently changed to other fatty acids.

The process of fatty acid synthesis is called **de novo synthesis.** In human beings, fatty acid synthesis occurs, primarily in the cytosol in the liver, and the lactating mammary glands, and to a lesser extent in the adipose tissue.

DE NOVO SYNTHESIS

Acetyl CoA, which is produced in the mitochondria, first comes out of the mitochondria to the cytosol, where fatty acid synthesis occurs. Mitochondrial membrane however, is impermeable to CoA. Thus, first step in fatty acid synthesis is the transfer of the acetate units, from mitochondria to the cytosol. For this purpose, **acetyl CoA condenses with oxaloacetate and forms citrate. Citrate is then translocated from mitochondria to the cytosol,** where it is cleaved **by the enzyme ATP-citrate lyase and releases acetyl CoA and oxaloacetate, in the cytosol** (Fig. 13.11).

Acetyl CoA is then converted to malonyl CoA and is used in fatty acid synthesis.

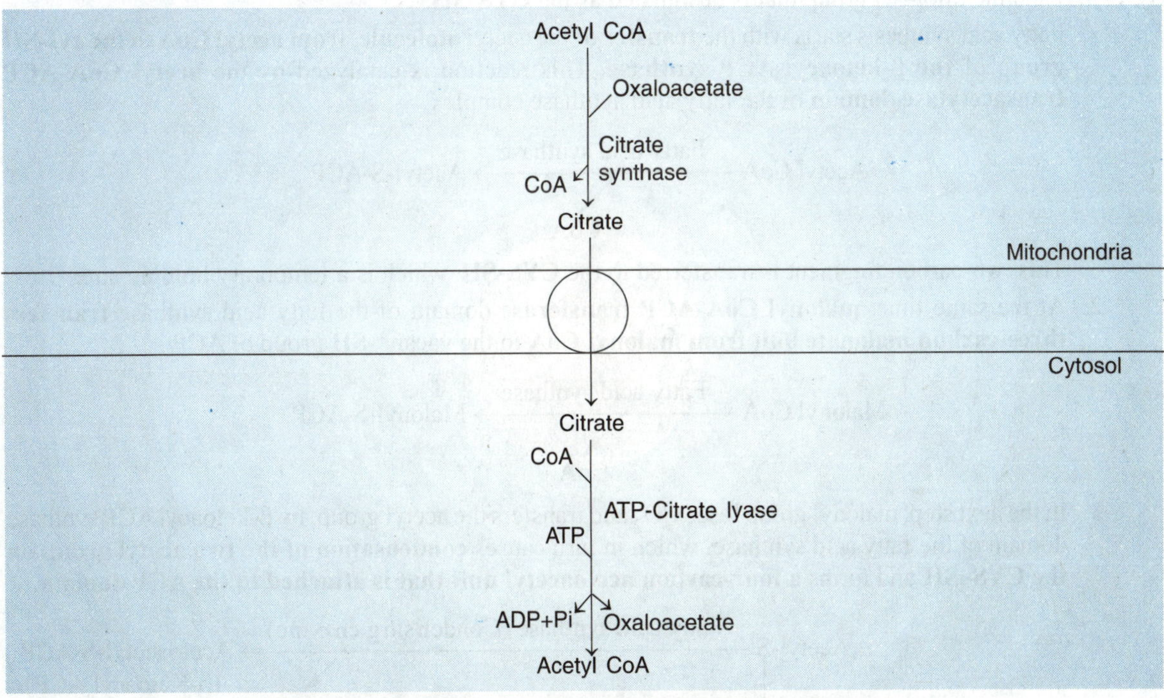

Fig. 13.11. Transport of acetyl CoA across the mitochondria.

Conversion of Acetyl CoA to Malonyl CoA

In the cytosol, **acetyl CoA** is carboxylated to **malonyl CoA** by a biotin-containing enzyme referred to as **acetyl CoA carboxylase.** This coenzyme is covalently linked to the lysyl residue of the enzyme, which requires ATP and CO_2 (HCO_3^-).

$$\text{Acetyl CoA} \xrightarrow[\text{CO}_2,\ \text{ATP},\ \text{Biotin},\ \text{Mn}^{2+}\ \rightarrow\ \text{ADP + Pi},\ \text{H}_2\text{O}]{\text{Acetyl CoA carboxylase}} \text{Malonyl CoA}$$

Prolonged consumption of high calories diet increases synthesis of the enzyme **acetyl CoA carboxylase** while fasting or low calories diet decreases its synthesis.

Synthesis of Palmitic Acid

An enzyme referred to as fatty acid synthase catalyzes the remaining reactions of fatty acid synthesis, in eukaryotes. It is a multifunctional, dimeric enzyme, composed of the two identical subunits. Its each monomer is a multicatalytic polypeptide with seven different enzyme activities plus a domain that covalently binds a molecule of 4′-phosphopantotheine.

In prokaryotes, fatty acid synthase consists of seven separate polypeptides. These include acyl carrier protein (ACP), besides six enzymes that are designated as **acetyl CoA-ACP transacetylase, malonyl CoA-ACP transferase,** β-ketoacyl-ACP synthase (**condensing enzyme),** β-keoacyl ACP **reductase,** β-hydroxyacyl ACP **dehydratase,** and enoyl-ACP **reductase. These enzyme activities** are separate catalytic domains that are present on each subunit of the multicatalytic fatty acid synthase complex.

Fatty acid synthase contains **two-SH groups,** called **pantotheinyl-SH group,** which is referred to as the **ACP-SH,** and the thiol-SH group that is designated as the **CYS-SH.**

1. Fatty acid synthesis starts with the **transfer of** the acetyl **molecule, from acetyl CoA to the cys-SH group of the β-ketoacyl-ACP synthase**. This reaction is catalyzed by the **acetyl CoA-ACP transacetylase domain** of the fatty acid synthase complex.

$$\text{Acetyl CoA} \xrightarrow[\rightarrow\ \text{CoA}]{\text{Fatty acid synthase}} \text{Acetyl-S-ACP}$$

   This two-carbon fragment is transferred to the **CYS-SH,** which is **a** temporary holding site.

2. At the same time, **malonyl CoA-ACP transferase** domain of the fatty acid synthase **transfers three-carbon malonate unit from malonyl CoA** to the vacant **-SH** group of ACP.

$$\text{Malonyl CoA} \xrightarrow[\rightarrow\ \text{CoA}]{\text{Fatty acid synthase}} \text{Malonyl-S-ACP}$$

3. In the next step, malonyl group loses CO_2 and transfers the acetyl group, by β-ketoacyl ACP synthase domain of the fatty acid synthase, which in turn causes **condensation of the two acetyl group on the CYS–SH** and forms **a four-carbon acetoacetyl unit that is attached to the ACP domain.**

$$\begin{array}{l}\text{Acetyl-S}\\ \quad |\\ \text{Malonyl-S-ACP}\end{array} \xrightarrow[\rightarrow\ \text{CO}_2]{\text{Fatty acid synthase (Condensing enzyme)}} \begin{array}{c}\text{Acetoacetyl-S-ACP}\\ (\beta\text{-Ketoacyl ACP})\end{array}$$

4. β-Ketoacyl ACP **reductase** domain of the fatty acid synthase reduces keto group of the **acetoacetyl-S-ACP to β-hydroxybutryl-S-ACP** (β-hydroxyacyl-S-ACP).

$$\underset{(\beta\text{-Ketoacyl ACP})}{\text{Acetoacetyl-S-ACP}} \xrightarrow[\text{NADPH + H}^+ \;\searrow\; \text{NADP}^+]{\text{Fatty acid synthase (Reductase)}} \underset{(\beta\text{-Hydroxyacyl-ACP})}{\beta\text{-Hydroxybutyryl-S-ACP}}$$

5. β-Hydroxyacyl-ACP **dehydratase domain** of the fatty acid synthase removes a molecule of H_2O from **β-hydroxyacyl-S-ACP** and introduces a double bond in it, to form crotonyl-S-ACP **(α, β-transbutenoyl-ACP** or α, β-unsaturated acyl-S-ACP).

$$\underset{(\beta\text{-Hydroxyacyl-ACP})}{\beta\text{-Hydroxybutyryl-S-ACP}} \xrightarrow[\searrow\; H_2O]{\text{Fatty acid synthase (Dehydratase)}} \underset{(\alpha,\beta\text{-Unsaturated acyl-S-ACP})}{\text{Crotonyl-S-ACP}}$$

6. **Crotonyl-S-ACP is reduced by the enoyl-ACP reductase domain** of the fatty acid synthase, and is converted **to butyryl-S-ACP** (acyl-S-ACP).

$$\underset{(\alpha,\beta\text{-Unsaturated acyl-S-ACP})}{\text{Crotonyl-S-ACP}} \xrightarrow[\text{NADPH + H}^+ \;\searrow\; \text{NADP}^+]{\text{Fatty acid synthase (Reductase)}} \underset{(\text{Acyl-S-ACP})}{\text{Butyryl-S-ACP}}$$

As a result of these reactions, a four-carbon compound is formed whose three terminal carbons are fully saturated and remain attached to ACP.

These steps are again repeated, beginning with the transfer of the butyryl chain to the CYS-SH. This cycle of the reactions is repeated five more times, each time incorporating two-carbon units that are derived from malonyl CoA, and are attached to the growing fatty acid chain at the carboxyl end. When the chain length reaches 16 carbons, the process is terminated with the formation of palmitoyl-S-ACP. Thereafter, **palmitoyl thioesterase cleaves the thioester bond with the release of palmitate** (Fig. 13.12).

$$\text{Palmitoyl-S-ACP} \xrightarrow{\text{Thioesterase}} \text{Palmitate}$$

Reducing equivalents (NADPH+H^+), which are used in the biosynthesis of fatty acids, are derived from the pentose phosphate pathway.

The overall reaction is:

$$\text{Acetyl CoA} + 7\ \text{Malonyl CoA} \xrightarrow[14\text{NADPH} + 14\text{H}^+ \;\searrow\; 14\text{NADP}^+]{\text{Fatty acid synthase}} \text{Palmitate} + 7CO_2 + 6H_2O + 8\text{CoA}$$

SYNTHESIS OF OTHER FATTY ACIDS

Palmitate, produced by the fatty acid synthase catalyzed reactions can be modified by:

- Chain elongation, and/or
- Desaturation.

Elongation

Chain elongation of a fatty acid occurs in the mammalian system by the addition of two-carbon units in the mitochondria and the endoplasmic reticulum.

In the Mitochondria

Chain elongation in the mitochondria takes place by the successive addition of acetyl CoA, as two carbon units, where both NADH as well as NADPH can be used as source of the reducing equivalents.

This is the process of the **reversal of β-oxidation** with the exception that NADPH-linked enoyl CoA reductase replaces FAD-linked acyl CoA dehydrogenase.

Firstly, **acyl CoA condenses with acetyl CoA** and **forms β-ketoacyl CoA,** which is subsequently reduced to β-hydroxyacyl CoA. Removal of a molecule of water converts β-hydroxyacyl CoA to α, β-unsaturated fattyacyl CoA (enoyl CoA), which is finally reduced to the higher member of the fatty acid (Fig. 13.13).

In the Endoplasmic Reticulum

The process of chain elongation in the endoplasmic reticulum is **similar to the process of de novo synthesis of fatty acid,** as occur in the cytosol. It utilizes malonyl CoA as a source of two-carbon unit but elongation occurs **as a CoA derivative of the fatty acid rather than the ACP-derivative.**

In most of the tissues, chain elongation in the endoplasmic reticulum converts palmitate to stearate.

Brain, however, has additional elongation capabilities, allowing it to produce very long chain fatty acids (up to 24-carbon atoms). These fatty acids are required for the synthesis of complex lipids, with in the brain.

Desaturation

Desaturation of a fatty acid (addition of the cis double bond) occurs in higher animals, in the endoplasmic reticulum, **by the enzyme desaturases,** which are the mixed function oxidases. Desaturation reaction requires NADPH and O_2 (Fig. 13.14).

Several polyunsaturated fatty acids can be synthesized through additional desaturation and

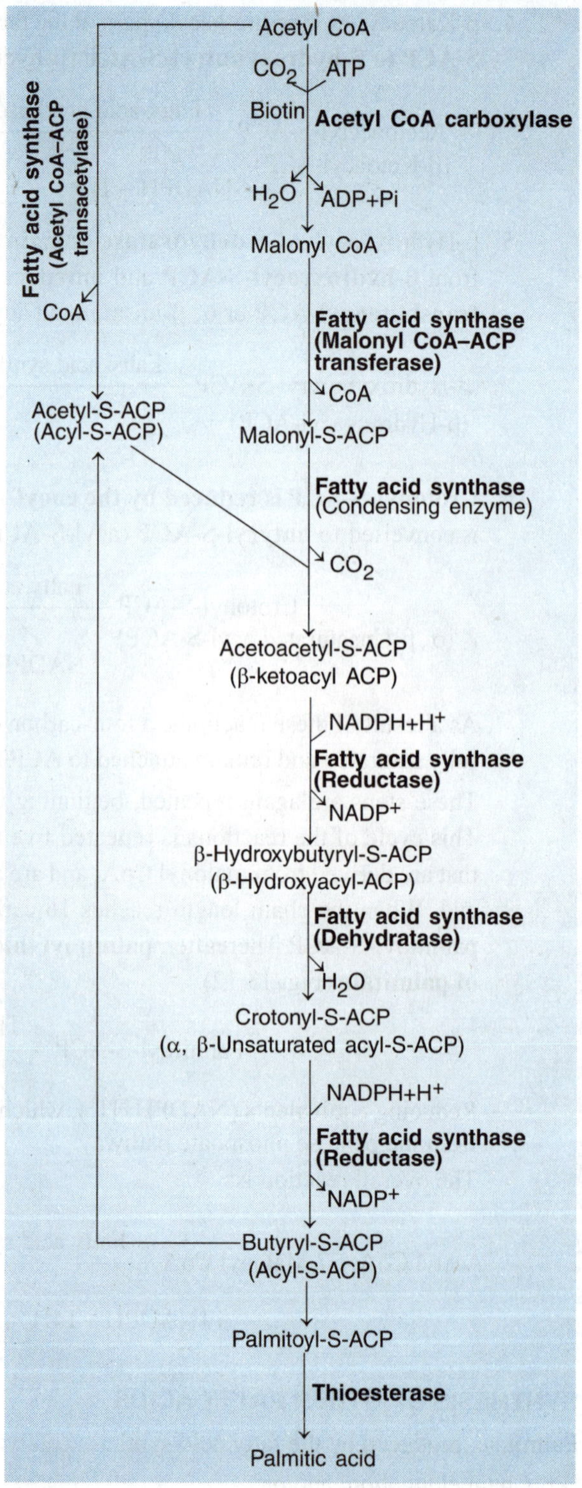

Fig. 13.12. De Novo synthesis of a fatty acid.

elongation. Human beings however, lack the ability to introduce a double bond prior to carbon-9, i.e. between carbon-9 and the ω-end of the chain.

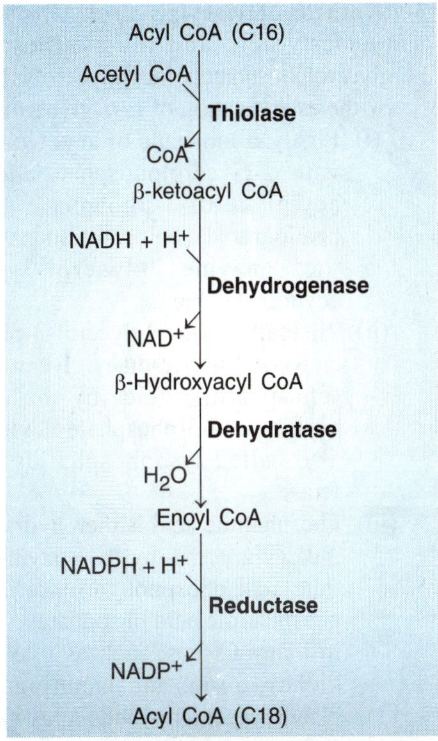

Fig. 13.13. Chain elongation of a fatty acid.

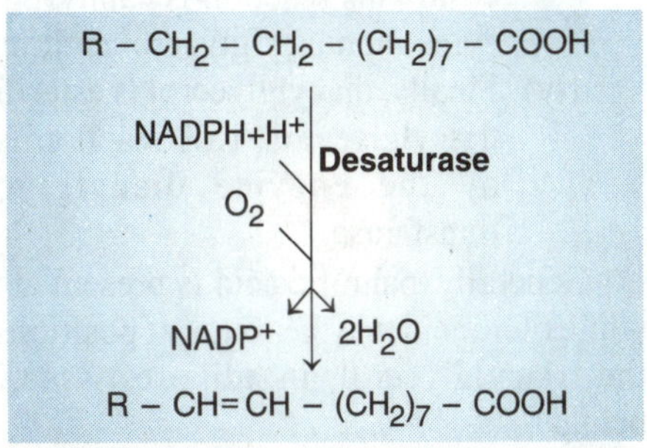

Fig. 13.14. Desaturation of a fatty acid.

REGULATION OF FATTY ACID SYNTHESIS

The rate-limiting step, in the synthesis of fatty acids, is the conversion of acetyl CoA to malonyl CoA. This reaction is catalyzed by the enzyme acetyl CoA carboxylase, which is stimulated by citrate.

Citrate, allosterically, **activates acetyl CoA carboxylase,** while a **long chain fattyacyl CoA** acts **as allosteric inhibitor.**

Insulin also **stimulates** activity of **this enzyme**. A high-carbohydrate diet increases production of acetyl CoA, which in turn increases the citrate pool. Thus, a high carbohydrate diet leads to increased fatty acid synthesis. Insulin also reduces cAMP level, inhibits activation of the hormone sensitive lipase, and favors lipogenesis.

On the other hand, **glucagon** increases cAMP level, activates lipase activity, and **inhibits fatty acid synthesis**. Glucagon thus, promotes release of fatty acids from the adipose tissue (lipolysis), and opposes lipogenesis.

Fatty acid synthase is the other key enzyme of the palmitate biosynthesis. **A high-carbohydrate diet** or a **fat-free diet stimulates** fatty acids synthase activity. On the other hand, **high fat diet, fasting,** and **glucagon** decrease enzyme synthesis.

Phosphorylated sugars, e.g. **glucose-6-phosphate**, also **activate** this enzyme.

LIPOGENESIS

Fatty acids are stored in the liver and adipose tissue in collaboration with glycerol, as triacylglycerols. The process of biosynthesis of triacylglycerol is called **lipogenesis.**

Lipogenesis occurs mainly, in the liver and the adipose tissue. It requires activation of free fatty acid and α-glycerolphosphate, and the re-esterification of glycerolphosphate (Fig.13.15).

1. **Activation of Fatty acid**: Free fatty acid, in the presence of ATP and CoA, is activated to fatty acyl CoA (Acyl CoA), by the family of fatty acyl CoA synthetases (thiokinases).
2. **Synthesis of glycerol phosphate**: There are two pathways for the production of glycerol phosphate:
   In the liver and the adipose tissue, L-α-glycerol-3-phosphate is formed by the reduction of dihydroxyacetonephosphate, an intermediate of the glycolytic pathway. This reaction is catalyzed by glycerol-3-phosphate dehydrogenase.
   Alternatively, in the tissue, such as liver, lactating mammary glands, kidney, and intestinal mucosa, glycerol is converted directly, to L-α-glycerol-3-phosphate, by the enzyme glycerol kinase.

3. **Synthesis of triacylglycerol**: After activation of the fatty acid and the synthesis of L-α-glycerolphosphate, triacylglycerol is synthesized by the esterification of L-α-glycerolphosphate:
   (i) Firstly, a molecule of acyl CoA combines with α-glycerolphosphate and forms 1-acylglycerol-3-phosphate (lysophosphatidic acid). This reaction is catalyzed by the enzyme glycerol-3-phosphate acyltransferase.
   (ii) Thereafter, 1-acylglycerol-3-phosphate is converted to 1,2-diacylglycerolphosphate (phosphatidic acid) by the enzyme 1-acylglycerol-3-phosphate acyltransferase, also called lysophosphatidylacyltransferase.
   (iii) Phosphatidic acid is then hydrolyzed to 1, 2-diacylglycerol by the enzyme phosphatidic acid phosphohydrolase, also called phosphatidic acid phsophatase.
   In many tissues, such as intestine, liver, kidney, aorta, and lactating mammary glands, especially in the intestinal mucosa, 1, 2–diacylglycerol is also formed from 2-monoacylglycerol, since monoacylglycerol is directly absorbed in the intestinal mucosa. This reaction is catalyzed by the enzyme monoacylglycerolacyltransferase.
   (iv) Finally, diacylglycerol is esterified to form triacylglycerol. This reaction is catalyzed by the enzyme diacylglycerolacyltransferase.

Generally, palmitic acid is present at position 1, while oleic acid may be found at positions 2 and 3 of the triacylglycerol, in adipose tissue, in human beings.

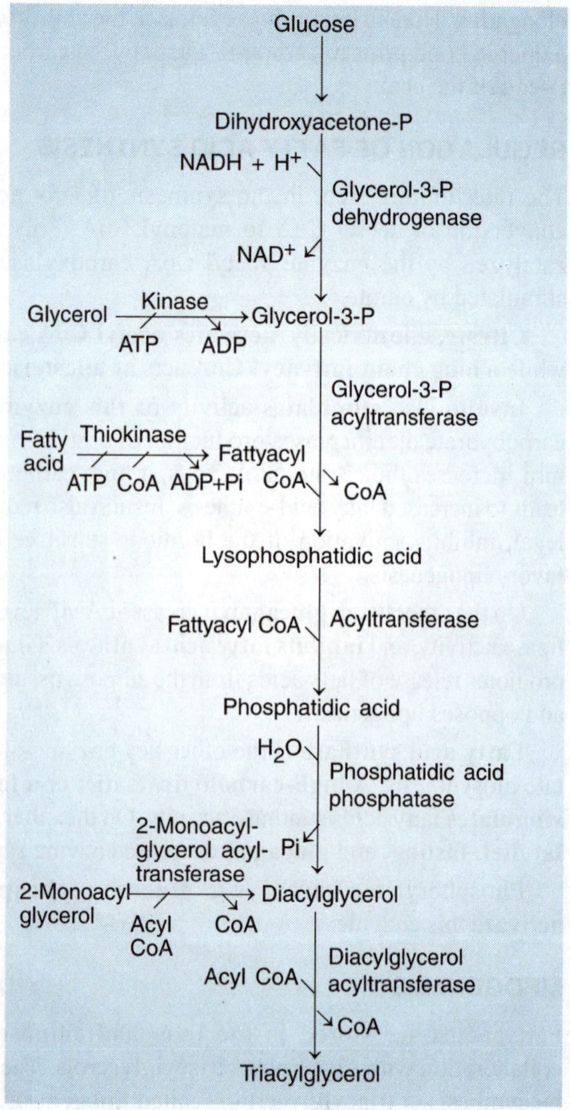

Fig. 13.15. Biosynthesis of triacylglycerol.

LIPOLYSIS

Only a little amount of triacylglycerol is stored **in the liver**. Most of it is exported, packaged with cholesteryl esters, cholesterol, phospholipids, and apolipoproteins, as very low-density lipoproteins.

Triacylglycerol is stored **in adipose tissue,** in the cytosol of the cell. It serves as depot fat, which is ready for mobilization, when body requires it as fuel.

Fatty acids that are stored in the adipose tissue in the form of **triacylglycerol are** mainly **oxidized for energy**. Mobilization of the stored fat requires hydrolytic release of the fatty acids and glycerol, from triacylglycerol. The enzyme called hormone-sensitive lipase, which removes fatty acids from carbon-1 and/ or 3 of a triacylglycerol, initiates this process. Additional lipases, which are specific for diacylglycerol and monoacylglycerol, remove the remaining fatty acids.

Utilization of these fatty acids, however, varies from tissue to tissue, depending upon the metabolic status of the tissue. Impairment in fatty acid oxidation may lead to hypoglycemia.

METABOLISM OF CHOLESTEROL

Cholesterol is derived **from diet**. It is **also synthesized in various tissues** in the body. About 50% of the normal intake of dietary cholesterol is absorbed by the small intestine while the rest of it is excreted in the feces.

Nearly 0.3 g of **cholesterol is absorbed** from the diet, daily. Ingested cholesterol is absorbed with other lipids and is incorporated into chylomicrons and VLDL. More than 80% of it is esterified in the intestinal mucosa and is transported with lipoproteins.

Cholesterol is **excreted from the body** either as fecal neutral sterol or as bile acid. About 600-750 mg of cholesterol is lost each day as bile acids, 500-600 mg in fecal neutral sterols, 75-100 mg is shed by the skin, and nearly 35-50 mg is converted into steroid hormones.

Cholesterol **content in normal human blood** varies from 130 to 220 mg/100 ml, being equally distributed between plasma and erythrocytes.

Only about 30% of the circulating cholesterol occurs **free**, while the remaining of it exists in the form of **cholesterol esters**. Usually, a long chain fatty acid is attached to the –OH group (by an ester linkage), on carbon 3 of the ring A of cholesterol.

CHOLESTEROL SYNTHESIS

A large quantity of cholesterol (about 1g/day) is synthesized in the extra-mitochondrial compartment of the cell. Important sites for cholesterol biosynthesis include liver, skin, intestine, adrenal cortex, and reproductive tissues, including ovaries, testes, and placenta.

All the carbon atoms of **cholesterol** are derived **from acetate** (acetyl CoA), which is obtained from several sources, such as oxidation of long chain fatty acids, ketogenic amino acids, and glucose (via pyruvate).

De novo synthesis of cholesterol takes place in the body, as shown in Fig. 13.16.

1. First, **two molecules of acetyl CoA** condense to **form acetoacetyl CoA.**

   This reaction is catalyzed by the enzyme **acetoacetyl CoA thiolase.**

   2 Acetyl CoA —(Thiolase)→ Acetoacetyl CoA + CoA

2. In the presence of the enzyme β-hydroxy-β-methylglutaryl CoA synthase **(HMG CoA synthase), acetoacetyl CoA** further **condenses with** another molecule of **acetyl CoA** and **forms** β-hydroxy-β-methylglutaryl CoA **(HMG CoA).**

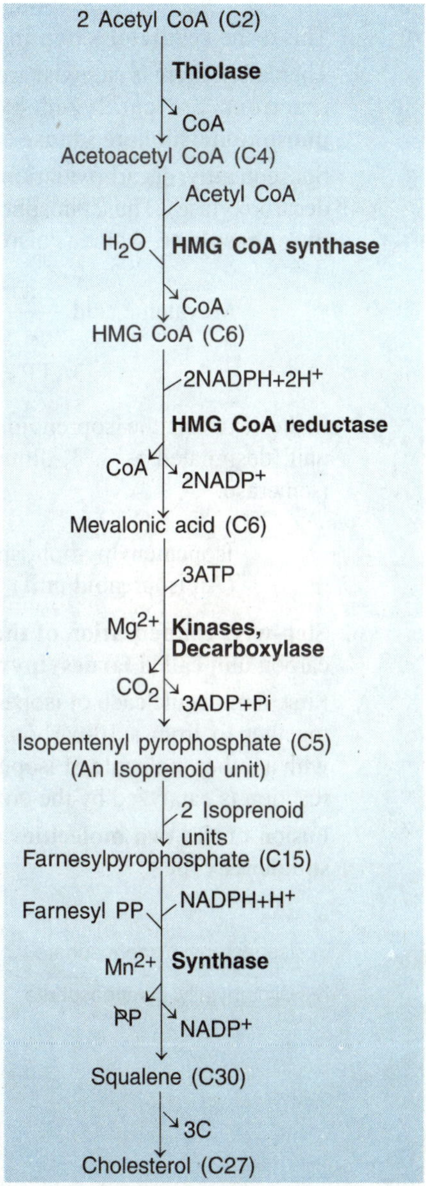

Fig. 13.16. Biosynthesis of cholesterol.

$$\text{Acetoacetyl CoA} + \text{Acetyl CoA} + H_2O \xrightarrow{\text{HMG CoA synthase}} \text{HMG CoA} + \text{CoA}$$

3. An NADPH dependent enzyme, **HMG CoA reductase**, converts HMG CoA to **mevalonic acid.**

$$\text{HMG CoA} + 2\text{NADPH} + 2H^+ \xrightarrow{\text{HMG CoA reductase}} \text{Mevalonic acid} + \text{CoA} + 2\text{NADP}^+$$

This is the **regulatory step** in cholesterol biosynthesis.

4. Thereafter, there is stepwise transfer of two γ-phosphate groups, from two molecules of ATP. These reactions are catalyzed by two kinases, called **mevalonate kinase** (enzyme I) and **phosphomevalonate kinase** (enzyme II).

   Subsequently, decarboxylation takes place by the enzyme decarboxylase (pyrophosphomevalonate decarboxylase). Thus, phosphorylation and decarboxylation of **mevalonic acid forms isopentenyl pyrophosphate,** which is also called as **active isoprenoid unit**.

$$\text{Mevalonic acid} + 3\text{ATP} \xrightarrow[Mg^{2+}]{\text{Kinases, decarboxylase}} \text{Isopentenylpyrophosphate (an isoprenoid unit; 5C)} + CO_2 + 3\text{ADP} + \text{Pi}$$

5. In the next step, the isoprenoid unit (isopentenyl pyrophosphate) is isomerised to another isoprenoid unit, designated as 3, 3,-dimethylallylpyrophosphate, by the enzyme isopentenylpyrophosphate isomerase.

$$\underset{\text{(An isoprenoid unit)}}{\text{Isopentenylpyrophosphate}} \xrightarrow{\text{Isomerase}} \underset{\text{(An isoprenoid unit)}}{\text{Dimethylallylpyrophosphate}}$$

6. **Step-wise condensation of the three-isoprenoid units (5C units)** leads to the formation of a 15-carbon unit called **farnesylpyrophosphate** (15C).

   First, a molecule each of isopentenylpyrophosphate and 3,3-dimethylallylpyrophosphate condense together to from a 10-carbon unit called geranylpyrophosphate (10C), which further condenses with another molecule of isopentenylpyrophosphate and forms farnesylpyrophosphate (15C). This reaction is catalyzed by the enzyme geranyltransferase (Fig. 13.17).

7. Fusion of the **two molecules of farnesylpyrophosphate forms a 30-carbon compound called squalence** (30C).

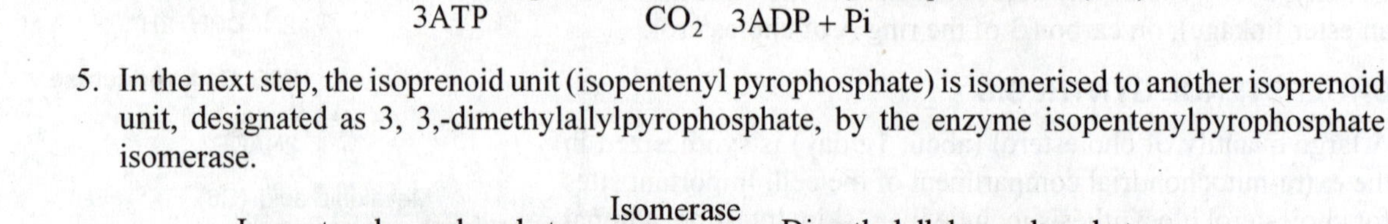

Fig. 13.17. Synthesis of farnesylpyrophosphate.

$$\text{2 Farnesylpyrophosphate} \xrightarrow[\text{NADPH + H}^+ \;\searrow\; 2PP \;\searrow\; NADP^+]{\text{Squalene synthase, } Mn^{2+}} \text{Squalene (30C)}$$

8. By ring closure and removal of the three methyl groups, **squalene is converted to cholesterol,** which has 27 carbons.

$$\text{Squalene} \xrightarrow[\searrow 3C]{} \text{Cholesterol (27C)}$$

Regulation of cholesterol synthesis

Dietary cholesterol, feedback inhibition, and its disposal from the liver regulate cholesterol synthesis.

Dietary cholesterol: Rate of de novo synthesis of cholesterol is inversely related to the amount of dietary cholesterol. When dietary cholesterol is reduced, cholesterol synthesis is increased in the liver and the intestine, to meet needs of the other tissues.

On the other hand, when dietary cholesterol is increased, its synthesis is reduced.

Feed back inhibition: Cholesterol inhibits its own synthesis, by feed back inhibition. The enzyme HMG CoA reductase regulates cholesterol synthesis. Cholesterol inhibits the activity of HMG CoA reductase, by suppressing its synthesis and promoting inactivation.

Disposal by the liver: In a normal healthy adult, on a low cholesterol diet, about 1300 mg of cholesterol is returned to the liver, each day.

Liver removes cholesterol by different processes:

(i) **Esterification of cholesterol:** Both, HDL and lecithin:cholesterol acyltransferase (LCAT) are important for the removal of cholesterol from the body.

LCAT is a plasma enzyme, which is produced mainly, by the liver. It transfers one fatty acid from carbon 2 of lecithin to the 3-hydroxyl group of cholesterol. This reaction is freely reversible and utilizes cholesterol, which is present in **HDL**.

$$\text{Cholesterol + Lecithin} \xleftrightarrow{\text{LCAT}} \text{Cholesterol ester + Lysolecithin}$$

Cholesterol esters so formed diffuse into the core of the HDL particle, where they are transported from the tissues and plasma, to the liver, which is the only organ that is capable of metabolizing and excreting cholesterol.

This is referred to as the **reverse transport of cholesterol** since HDL provides the vehicle for the transport of cholesterol, from the peripheral tissues to the liver.

(ii) **Excretion of cholesterol**: Free cholesterol as well as bile acids/salts are excreted in the bile.

(iii) **Incorporation of cholesterol into VLDL:** In the liver, cholesterol is incorporated into VLDL and is secreted into circulation.

CHOLESTEROL UTILIZATION

Free cholesterol is present in abundance, **in bile.** It is also present in large amounts **in the myelin structure in the brain.** Cholesterol also occurs in the esterified form **in the cell membrane.**

Cholesterol is also a precursor of the **bile acids, steroid hormones,** and **vitamin D** (Fig. 13.18).

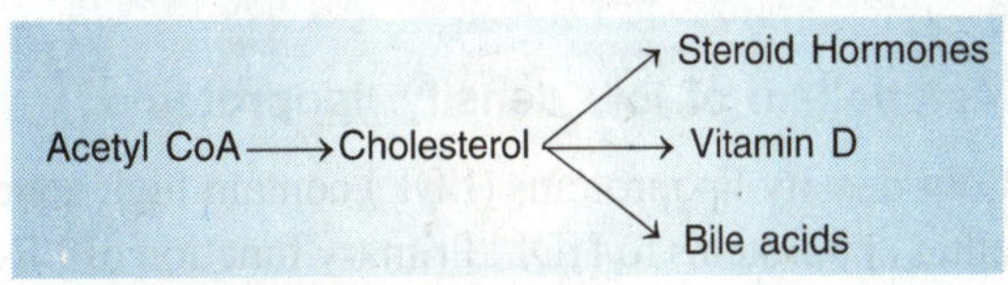

Fig. 13.18. Metabolic fates of cholesterol.

METABOLISM OF LIPOPROTEINS

Metabolism of chylomicrons

Chylomicrons are triglyceride rich particles that are assembled in the intestinal mucosal cells. They carry dietary triacyglycerols, cholesterol, and cholesteryl esters to peripheral (extrahepatic) tissues.

Intestinal mucosal cells release nascent chylomicrons, which contain apo B-48, which is synthesized in the intestine. These nascent chylomicrons **receive apo E and apo C from** the circulating **HDL**. Apo CII in turn activates lipoprotein lipase and hydrolyzes triacylglycerols to monoacylglycerols, free fatty acids, and glycerol. As a result of **hydrolysis of triacylglycerol, by lipoprotein lipase**, chylomicrons decrease in size and increase in density. Thereafter, **apo C is returned to HDL** and the **leftover particles are called chylomicron remnants** (Fig. 13.19).

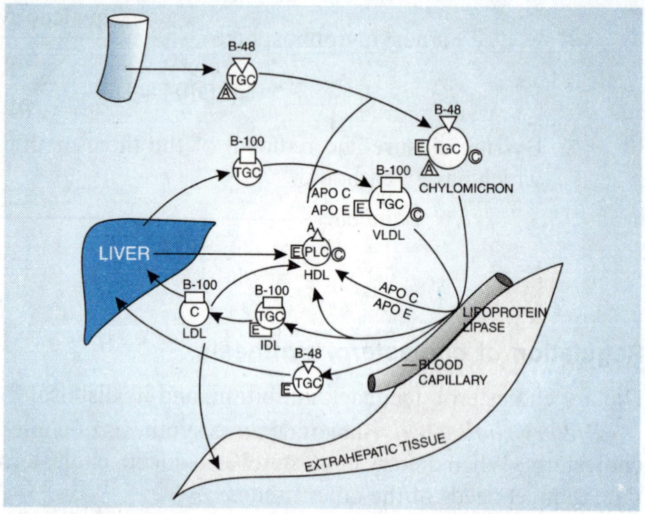

Fig. 13.19. Metabolism of various lipoproteins.

Chylomicron remnants bind to apo E receptors on hepatocytes. They are then internalized and their lipids, including cholesteryl esters, are either utilized or stored, intracellularly.

A small amount of the released free fatty acids enters the circulation and contributes to plasma free fatty acids pool.

Metabolism of very low density lipoproteins

Very low-density lipoproteins (VLDL), also called pre β-lipoproteins, are composed of triacylglycerols, like chylomicrons but their function is to transport lipids from liver to the peripheral tissues.

VLDL is **released from the liver as nascent VLDL,** similar to the release of nascent chylomicrons from the intestinal mucosa. Nascent VLDL particles contain apo B-100 and apo A-1. Subsequently, they **acquire apo C-II and apo E from the circulating HDL.**

During circulation, **lipoprotein lipase hydrolyses triacylglycerols and releases free fatty acids,** which are taken up by the peripheral tissues. **Apo C and apo E are transferred to HDL**. In addition, cholesteryl esters, which are synthesized in the plasma, as a result of the action of lecithin cholesterol acyltransferase (LCAT) on HDL, are transferred from HDL to VLDL and IDL via cholesteryl ester transfer protein (CETP). As a result of it,, their particle size is reduced and density is increased. **VLDL particles** are hence **converted into VLDL remnants**, which are also designated as **intermediate density lipoproteins (IDL).**

IDL particles are removed by the liver and converted to the LDL.

Metabolism of low density lipoproteins

Low-density lipoproteins (LDL) contain high concentration of cholesterol. They retain apo B-100 and lose other apoproteins to HDL. Primary function of LDL is to transport cholesterol from liver to the extrahepatic tissues.

LDL bind to its receptor, which are present in the cell membrane. The LDL receptors are negatively charged glycoproteins that are clustered in the pits on the cell membrane and recognize apo B-100, which in turn acts as a ligand between the IDL and its receptor. The intracellular side of the pit is coated with a protein called clathrin, which stabilizes shape of the pit.

Ability of the tissue to take up LDL depends upon the rate of transcapillary transport as well as the number of receptors. The number of these receptors is regulated by cholesterol content of the cell.

After binding, LDL particles are **internalized by endocytosis**, in the form of vesicles. These **vesicles** rapidly loose clathrin coat, **fuse with the other vesicles,** and **form endosomes** (large vesicles). This in turn results in **separation of LDL particles from their receptors**.

Receptors are recycled whereas **endosomes contents are degraded;** resulting in **release of cholesterol,** free fatty acids, phospholipids, and amino acids.

Free cholesterol is used for membrane biosynthesis, or is converted to steroid hormones. Excess of the cholesterol, however, is re-esterified by acylcholesterol acyltransferase (ACAT), and is stored.

In man, 70-80% of LDL is removed by LDL receptors while rest of it is removed by the nonspecific endocytosis via the scavenger pathway. The latter is also a receptor-mediated process involving phagocytic cells, in the reticuloendothelial system.

Metabolism of high density lipoproteins

High density lipoprotein (HDL) particles are synthesized in the liver and **are released into the blood stream,** by exocytosis.

These secretary HDL particles are called **nascent HDL** and are discoid in shape. Nascent HDL is composed of apo A, apo E, phospholipids, and free cholesterol.

There also occurs **transfer of apo C** from the chylomicrons and VLDL **to nascent HDL,** which are converted to **mature HDL, called HDL_3.**

From HDL_3, cholesteryl esters (produced by the action of LCAT) are shifted to VLDL and IDL. At the same time, HDL_3 acquires triacylglycerols and is converted to **HDL_2**.

This is an important mechanism for the removal of excess cholesterol from the peripheral tissues and is referred to as the **reverse transport of cholesterol.**

HDL performs several functions:

1. HDL serves as a circulating reservoir of apo C-II, which in turn is transferred to the chylomicrons and VLDL as an activator of lipoprotein lipase.
2. It removes free cholesterol from the extrahepatic tissues and esterifies it with the help of lecithin cholesterol acyltransferase (LCAT), which is present in plasma. HDL thus, transports cholesterol from the extrahepatic tissues to liver.
3. HDL transfers cholesteryl esters to VLDL and LDL, in exchange of triacyglycerols and phospholipids from there.
4. HDL also carries cholesteryl esters to the liver.

In the liver HDL is degraded and releases cholesterol, which is either repacked in the lipoproteins or is converted to bile acids and secreted into bile, for its removal from the body. Elevated levels of HDL in plasma thus, protect against atherosclerosis.

ATHEROSCLEROSIS

Atherosclerosis (arteriosclerosis) is a disease of arterial wall. It is characterized by the accumulation **of cholesterol** and its ester in cells, which are derived from monocyte-macrophage line smooth muscle cells. This in turn results in the formation of **atherosclerotic plaque, which narrows the blood vessels** and serves as the site of thrombus formation.

High caloric diet or diet rich in saturated fat and cholesterol, hypercholesterolemia, sedentary life style, stress and strain, obesity, hypertension, and smoking are important contributory factors, favorable in the development of atherosclerosis.

Risk of developing the disease is directly related to the concentration of the LDL-cholesterol, in plasma. It is also inversely related to the plasma concentration of HDL-cholesterol. Therefore, **LDL-cholesterol is called as the bad cholesterol** while **HDL-cholesterol** is referred to as **good cholesterol**.

Drugs like **cholestyramine** bind bile salts and promote their excretion in stool. This in turn **increases the rate of bile salt synthesis** and LDL uptake by the liver. **Lovastatin**, the drug that is used in the treatment of **hyperlipidemia**, is an **inhibitor of the enzyme HMG CoA reductase**. Hence, it decreases endogenous synthesis of cholesterol and stimulates LDL uptake (via LDL receptors) by the tissues.

APPROACH TO TREATMENT

Dietary recommendations

1. Reduce the total amount of fat. Not more than 30% of total energy intake should come from fat.
2. Reduce the use of animal fat. Not more than one third of the total fat (less than 10% calories/day) should come from saturated animal fat, with the remainder coming from unsaturated (plant) fat.
3. Reduce the intake of cholesterol. Dietary cholesterol should be less than 300 mg/day.
4. Trans-fatty acids intake should limit to less than 1% calories/day.
5. Increase omega-3 fatty acid intake from dietary or supplementary fish oils.
6. Eat five or more servings of fruits and vegetables/day.
7. Reduce salt intake.

OTHER LIFE-STYLE INTERVENTIONS

In addition to dietary advice, other life-style interventions include:

- Promotion of physical activity, e.g. adults should perform at least 30 minutes of moderate activity (brisk walking), at least 5 days per week. Maintaining ideal body weight emphasizes activity.
- Limit sedentary activities and give up smoking.

LIPOPROTEINS DISORDERS

Hyperlipoproteinemias

Increased rate of synthesis or reduced clearance of lipoproteins from blood may result in a group of disorders, referred to as hyperlipidemias or hyperlipoproteinemias.

Usually, they are detected by measuring plasma triacylglycerol and cholesterol (Table 13.1).

Hypolipoproteinemias

Abetalipoproteinemia: This is **due to** the **absence of apo B**. As a result of it, all the plasma lipids, particularly, triacyglycerols are reduced. Fat malabsorption is present from birth. There is also poor appetite, vomiting, diarrhea, and failure to thrive in neonates.

Table 13.1. Primary hyperlipoproteinemias

Type		*Elevated lipoprotein fraction*
I	Exogenous hyperlipidemia (Exogenous hypertriglyceridemia)	Chylomicron
IIa	Hypercholesterolemia	LDL
IIb	Combined hyperlipidemia	LDL + VLDL
III	Remnant hyperlipidemia	Remnant VLDL
IV	Endogenous hyperlipidemia	VLDL
V	Mixed hyperlipidemia	VLDL + chylomicrons

Familial Hypobetalipoproteinemia: **Low level of apo B** results in moderate reduction of plasma lipids. VLDL and LDL are low while HDL concentrations are variable.

Tangier Disease: It is the HDL deficiency state where plasma triacylglycerol and VLDL levels are normal or moderately increased. LDL is rich in triacylglycerols. Plasma total cholesterol as well as LDL-cholesterol levels are reduced by about 2/3rd while HDL-cholesterol is extremely low. Apo AI is around 1% of the concentration normally found in plasma and apo AII about 5-8% of the normal. Besides apo AI and apo AII, there is also a moderate **reduction in** other **apoproteins.**

SERUM LIPID PROFILES

Serum lipids and lipoproteins **should be measured after a 10 hours fast** because chylomicrons normally may be present in plasma up to 10 hours after a meal.

Serum may appear hazy when the level of triglycerides exceeds 200 mg/dl. Chylomicrons can be readily detected, because they form a white supernatant layer after refrigeration. **For differentiation of disorders of lipoproteins, triglycerides and total cholesterol are routinely measured.** The measurement of plasma total cholesterol is a first line-screening test. **Most of the cholesterol present in the plasma is in the LDL.** Similarly, **plasma triglyceride concentrations** are a matter of the **sum of total of VLDL and IDL.** To obtain a more accurate picture of lipid metabolism, we measure/calculate cholesterol present in the LDL and HDL fractions.

The fasting lipid profile, i.e. the **concentration of total cholesterol, LDL-cholesterol, HDL-cholesterol and triglycerides,** provides information about the main **lipid markers of cardiovascular risk.** The **LDL cholesterol to HDL cholesterol ratio** indicates the balance between cholesterol transport to and from peripheral tissues. A **ratio above 5 indicates an increased cardiovascular risk.**

Dividing the value of triglyceride by 5 gives the concentration of VLDL-cholesterol in plasma.

VLDL–Cholesterol (mg/dl) = Triglyceride/5

LDL–Cholesterol concentration in plasma can also be calculated from the value of total cholesterol, triglycerides and HDL-cholesterol as follows:

LDL cholesterol (mg/dl) = Total cholesterol – [HDL cholesterol + Triglyceride/5]

A large number of specialized investigations including ultracentrifugation, apolipoproteins and enzyme studies and molecular genetic studies may occasionally be helpful. **Other biochemical** cardiovascular risk factors or **markers include troponin, myoglobin, homocysteine and C-reactive protein.**

In about 95% of the patients with **primary hypercholesterolemia, plasma cholesterol concentration is** usually **raised**, as the abnormality is due to a combination of dietary factors and a number of genetic abnormalities in handling cholesterol.

In-patients with familial hypertriglyceridemia plasma triglyceride (VLDL) concentration is increased since this condition is associated with defects either in the production or in the catabolism of VLDL.

In familial combined hyperlipidemia, there may be **increased plasma LDL only, increased plasma VLDL only, or increase in both**

SOME IMPORTANT QUESTIONS

1. Outline β-oxidation of fatty acids. How much energy is produced when a molecule of palmitic acid is oxidized to acetyl CoA?
2. Outline de novo synthesis of fatty acid. What is the source of reducing equivalents? How de novo fatty acid synthesis differs from fatty acid elongation in the microsomes and the mitochondria.
3. Outline cholesterol synthesis. Add a note on its relationship with atherosclerosis.
4. Describe briefly:
   - (i) Role of carnitine in fatty acid oxidation
   - (ii) Degradation of cholesterol
   - (iii) Process of β-oxidation of fatty acid
   - (iv) Synthesis of cholesterol and its regulation
   - (v) Oxidation of fatty acids containing odd number of carbon atoms
5. Write notes on:
   - (i) Ketone bodies
   - (ii) ω-oxidation
   - (iii) Atherosclerosis
   - (iv) De novo synthesis of fatty acids
   - (v) Sudden infant death syndrome
   - (vi) α-oxidation of fatty acids
   - (vii) Refsum disease
   - (viii) Lipofuscin
   - (ix) Metabolic fates of acetyl CoA
   - (x) Metabolic fates of cholesterol
   - (xi) LCAT
   - (xii) Diabetic ketoacidosis

CHAPTER

14

Metabolism of Proteins

Proteins are degraded to amino acids, which contribute to the amino acid pool. They are used for protein biosynthesis. Excess of them is also used for energy. They are also the important source of nitrogen for the body.

PHYSIOLOGICAL FUNCTIONS OF AMINO ACIDS

Amino acids perform several important functions in the body:

1. Amino acids are used as a source of energy. Some of the amino acids are glucogenic while others are ketogenic in nature, which are used for energy.
2. All amino acids are degraded to release ammonia, which is excreted as urea.
3. Some of the amino acids are used in the synthesis of various specialized products, such as phosphocreatine.
4. Amino acids like methionine are used in transmethylation reactions.
5. Aromatic amino acids are used for the synthesis of amines, such as dopamine.
6. Several amino acids are important in one-carbon transfer, such as glycine, histidine, etc.
7. Some of the amino acids, such as glycine and glutamine, are important in detoxification.

PROTEIN UTILIZATION FOR ENERGY

Catabolism of amino acids involves removal of α-amino groups followed by breakdown of the resulting carbon skeletons. These pathways form various intermediate products, which directly enter different metabolic pathways, resulting either in the synthesis of glucose or lipid, or in the production of energy through their oxidation to CO_2 and water by the citric acid cycle.

A large proportions of the amino acids, within the cells, are incorporated into proteins, which are constantly being synthesized and degraded. Excess of these dietary amino acids are not simply excreted but are degraded to common metabolites and are used as metabolic fuels.

GLUCOGENIC AND KETOGENIC AMINO ACIDS

Carbon skeletons of amino acids, after the removal of α-amino group as ammonia, **form amphibolic intermediates, which** can be **converted to** either **glucose or ketone bodies.** For example, transamination of **alanine, glutamate, and valine** forms pyruvate, α-ketoglutarate, and succinyl CoA, respectively. As these are the **intermediates of the citric acid cycle** and can be converted to glucose by gluconeogenesis, these amino acids are called **glucogenic amino acids.**

Catabolism of some other amino acids, such as phenylalanine, in addition to an intermediate of the citric acid cycle, also **forms acetyl CoA or acetoacetyl CoA**, which are the precursors of the ketone bodies. Therefore, **these amino acids are** referred as **both, glucogenic and ketogenic.**

Leucine is purely a ketogenic amino acid as the end products of its catabolism are acetyl CoA and acetoacetyl CoA. Lysine is also a ketogenic amino acid as the end product of its catabolism is acetoacetyl CoA.

End products of the catabolism of different amino acids and their metabolic fates are shown in Table 14.1.

Table 14.1. Metabolic fates and end products of the catabolism of different amino acids

Metabolic fates of amino acids	*End products of their catabolism*
Glucogenic	
Gly, Ala, Ser, Cys, HO-Pro	Pyruvate
Glu, Gln, Pro, Arg, His	α-Ketoglutarate
Val, Met	Succinyl CoA
Asp, Asn	Oxaloacetate
Glucogenic and ketogenic	
Ile	Succinyl CoA and Acetyl CoA
Phe and Tyr	Fumarate and Acetoacetyl CoA
Trp	Pyruvate and Acetoacetyl CoA
Thr	Pyruvate and Acetyl CoA
Ketogenic	
Leu	Acetyl CoA and Acetoacetyl CoA
Lys	Acetoacetyl CoA

AMMONIA METABOLISM

There are two processes by which the α-**amino group can be removed** from amino acids. These are referred to as **transamination** and **deamination.**

TRANSAMINATION

Transamination is a process of **transfer of the α-amino group** from an **amino acid to a keto acid.** As a result of it, the **amino acid is converted to a keto acid** while the **keto acid is converted to an amino acid** (Fig. 14.1).

Enzymes, which catalyze transamination, are called **transaminases (aminotransferases).**

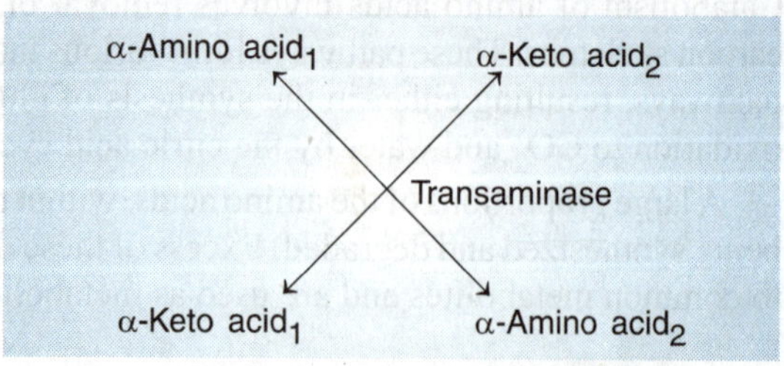

Fig. 14.1. Process of transamination.

Although liver contains transaminases for all the amino acids (except for threonine and lysine), most important of these transaminases are glutamate pyruvate transaminase (GPT, also called alanine **amino-transferase** or ALT) and glutamate oxaloacetate transaminase (GOT, also called **aspartate aminotransferase** or AST). These two transaminases catalyze the following reactions:

$$\text{Alanine} + \alpha\text{-Ketoglutarate} \underset{B_6}{\overset{GPT}{\longleftrightarrow}} \text{Pyruvate} + \text{Glutamate}$$

$$\text{Aspartate} + \alpha\text{-Ketoglutarate} \underset{B_6}{\overset{GOT}{\longleftrightarrow}} \text{Oxaloacetate} + \text{Glutamate}$$

An obligate amino acid or the α-keto acid, which participates in these reactions, is either glutamate or α-ketoglutarate.

During the process of transamination, the amino acid first reacts with the coenzyme pyridoxal-5-phosphate (PLP), and forms **Schiff's base**. Coenzyme in turn becomes protonated and is subsequently hydrolyzed to release the α-keto acid of the corresponding amino acid while retaining the α-amino group ($-NH_2$). Pyridoxal-5-phosphate thus gets aminated and is converted to pyridoxamine-5-phosphate. Thereafter, a α-keto acid combines with the coenzyme bound amino group (pyridoxamine-5-phosphate) which in turn releases the keto acid as a new amino acid and regenerates the coenzyme (Fig. 14.2).

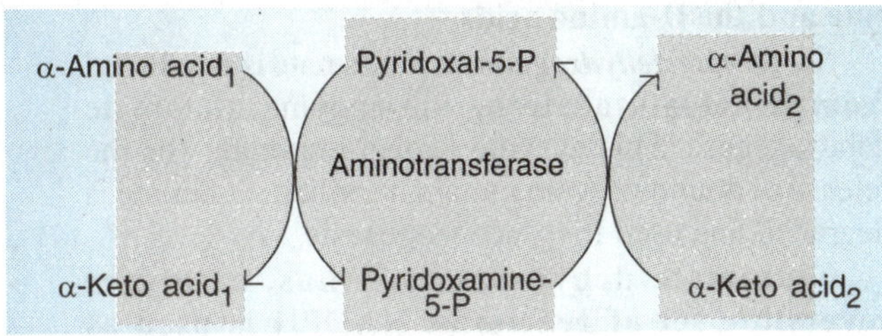

Fig. 14.2. Role of pyridoxal-5-phosphate in transamination.

DIAGNOSTIC SIGNIFICANCE OF TRANSAMINASES

Serum GOT and GPT have diagnostic significance. They are present in large amounts in cardiac muscle and liver, respectively. Although serum levels of both the enzymes are raised in heart as well as liver diseases, **SGOT is markedly raised in myocardial infarction** while **SGPT is more increased in liver disorders,** such as viral hepatitis or toxic liver necrosis (Table 14.2).

Table 14.2. Diagnostic significance of transaminases

Enzyme	*Comparatively more raised in*
SGOT	Cardiac disorders, e.g. myocardial infarction
SGPT	Liver disorders, e.g. viral hepatitis

DEAMINATION

Process of removal of the α-amino group from amino acids is referred as deamination. Liver and kidney are the main organs, which are responsible for the deamination of amino acids. Deamination may take place either by oxidative or nonoxidative process.

Oxidative Deamination

Liver and kidney contain several **enzymes, which catalyze deamination** of amino acids, such as amino acid oxidases, glutamate dehydrogenase, etc.

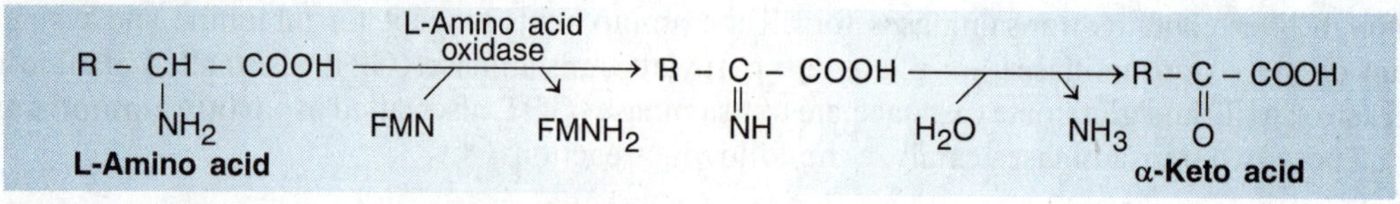

Fig. 14.3. Oxidative deamination.

Amino acid oxidases: L-amino acid oxidase is linked to FMN (the prosthetic group) and catalyzes the oxidation of an L-amino acid producing α-keto acid, ammonia, and water as the final products (Fig. 14.3).

Some of the tissues also contain **FAD-linked D-amino acid oxidases,** which **catalyze oxidation of glycine and the D-amino acids.**

Glutamate dehydrogenase: Glutamate **is produced from α-ketoglutarate** by the enzyme glutamate dehdrogenase. This enzyme is also important for the release of ammonia from glutamate, when glutamate is degraded and used for gluconeogenesis.

Glutamate dehydrogenase thus, catalyzes reversible set of reactions. NADPH is used as coenzyme in the synthetic reaction while NAD^+ is used in the degradative reaction (Fig. 14.4).

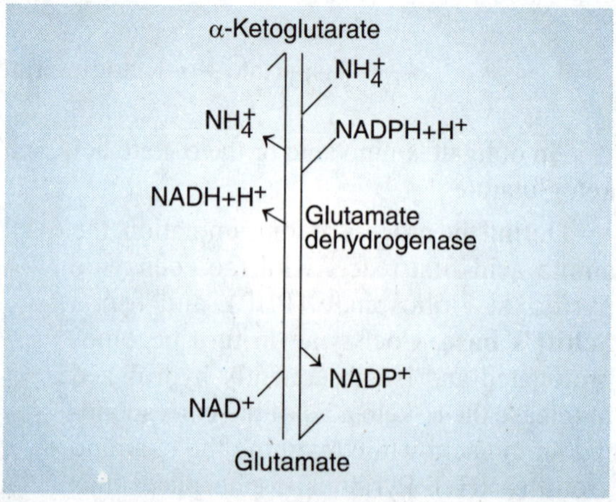

Fig. 14.4. Glutamate dehydrogenase reactions.

Nonoxidative Deamination

Dehydratase, sulfhydrase and histidase catalyze deamination of some of the amino acids, such as serine, cysteine and histidine, respectively. They catalyze dehydration followed by nonoxidative deamination of the amino acid, spontaneously, (Fig. 14.5).

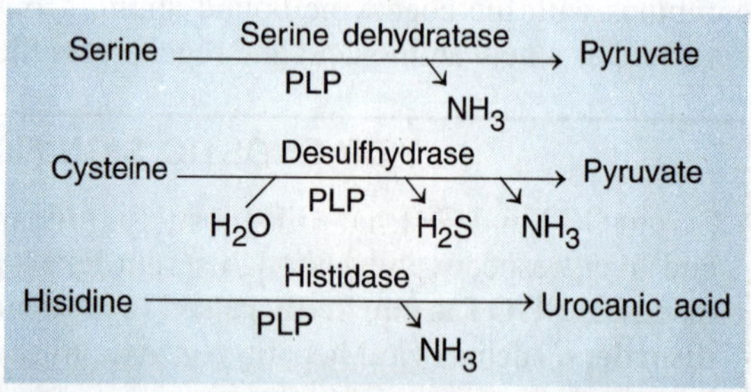

Fig. 14.5. Nonoxidative deamination of amino acids.

Metabolic Fates of Ammonia

Ammonia is removed as glutamine from the brain or converted to urea by urea cycle in the liver.

FORMATION OF GLUTAMINE

From the brain, ammonia is removed as glutamine. This reaction is catalyzed by the enzyme **glutamine synthetase.**

Glutamine is transported to the kidney, where **glutaminase** removes the amide group from glutamine as ammonia, which is excreted in the urine (Fig. 14.6).

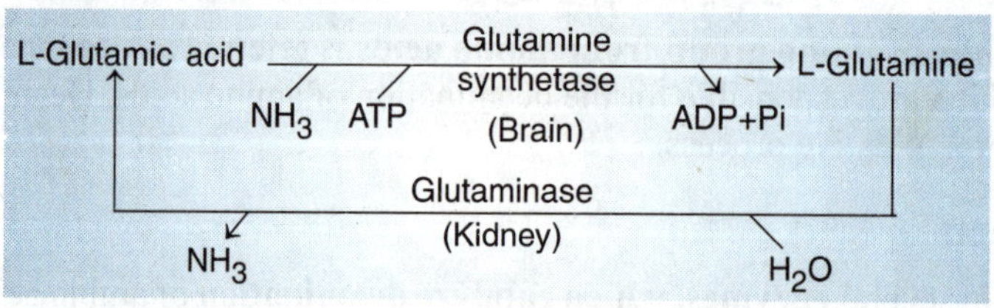

Fig. 14.6. Formation and disposal of glutamine.

UREA FORMATION

Urea cycle is the process by which ammonia that is a highly toxic substance, is converted to urea, which is a less toxic, water-soluble, excretory waste product, in the liver (Fig. 14.7).

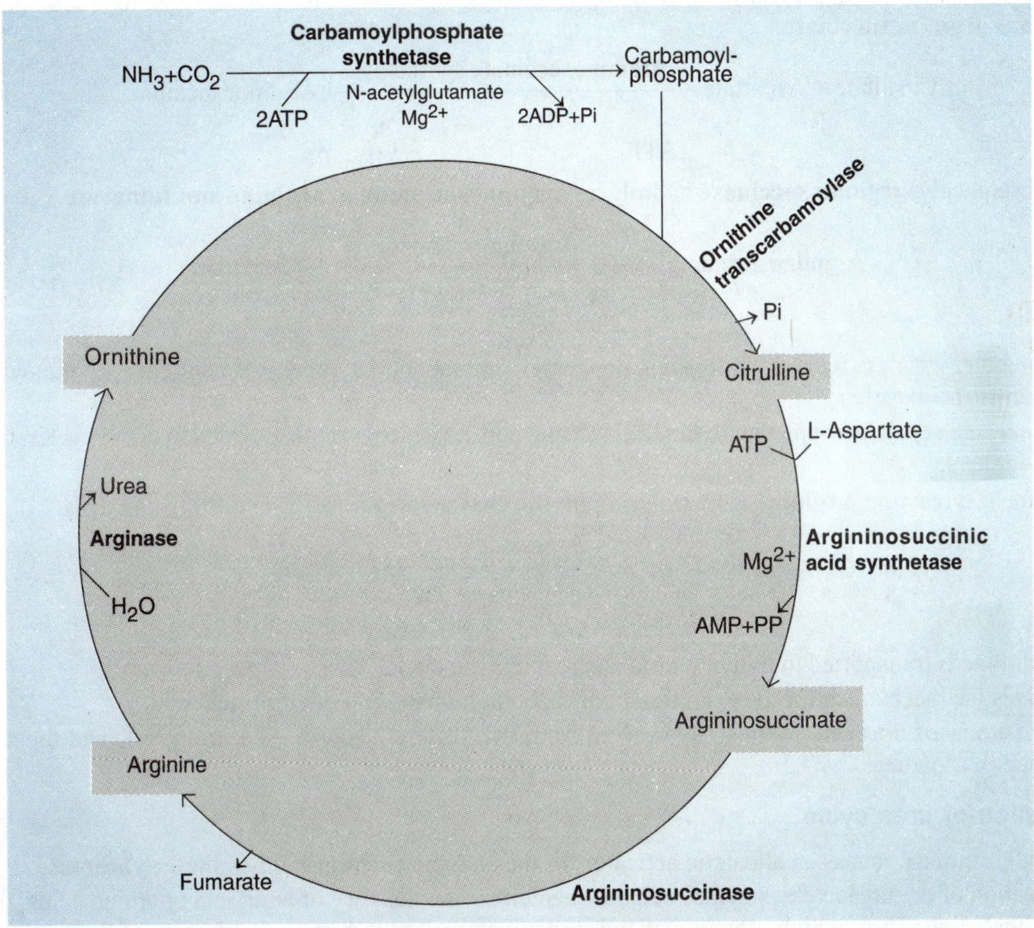

Fig. 14.7. The process of urea cycle.

1. In the first step, **ammonia reacts with carbon dioxide** and **forms carbamoylphosphate,** in the mitochondria.
   This reaction is catalyzed by the enzyme **carbamoylphosphate synthetase** (CPS), which requires N-acetylglutamate as coenzyme.

$$CO_2 + NH_3 \xrightarrow[\text{N-Acetylglutamate}]{\text{CPS}} \text{Carbamoylphosphate}$$
$$\text{(2ATP} \rightarrow \text{2ADP + Pi)}$$

2. **Thereafter, ornithine transcarbamoylase transfers carbamoyl group from carbamoylphosphate to ornithine,** and forms **citrulline.**

$$\text{Carbamoylphosphate} + \text{Ornithine} \xrightarrow{\text{Ornithine transcarbamoylase}} \text{Citrulline} + \text{Pi}$$

3. In the presence of the enzyme **argininosuccinate synthetase, citrulline** combines with L-aspartate, and **forms argininosuccinate.**

$$\text{Citrulline} + \text{Aspartate} \xrightarrow[\text{ATP} \;\rightarrow\; \text{AMP + PP}]{\text{Argininosuccinate synthetase}} \text{Argininosuccinate}$$

4. Subsequently, **argininosuccinase** hydrolyzes **argininosuccinate** to **arginine and fumarate.**

$$\text{Argininosuccinate} \xrightarrow{\text{Argininosuccinase}} \text{Arginine} + \text{Fumarate}$$

Fumarate, which is released in this reaction, enters mitochondria where it is converted to oxaloacetate via citric acid cycle.

Hence, urea cycle is coupled with the Krebs cycle, both of which were discovered by Sir Hans Krebs and Coworkers.

5. In the last reaction, **arginine** is hydrolyzed, **by the enzyme arginase,** to **ornithine** and **urea**.

$$\text{Arginine} \xrightarrow[H_2O]{\text{Arginase}} \text{Ornithine} + \text{Urea}$$

Ornithine is transported to mitochondria and reenters the cycle.

This is the mechanism for the excretion of nitrogen in humans and other primates.

Two atoms of nitrogen, in urea, are derived from two different sources, i.e. from NH_3 and the amino group of aspartate.

Regulation of urea cycle

N-acetylglutamate acts as an allosteric activator for the enzyme **carbamoylphosphate synthetase**.

Induction of the urea cycle enzymes occurs when either the delivery of ammonia or amino acids, to the liver, is increased. Thus, a high protein diet and starvation result in induction of enzymes of the urea cycle.

Inborn errors of urea cycle

Inborn errors of various enzymes of the urea cycle have been reported (Table 14.3).

Since ammonia is very toxic, a metabolic disorder of urea cycle may result in coma and may be potentially fatal.

Table 14.3. Inborn errors of Urea Cycle

Enzyme	*Disorder*
Carbamoylphosphate synthetase	Hyperammonemia type I
Ornithine transcarbamoylase	Hyperammonemia type II
Argininosuccinate synthetase	Citrullinemia
Argininosuccinase	Argininosuccinic aciduria
Arginase	Hyperargininemia

METABOLISM OF AROMATIC AMINO ACIDS

METABOLISM OF PHENYLALANINE

As men and most animals cannot synthesize aromatic ring hence, phenylalanine is dietary essential. Under normal conditions, dietary phenylalanine that is not incorporated into proteins is converted to tyrosine.

CONVERSION TO TYROSINE

Conversion of phenylalanine to tyrosine is catalyzed by phenylalanine hydroxylase (Fig. 14.8).

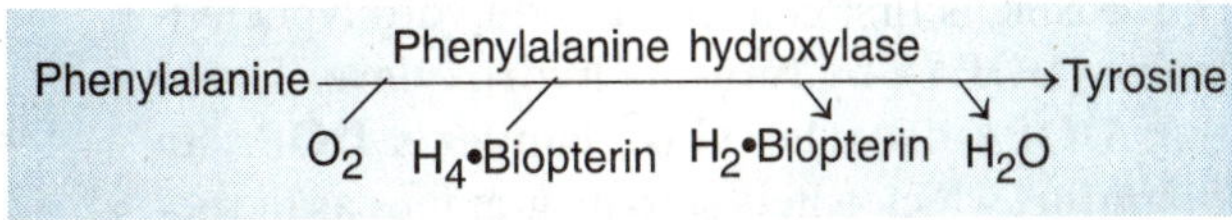

Fig. 14.8. Conversion of phenylalanine to tyrosine.

METABOLISM OF TYROSINE

As tyrosine can be synthesized from phenylalanine, tyrosine is dietary nonessential.

In the liver, tyrosine, is transaminated **to p-hydroxyphenylpyruvate, by tyrosine aminotransferase** (tyrosine transaminase). It is an inducible enzyme whose synthesis is increased by gluco-corticoids as well as phenylalanine/tyrosine.

In the next step, a copper containing enzyme **p-hydroxyphenylpyruvate oxidase, converts p-hydroxyphenylpyruvate to homogentisic acid.**

p-Hydroxyphenylpyruvate oxidase is a complex which requires ascorbic acid and catalyses decarboxylation, oxidation, migration of the side chain as well as its hydroxylation.

Subsequently, an iron-containing enzyme, **homogentisic acid oxidase, oxidizes homogentisic acid.**

Subsequent reactions, catalyzed by **maleylacetoacetate isomerase** and **fumarylacetoacetate hydrolase, result in the formation of the end product** of tyrosine catabolism, i.e. **fumarate and acetoacetate** (Fig. 14.9).

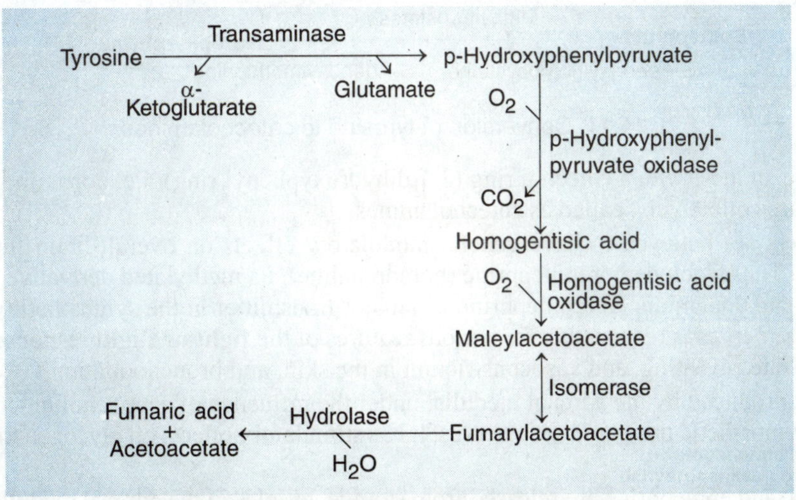

Fig. 14.9. Degradation of tyrosine in the liver.

METABOLIC FATES OF PHENYLALANINE/TYROSINE

Phenylalanine and tyrosine serve as precursors for a number of biologically active compounds, in different tissues (Fig. 14.10).

Synthesis of Catecholamines

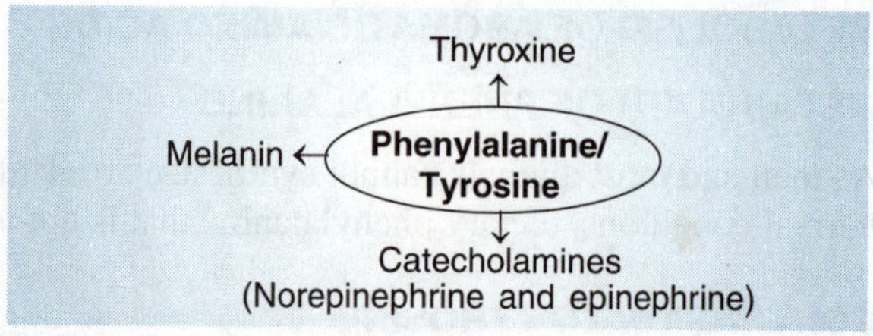

Fig. 14.10. Metabolic fates of phenylalanine/tyrosine.

In the adrenal medulla, tyrosine is converted to norepinephrine (noradrenaline) and epinephrine (adrenaline), which are the two hyperglycemic hormones, secreted by the gland.

Tyrosine is first converted to dihydroxyphenylalanine **(DOPA), by tyrosine hydroxylase.** Thereafter, **DOPA-decarboxylase converts DOPA to dopamine,** which enters storage granules as the active neurotransmitter. **Dopamine is** then **converted to norepinephrine, by dopamine-β-hydroxylase.**

Norepinephrine is a hormone, present in sympathetic nerve endings. Its synthesis is regulated by plasma tyrosine in the brain.

Methylation of norepinephrine, by phenylethanolamine-N-methyltransferase (PNMT), **forms epinephrine**. In this reaction active methionine (S-adenosylmethionine) is used as a methyl donor (Fig. 14.11).

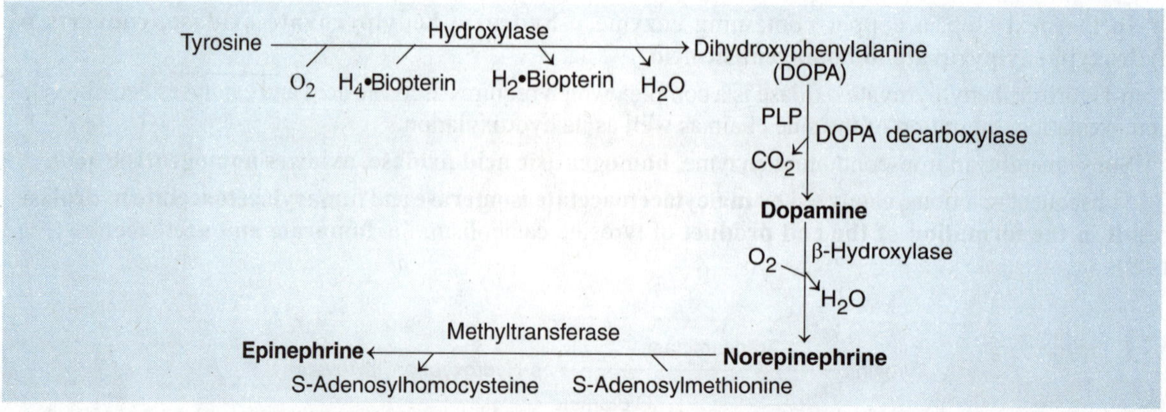

Fig. 14.11. Conversion of tyrosine to catecholamines.

These aromatic amines, with a catechol ring (3,4-dihydroxyphenyl ring), i.e. dopamine, norepinephrine and epinephrine, are collectively, called as catecholamines.

Catecholamines are believed to have general modulatory effects on overall brain functions, such as mood and arousal. These include norepinephrine (noradrenaline), its methylated derivative, called epinephrine (adrenaline), and dopamine. Norepinephrine is a major transmitter in the sympathetic nervous system. Stimulation of these nerves is responsible for various features of the **fight or flight** response, such as stimulation of the heart rate, sweating, and vasoconstriction in the skin, and bronchodilation.

Epinephrine is produced by the adrenal medulla, under the influence of acetylcholine-containing nerves analogous to the sympathetic pre-ganglionic nerves. It has stimulatory effects on glycogen metabolism in the liver.

Norepinephrine and epinephrine are released from storage vesicles in the adrenal medulla, in response to stress, exercise, cold, and low levels of blood glucose. They increase degradation of glycogen and triacylglycerol as well as increase blood pressure and the output of the heart.

Dopamine is an intermediate in the synthesis of norepinephrine. It is a neurotransmitter in nerves that interconnect the nuclei of the basal ganglia in the brain, and controls voluntary movement. Damage to these nerves causes Parkinson's disease, which is characterized by tremors and difficulties in initiating and controlling movement.

Synthesis of Melanin

In the melanocytes, tyrosine is converted to melanin.

Tyrosine is first converted to DOPA, and **then to dopaquinone,** by the enzyme **tyrosinase** (a copper-containing protein). Subsequently, dopaquinone **forms melanin,** a brown-black pigment, which is found in the skin, hair and retina (Fig. 14.12).

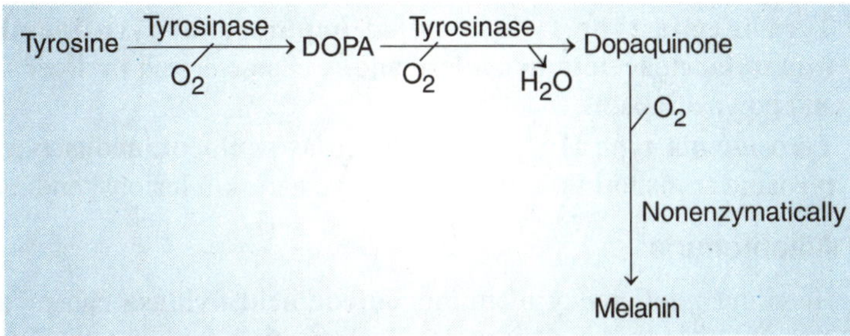

Fig. 14.12. Conversion of tyrosine to melanin.

Synthesis of Thyroid Hormones

In the thyroid gland, iodination of tyrosyl- residues of the thyroglobulin results in the synthesis of thyroid hormones.

Various inborn errors of phenylalanine/tyrosine metabolism are shown in Table 14.4.

Table 14.4. Inborn errors of phenylalanine/tyrosine metabolism

Metabolic Disorder	Deficient Enzyme
Phenylketonuria	Phenylalanine hydroxylase
Tyrosinemia type I	Fumarylacetoacetate hydrolase
Tyrosinemia type II	Tyrosine transminase
Alkaptonuria	Homogentisic acid oxidase
Albinism	Tyrosinase

INBORN ERRORS OF PHENYLALANINE/TYROSINE METABOLISM

Phenylketonuria

Autosomal recessive deficiency of hepatic **phenylalanine hydroxylase** results in a condition called **phenylketonuria.**

The alternative pathway catabolizes excess of phenylalanine, which cannot be converted to tyrosine. It is transaminated to phenylpyruvic acid, which is subsequently reduced to phenyllactic acid as well as decarboxylated to phenylacetic acid (Fig. 14.13).

Due to increased urinary excretion of phenylpyruvic acid (a phenylketone), this disease is called as phenylketonuria. Increased levels of phenylketoacids in the blood cause mental retardation and convulsions.

Such infants are given low phenylalanine diet and under these conditions tyrosine becomes dietary essential.

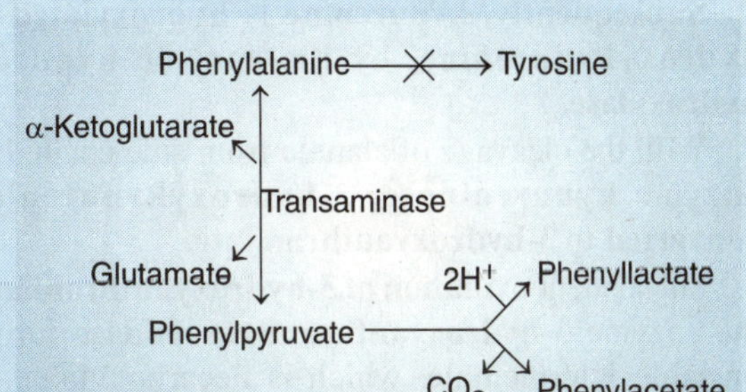

Fig. 14.13. Metabolism of phenylalanine in phenylketonuria.

Tyrosinemias

A complete or partial **deficiency of tyrosine aminotransferase** may result in **tyrosinemia,** which in turn leads to accumulation and excretion of tyrosine and its metabolites. Tyrosinemias are of two types:

Tyrosinemia type I: It is called **hepatorenal tyrosinemia**. It is caused by the **deficiency of fumarylacetoacetate hydrolase** and is characterized by liver failure, renal tubular dysfunction, rickets and polyneuropathy.

Tyrosinemia type II: It is also called as **oculocutaneous tyrosinemia**. It is due to the **deficiency of tyrosine transaminase.** It results in eye and skin lesions, and mental retardation.

Alkaptonuria

Hereditary **deficiency of homogentisic acid oxidase** causes **alkaptonuria.** Such individuals excrete homogentisic acid in their urine. Homogentisic acid, in turn, gets auto-oxidized and polymerized to form intensely dark substance, referred to as **alkapton**.

Dark urine is the only consequence of this condition, in early life. Homogentisate is slowly oxidized and deposited in the bone, connective tissue and other organs. This condition is called as **ochronosis** because of ochre color of the pigment.

Albinism

Lack of tyrosinase, in the melanocytes, affects the synthesis of melanin and leads to the formation of white patches on the skin and iris in the eyes. This condition is referred to as **albinism**.

Lack of the pigment in the skin makes these albinos more sensitive to sunlight and increases the risk of carcinoma of skin. Lack of the pigment in the eyes contributes to photophobia.

METABOLISM OF TRYPTOPHAN

Tryptophan is an **essential** amino acid, containing an **indole ring.**

The major pathway for degradation of tryptophan is called as the **kynurenine-anthranilate pathway.**

Degradation of tryptophan begins with the opening of the indole ring, which in turn results in the formation of **N-Formylkynurenine.** This reaction is catalyzed by a heme containing enzyme **tryptophan pyrrolase,** also called as **tryptophan oxygenase,** which is a dioxygenase. This enzyme is found in the liver, and is induced by glucocorticoids and glucagon.

With the removal of the formate, **formylkynurenine is converted to kynurenine,** by the enzyme **formylase.**

Subsequently, kynurenine is **hydroxylated to 3-hydroxykynurenine, by** the enzyme **kynurenine hydroxylase.**

With the cleavage of alanine from side chain, by the enzyme **kynureninase, 3-hydroxykynurenine is converted to 3-hydroxyanthranilate.**

Subsequent **oxidation of 3-hydroxyanthranilate,** by the enzyme **3-hydroxyanthranilate oxidase** forms an unstable intermediate, which is decarboxylated to **2-amino-3-carboxymuconate-6-semialdehyde**. Through a number of steps, it is then **converted to acetoacetyl CoA** (Fig. 14.14).

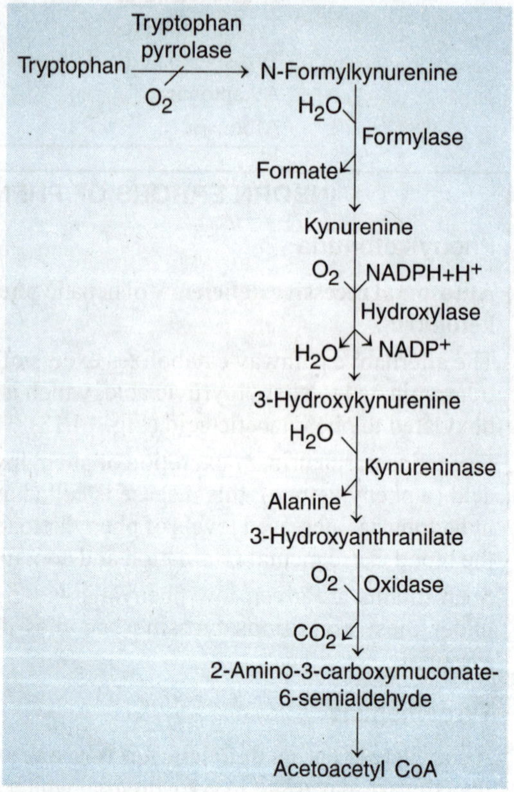

Fig. 14.14. Degradation of tryptophan in the liver.

METABOLIC FATES OF TRYPTOPHAN

Metabolic fates of tryptophan are shown in Fig. 14.15.

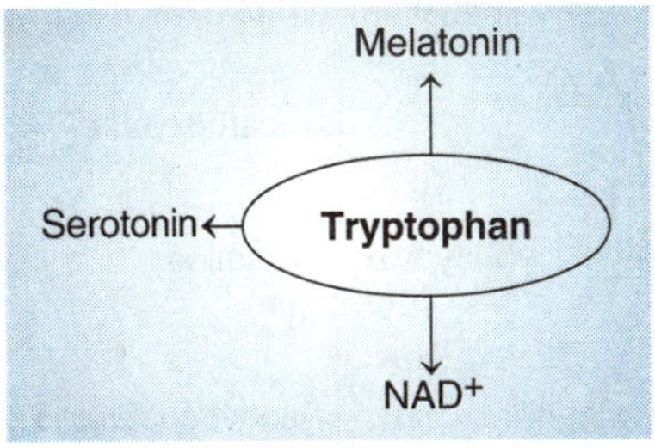

Fig. 14.15. Metabolic fates of tryptophan.

Synthesis of NAD

Kynurenine-anthranilate pathway is also important for the synthesis of NAD^+. In the liver and some other tissues, tryptophan is catabolized to an unstable intermediate referred to as 2-acroleyl-3-aminofumarate. Nonenzymatic **cyclization of it forms quinolinic acid.** Thereafter, **quinolinate phosphoribosyltransferase (QPRT) transfers a ribonucleotide moiety from phosphoribosylpyrophosphate** (PRPP) and **leads to the synthesis of nicotinate mononucleotide**, which is finally converted to NAD^+ (Fig. 14.16).

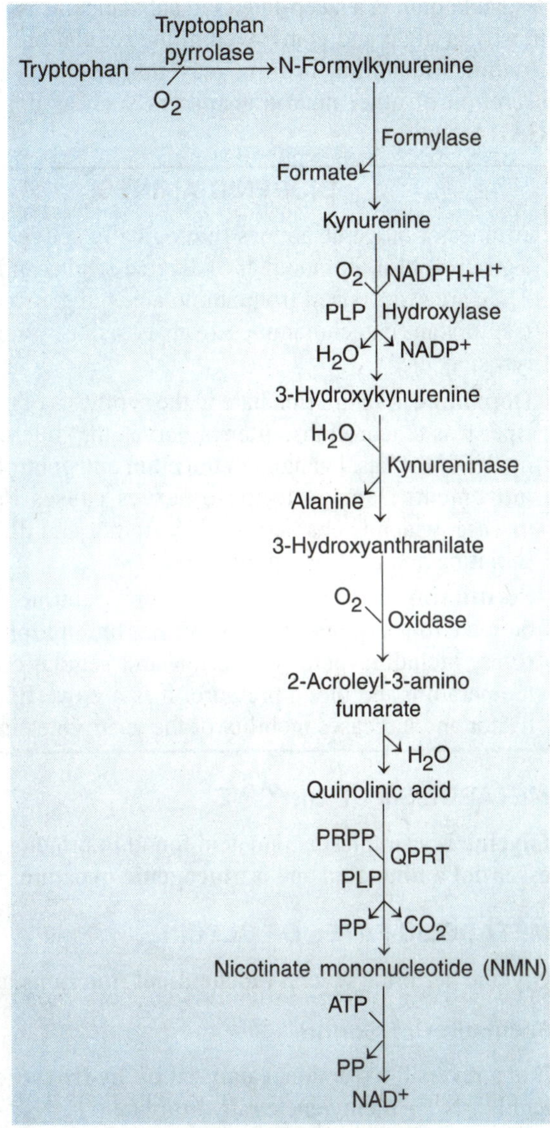

Fig. 14.16. Synthesis of NAD^+.

Synthesis of Serotonin

In platelets, brain and intestinal epithelium **tryptophan is hydroxylated by tryptophan hydroxylase to 5-hydroxytryptophan,** which is subsequently **decarboxylated to 5-hydroxytryptamine** (serotonin), **by a decarboxylase** (Fig. 14.17).

Serotonin is a neurotransmitter and causes contraction of smooth muscle of arterioles and bronchioles.

Synthesis of Melatonin

Acetyltransferase, present **in the pineal gland** and the retina, **synthesizes melatonin** (N-acetyl-5-methoxytryptamine) **from tryptophan** (Fig. 14.18).

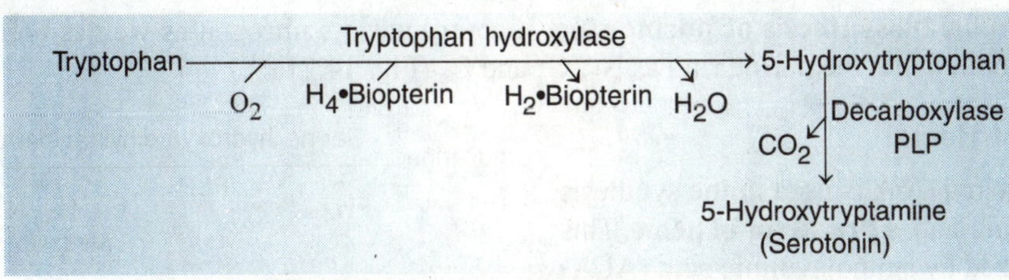

Fig. 14.17. Conversion of tryptophan to serotonin.

Melatonin is a sleep-inducing substance. It is synthesized mostly at night and is involved in the regulation of circadian rhythm. Melatonin, in turn, may inhibit the synthesis and secretion of other neurotransmitters such as dopamine and GABA.

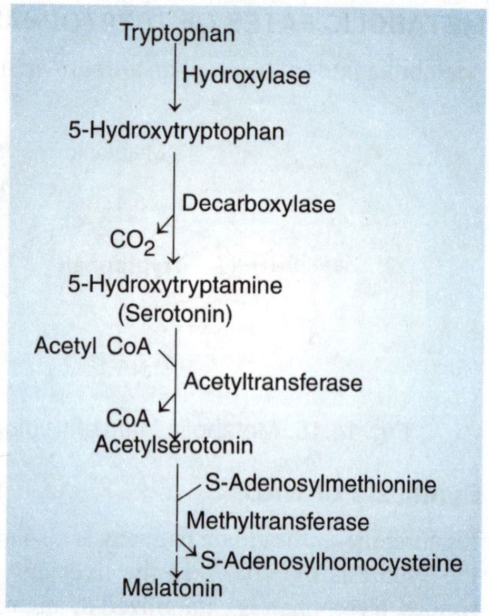

Fig. 14.18. Synthesis of melatonin.

BIOGENIC AMINES

Amines or biogenic amines (biologically active amines) are a group of basic compounds of diverse origins and functions. They are synthesized from amino acids, e.g. serotonin from tryptophan, catecholamines from tyrosine, tyramine from tyrosine, etc.

Dopamine is an intermediate in the synthesis of norepinephrine. It is a neurotransmitter in nerves that interconnect the nuclei of the basal ganglia in the brain and control voluntary movement. Damage to these nerves causes Parkinson's disease, which is characterized by tremor and difficulties in initiating and controlling movement.

Serotonin, also called 5-hydroxytryptamine (5-HT), is derived from tryptophan. Serotonin has multiple physiological roles, including pain perception and regulation of sleep, temperature and blood pressure. It is a powerful vasoconstrictor and increases mobility of the gastrointestinal tract.

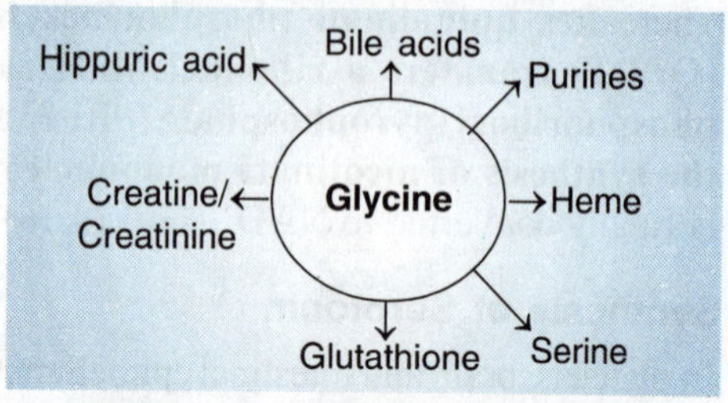

Fig. 14.19. Metabolic fates of glycine.

METABOLISM OF GLYCINE

Glycine is a simplest amino acid found in proteins. It is **non-essential amino acid** and is **glucogenic** in nature.

METABOLIC FATES OF GLYCINE

Glycine performs several **biochemical functions** as it is a precursor of various compounds (Fig. 14.19).

Formation of Serine

It is a reversible reaction, catalyzed **by hydroxymethyltransferase,** which requires pyridoxal-5-phosphate and N^5, N^{10} – methylenetetrahydrofolate (N^5, N^{10} –methylene. FH_4).

Need of the body for glycine or serine, and the availability of N^5, N^{10}–methylene.FH_4 determine the direction of reaction (Fig. 14.20).

Biosynthesis of Purine Ring

Glycine is used in the **biosynthesis of purine ring.** It contributes its nitrogen as well as both the carbons, which are incorporated into the purine ring as N_7, C_4 and C_5 (Fig. 14.21).

Biosynthesis of Heme

Glycine with succinyl CoA is used in the synthesis of δ-aminolevuilinic acid, **a precursor of heme.** This reaction is catalyzed by aminolevulinic acid (ALA) synthase.

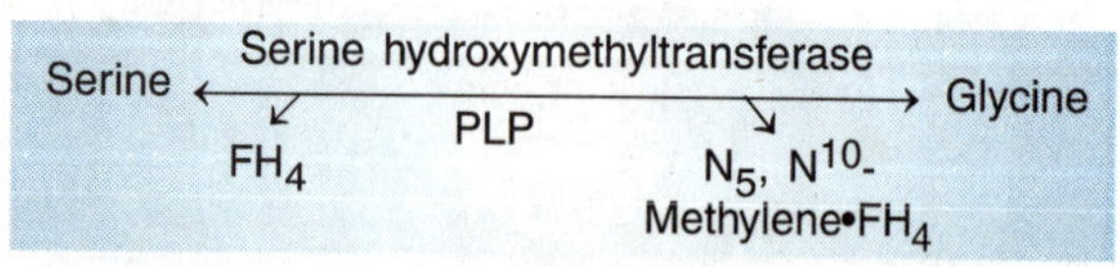

Fig. 14.20. Interconversion of glycine and serine.

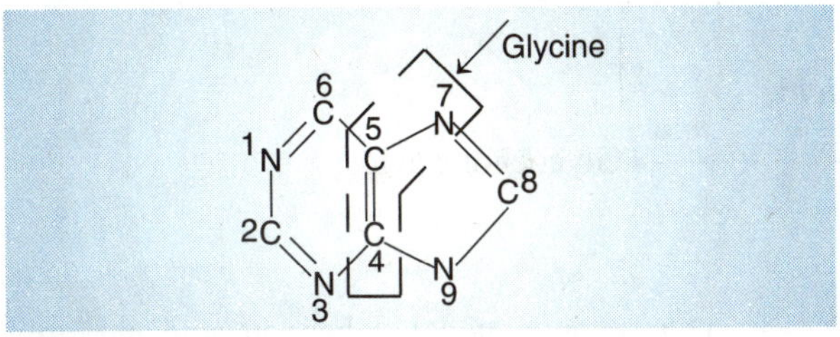

Fig. 14.21. Incorporation of glycine in the purine ring.

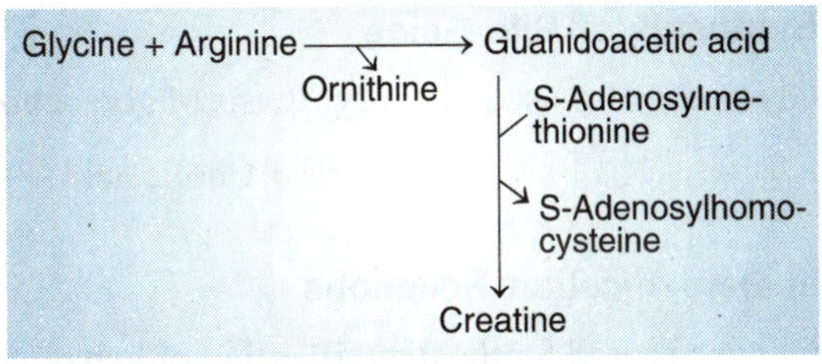

Fig. 14.22. Synthesis of creatine.

$$\text{Glycine} + \text{Succinyl CoA} \xrightarrow{\text{ALA synthase}} \delta\text{-Aminolevulinic acid} \rightarrow \text{Heme}$$

Synthesis of Phospho-creatine

Glycine is also used in the **synthesis of creatine** (Fig. 14.22).

Three amino acids, i.e. **glycine, arginine, and methionine,** are used for the **synthesis of creatine** in the liver, which is stored in the muscle as **phosphocreatine**.

First, the **guanidino group of arginine is transferred to glycine** and forms guanidoacetate. This reaction is catalyzed by the enzyme arginine-glycine transaminidase, in the kidney.

Subsequently, guanidoacetatemethyltransferase transfers **methyl group from S-adenosylmethionine,** in the liver.

Simultaneously, a high-energy phosphate group is transferred from ATP and forms **creatine- phosphate** (phospho-creatine). It is the form in which energy is stored in the muscle. **During exercise, ATP is** used as a source of energy and is **hydrolyzed to ADP and Pi**.

Subsequently, **creatine-phosphate** is utilized to **phosphorylate ADP** to regenerate ATP, while creatine is converted to **creatinine**. This reaction is called Lohmann's reaction and is catalyzed by **creatine kinase (creatine phosphokinase or CPK).**

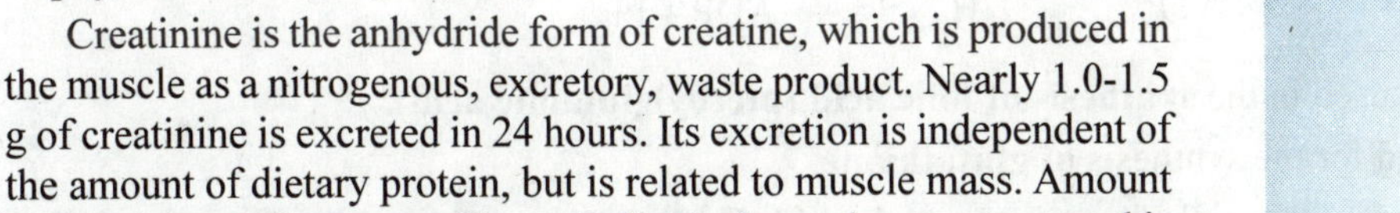

Only the traces of creatine are normally excreted in the urine. Large quantities of it may be excreted in conditions, such as muscular dystrophy, starvation, or pregnancy.

Creatinine is the anhydride form of creatine, which is produced in the muscle as a nitrogenous, excretory, waste product. Nearly 1.0-1.5 g of creatinine is excreted in 24 hours. Its excretion is independent of the amount of dietary protein, but is related to muscle mass. Amount of creatinine daily excreted by an individual remains constant, and is used as an index to determine daily urinary output.

Thus, creatine is stored in the muscle as creatine phosphate. After phosphrylation of ADP, creatine phosphate is converted to **creatinine,** which is excreted in the urine.

Biosynthesis of Glutathione

Glycine is also used in the synthesis of **glutathione** (Fig. 14.23).

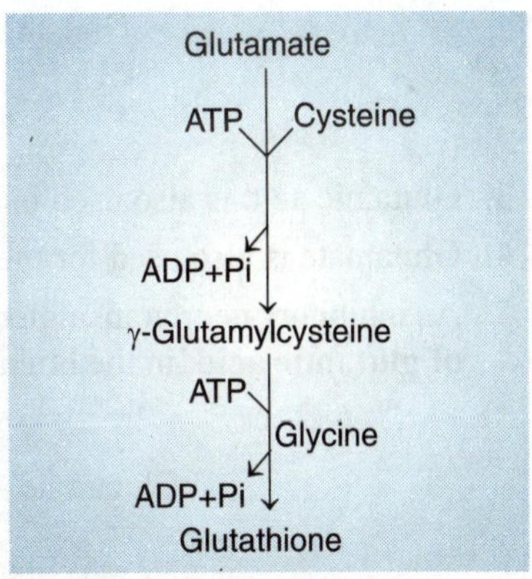

Fig. 14.23. Synthesis of glutathione.

Synthesis of Bile Acids

Glycine is also used in the **synthesis of glycocholic acid.**

$$\text{Glycine} + \text{Cholic acid} \longrightarrow \text{Glycocholic acid}$$

In Detoxification Reactions

Glycine is used for the **detoxification of benzoic acid**. Glycine gets conjugated with benzoic acid and forms benzoylglycine (hippuric acid), which is excreted in the urine.

$$\text{Glycine} + \text{Benzoic acid} \longrightarrow \text{Hippuric acid}$$

METABOLISM OF GLUTAMIC ACID

Glutamic acid is a nonessential amino acid. It is acidic in nature and is a glucogenic amino acid.

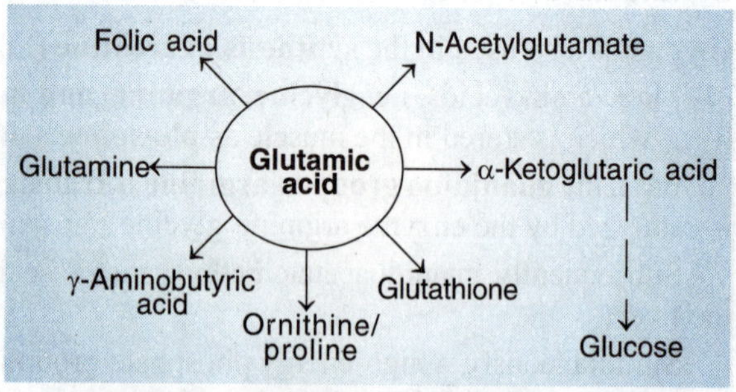

Fig. 14.24. Metabolic fates of glutamic acid.

METABOLIC FATES OF GLUTAMIC ACID

Glutamic acid is a precursor of several, biologically active, compounds (Fig. 14.24):

1. By a reversible reaction, catalyzed **by glutamate dehydrogenase, glutamic acid is formed in the liver** from α-ketoglutaric acid and ammonia as well as glutamate is used as a source of α-ketoglutarate, for gluconeogenesis.

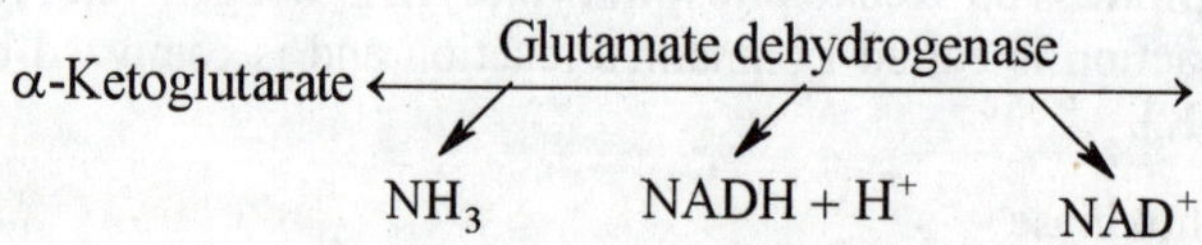

2. Glutamic acid, in the presence of glutamine synthetase, reacts with ammonia and **forms glutamine,** in the brain.

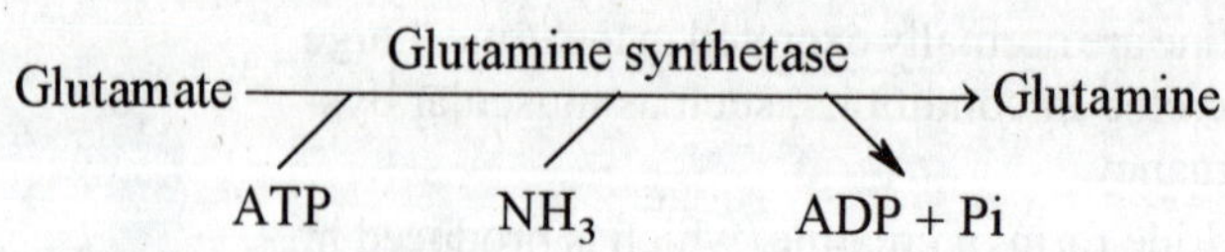

3. Glutamic acid is also used in the **synthesis of folic acid (pteroylglutamic acid).**
4. Glutamate is also used for the synthesis **of glutathione.**
5. An inhibitory neurotransmitter, called **γ-aminobutyric acid (GABA), is also formed by decarboxylation of glutamic acid,** in the brain.

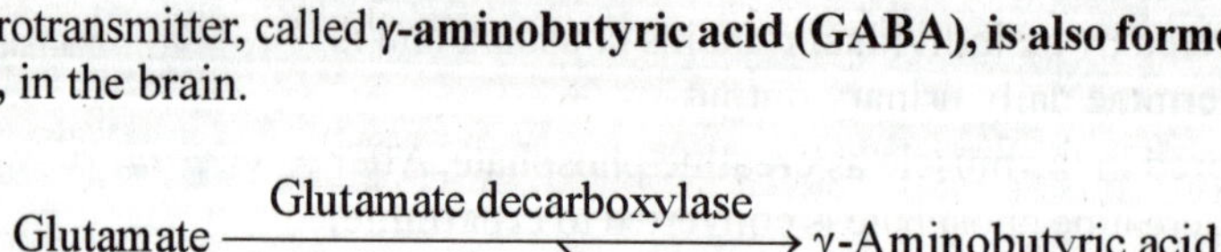

6. Glutamic acid is also **reversibly converted to ornithine** and/or **proline.**

7. With acetyl CoA, glutamate also **forms N-acetylglutamate**, which is required as a coenzyme in urea cycle.

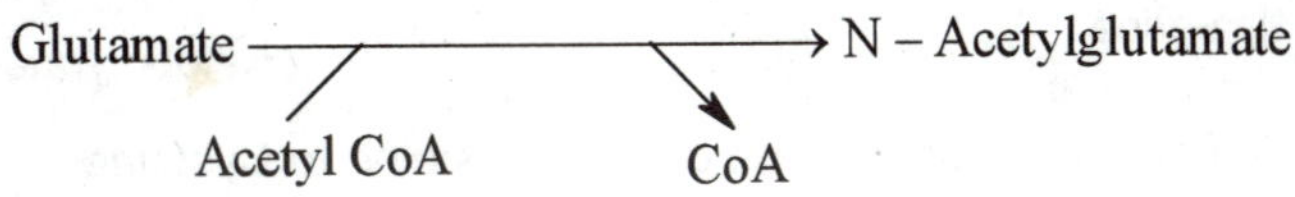

METABOLISM OF METHIONINE

Methionine is sulfur containing amino acid that forms succinylCoA and thus, is glucogenic in nature.

Degradation of methionine begins with its reaction with ATP to form S-adenosylmethionine (SAM)

ROLE OF METHIONINE IN TRANSMETHYLATION

Methionine condenses with ATP and with the hydrolysis of all the three phosphate bonds of ATP, S-adenosylmethionine is formed. Since it has a highly reactive methyl group, it is also called as active methinionine.

S-Adenosylmethionine is the major methyl group donor in one-carbon metabolism and is used for methylation of several compounds, such as in the synthesis of phosphatidylcholine from phosphatidylethanolamine.

After donation of the methyl group, S-adenosylmethionine forms S-adenosylhomocysteine, which is hydrolysed to homocysteine and adenosine (Fig. 14.25).

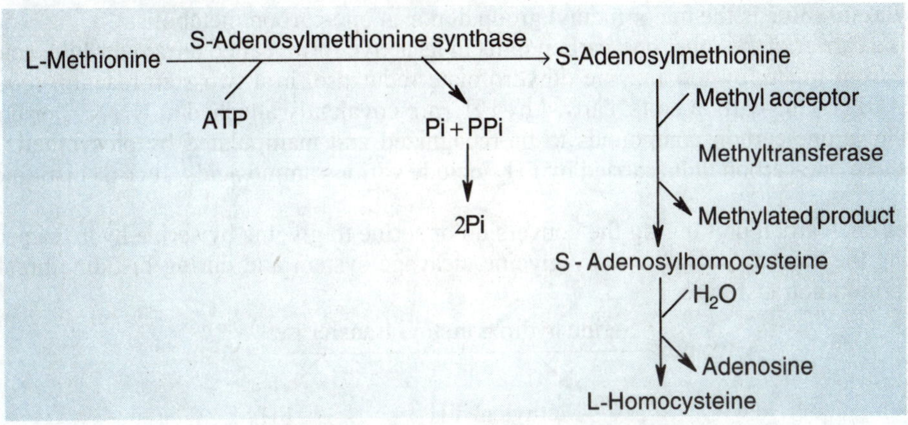

Fig. 14.25. Role of Methionine in Transmethylation

Homocysteine can be methylated to methionine by accepting methyl group from N^5-methyltetrahydrofolate. This reaction is catalyzed by the enzyme homocystine methyl- transferase (Fig. 14.26).

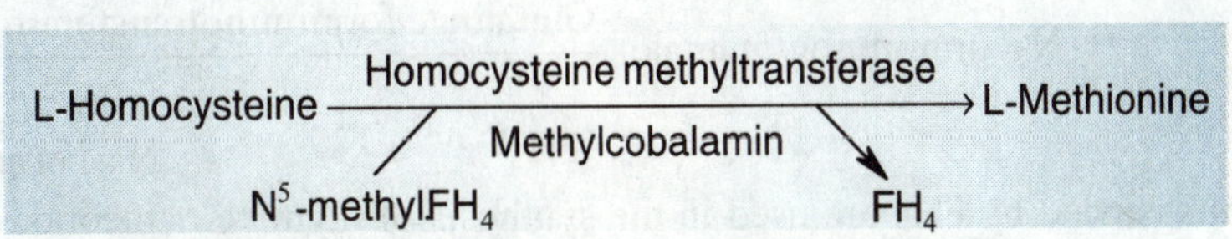

Fig. 14.26. Conversion of Homocysteine to Methionine

Alternatively, homocysteine combines with serine and forms cystathionine, which is hydrolyzed to cysteine and α-ketobutyrate (Fig. 14.27).

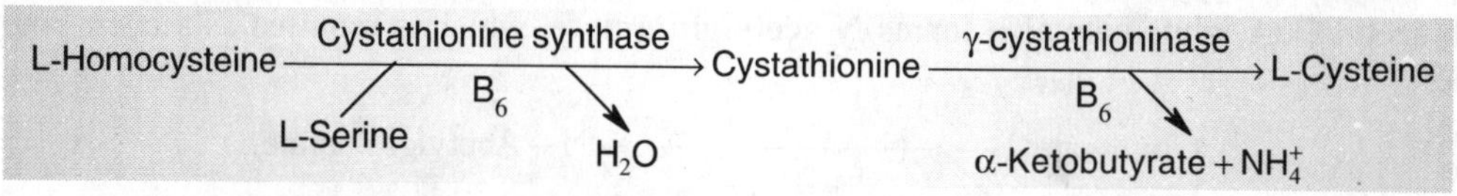

Fig. 14.27. Conversion of Homocysteine to Cysteine

Homocysteine has been shown to be associated with atherosclerotic vascular disease. Patients with high serum levels of homocysteine and homocystinuia, experience premature vascular disease and usually die of myocardial infarction, stroke or pulmonary problems.

ONE-CARBON TRANSFER

In most of the carboxylation reactions, which are catalyzed by pyruvate carboxylase, carbonic acid (the hydrated form of CO_2) that is carried by the vitamin biotin, is used. This is however, not considered as one-carbon transfer.

On the other hand, there are many biosynthetic pathways, which involve the addition of a single carbon group as a one-carbon (1-C) unit to a metabolic precursor. These one-carbon units can exist in a variety of oxidation states, which include **formyl** (–CHO), **formate** ($-HCOO^-$), **methenyl** (=CH–), **methylene** ($-CH_2-$), **methyl** ($-CH_3$), **hydroxymethyl** ($-CH_2OH$), or **formimino** (–CH=N–) groups.

It is possible to incorporate these one-carbon units into an acceptor organic compound. These single carbon units can be transformed from the carrier compounds, such as tetrahydrofolic acid and S-adenosylmethionine, to a specific molecule that is being synthesized or modified. Single carbon units attached to this group of carriers are referred to as one-carbon pool.

S-Adenosylmethionine is the major methyl group donor in one-carbon metabolism.

Folic acid is a carrier of the other one-carbon units in its active form, called tetrahydrofolic acid (FH_4). It is produced from folate, by the enzyme dihydrofolate reductase, in a two step reaction requiring two moles of NADPH. One-carbon units, carried by FH_4, are covalently attached at N^5, N^{10}, or both N^5 and N^{10}. FH_4 allows one-carbon compounds to be recognized and manipulated by biosynthetic enzymes. Sources of these one-carbon units carried by FH_4 include various amino acids, such as histidine, glycine, and serine.

FH_4 acquires one-carbon unit during the conversion of serine to glycine by serine hydroxymethyl transferase, during the cleavage of glycine by glycine-cleavage system and during histidine breakdown by glutamate formiminotransferase.

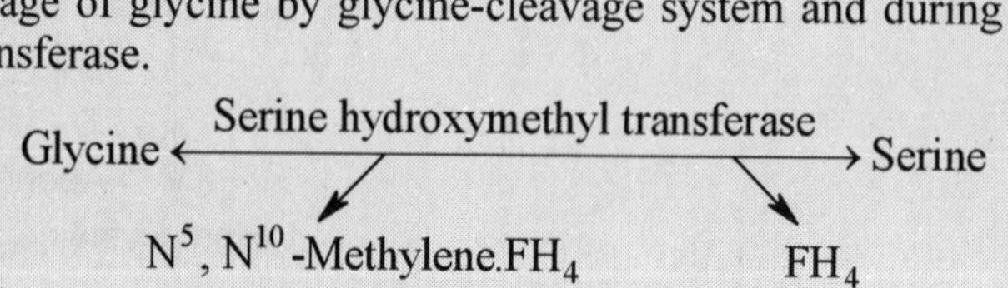

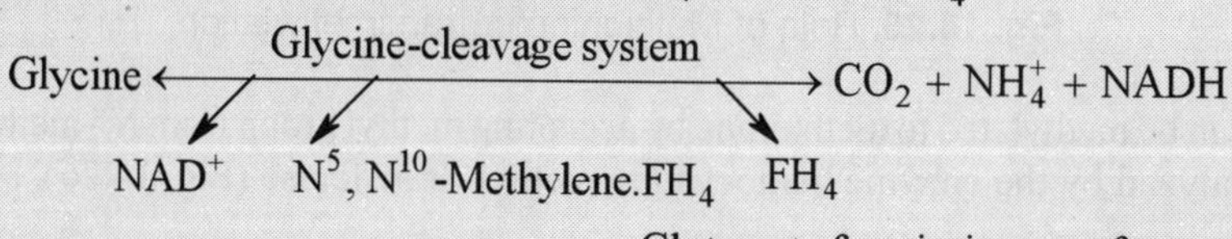

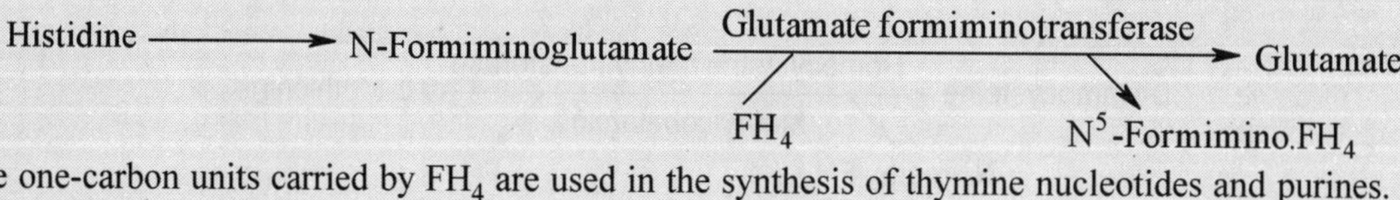

The one-carbon units carried by FH_4 are used in the synthesis of thymine nucleotides and purines. It is also used in the synthesis of methionine from homocysteine.

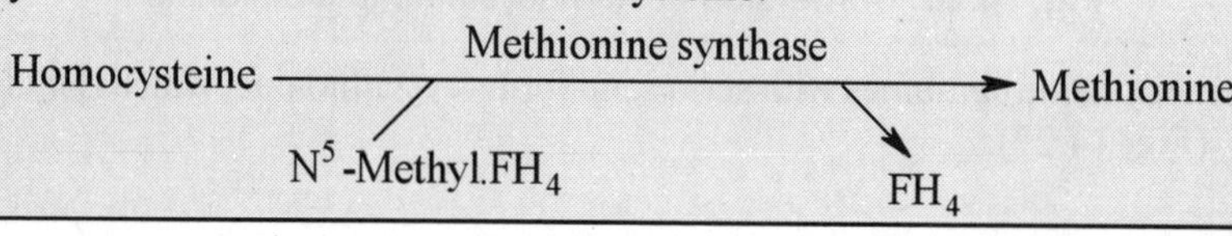

ROLE OF AMINO ACIDS IN DETOXICATION

Drugs and xenobiotics (chemicals that are foreign to the body) are metabolized primarily via two pathways, i.e. phase I (oxidative) and phase II (biosynthetic reactions). They may be metabolized by either or both the pathways.

In phase I metabolism, a functional group, such as a hydroxyl group, is introduced into or exposed by cytochormes P_{450}. The enzymes in **phase II metabolism** then connect this functional group to an endogenous species, such as sulfate, acetate, glutathione or amino acid. The net effect of either or both of these modifications is to make the foreign compound more water soluble and thus easier to excrete, generally, through the kidneys but also through the intestine, via excretion into bile.

Several drugs are metabolized and detoxicated after conjugation with glycine or glutamine.

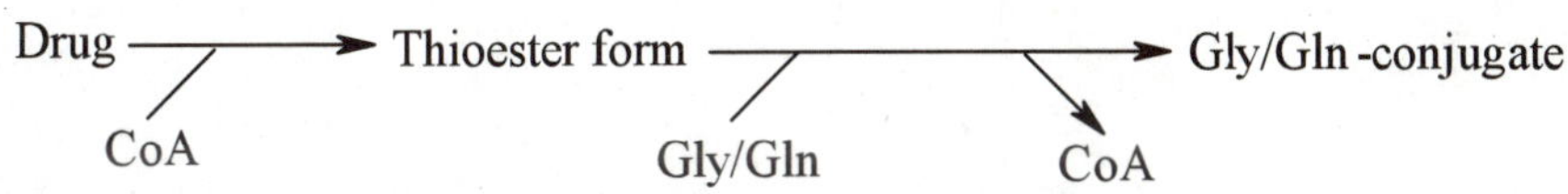

For example, benzoic acid after conversion to benzoyl CoA is conjugated with glycine and excreted as hippuric acid (benzoylglycine).

SOME IMPORTANT QUESTIONS

1. Outline urea cycle. What is the site of urea synthesis? What is the need for urea synthesis in the body?
2. Describe various mechanisms of the removal of ammonia from amino acids.
3. How is ammonia removed from the body?
4. Explain how tyrosine is metabolized. Describe biologically important compounds derived from it?
5. Describe various fates of phenylalanine in the body.
6. Name enzymes and coenzymes of the following reactions :
   (i) Synthesis of carbamoylphosphate
   (ii) Conversion of phenylalanine to tyrosine.
7. Name important biologically active compounds derived from:
   (i) Glutamic acid
   (ii) Tryptophan
8. Discuss briefly:
   (i) Biosynthesis of phospho-creatine
   (ii) Metabolic fates of glycine
   (iii) Reactions of urea cycle
   (iv) Synthesis of urea and its abnormalities
   (v) Two inborn errors of amino acid metabolism
   (vi) Transamination and its importance
   (vii) Metabolism of phenylalanine
   (viii) Processes of the removal of NH_3 from amino acids

9. Write notes on:
   - (i) Alkaptonuria
   - (ii) Catabolism of tyrosine
   - (iii) Phenylketonuria
   - (iv) Disposal of ammonia from the body
   - (v) Deamination
   - (vi) Active methionine
   - (vii) One-carbon transfer
   - (viii) Role of amino acids in detoxication

CHAPTER

15

Integration of Metabolism

Several metabolic pathways which are concerned with the oxidation of fuel for the production of ATP, such as glycolysis, gluconeogenesis, citric acid cycle, fatty acid oxidation, lipogenesis, amino acid oxidation, protein synthesis and proteolysis, etc., do not operate in every tissue at all the times. These various metabolic processes are integrated and have interdependence of several tissues of the body.

Five major organs, i.e. liver, adipose tissue, muscle, brain and kidney, play a dominant role in fuel metabolism. These tissues contain unique sets of enzymes, in such a way that each organ is specialized for the storage, use and generation of specific fuel. These tissues do not function in isolation but are interdependent on each other, in which one tissue may provide substrates to another or process the compounds produced by the other organs. Metabolites flow between these organs in well-defined pathways in which flux also varies with the nutritional state of the animal. Communication between the tissues is mediated by the nervous system, by the availability of circulating substrates, and by variations in the levels of plasma hormones. For example, immediately following meal, glucose, amino acids and fatty acids are directly available from the intestine. Glucose passes from the intestinal epithelial cells, via the portal vein, to the liver. Amino acids are partially metabolized in the gut before being released into portal blood. Chylomicrons containing triacylglycerol are secreted by the intestinal epithelial cells into lymphatic and via thoracic duct are delivered to the rest of the body. This integration of energy metabolism is controlled primarily by insulin and the opposing actions of glucagon and epinephrine.

ROLE OF LIVER

The liver is referred to as the central metabolic clearing house of the body, as it maintains the proper levels of the circulating fuels for use by the brain, muscles and other tissues. Moreover, all the nutrients absorbed by the intestine except fatty acids, directly reach the liver via portal vein.

GLUCOSE

One of the major functions of the liver is to act as a buffer for blood glucose. It takes up and releases glucose in response to hormones and to the circulation (blood glucose). When the blood glucose concentration is high, such as after a carbohydrate containing meal, liver takes up glucose and converts it to glucose-6-phosphate, by the enzyme glucokinase. Glucose-6-phosphate thereafter has several fates in the liver:

- It can be converted to glucose (by glucose-6-phosphatase) for transport to the peripheral organs when blood glucose concentration is reduced.
- It can be converted to glycogen, when the demand of the body for glucose is low.
- Glucose-6-phosphate can be converted to acetyl CoA via glycolysis, which (if not oxidized via citric acid cycle for the generation of ATP) can be used to synthesize fatty acids (triacylglycerols) and cholesterol.
- It can also be degraded via the pentose phosphate pathway to generate NADPH, which is required for the biosynthesis of fatty acids, cholesterol and other compounds.

TRIACYLGLYCEROL

The liver can synthesize or degrade triacylglycerol. Under conditions of high metabolic demand, fatty acids are degraded to acetyl CoA and then to ketone bodies. The liver generates ATP from acetyl CoA and exports ketone bodies to the peripheral tissues, to be used there as fuel.

When the demand for metabolic fuel is low, fatty acids are incorporated into triacylglycerol that are secreted into the blood stream as VLDL.

AMINO ACIDS

The liver degrades amino acids to a variety of metabolic intermediates that can be completely oxidized to CO_2 and H_2O, or converted to glucose or ketone bodies.

Immediately after food, when amino acids are present in high concentration in the blood, their oxidation provides a significant fraction of metabolic energy.

During a fast glucose is produced from amino acids, which mostly arise from degradation of muscle protein (Fig. 15.1).

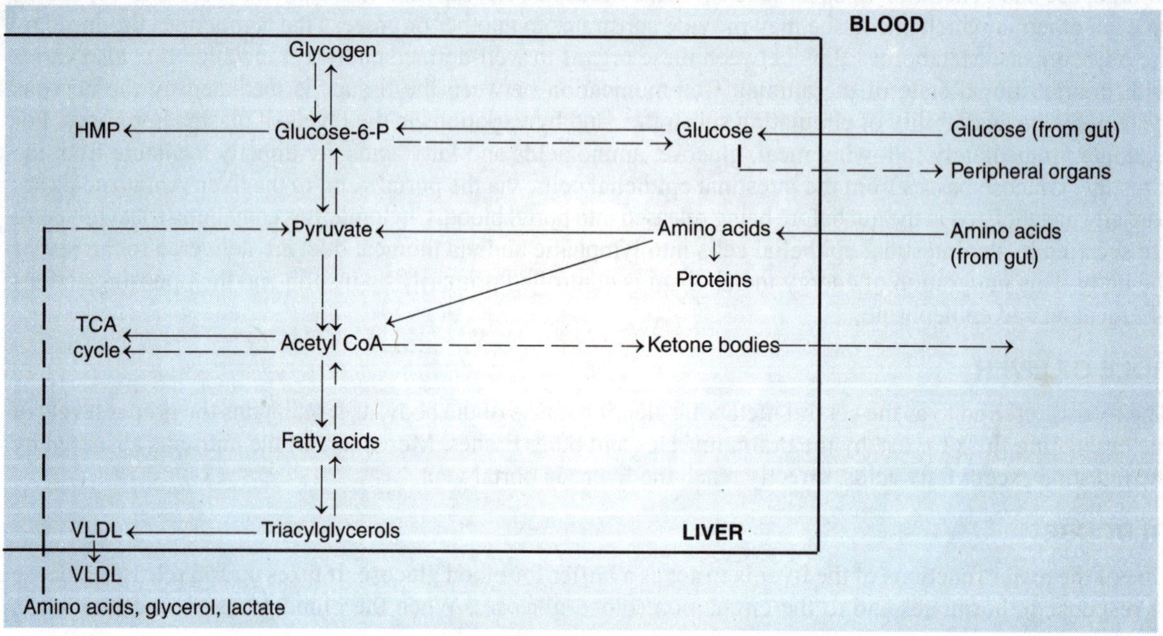

Fig. 15.1. Major metabolic pathways in the liver.
——→ In the absorptive state —–→ During starvation

ROLE OF BRAIN

Brain tissue has a very high respiration rate and requires a steady supply of glucose from the blood, which is its primary fuel. During prolonged fast, the brain gradually switches to ketone bodies (Fig. 15.2).

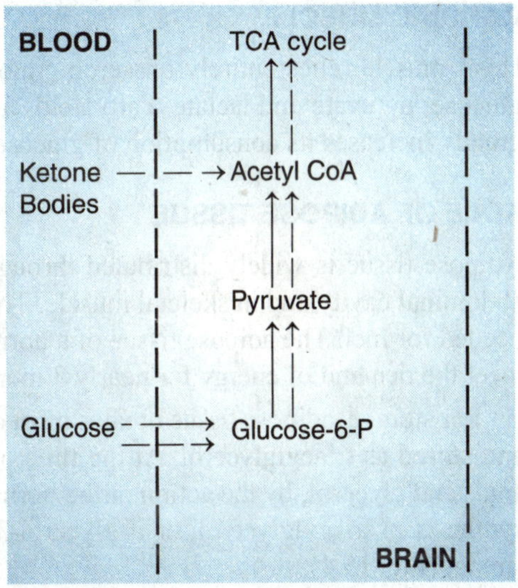

Fig. 15.2. Major metabolic pathways in the brain.

⟶ In the absorptive state

- - → During starvation

ROLE OF MUSCLE

Major fuels for muscle are glucose, fatty acids and ketone bodies.

Glycogen is converted to glucose-6-phosphate for entry into glycolysis, for use within the muscle only. Muscle contraction is driven by ATP hydrolysis.

SKELETAL MUSCLE

About 30% of the O_2 consumed by the human body is used by skeletal muscle at rest, which is increased by several folds in response to a heavy work load. In resting muscle, ATP is used to phosphorylate creatine and is stored as phosphocreatine. During the initial stage of exercise ATP is regenerated by the reaction of phosphocreatine with ADP. With the increasing intensity of exercise, muscle shift to ATP production via glycolysis and most of the glucose-6-phosphate is then degraded anaerobically.

During exercise in humans, the supply of endogenous ATP is made available for a few seconds by phosphocreatine after which anaerobic glycolysis generates ATP. Subsequently after about 90 seconds, the shift from anaerobic to aerobic metabolism occurs (Fig. 15.3).

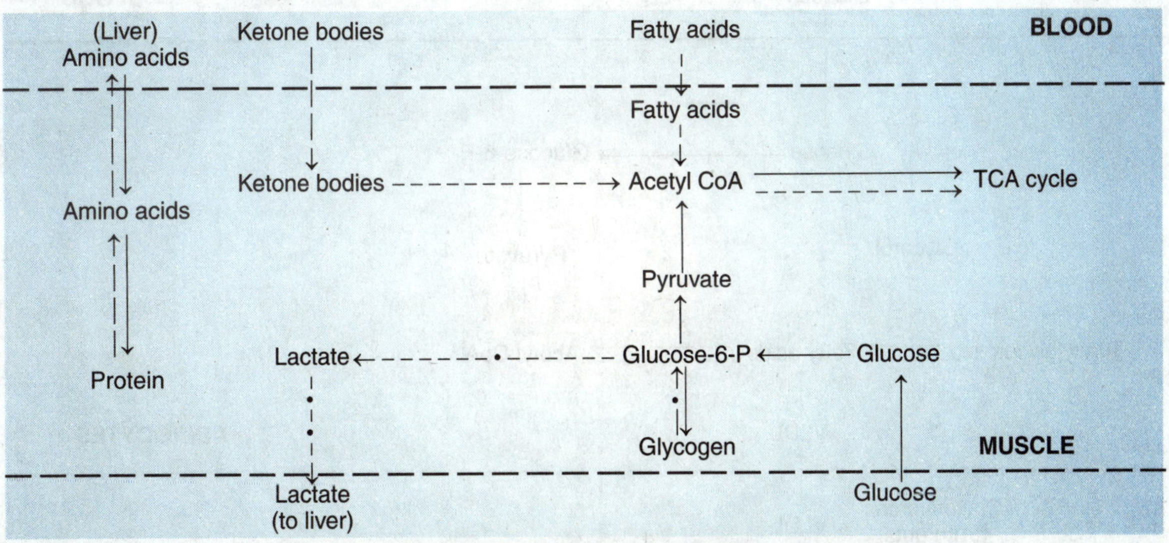

Fig. 15.3. Major metabolic pathways in the skeletal muscle.

⟶ In the absorptive state

— — → During starvation

—•→ During exercise

CARDIAC MUSCLE

Heart muscle relies entirely on aerobic metabolism. The heart can metabolize fatty acids, ketone bodies, glucose, pyruvate and lactate. Fatty acids are used by the resting heart while during heavy work; the heart greatly increases its consumption of glucose.

ROLE OF ADIPOSE TISSUE

Adipose tissue is widely distributed throughout the body but occurs most prominently under skin, in the abdominal cavity and in skeletal muscle. The function of adipose tissue is to store and release fatty acids as needed for fuel. The adipose tissue of a normal 70 kg man contains about 15 kg of fat, which is sufficient to meet the demand of energy for nearly 3 months.

For storage, adipose tissue obtains most of its fatty acids from circulating lipoproteins. They are activated and stored as triacylglycerol. At the time of metabolic need, adipocytes hydrolyze triacylglycerol to fatty acids and glycerol, by the action of the hormone-sensitive lipase. Fatty acids may be either reutilized for the synthesis of triacylglycerol, or if glycerol-3-phosphate is in short supply, they are released into the blood stream (Fig. 15.4).

ROLE OF KIDNEY

The kidney filters urea and other waste products from the blood. It also maintains pH of the blood. It also regulates important metabolites, such as glucose. Kidney also generates glucose by gluconeogenesis particularly, during starvation.

The complexity of the mechanisms that regulate mammalian fuel metabolism permits the body to response efficiently to changing energy needs in response to the changes in the availability of various fuels, maintaining

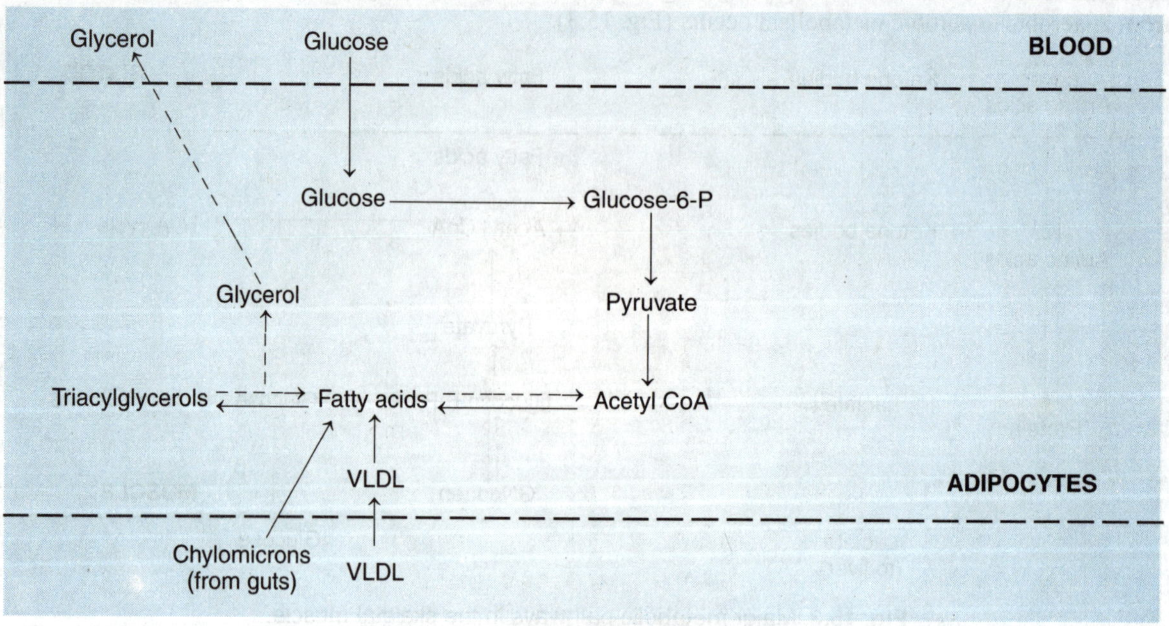

Fig. 15.4. Major metabolic pathways in the adipose tissue.
——→ In the absorptive state
– – → During starvation

reasonable balance between energy inflow and output, such as during starvation or disorders of fuel metabolism, like diabetes and obesity.

METABOLISM DURING STARVATION

After a meal is digested, nutrients are catabolised to small units for absorption by the intestinal mucosa, from where they pass through the circulation to the rest of the body. Glucose uptake, and glycogen and fatty acid biosynthesis are stimulated by insulin, whose concentration in the blood increases in response to high blood glucose concentration.

As tissues take up and metabolize glucose, blood glucose concentration drops, thereby causing the release of glucagon by the α cells of the pancreas. This in turn stimulates glycogen break down and release of glucose from the liver. It also promotes gluconeogenesis from amino acids and lactate. After an overnight fast, combination of increased glucagon and decreased insulin secretion promotes mobilization of fatty acids from adipose tissue. The diminished insulin also inhibits glucose uptake by muscle tissue. Muscle therefore; switch from glucose to fatty acids metabolism for energy production.

When the fast is prolonged, the liver glycogen store becomes depleted and the rate of gluconeogenesis increases. After several days of starvation, liver directs acetyl CoA, which is derived from fatty acids, to the synthesis of ketone bodies that are released into the blood. The brain gradually adapts to the use of ketone bodies as fuel.

SOME IMPORTANT QUESTIONS

1. Discuss the role of liver in the integration of metabolism.
2. Briefly describe the process of fuel metabolism during starvation.
3. Discuss the role of various tissues in fuel metabolism.

CHAPTER

16

Oxygen Toxicity

The elemental oxygen (O_2), as we all know, is essential for life. About 90% of it is used via oxidative phosphorylation while the other 10% in enzymatic hydroxylation and oxygenation reactions. A small fraction of the oxygen is converted to inherently toxic forms, such as superoxide and hydrogen peroxide, etc. These are the highly reactive forms of oxygen and are referred to as reactive oxygen species (ROS). They are a source of chronic damage to biomolecules, within the tissues.

REACTIVE OXYGEN SPECIES

In biological redox reactions involving O_2, oxygen is activated by redox active metal ions, such as iron and copper, which are present in metallo-enzymes and other proteins, e.g. hemoglobin, myoglobin, etc. These metal ions provide one electron at a time to oxygen and activate it to strong oxidizing forms. As shown in fig. 16.1, a number of reactive oxygen species, also called free radicals, are formed from partial reduction of molecular oxygen. The first product is the anion radical called, superoxide (O_2). Reduction of superoxide yields hydroperoxide in the form of H_2O_2. Reduction of H_2O_2 causes a cleavage reaction that releases hydroxyl radical ($OH^{\cdot}$). The end product of complete reduction of oxygen is water.

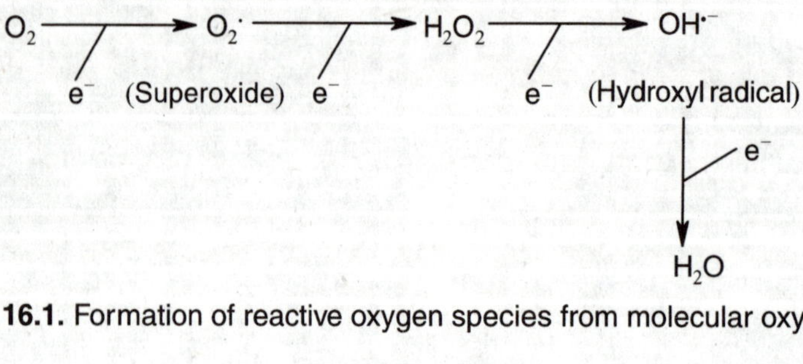

Fig. 16.1. Formation of reactive oxygen species from molecular oxygen

ROS are formed by three mechanisms in vivo, i.e. by reaction of oxygen with decompartmentalised metal ions, as a side reaction of electron transport, or by normal enzymatic reactions of electron transport, e.g. monoamine oxidase (in dopamine metabolism), fatty acid oxidases (in the peroxisomes), etc.

OXIDATIVE STRESS

Various reactive oxygen species are formed continuously as by-products of aerobic metabolism, through reactions with drugs and environmental toxins. When their level is inreased or the level of antioxidants is diminished, this in turn creates a condition called **oxidative stress.** Reactive oxygen species can cause serious chemical damage to DNA, proteins and unsaturated lipids and can lead to cell death. ROS have also been implicated in a number of pathological processes, including reperfusion injury, cancer, inflammatory disease, and ageing.

Nature of Oxygen Radical Damage

Among the family of reactive oxygen species, hydroxyl radical ($OH^{\cdot}$) is the most reactive and damaging. Its half life is measured in nanoseconds. It reacts with biomolecules primarily by hydrogen abstraction and addition reactions. One of the most sensitive sites of free radical damage is the cell membrane, which is rich in readily oxidized polyunsaturated fatty acids.

The hydroxyl radical extracts a hydrogen atom from a polyunsaturated fatty acid, setting off a chain of lipid peroxidation reactions. Lipid peroxides formed in this reaction degrade, to form characteristic products, such as malondialdehyde (MDA). These compounds react with proteins to form adducts and cross links, known as advanced lipoxidation end-products (ALE).

ROS also react with carbohydrates to form dicarbonyl compounds that react with protein to form cross links and adducts, known as glycoxidation products or advanced glycation end-products (AGE). ROS also cause some residual damage to the genome, in the form of mutations in DNA. As a result of oxidative stress, MDA adducts ALE and AGE increase in several chronic conditions, such as atherosclerosis, Alzeheimer's disease and diabetes.

Antioxidant Defenses

There are several levels of protection against oxidative damage by antioxidant enzymes and vitamins:

Enzymatic Defenses

There is a group of enzymes that act to detoxify the precursors of hydroxyl radicals. These include catalase, superoxide dismutase (SOD), and glutathione peroxidase (GP_x).

Catalase detoxifies H_2O_2 and is found in large amount in peroxisomes:

$$2H_2O_2 \xrightarrow{\text{Catalase}} O_2 + 2H_2O$$

SOD detoxifies superoxides:

$$O_2^{\cdot} \xrightarrow{\text{SOD}} O_2 + H_2O$$

There are two classes of SOD. One is Mn.SOD, which is found in the mitochondria while the other is Cu-Zn.SOD, which is widely distributed in all compartments of the cell.

Glutathione peroxidase (GPx) reduces both, H_2O_2 and lipid hydroperoxides to water and a lipid alcohol, respectively. GPx requires reduced glutathione (GSH) as a co-substrate.

$$H_2O_2 + 2GSH \xrightarrow{\text{GPx}} 2H_2O + GSSG$$

GSH is tripeptide-thiol (γ-glutamylcysteinylglycine) containing glutamate, cysteine and glycine. It is found in all the cells and can chemically detoxify H_2O_2. This reaction is catalyzed by GPx, which is a selenium containing enzyme. In this reaction, GSH is oxidized to GSSG (oxidized glutathione), which is not protective. The cell regenerates GSH from GSSG by an NADPH-dependent enzyme, called glutathione reductase. NADPH is produced by the pentose phosphate pathway.

ANTIOXIDANT DEFENSES IN ERYTHROCYTES

ROS are formed continuously in the erythrocytes and initiate lipid peroxidation reaction, which can lead to loss of membrane integrity, causing cell lysis. They are well protected against oxidative stress, as the cell has high concentration of GSH. Moreover, erythrocytes are totally dependent on the pentose phosphate pathway for the supply of NADPH.

ANTIOXIDANT VITAMINS

Three vitamins, i.e. **vitamin A, C, and E,** provide the other line of defense against oxidative damage and are called antioxidant vitamins.

Vitamin C (ascorbate) in the aqueous phase while **vitamin E** (α- and γ-tocopherols) in the lipid phase, act as chain-breaking antioxidants. Vitamin C reduces superoxide and lipid peroxyl radicals. It also has a role in reduction and recycling of vitamin E. In response to severe oxidative stress, vitamin E is maintained at constant concentration in the lipid phase until all the vitamin C is consumed. Thus, they do not propagate radical damage and are recycled.

Vitamin A is a lipophilic antioxidant. It is a potent singlet oxygen scavenger and protects against damage from sunlight in the retina and skin. Consumption of food rich in ascorbate, vitamin E, and β-carotene, has been correlated with a reduced risk for certain types of cancers and decreased frequency of certain other chronic health problems.

SOME IMPORTANT QUESTIONS

1. What is oxidative stress?
2. Write notes on:
   - (i) Reactive oxygen species
   - (ii) Oxidative stress
   - (iii) Free radicals
   - (iv) Antioxidant defenses
   - (v) Antioxidant vitamins

CHAPTER

17

Biochemical Genetics and Protein Synthesis

All cells can synthesize nucleotides either by the biosynthetic process, called **de novo synthesis,** or from the degradation products of the nucleic acids, i.e. free bases and nucleosides, by the process referred as the **salvage pathway.**

METABOLISM OF NUCLEOTIDES

FORMATION OF PURINE NUCLEOTIDES

De novo synthesis

The process of the **biosynthesis of the end product** in a pathway, **from the precursor molecules** is called **de novo synthesis.**

A purine ring is synthesized in mammalian cells by utilizing **three amino acids, i.e. aspartate, glutamine and glycine,** which serve as carbon and nitrogen donors, besides the **respiratory CO_2** (HCO_3^-). and the **one-carbon moiety** that is transferred via FH_4.

In the purine ring, **nitrogen at position 1** is obtained **from the amino group** ($-NH_2$) **of aspartate. One-carbon moiety, via tetrahydrofolate (FH4), forms carbons at positions 2 and 8. The amide nitrogen** ($-CO.NH_2$) **of glutamine forms nitrogen** that are present at positions **3 and 9,** while **carbon at position 6** is obtained **from CO_2**. Glycine is incorporated as a whole and forms carbon at positions **4 and 5 and nitrogen at position 7** (Fig. 17.1).

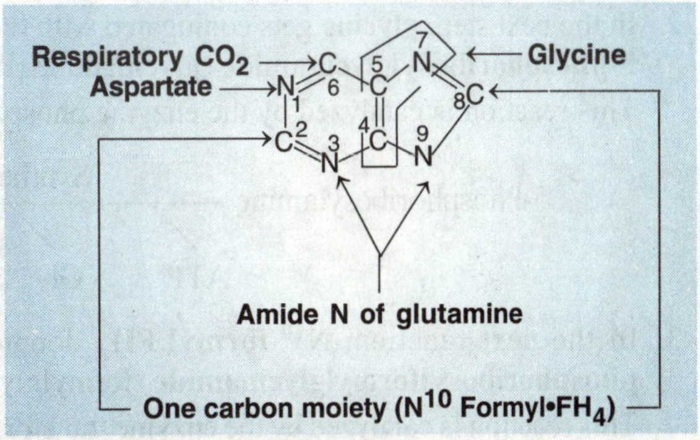

Fig. 17.1. Sources of the carbon and nitrogen atoms in a purine ring.

The purine ring is synthesized, by a series of

reactions, with the addition of various carbon and nitrogen atoms at ribose-5-phosphate, which forms a part of the nucleotide and not a free base.

Starting material for the synthesis of the purine ring is **phosphoribosylpyrophosphate** (PRPP) and the first purine nucleotide, which is synthesized by this process, is called IMP.

Synthesis of PRPP

PRPP is **synthesized** by the addition of pyrophosphate, **from ATP**, on to **ribose-5-phosphate,** which is produced in the pentose phosphate pathway. This reaction is catalyzed by the enzyme **phosphoribosylpyrophosphate synthetase (PRPP synthetase).**

Ribose-5-P —(PRPP synthetase; ATP in, AMP out; Mg^{2+})→ 5-Phosphoribosyl-1-pyrophosphate (PRPP)

PRPP is used as the starting material, not only for the synthesis of the purines but also for pyrimidines. PRPP is also used in utilization of the purine and pyrimidine bases, by the salvage pathway.

Synthesis of IMP

De novo pathway for the synthesis of the **purine nucleotides** leads to the **synthesis of** the nucleotide of hypoxanthine, called **inosine-5′-monophosphate** (IMP), which in turn also serves as a **precursor** for the synthesis of **AMP** and **GMP**.

1. First step in the biosynthesis of IMP is the formation of **5′-phosphoribosylamine.**
   This reaction is catalyzed by the enzyme **amidotransferase**. The pyrophosphate group in PRPP is replaced by the **amide nitrogen of glutamine**.

   5-Phosphoribosylpyrophosphate —(Amidotransferase; Glutamine in; Mg^{2+}; PPi and Glutamate out)→ 5-Phosphoribosylamine

   This in turn results in the acquisition of **nitrogen-9** of the purine ring.
   It is a committed step in this pathway. Rate of the reaction is controlled by the intracellular concentration of both the substrates, i.e. glutamine as well as PRPP.
2. In the next step, **glycine** gets conjugated with the amino group of the **phosphoribosylamine,** and forms **5-phosphoribosylglycinamide** (glycinamide ribotide).
   This reaction is catalyzed by the enzyme phosphoribosylglycinamide **synthetase**.

   5-Phosphoribosylamine —(Synthetase; ATP and Gly in; ADP + Pi out)→ 5-Phosphoribosylglycinamide

3. In the next reaction, **N^{10}-formyl.FH_4** donates formyl group and results in the formation of **5-phosphoribosylformylglycinamide** (formylglycinamide ribotide).
   This reaction is catalyzed by the enzyme transformylase (**phosphoribosylglycinamide transformylase).**

   5 – Phosphoribosylglycinamide (Glycinamide ribotide) —(Transformylase; N^{10}-Formyl.FH_4 in; FH_2 out)→ 5 – Phosphoribosylformylglycinamide (Formylglycinamide ribotide)

4. Thereafter, **IMP is synthesized** through a series of reactions (Fig. 17.2)

   Various enzymes, which are involved in the synthesis of the purine nucleotide, are found in the cytosol of the cell, whereas energy that is required to drive some of these reactions is obtained from the hydrolysis of ATP. During this process, six molecules of ATP are utilized per molecule of IMP synthesized.

Conversion of IMP to AMP and GMP

IMP serves as a common **precursor for** the synthesis of **AMP** as well as **GMP** (Fig. 17.3).

Conversion of IMP to AMP: IMP reacts with **aspartate** and forms **adenylosuccinate** (AMPS). This reaction is catalyzed by the enzyme **adenylosuccinate synthetase.**

This is the rate-limiting step. AMP inhibits this reaction. GTP is used in this reaction as a source of energy.

Subsequently, **adenylosuccinase** (adenylosuccinate lyase) removes **fumarate** from AMPS, which is converted to **AMP**.

Conversion of IMP to GMP: First, the enzyme IMP dehydrogenase converts IMP to xanthosine-monophosphate (XMP).

IMP dehydrogenase is the rate-limiting enzyme for which GMP acts as a competitive inhibitor.

Subsequently, **GMP synthetase** converts **XMP** to **GMP**. This reaction requires ATP.

REGULATION OF THE BIOSYNTHESIS OF THE PURINE NUCLEOTIDES

Biosynthesis of IMP is regulated at the first step of the pathway. The reaction, which is catalyzed by the enzyme **amidotransferase**, is a **committed step.** This enzyme is regulated allosterically, by the end products of the pathway, i.e. by **IMP, GMP, and AMP,** which serve as the **negative effectors**. On the other hand, **PRPP** acts as **positive effector** for this enzyme.

Biosynthesis of AMP and GMP, from IMP, is also **regulated**. Both, AMP and GMP act as competitive inhibitors in their own synthesis.

In the conversion of IMP to GMP, **IMP dehydrogenase** is the rate-limiting enzyme. It is regulated by **GMP,** which acts as **competitive inhibitor**. **Adenylosuccinate synthetase** is the rate-limiting enzyme in the conversion of IMP to AMP, where **AMP** acts as **competitive inhibitor.**

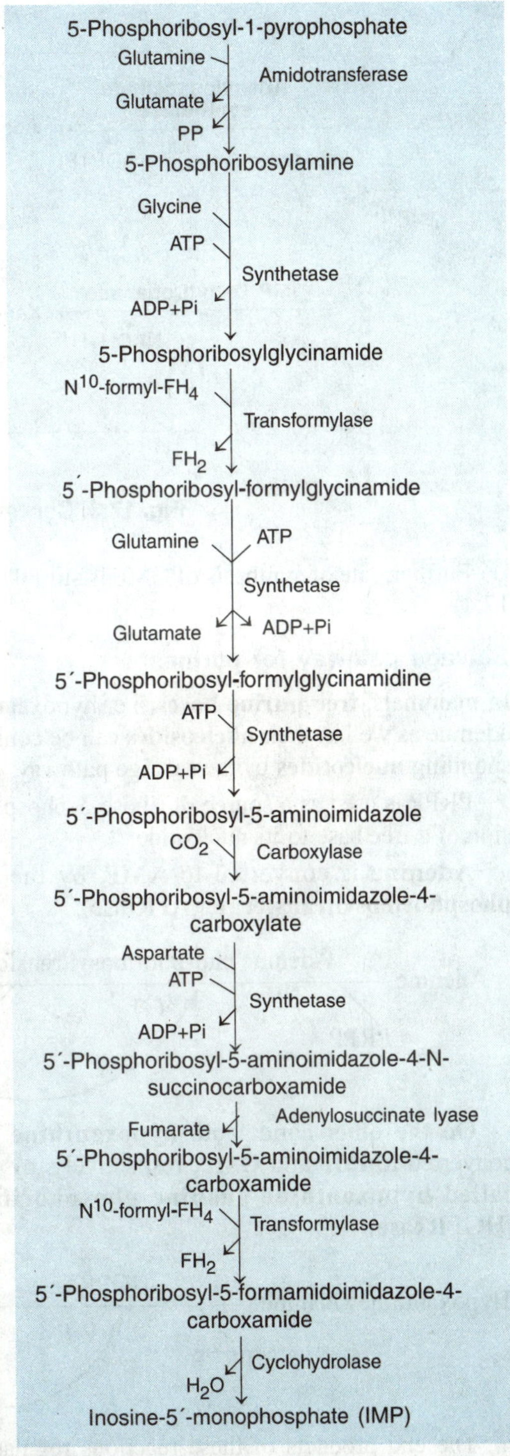

Fig. 17.2. De Novo synthesis of Inosine-5′-Monophosphate (IMP).

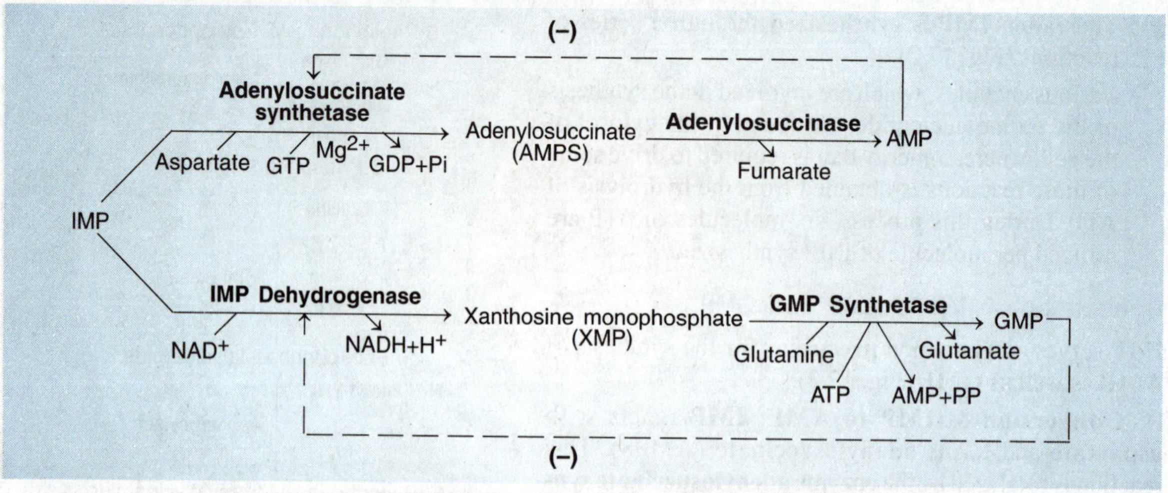

Fig. 17.3. Conversion of IMP to AMP and GMP.

Further, rate of synthesis of GMP is stimulated by ATP while GTP stimulates the synthesis of AMP (Fig. 17.4)

Salvage pathway for purines

In mammals, **free purine bases,** i.e. hypoxanthine, guanine and adenine as well as their **nucleosides** can be converted to the corresponding **nucleotides** by the salvage pathway.

PRPP is used as a source of ribose-5-phosphate in the conversion of a free base to its nucleotide.

Adenine is converted to **AMP,** by the enzyme **adenine phosphoribosyltransferase** (APRTase).

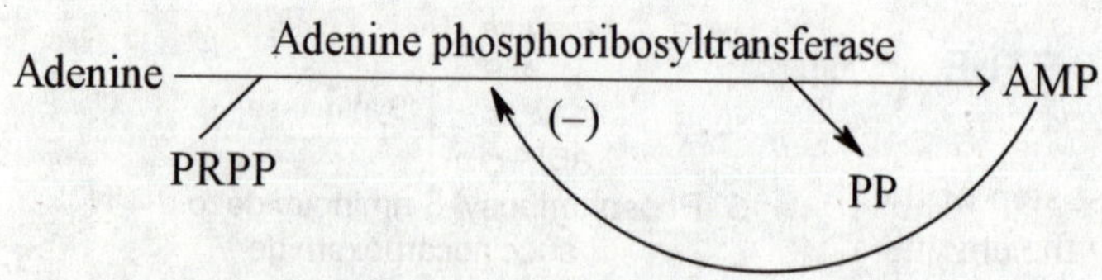

On the other hand, both **hypoxanthine** and **guanine** are converted to **IMP** and **GMP**, respectively, by the same enzyme, called **hypoxanthine-guanine phosphoribosyltransferase (HGPRTase).**

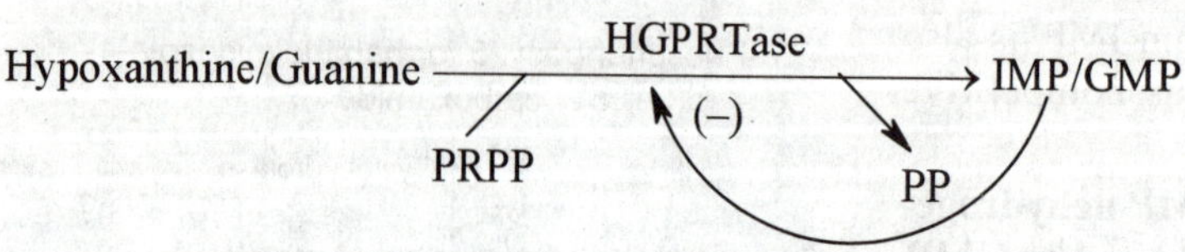

The end products of these reactions regulate these enzymes, i.e. AMP acts as a competitive inhibitor for APRTase, whereas IMP and GMP competitively inhibit HGPRTase activity.

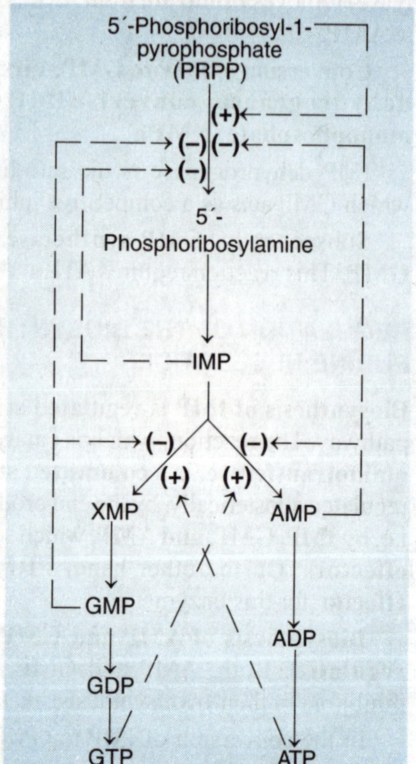

Fig. 17.4. Regulation of the synthesis of purine nucleotides [(+) = stimulation; (–) = Inhibition].

Lack of the HGPRTase activity results in a condition called **Lesch-Nyhan syndrome**.

> **LYSCH-NYHAN SYNDROME**
>
> Inability of the body to salvage hypoxanthine and guanine, due to marked **deficiency of** the enzyme **HGPRTase** leads to the condition called **Lesch-Nyhan syndrome**. Since these nitrogenous bases can not be salvaged, they are degraded and cause **excessive production of uric acid.**
> Hyperuricemia, mental retardation and self-mutilation characterize Lesch-Nyhan syndrome.

Salvage reactions conserve energy and are important in cells, such as erythrocytes, which lack amidotransferase and can not synthesize purines.

Nucleosides can also be salvaged and converted to their corresponding nucleotides, **by** the respective **nucleoside kinases**. For example, adenosine is salvaged by the enzyme adenosine kinase and converted to AMP.

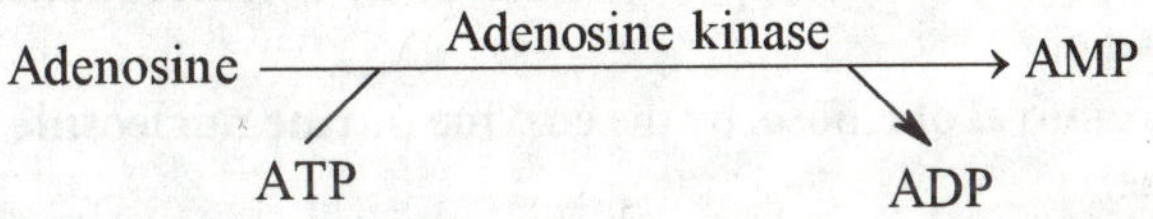

DEGRADATION OF PURINE NUCLEOTIDES

Degradation of the purine nucleotides leads to the formation of uric acid, in human beings (Fig 17.5).

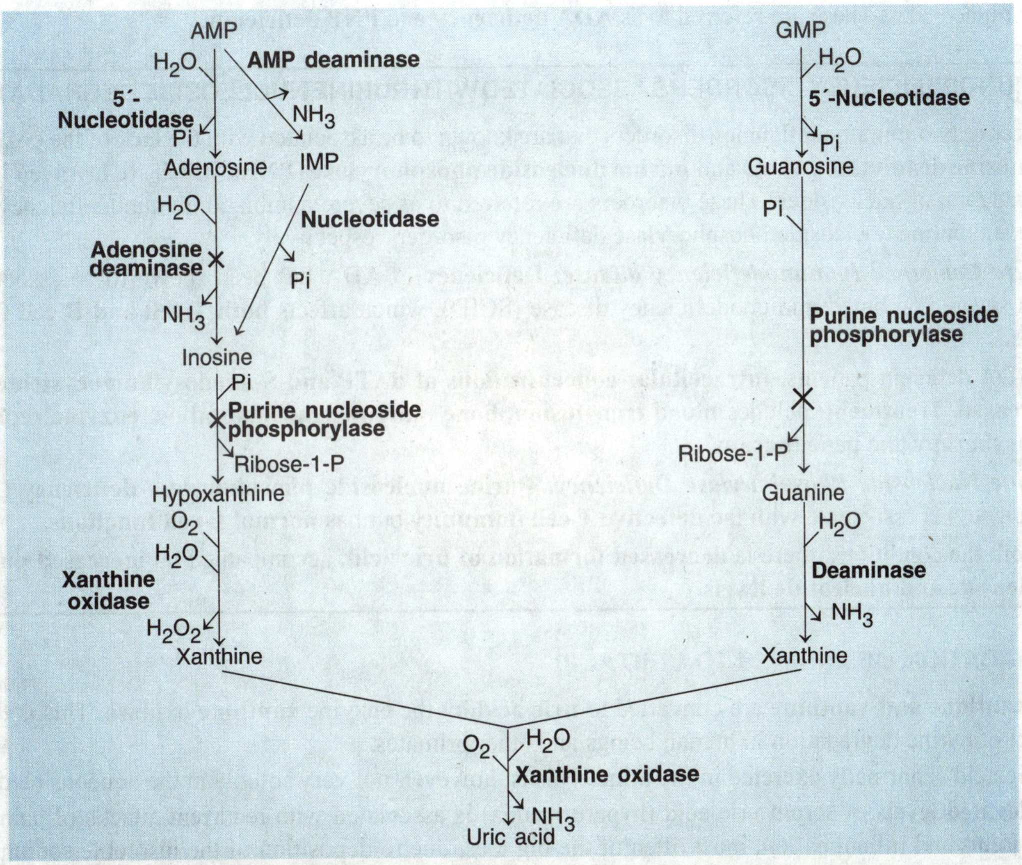

Fig. 17.5. Degradation of purine nucleotides. (X = enzyme deficient in severe combined immunodeficiency disease).

Degradation of AMP

1. **AMP is converted to adenosine by the enzyme 5′-AMP nucleotidase,** which has high specificity for its substrate.
   Thereafter, **adenosine deaminase (ADA) converts adenosine to inosine.**
   Alternatively, **AMP deaminase removes ammonia** and **converts it to IMP.** Subsequently, nucleotidase removes phosphoric acid and **forms inosine.**
2. Thereafter, **purine nucleoside phosphorylase** (PNP) **removes ribose** from inosine and **converts it to hypoxanthine**.

Degradation of GMP

1. In the first step, **phosphoric acid is removed by the enzyme 5′-nucleotidase,** as a result of which **GMP is converted to guanosine.**
2. Subsequently, with the **removal of ribose,** by the enzyme **purine nucleoside phosphorylase, guanosine is converted to guanine.**
3. **Deaminase** (an aminohydrolase) thereafter, removes the amino group from **guanine** and converts it to **xanthine.**

Two **immunodeficiency diseases** have been shown to be associated with defects in degradation of the purine nucleosides. These are referred to as **ADA deficiency** and **PNP deficiency.**

IMMUNODEFICIENCY DISORDERS ASSOCIATED WITH PURINE NUCLEOSIDE DEGRADATION

There are two immunodeficiency disorders that are known to be associated with the lack of the enzymes **adenosine deaminase (ADA)** and **purine nucleoside phosphorylase (PNP),** which are involved in the degradation of nucleosides. These disorders are referred to as severe combined immunodeficiency disease and purine nucleoside phosphorylase deficiency disorder, respectively.

Severe Combined Immunodeficiency disease: **Deficiency of ADA** has been shown to be associated with severe combined immunodeficiency disease (SCID), which affects **both T cell and B cell functions.**

In ADA deficient patients, **intracellular concentrations of dATP and S-adenosylhomocysteine are increased. Treatment** includes **blood transfusion, bone marrow transplantation, enzyme replacement therapy** and **gene therapy.**

Purine Nucleoside Phosphorylase Deficiency: **Purine nucleoside phosphorylase deficiency** (PNP deficiency) is associated with the **defective T cell immunity** but has **normal B cell functions.**

In both the conditions, there is **decreased formation of uric acid,** accompanied by **increased purine nucleoside and nucleotide levels.**

DEGRADATION OF PURINES TO URIC ACID

Hypoxanthine and xanthine are converted to **uric acid** by the enzyme **xanthine oxidase**. This is the end product of purine degradation in human beings and other primates.

Uric acid is normally excreted in the urine. This is, however, not very soluble in the aqueous medium.

Elevated levels of serum uric acid (hyperuricemia) is associated with recurrent attacks of painful arthritic joints and inflammation, most often of the big toes, due to deposition of the insoluble sodium urate crystals, called **tophi,** in a clinical condition referred to as **gout**.

GOUT

Gout is a disease, which is characterized by the **elevated level of uric acid in the blood (hyperuricemia)** and its **increased excretion in the urine (uric aciduria)**, due to variety of metabolic abnormalities.

Hyperuricemia may be due to the **overproduction of uric acid**. This is called as **primary hyperuricemia.** Hyperuricemia may also be a result of some **kidney disease** or **excessive cell death**, e.g. during radiation therapy. This is referred to as **secondary hyperuricemia.**

Primary Hyperuricemia

This is due to some metabolic defect that results in increased synthesis of purine nucleotides, such as:

1. **Increased PRPP synthetase activity:** This results in **increased intracellular concentration of PRPP,** which acts as a positive effector for the enzyme amidotransferase. This in turn leads to **increased synthesis of purine nucleotides** as well as their **degradation to uric acid.**
2. **HGPRTase deficiency:** Complete or partial **deficiency of** the enzyme **HGPRTase** (Lesch-Nyhan syndrome), causes a **decrease in utilization of** hypoxanthine and guanine, in the **salvage pathway**. This in turn **spares PRPP,** which is **used in the de novo synthesis of purine nucleotides,** thereby **resulting in their overproduction** and subsequent **degradation to uric acid.**
3. **Glucose-6-phosphatase deficiency: Glucose-6-phosphatase deficiency (Von Gierke's disease,** also called **glycogen storage disease I)** results in **increased levels of glucose-6-phosphate,** which is diverted towards the pentose phosphate pathway. This in turn **increases** availability of **ribose-5-phosphate** and enhances **generation of PRPP.**

Raised levels of PRPP in turn, increase de novo synthesis of purines and subsequently, over-production of uric acid.

Allopurinol decreases both uric acid formation as well as de novo synthesis of purine nucleotides and thus is used in the treatment of gout.

Secondary Hyperuricemia

Hyperuricemia is secondary to **some disease other than a metabolic disorder,** such as a **kidney disease** or some disease that is associated with the **excessive cell turnover,** e.g. **leukemia** or **psoriasis.**

METABOLISM OF PYRIMIDINE NUCLEOTIDES

FORMATION OF PYRIMIDINE NUCLEOTIDES

De Novo Synthesis of Pyrimidine Nucleotides

A **pyrimidine ring** is synthesized, in mammalian cells, from **two amino acids, i.e. aspartate and glutamine,** which are used as the sources of carbon and nitrogen along with the **respiratory $CO_2(HCO_3^-)$** as a carbon donor.

As shown in Fig. 17.6, **nitrogen** at position **1 and carbons at positions 4, 5 and 6 of the pyrimidine ring** are derived **from aspartate, carbon at position 2 from HCO_3^-** and **nitrogen at position 3 from glutamine.**

In de novo synthesis of the pyrimidine nucleotides, a **pyrimidine ring is formed** first. Thereafter, **ribose-5-phosphate is added,** via PRPP, which in turn leads to **synthesis of UMP** that serves as precursor for the synthesis of both, **CMP and TMP.**

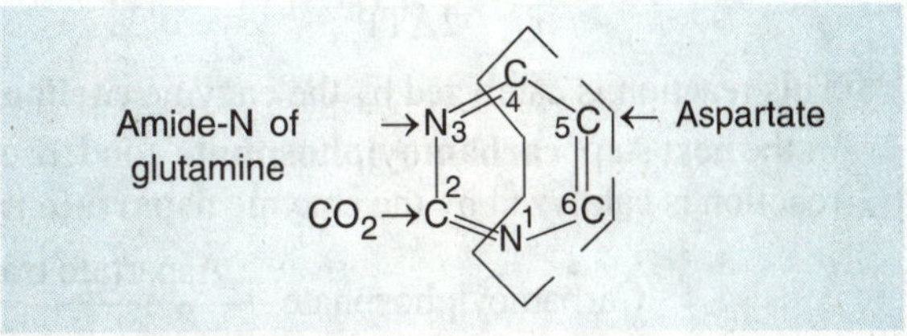

Fig. 17.6. Sources of carbon and nitrogen atoms in a pyrimidine ring.

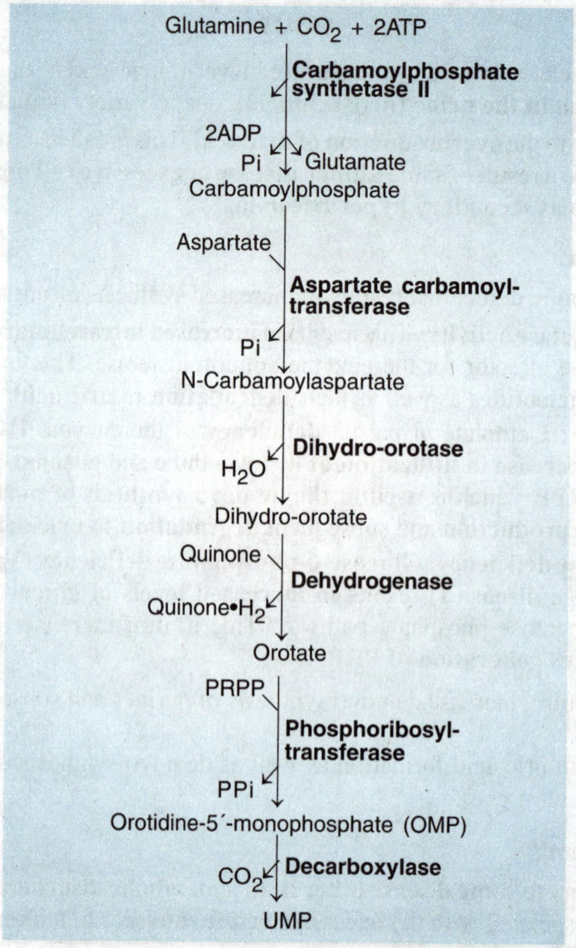

Fig. 17.7. De Novo synthesis of UMP.

Synthesis of UMP

De novo synthesis of UMP is shown in Fig. 17.7

1. The first step, in the synthesis of UMP is **synthesis of carbamoylphosphate**, from **glutamine** and **HCO_3^-**.

$$HCO_3^- + \text{Glutamine} \xrightarrow[2ATP \;\; \searrow 2ADP + Pi]{\text{Carbamoylphosphate synthetase II}} \text{Carbamoylphosphate + Glutamate}$$

This reaction is catalyzed by the enzyme **carbamoylphosphate synthetase II (CPS II), in the cytosol.**

2. In the next step, **carbamoylphosphate** condenses with **aspartate** and forms **carbamoylaspartate**. This reaction is catalyzed by the enzyme **aspartate transcarbamoylase**.

$$\text{Carbamoylphosphate} \xrightarrow[\text{Aspartate} \;\; \searrow Pi]{\text{Aspartate transcarbamoylase}} \text{Carbamoylaspartate}$$

This is a **committed step,** in the synthesis of pyrimidine nucleotides.

3. Subsequently, **dihydro-orotase** results in ring closure, and **forms dihydro-orotate.**

$$\text{Carbamoylaspartate} \xrightarrow[\searrow H_2O]{\text{Dihydro-orotase}} \text{Dihydro-orotate}$$

Activities of the above **3 enzymes**, i.e. **CPS II**, **aspartate transcarbamoylase** and **dihydro-orotase** are present on **a single trifunctional protein,** which is termed as **CAD.**

4. Thereafter, **dihydro-orotate dehydrogenase** oxidizes **dihydro-orotate** to **orotate.**

$$\text{Dihydroorotate} \xrightarrow[\text{Quinone} \nearrow \quad \searrow \text{Quinone.}H_2]{\text{Dihydroorotate dehydrogenase}} \text{Orotate}$$

5. In the next step, **orotate phosphoribosyltransferase** transfers **ribose-5-phosphate from PRPP** and converts **orotate** to **orotidine monophosphate (OMP).**

$$\text{Orotate} \xrightarrow[\text{PRPP} \nearrow \quad Mg^{2+} \quad \searrow \text{PPi}]{\text{Orotate phosporibosyltransferase}} \text{Orotidine-5}'\text{-monophosphate (OMP)}$$

6. **OMP** is subsequently converted to **UMP**, by the enzyme **OMP decarboxylase.**

$$\text{OMP} \xrightarrow[\searrow CO_2]{\text{OMP Decarboxylase}} \text{UMP}$$

Orotate phosphoribosyltransferase and **OMP decarboxylase** activities are present on a **single bifunctional protein, which is** termed as **UMP synthase.**

> **OROTIC ACIDURIA**
>
> A **defect in** the de novo **synthesis of pyrimidine nucleotides** results in a condition, which is referred to as **orotic aciduria.**
>
> This is due to genetic deficiency of the bifunctional protein **UMP synthase,** or the individual enzymes, i.e. **orotate phosphoribosyltransferase and/or OMP decarboxylase.**
>
> Severe anemia, growth retardation and high levels of orotic acid in urine characterize orotic aciduria.

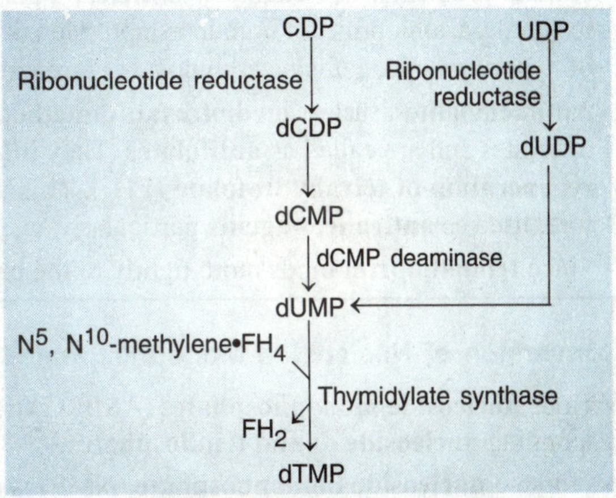

Fig. 17.8. Synthesis of TMP.

Synthesis of TMP

Both, UTP and CTP serve as precursors of TMP. They are hydrolyzed to the corresponding diphosphates (CDP and UDP) and serve as the precursors of dUMP.

TMP is thereafter synthesized by the methylation of dUMP. This reaction is catalyzed **by** the enzyme **thymidylate synthase.** In this reaction, N^5, N^{10}-methylenetetrahydrofolate (N^5, N^{10}-methylene.FH_4) is used as a source of the methyl group (Fig. 17.8).

DEGRADATION OF PYRIMIDINE NUCLEOTIDES

Pyrimidine nucleotides, released as a result of hydrolysis of nucleic acids, are converted to the corresponding nucleosides by the nonspecific phosphatases. Thereafter, cytidine and deoxycitidine are converted to uridine and deoxyuridine by the enzyme pyrimidine nucleoside deaminase. The nucleosides are then converted to free bases by the enzyme uridine phosphorylase.

Uracil and thymine are subsequently converted to β-alanine and β-aminoisobutyric acid, respectively (Fig. 17.9).

β-Aminoisobutyric acid is excreted in urine and is a measure of turnover of DNA (thymine nucleotides). Its excretion is increased in-patients undergoing cancer therapy, due to increased degradation of DNA.

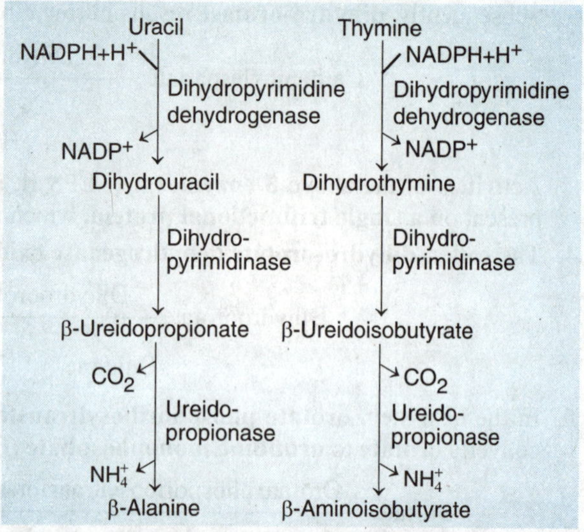

Fig. 17.9. Degradation of pyrimidine bases.

ANTIMETABOLITES

Antimetabolites are usually structural analogs of purine and pyrimidine bases or nucleosides that interfere with very specific metabolic reactions. These compounds are relatively specific inhibitors of enzymes involved in nucleotide synthesis or interconversions and have proved to be useful in therapy of diverse clinical problems. For example, 6-mercaptopurine and 6-thioguanine used in the treatment of acute leukemia, azathioprine for immunosuppression in patients with organ transplants, allopurinol for treatment of hyperuricemia; cytosine arabinoside in treatment of several forms of human cancer, etc.

Antimetabolites, such as **methotrexate (amethopterin), aminopterin and trimethoprim,** are the analogs of folates and are called as **antifolates**. They **inhibit the enzyme dihydrofolate reductase** and **blocks regeneration of tetrahydrofolate (FH_4).** This in turn affects dTMP synthesis**.** These drugs are, therefore, used as **anticancer agents** particularly, against childhood leukemia.

Since **trimethoprim** binds more tightly to the bacterial enzyme, it is used as an **antibacterial agent.**

Conversion of Nucleoside Monophosphates to Di and Triphosphates

Various **nucleoside monophosphates** (AMP, GMP, CMP and UMP) are sequentially converted to their corresponding **nucleoside di and triphosphates.**

First, a **nucleoside monophosphate** (NMP) is converted to the **nucleoside diphosphate** (NDP), by the specific **nucleoside monophosphate kinase**. Thereafter, the enzyme **nucleoside diphosphate kinase** converts the **nucleoside diphosphate** to **nucleoside triphosphate** (Fig. 17.10).

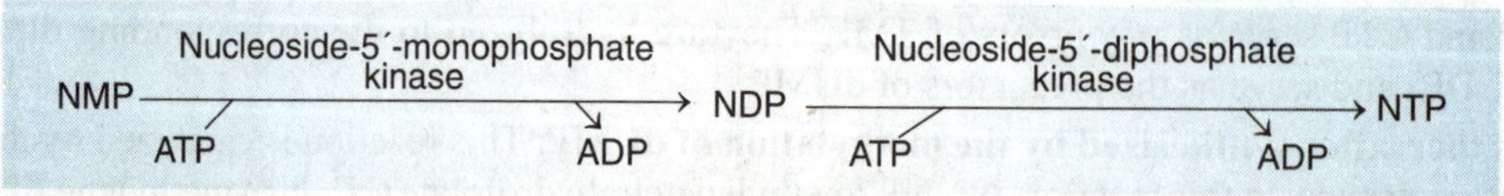

Fig. 17.10. Conversion of nucleosidemonophosphate to di and triphosphates.

Conversion of Ribonucleotides to Deoxyribonucleotides

Purine and pyrimidine ribonucleotides are converted to their corresponding deoxyribonucleotides, during DNA replication, at the level of diphosphates.

Ribonucleoside diphosphates (NDPs), i.e. ADP, GDP, CDP and UDP are reduced at carbon 2, to their deoxy forms, i.e. dADP, dGDP, dCDP and dUDP, by the enzyme **ribonucleotide reductase** (Fig. 17.11).

dATP is a potent inhibitor in the reduction of the four nucleoside diphosphates. On the other hand, dGTP inhibits the reduction of CDP, UDP and GDP, while dTTP inhibits the reduction of CDP, UDP and ADP.

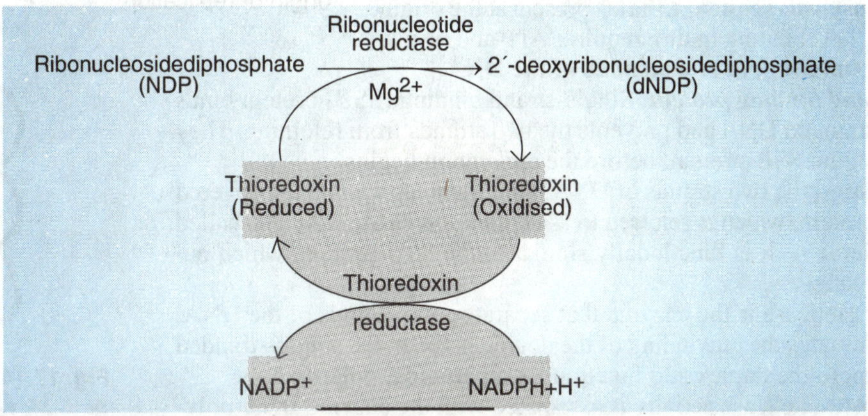

Fig. 17.11. Conversion of a ribonucleotide to deoxyribonucleotide.

Phosphorylation of the **dNDPs** produces **dNTPs,** which in turn are used in the synthesis of DNA. This reaction is catalyzed by the enzyme **nucleoside diphosphate kinase**. Among the four NTPs or dNTPs, any one of them can be used as the phosphate donor for this reaction.

$$\text{dNDP} \xrightarrow[\text{ATP} \;\to\; \text{ADP}]{\text{Nucleoside diphosphate kinase}} \text{dNTP}$$

DNA REPLICATION

The **process of DNA synthesis** is called **replication**. During replication, **each strand** of the double-stranded **DNA serves as template for** the synthesis of the **new strand** in a very accurate manner. Since **both the strands** of the parent DNA serve as templates and produce two daughter strands therefore, after each round of the replication, the newly formed double-stranded DNA contains one **strand from the parent DNA** while the other **one is the newly synthesized** complementary strand. This process of DNA replication is called **semiconservative replication** (Fig. 17.12)

The site, where DNA replication begins is called **origin of replication,** which is **AT-rich** region.

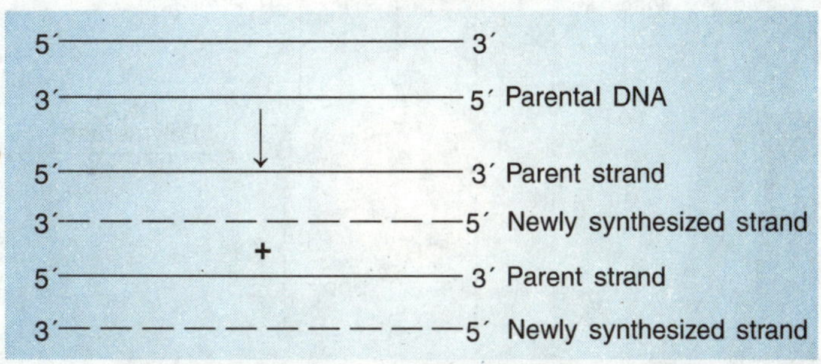

Fig. 17.12. Semiconservative replication of DNA.

Separation of the two strands, of the parental DNA, is essential for the initiation of replication. For the initiation of unwinding of the double helix and continuation of separation of the two strands various proteins and enzymes are required. **These include:**

DnaA: DnaA is a protein that binds at the origin of replication. It is also called as the **origin-binding protein** (Fig. 17.13).

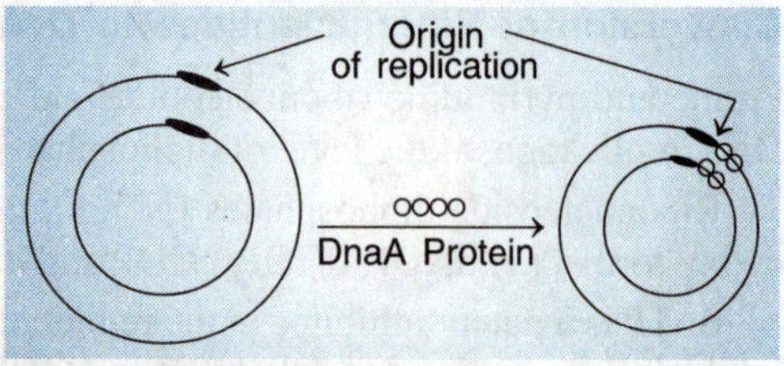

Fig. 17.13. Binding of DnaA protein at the origin of replication.

Nearly **20-50 monomers of DnaA bind** at the specific **nucleotide consensus sequence that** is present at the origin of replication. This binding in turn requires ATP and results in **separation (melting) of two strands of the DNA.**

Single-strand binding protein: Single-strand binding (SSB) protein binds to the single-stranded DNA and prevents the two strands from rejoining. They are stripped-off the SSB-protein, before the replication begins.

In eukaryotes, the two strands of DNA, after their separation, are covered with another protein, which is referred to as **replication protein A,** also called **replication factor A**. It is functionally similar to the SSB-protein, which occurs in prokaryotes.

Helicases: Helicase is the enzyme that separates two strands of the DNA. This enzyme initiates the unwinding of the double helix, at the single-stranded region, adjacent to the duplex and functions in a particular polarity only.

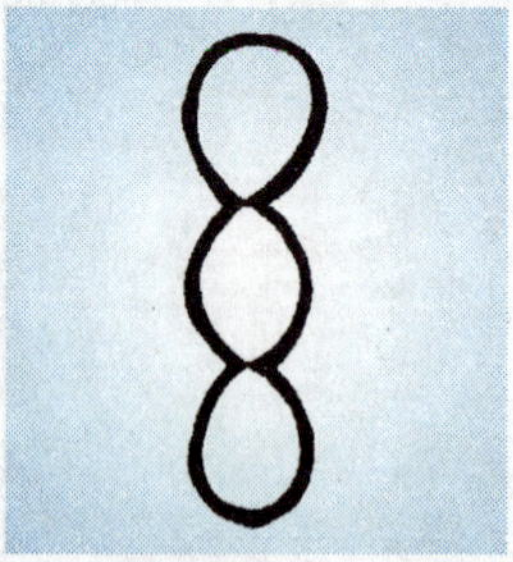

Fig. 17.14. Supercoils.

In eukaryotes, helicase activity is associated with the enzyme **DNA polymerase δ.**

Topoisomerases : As we know, chromosomes of many bacteria and viruses are the circular molecules of the double helix DNA and have a peculiar twisted appearance. This is referred as **super-coiling** or **superhelicity** (Fig. 17.14).

The group of enzymes, called topoisomerases overcomes supercoiling. They are endonucleases, which **alter topological coiling of the circular DNA.** They introduce nicks in one or both the strands, remove supercoils, and reseal the ends.

If the topological problems are not corrected, it may stop unwinding of the parent DNA and hence, DNA replication.

DNA polymerases: DNA polymerases (DNA dependent-DNA polymerases) are the enzymes that catalyze the synthesis of the complementary strand, on the single-stranded DNA template. They add nucleotides at the free 3′-OH group and extend the chain in 5′→ 3′ direction (Fig.17.15).

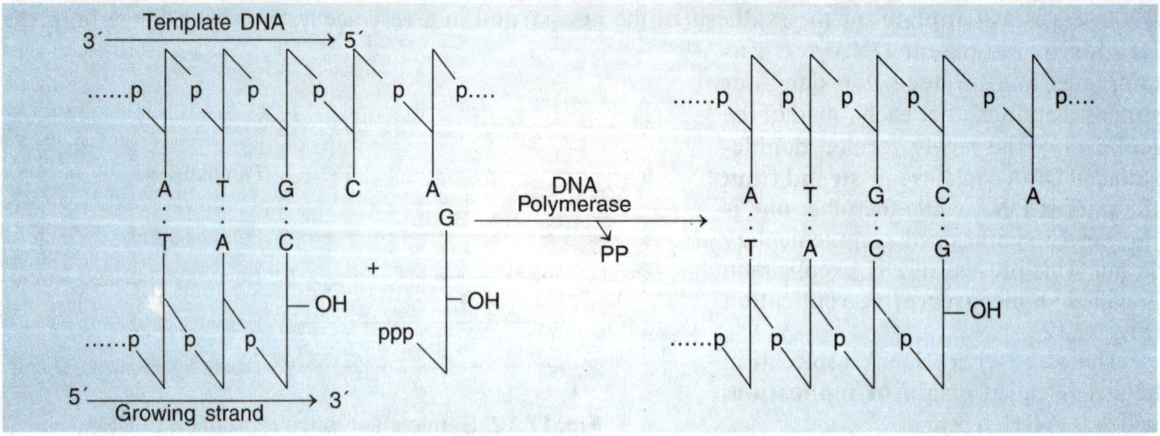

Fig. 17.15. Action of DNA polymerase.

DNA POLYMERASES

Different types of the enzymes are found in prokaryotes and eukaryotes.

In Prokaryotes

Three distinct forms of the enzyme are found in prokaryotes. These are designated as DNA polymerase I, II, and III.

DNA Polymerase I: **DNA Polymerase I (pol I)** has **three distinct activities,** i.e. it has $5' \rightarrow 3'$ **polymerase (synthetic) activity** and both, $3' \rightarrow 5'$ and $5' \rightarrow 3'$ **exonuclease (hydrolytic) activity.**

The enzyme has two fragments, which are referred to as the large fragment and the small fragment.

Its large fragment is designated as **Klenow fragment**. It has $5' \rightarrow 3'$ **polymerase** and $3' \rightarrow 5'$ **exonuclease activities,** whereas the **small fragment** has $5' \rightarrow 3'$ **exonuclease activity.**

DNA polymerase I also **edit mistakes** and its **proof reading action** suggests that the enzyme has high fidelity in DNA replication. It is also important in the repair of the damaged DNA.

DNA Polymerase II: **DNA Polymerase II (pol II)** has $5' \rightarrow 3'$ **polymerase** activity along with the $3' \rightarrow 5'$ **exonuclease activity** but lacks $5' \rightarrow 3'$ exonuclease activity. It mainly participates in the process of DNA repair.

DNA Polymerase III: DNA Polymerase III (pol III) is a more complex enzyme as it consists of atleast **ten different subunits. All the subunits** together form a labile multisubunit enzyme, known as **pol III holoenzyme**. It **polymerizes** DNA and **edits mistakes** but lacks nick-translation.

In Eukaryotes

Five different types of DNA polymerases are found in eukaryotes. These are designated as DNA polymerase α, β, γ, δ and ε.

All have $5' \rightarrow 3'$ **synthetic activities**. With the exception of the polymerase γ, which occurs in mitochondria, they are involved in the chromosomal DNA synthesis as well as its repair.

DNA polymerase α: **DNA polymerase (pol α)** has $5' \rightarrow 3'$ **polymerase activity** but lacks proof reading (exonuclease) activity. Thus, **it can replicate DNA** but **can not correct its mistakes**. It also has tightly **associated primase activity,** which is concerned with the priming (initiation) of replication. It is also called as the **lagging strand replicase.**

DNA polymerase δ: **DNA polymerase δ (pol δ) has** $5' \rightarrow 3'$ **polymerase activity** and $3' \rightarrow 5'$ **exonuclease (proof reading) activity.**

Pol δ has a very **high processivity when associated with a protein** called **proliferating cell nuclear antigen** (PCNA). The **pol δ-PCNA complex** is designated as the **leading strand replicase.**

DNA polymerase ε: **DNA polymerase ε (pol ε)** though resembles pol δ but is **highly processive even in the absence of the factor PCNA.** It also has $3' \rightarrow 5'$ **exonuclease activity** and is involved in repairing the damaged nuclear DNA.

DNA polymerase β: **DNA polymerase β (pol β)** is a small polypeptide. Its biological function is not yet known.

DNA polymerase γ: **DNA polymerase γ (pol γ) occurs exclusively in mitochondria** and is involved in the mitochondrial DNA replication only.

Reverse Transcriptase

RNA-dependent DNA polymerase, designated as **reverse transcriptase**, is also a member of the **polymerase family of enzymes**. It is found in **retroviruses** (RNA-containing eukaryotic viruses), such as **human immunodeficiency virus (HIV)**, which is the causative agent of the **acquired immunodeficiency syndrome (AIDS).**

Reverse transcriptase **catalyzes synthesis of the double-stranded DNA, from the single-stranded RNA template.**

THE PROCESS OF DNA SYNTHESIS IN PROKARYOTES

DNA Replication is a complex process, which involves initiation, elongation and termination.

Initiation

Initiation of DNA replication involves formation of the replication fork and synthesis of the RNA primer.

Formation of the Replication Fork

Replication starts at the origin, which is referred as ori C in *E.coli*.

Initiation of replication begins with the **binding of the DnaA,** which in turn **promotes unwinding of DNA strands at the A.T-rich region.**

When two strands of the parental DNA get separated, the **circular chromosome** exhibits a bubble like structure, called **replication bubble (replication eye).**

The **branch point in the replication bubble**, at which DNA synthesis begins, is called replication **fork.**

A replication bubble may contain one replication fork, called unidirectional replication, or two replication forks, which is referred to as bi-directional replication.

Formation of the replication fork initiates step wise assembly of all the proteins and enzymes, which are necessary to carry out the process of DNA replication (Fig. 17.16)

As the enzyme helicase moves, in advance of each fork, **two-single stranded regions are generated.** The SSB-protein soon covers them. This in turn helps in keeping the two strands apart from each other.

In the process of replication, two antiparallel strands of the DNA are simultaneously replicated at the two advancing replication forks in **5′→ 3′** directions, but differently. One of the strands is **synthesized continuously,** in the direction of the movement of the replication fork. It is called as the **leading strand**.

On the other hand, the **other strand** though is also synthesized in its **5′→ 3′** direction but **discontinuously**, i.e. it is synthesized in small fragments. This strand is called as the **lagging strand,** while these **fragments** are called **Okazaki fragments**.

Okazaki fragments vary in size from about 100-200 deoxyribonucleotides, in eukaryotes, to nearly 1000-2000 deoxyribonucleotides, in prokaryotes.

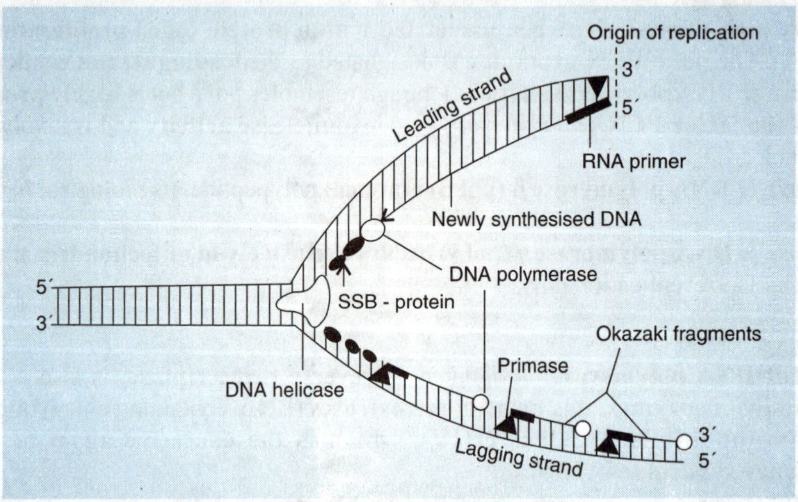

Fig. 17.16. A replication fork.

Synthesis of the RNA Primer

Synthesis of RNA primer begins with the formation of a complex, called **prepriming complex** (pre-priming assembly), which consists of **DnaB-DnaC complex along with four more proteins that are referred to as n, n′, n″ and i**. Association of the enzyme primase (RNA polymerase) to the pre-priming complex results in formation of the primosome (the priming complex).

The primosome interacts with the template, at the replication fork and begins synthesis of the RNA primer. Whereas, only **one priming complex** is required to **initiate synthesis of the leading strand, multiple copies of the complex** are required **for the synthesis of the lagging strand.**

Once the site for the primer initiation has been recognized, SSB-proteins are displaced and the primase lays down the primer.

Elongation

The entire assembly, which carries out the process of elongation, is called **replisome (replicase system).**

Various components of the replisome are shown in Table 17.1.

Table 17.1. Components of the replisome

Component protein/enzyme	*Functions*
DnaA	Unwinding of the two strands of DNA at the origin of replication
DnaB	Helicase activity, unwinds DNA for creation of the initiation bubble
Topoisomerase II	Removal of the supercoils
SSB-protein	Binds to single-strands of the DNA, to keep the two strands apart from each other
DnaC	Binding with the SSB-protein at the origin of replication
Primase	Synthesis of the RNA primer
n, n′, n″, and i proteins	Primosome assembly
DNA polymerase III	Chain elongation on the 3′-OH group of the primer
DNA polymerase I	Excision of the primer and gap-filling
DNA ligase	Ligation of the polynucleotide fragments

A replisome exists only as a protein complex, associated with the particular structure that DNA takes at the replication fork.

A replisome, which contains two polymerase III holoenzymes, synthesizes the leading strand as well as the lagging strand. It moves, as a single unit, in the 5′→ 3′ direction along the leading strand, whereas the lagging strand template loops around to permit the holoenzyme to extend the primed lagging strand. After completing the synthesis of an Okazaki fragment, holoenzyme (on the lagging strand) is relocated to the new primer, near the replication fork and extends the RNA primer to form a new Okazaki fragment.

At each location, DNA polymerase uses RNA primer, for the synthesis of DNA. After the polymerase reaches the end of the single-stranded template, it takes over the next primer that is annealed to the template, as DNA-RNA hybrid.

In **eukaryotes, the primers may be formed at several locations, which** are determined by nucleosome spacing. This in turn results in continuous synthesis of the leading strand and several RNA primed Okazaki fragments, which are separated from each other by the single-stranded nicks, on the lagging strand.

In this process, synthesis of the leading strand is always ahead of the synthesis of the lagging strand.

DNA polymerase I replaces ribonucleotides (from RNA primer) with the deoxyribonucleotides and finally, the **nicks are sealed by the DNA ligase.**

Termination

A protein, designated as the **Tus protein** (terminator utilization substance), **arrests movement of the replication fork** and **terminates DNA synthesis.** It acts as a **contrahelicase** and **binds** to the region called **ter site,** which has **G.T rich sequence.** This in turn **prevents advancement of the replication fork**, by arresting the action of **DnaB.** Finally, **delinking of the parent strands,** from the daughter strands, is catalyzed by the enzyme topoisomerase.

DIFFERENCES IN DNA REPLICATION BETWEEN PROKARYOTES AND EUKARYOTES

As shown in Table 17.2, DNA replication in **eukaryotes differs from** the process in **prokaryotes** in several ways:

Table 17.2. Differences in DNA replication between prokaryotes and eukaryotes

Prokaryotes	*Eukaryotes*
Replication begins at the origin	Replication begins at multiple sites, simultaneously
SSB-protein keeps two strands separate	Replication protein A keeps two strands separate
Only negative supercoils are relaxed	Both, negative and positive supercoils are relaxed
There are 3 types of DNA polymerases, called polymerase I, II and III.	There are 5 types of DNA polymerases, called polymerase α, β, γ, δ and ε
Helicase is a specific enzyme	Helicase activity is associated with DNA polymerase δ
Primase is a specific RNA polymerase	Primase activity is present in DNA polymerase α
Both the DNA strands are synthesized by DNA polymerase III	Leading strand is synthesized by DNA polymerase δ while lagging strand is synthesized by DNA polymerase α
Very long Okazaki fragments are synthesized	Small-sized Okazaki fragments are synthesized
The process is simple, rapid and error-prone	The process is complex, slow but accurate

1. The amount of DNA present in the eukaryotic cell is much more than the prokaryotic cell.
2. **Eukaryotic cell contains large number of the DNA polymerase molecules** (often more than 20,000) as compared to the small number (a few dozens), that occur in a prokaryotic cell.
3. **Origin of replication** in eukaryotes has specific sequences, termed **autonomous replicating sequences (ARS)**. Each such sequence is 100-200 base-pair (bp) in size and has **A.T-rich region**. It is the 11-bp element and is designated as **ARS- consensus sequence.**
4. Initiation of the **DNA replication occurs at several origins of replication,** simultaneously, in eukaryotes. DNA segment between the two origins of replication is termed as **replicon**. An average human chromosome may contain about 100 replicons hence; replication may proceed at nearly 200 forks, simultaneously.
5. **Eukaryotic DNA synthesis requires a protein,** called **replication protein A** (replication factor A), which is functionally same as the SSB-protein in prokaryotes.

6. In eukaryotes, **helicase** activity is associated with the DNA **polymerase δ.**
7. **Eukaryotic DNA is packed** along with the histones, **as chromatin, in the nucleosomes.** The DNA gets separated from histones, prior to its replication, just ahead of the replication fork.

   After replication, histones again **get associated** with the upcoming daughter duplexes and form nucleosomes.
8. Cyclins and cyclin-dependent kinases regulate initiation of DNA synthesis in eukaryotes.

   Moreover, DNA synthesis in eukaryotes is confined to the synthetic phase **(S-phase)** only. This is followed by the gap period (G_1). Thereafter, cell division occurs during mitosis (M- phase), which again follows a gap period (G_2).

   On the other hand, DNA is replicated through most of the cell cycle in prokaryotes and the cell division occurs immediately after the DNA synthesis has ceased.
9. In eukaryotes, **synthesis of the leading strand** and the **lagging strand** is carried out **by different enzymes.**

   In prokaryotes, DNA synthesis is catalyzed by two similar but distinct subunits of the same enzyme, i.e. DNA polymerase III.
10. **Ends of the eukaryotic chromosomes have unusual structures,** called **telomeres,** which are also replicated.

MUTATIONS

Mutations are **inheritable alterations** of the **genetic information,** which can not be repaired but cause drastic **changes in the DNA sequence.**

A mutation can be defined as a **permanent change in the DNA segment of a gene,** which may be **expressed as a phenotypic change** in the organism.

Mutations may arise by a number of means, such as due to **errors in replication** during proofreading, by **UV or ionizing radiation** (X-rays or γ-rays), or by a **chemical mutagen** (such as an alkylating agent). **Besides,** DNA may also undergo **certain spontaneous changes,** such as the deamination of cytosine to uracil, depurination etc. Whatever the cause may be, mutations occur at random.

They are classified into two categories as point mutation and frame shift mutation.

POINT MUTATION

A point mutation occurs due to a change in the single base pair in DNA, which in turn results in the single base change in the corresponding mRNA. This type of the mutation is also referred to as **base substitution mutation**.

Base substitution may be a result of transition or transversion (Fig. 17.17)

Transition

This is a type of **substitution** where **another such pair replaces a purine-pyrimidine** pair. This type of mutation **may occur spontaneously, induced chemically by a base analog,** e.g. 5-bromouracil, or by a **mutagen,** such as nitrous acid. For example, if 5-bormouracil gets incorporated into DNA, in place of thymine, this in turn may induce transition from AT → GC.

Transversion

This is a type of **substitution** where a **pyrimidine-purine pair replaces a purine-pyrimidine pair**. This **occurs spontaneously** and is common in human beings.

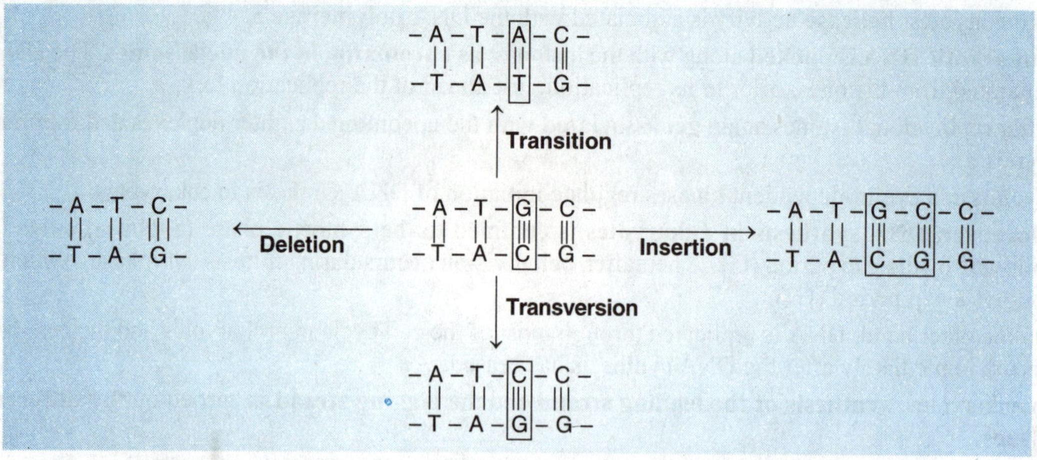

Fig. 17.17. Mutations.

FRAME SHIFT MUTATION

Frame shift mutation may be a result of either **deletion** or **insertion of a base pair.**

Deletion

Deletion of a base pair from the sequence of the gene may **change its reading frame** and result in a nonfunctional gene product. A frame shift mutation, due to base deletion, may result in the production of abnormal hemoglobin, such as hemoglobin Wayne.

Insertion

Insertion of a base pair into the gene sequence can lead to the synthesis of abnormal chain length of the protein.

A mutation may be visible (expressed) or phenotypically silent **(hidden)**. It can be detected by gene sequence determination.

Visible mutation

A visible mutation may result in missense mutation or nonsense mutation.

Missense mutation: It is the result of **a base change that causes incorporation of a different amino acid** in the encoded protein. Most common missense mutation is due to change in the second base of the codons in GAA or GAG, which code for glutamate, in the sixth position of the β-chain of hemoglobin. The change, from A to U, in turn results in different codons, GUA or GUG, which code for valine and causes sickle-cell anemia, the most common form of hemoglobinopathies.

Nonsense Mutation: It may be a result of the **change** in the base of a codon, which in turn may change the **codon to generate a termination codon, or cause destruction of the termination codon to a codon that codes for an amino acid.**

Generation of a termination codon: Generation of a termination codon, from the one that codes for an amino acid, **will result in premature termination** of the protein chain and thus **reduces its chain length**. For example UAU or UAC, which normally codes for tyrosine that is present as the 145th amino acid in the β-chain of hemoglobin. A single base mutation, from UAU to UAA, or UAC to UAG, results in a termination codon, which in turn causes immature termination of the protein and reduces its chain length from 146 to 144 amino acids. This results in the synthesis of a type of the abnormal hemoglobin, called hemoglobin McKees Rocks, which has high oxygen affinity with reduced oxygen delivery.

Change in termination codon to a codon that codes for an amino acid: Mutation of a base in the termination codon to a codon that codes for an amino acid results in a protein with increased chain length. For example, α-globulin chain in hemoglobin has 141 amino acids. When the stop codon UAA mutates, it results in the incorporation of an amino acid at the 142nd position and thus increases the chain length of the protein to 172 amino acids, i.e. until another stop codon is available. Abnormally, longer α-globulin chain has been shown to result in many instances of α-Thalassemia.

Silent mutation

A silent mutation is the result of the **base change** that occurs at **the third position of the codon**, e.g. from UUA to UUG. Since they both code for leucine, there is **no change in the specified amino acid.**

RNA TRANSCRIPTION

The **process of RNA synthesis,** by which a DNA sequence is transcribed into the RNA transcript, **is referred to as transcription.**

Transcription is a strand selective process since during this process only **one strand of the DNA,** i.e. the template strand, is **transcribed into RNA**. The sequence of ribonucleotides in RNA is **complementary** to the sequence of deoxyribonucleotides that is found in the **template strand of DNA.**

DNA strand that serves as the template for RNA synthesis is **called as the antisense strand.** Conventionally, this **strand** is the **bottom strand of the double-stranded DNA.**

The other strand is referred to as the **coding strand,** as with the exception of T for U, it **exactly corresponds to the sequence of the primary RNA script.** The coding strand is **also referred to as** the **sense strand** (Fig. 17.18).

Enzymes that catalyze the process of transcription are called **RNA polymerases**. They do not require a primer.

In some **viruses,** instead of DNA, the genetic information is present in the form of **RNA,** which is first **transcribed into DNA,** by the **process called reverse transcription**. This process is **important in** the life cycle of some viruses, called **retroviruses. Enzyme** that catalyzes the process of reverse transcription is called **reverse transcriptase.**

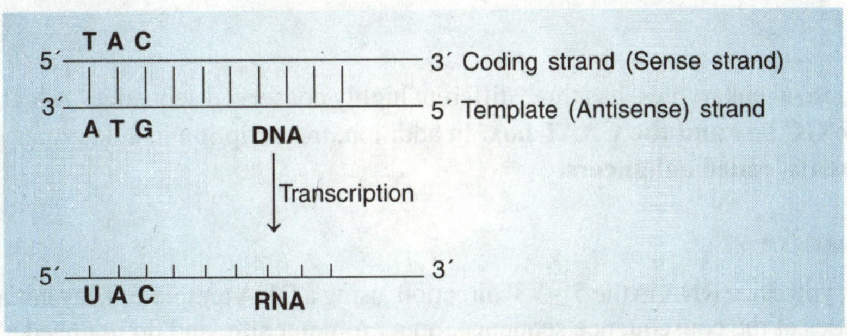

Fig. 17.18. Sense and antisense strands.

The process of RNA synthesis requires an appropriate sequence of **DNA as a template,** and the enzymes called **RNA polymerases.**

DNA Template

Each cycle of the transcription process begins as well as ends with the recognition of some **specific sites in the DNA template.**

The site, where **RNA polymerase binds** is called **promoter.**

The **nucleotide in the promoter region is assigned a negative number if, it is present towards the 5′-site,** i.e. **prior to the transcription start site.** This position is also referred as the **upstream.**

A nucleotide is assigned a **positive number if,** it is present **towards the 3′-site,** i.e. **after the transcription start site.** This position is called as the **downstream.**

The **first nucleotide at the transcription start site is** referred to as **+1.**

Certain conserved sequences have been shown to **occur in the promoter region** both, in prokaryotes and eukaryotes.

In Prokaryotes

The RNA polymerase binds at the site, which is extending nearly **45 base pair** (bp) **upstream** and **10 bp downstream,** of the transcription start site. With in this region, **there are two highly conserved short (oligonucleotide) sequences,** called **pribnow box** or **-10 sequence** and **-35 sequence** (Fig. 17.19).

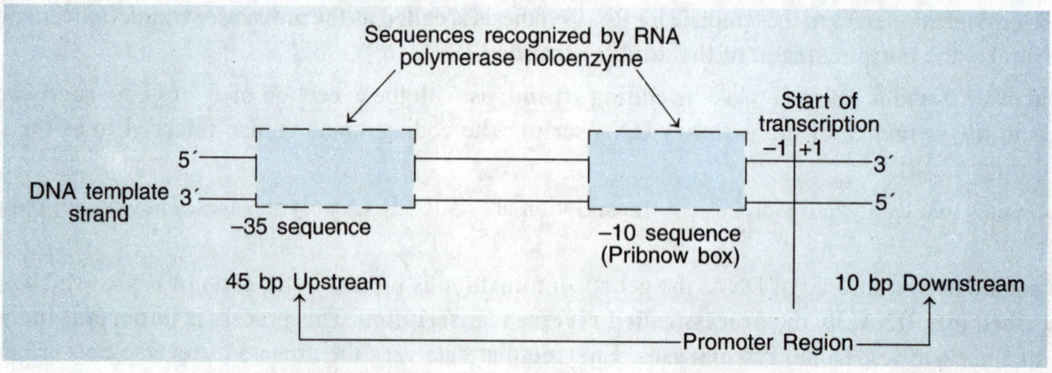

Fig. 17.19. Promoter region in prokaryotes.

In Eukaryotes

The promoters region, in eukaryotes, has three different highly conserved sequences, which are referred to as the **TATA box, tne GC box and the CAAT box.** In addition, transcription in eukaryotes is also affected by certain **other elements, called enhancers.**

RNA Polymerases

RNA polymerases synthesize RNA in the $5' \rightarrow 3'$ direction, using a DNA template. They initiate polymerization of the ribonucleotides at the consequence sequence, on a promoter site, and do not need a primer.

Different types of RNA polymerases are found in prokaryotes and eukaryotes.

In Prokaryotes

A single type of the **RNA polymerase** synthesizes all types of RNAs, in bacteria. It is a **multienzyme complex**. The core enzyme **consists of** four peptides, i.e. it has **two α, one β,** and **one β′** subunits. It can not recognize the promoter region, on the DNA template, without the addition of another protein, i.e. the fifth subunit, which is designated as the sigma (σ) factor. The binding of the σ factor with the core enzyme results in the formation of the holoenzyme, which in turn initiates the synthesis of RNA.

In Eukaryotes

Three different **types of the RNA polymerases** have been identified in eukaryotes. These are referred to as RNA polymerase I, II and III.

RNA polymerase I transcribes **ribosomal RNA (rRNA)**, genes for which are located with in the nucleolus.

RNA polymerase II transcribes **mRNA**. It synthesizes large RNA particle, which is the precursor of the mRNA and the small nuclear RNAs (snRNAs).

RNA polymerase III produces small RNA molecules, which are processed to give various types of tRNA, and some snRNAs.

In addition to the above three types of RNA polymerases, eukaryotes also have another type of RNA polymerase, called mitochondrial RNA polymerase (mtRNA polymerase), which is responsible for the synthesis of mRNA, tRNA and rRNA with in the mitochondria.

THE PROCESS OF RNA SYNTHESIS IN PROKARYOTES

The process of RNA synthesis occurs in 3 steps, which are referred to as initiation, elongation, and termination.

Initiation

RNA polymerase holoenzyme binds to the DNA template and locates a promoter. After the holoenzyme (RNA polymerase with the sigma factor) has recognized the promoter, it binds there and forms a complex. This in turn results in unwinding of nearly 10 nucleotide base pairs of the DNA double helix. The unwound DNA then binds to the initiating ribonucleotidetriphosphate, usually a purine ribonucleotide (GTP or ATP), and the holoenzyme forms the first phosphodiester bond.

Elongation

After the initiation of the process, RNA polymerase translocates to the next position and continues the synthesis. After the enzyme has begun to synthesize the RNA transcript, its σ subunit is released and the core enzyme continues the process.

The template strand gets attached to the growing RNA chain, by base pairing. The enzyme topoisomerase, which is a component of the transcription complex, helps in the process of unwinding and restoring the DNA double helix (Fig. 17.20)

Termination

RNA polymerase complex also recognizes the termination sequence, which is present at the end of the gene, and terminates the process.

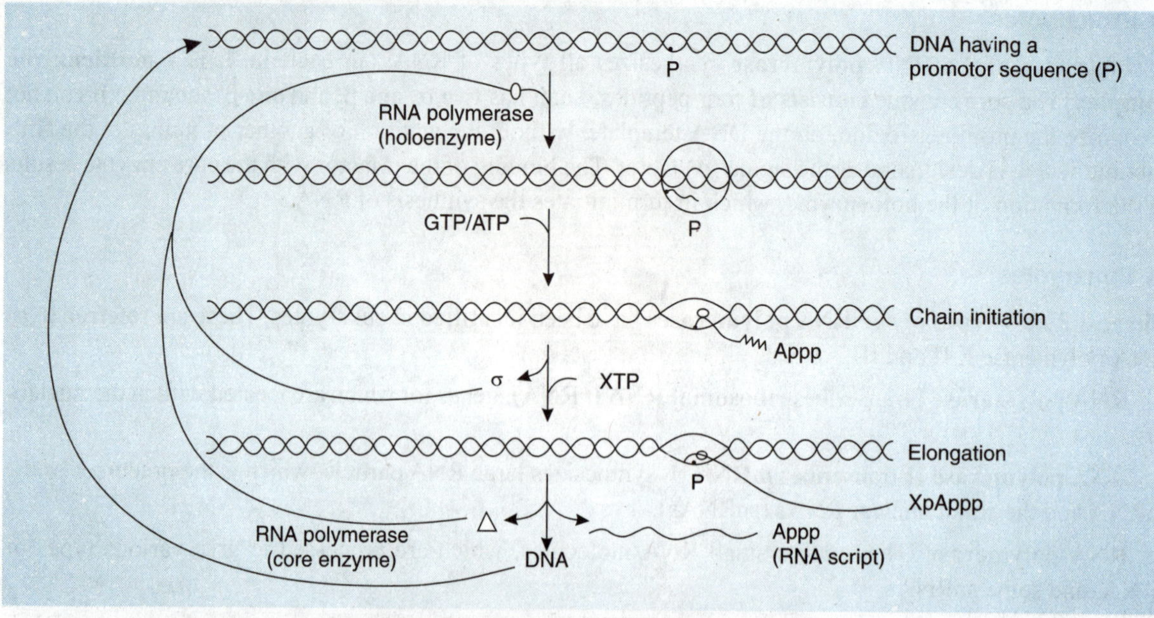

Fig. 17.20. The process of RNA transcription.

Termination of the transcription process can occur in either of the two modes. Either, the enzyme itself recognizes the termination region on the DNA template, by the process which is referred to as **rho (ρ) independent termination.** Alternatively, termination of the process may require an additional protein, which is designated as ρ factor, for the release of the RNA transcript. This is termed as the **ρ-dependent termination.**

DIFFERENCES IN TRANSCRIPTION PROCESS BETWEEN PROKARYOTES AND EUKARYOTES

Transcription in eukaryotes is more complex than prokaryotes. Whereas, transcription in prokaryotes requires only an appropriate sequence of the DNA as a template, the enzyme RNA polymerase (holoenzyme) and ribonucleosidetriphosphates as the substrates, initiation of the process in **eukaryotes requires several additional molecular events:**

1. Chromatin, though is organized in the nucleosomes however, some of its part, which is containing the promoter sequences, is not well organized and is not accessible to the transcription machinery. Such a nucleosomal organization requires **DNase activity** for proper access by the transcription machinery.
2. Certain gene specific sequences, referred to as **enhancers,** are also needed. These sequences stimulate transcription as well as binding of various transcription factors.
3. Besides RNA polymerases, certain additional proteins, called **transcription factors,** are required. They bind to some sequences in the promoter region, for the initiation of the process. These transcription factors also facilitate binding of the RNA polymerase.
4. Eukaryotes have **three distinct types of RNA polymerases**, each one of which is specific for the particular class of RNA.

Differences in the process of transcription between prokaryotes and eukaryotes are shown in Table 17.3.

Table 17.3. Differences in the process of RNA synthesis between prokaryotes and eukaryotes

Prokaryotes	*Eukaryotes*
No nucleosomal organization is required and chromatin is easily accessible to the transcription machinery	Nucleosomal organization is required, which is done by the enzyme DNase. This is essential for proper access by the transcription machinery
Promoter region, for the binding of the RNA polymerase, is simple.	Promoter region is complex, and binds RNA polymerase with other transcription factors
There is only one type of RNA polymerase	There are three distinct forms of the enzyme RNA polymerase, one for each class of the RNA. These are referred to as RNA polymerase I, II, and III
Introns are rarely found in the primary transcript	Introns very commonly occur in the primary transcript
Post-transcriptional modifications are restricted to tRNA and rRNA only	Post-transcriptional modifications take place in all the three types of RNAs

POST-TRANSCRIPTIONAL MODIFICATIONS

The primary transcripts of the **tRNA and rRNA are processed** post-transcriptionally **both, in prokaryotes and eukaryotes.**

Prokaryotic mRNA is generally, identical to its primary transcript and does not require modifications. **In eukaryotes, mRNA** genes are transcribed as pre-mRNA primary transcripts, which are extensively **modified post-transcriptionally.**

mRNA

RNA polymerase II synthesizes the primary mRNA transcript. It is called **pre-mRNA**. It is processed post-transcriptionally, as follows:

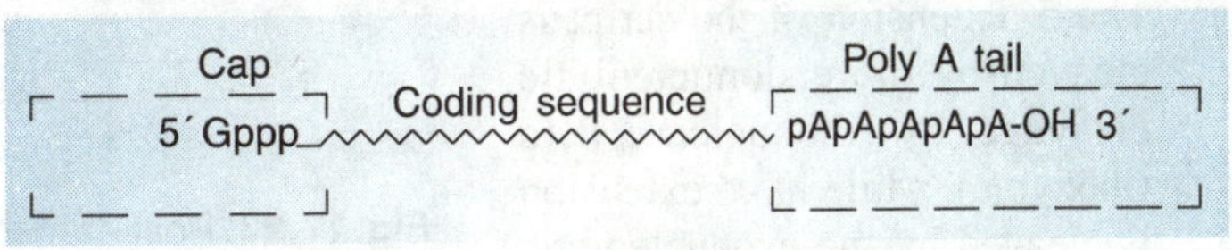

Fig. 17.21. Eukaryotic mRNA with Poly A tail.

1. The poly A tail of 40-200 adenine nucleotides is added to the free 3′-end, by a polymerase. This polyadenylation does not require a template (Fig. 17.21).

   The poly A tail helps in stabilizing the mRNA and facilitates its exit from the nucleus.
2. The primary transcript contains several terminal as well as internal sequences. These non-coding sequences are present with in pre-mRNA molecules but not in mature **mRNA** and are called **intervening sequences or introns.**

The other sequences, which are expressed or retained, are called **exons.**

As pre-mRNA is extruded from the RNA polymerase complex, it is rapidly bound by the small nuclear ribonucleoproteins (snRNPs or snrnps). Different snrnps bind to the RNA precursor and form a large complex, termed spliceosome. This in turn carries out dual steps of the RNA splicing, i.e. breaking of the introns at the 5′ site, and joining of the exon sequences together.

After removal of the introns, fully functional mature mRNA leaves the nucleus and passes into the cytosol (Fig. 17.22).

Primary RNA transcrips (pre mRNAs) are called **heterogenous nuclear RNAs (hnRNAs).**

Mutations in the β-globin gene interfere with introns removal and lead to a condition called β-Thalassemia.

rRNA

Ribosomal RNAs are synthesized from the long precursor molecules, called pre-rRNAs or 45S RNA, which contain sequences for 28S, 5.8S and 18S rRNAs. Each pre-rRNA is cleaved to yield the required rRNA species (Fig. 17.23).

Some of the proteins, which are destined to become components of ribosomes, also get associated with the pre-rRNAs, prior to and during post-transcriptional modifications, in the nucleolus.

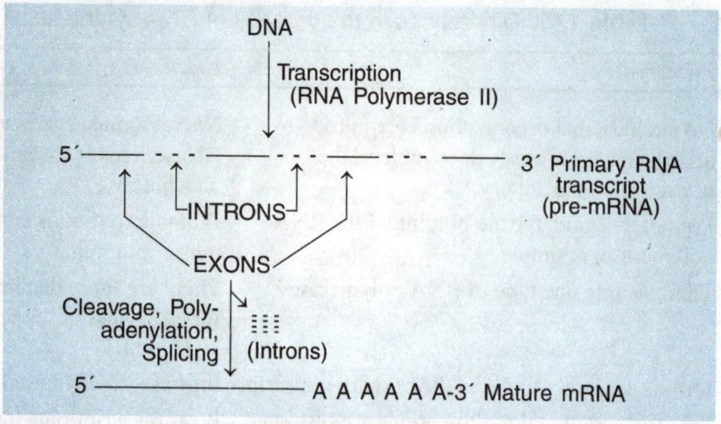

Fig. 17.22. Post-transcriptional Processing of mRNA in Eukaryotes.

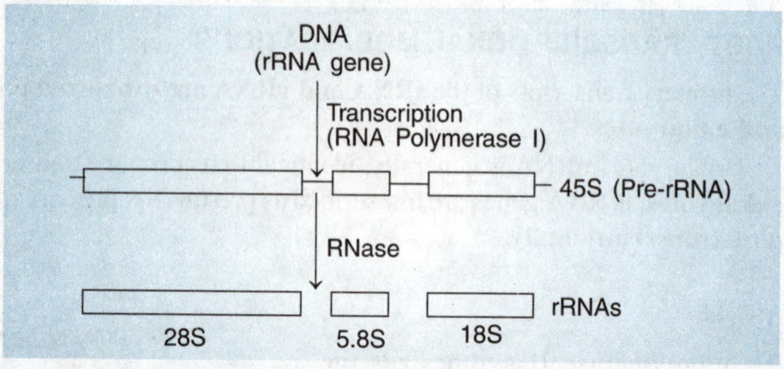

Fig. 17.23. Post–transcriptional Processing of rRNA in Eukaryotes.

tRNA

1. The primary transcript of tRNA gene has large number of extra nucleotide sequences, on both the ends. This script is trimmed, nonspecifically.

   The 5′ extension of the script is cleaved by the endonucleolytic cleavage, by ribonuclease P (a ribozyme), while its 3′ extension is cleaved by the exonucleolytic cleavage.

   Sometimes, the primary transcript may contain introns, which are removed by the two-component enzyme system, while one of the enzymes removes introns, the other rejoins the remaining exon chains.
2. Each functional tRNA, both in the cytosol and the mitochondria, has a sequence of three nucleotides, i.e. CCA at the 3′ terminus. These three nucleotides are added sequentially, by the enzyme tRNA-nucleotidyltransferase.
3. Each tRNA molecule also has several modified nitrogenous bases.

These modifications are completed before the tRNA precursors are cleaved to mature tRNA by various enzymes. Most of these enzymes are either site specific or nucleotide-sequence specific.

Antibiotics that Interfere in Transcription

Antibiotic rifampicin, used in treating tuberculosis, inhibits the RNA polymerase of a variety of bacteria. Rifampicin inhibits the transcriptional machinery of bacteria, inhibiting the β-subunit of bacterial RNA polymerase without great toxicity to the host.

PROTEIN SYNTHESIS

The **process of protein biosynthesis** is called translation. It is the **biochemical translation of the genetic information, from the four-letter language of nucleotides to the twenty-letter language of amino acids.**

THE GENETIC CODE

Genetic code is **a dictionary** that gives a correspondence between the **sequences of four nucleotide bases** that are found in mRNA to the **sequence of twenty amino acids,** which occur in peptides.

Each word of the genetic **code is composed of three letters (nucleotide bases)** and is referred to as **codon**. This is due to the reason that if **one nucleotide** encodes **for an amino acid**, four nucleotides will code for (4^1), i.e. **four amino acids**, only. If there are **two nucleotides in a code**, it will translate (4^2), i.e. **16 amino acids**, only. Hence, a **3:1 correspondence of nucleotides to amino acids** with (4^3), i.e. 64 combinations, is there to encode **all the 20 amino acids.**

Codons are present on the mRNA as the nucleotides (U, C, A and G), and are written in a sequence of three bases from the 5′-end to the 3′-end. These 64 combinations, of three bases each, define genetic code (Table 17.4).

Codons are thus, permutations of four bases, which are taken in the sets of three.

Salient features of the genetic code are shown in Table 17.5.

Table 17.4. Genetic code

	Middle-base								
5′-Base	*U*		*C*		*A*		*G*		*3′-Base*
U	UUU		UCU		UAU		UGU		U
	UUC	Phe	UCC		UAC	Tyr	UGC	Cys	
	UUA		UCA		UAA		UGA	Stop	
	UUG		UCG	Ser	UAG	Stop	UGG	Trp	
C	CUU		CCU		CAU		CGU		C
	CUC		CCC		CAC	His	CGC		
	CUA		CCA		CAA		CGA		
	CUG	Leu	CCG	Pro	CAG	Gln	CGG	Arg	
A	AUU		ACU		AAU		AGU		A
	AUC		ACC		AAC	Asn	AGC	Ser	
	AUA	Ile	ACA		AAA		AGA		
	AUG	Met/Start	ACG	Thr	AAG	Lys	AGG	Arg	
G	GUU		GCU		GAU		GGU		G
	GUC		GCC		GAC	Asp	GGC		
	GUA		GCA		GAA		GGA		
	GUG	Val	GCG	Ala	GAG	Glu	GGG	Gly	

Table 17.5. Salient features of the genetic code

Degeneracy	Multiple codons code for same amino acid
Unambiguous	A specific codon codes for only a single amino acid
Non-overlapping	Reading of the genetic code occurs with out overlapping
Punctuation	Message is read continuously without any break between the sequence of codons until a nonsense codon is reached
Universality	The same codon is used in all the living organisms, with only few exceptions in the mitochondria

WOBBLE HYPOTHESIS

Each tRNA carries a specific amino acid only, which has specific three bases anticodon sequence. However, there are 61 codons, which designate an amino acid while most of the cells have nearly 50 tRNA species. This in turn suggests that certain variations from the standard base pairing in codon-anticodon interaction occurs and that all the codons may not be being used, equally. Some codons may be read more efficiently by an anticodon, while some of the codons may be used less efficiently. This suggests that many amino acids can be carried by more than one tRNA species and it is also possible that the degenerate codon can be read by more than one tRNA.

The possibility by which one anticodon recognizes more than one codon for the specific amino acid is described by the hypothesis that was given by Crick, and is referred to as **Wobble hypothesis.** This explains that a **base at the 5′-end of the anticodon** (the first base of the anticodon or the third base of the codon) **is not as well defined, with respect to its spatial configuration, as the other two bases.** Thus, first two positions of the codon predominate in tRNA selection, and that the third position, called degenerate position, is wobbling, i.e. less important in this regard.

TRANSLATION

Protein synthesis (translation) requires mRNA, several tRNAs, ribosomes, and various protein factors.

Besides the activation of amino acids, the process of protein synthesis occurs in three stages, i.e. **initiation, elongation and termination,** along with the release of a polypeptide.

Activation of amino acids

For their incorporation into the polypeptide chain, amino acids are activated and attached to the appropriate tRNA carrier. **Linkage of the amino acid to its tRNA** requires ATP and is catalyzed by the enzyme aminoacyl-tRNA synthetase.

Aminoacyl-tRNA synthetase is a group of enzymes, each one of which is specific for an amino acid and its appropriate tRNA.

During the process of amino acid activation, a high-energy complex (**amino acid-AMP-enzyme complex)** is formed as the intermediate. Each synthetase then recognizes the tRNA and transfers amino acid from the amino acid-AMP-enzyme complex to the corresponding tRNA (Fig. 17.24).

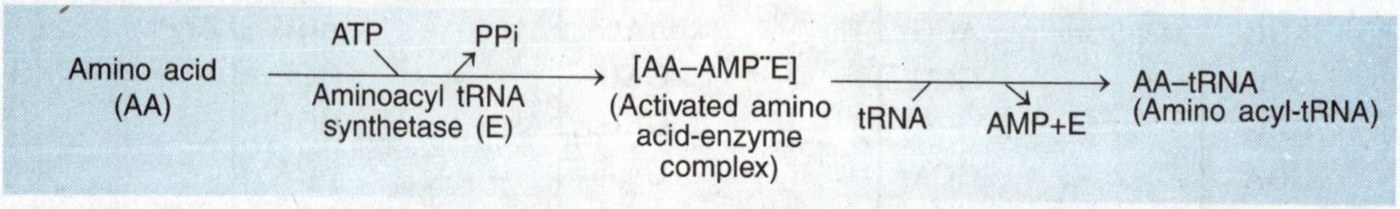

Fig. 17.24. Activation of an amino acid.

Aminoacyl **tRNA synthetase** not only carries a correct amino acid but **also edits protein synthesis,** since wrong acylated-tRNA is recognized by the enzyme and is removed.

During translation **mRNA sequence is** read **in 5′→ 3′ direction** whereas, due to codon-anticodon interaction, **amino acids are incorporated from the amino terminal end to the carboxy terminal end.**

Initiation of translation

Initiation of protein synthesis, in eukaryotes, **involves assembly of various components of the translation system,** i.e. **two ribosomal subunits, mRNA, aminoacyl-tRNA** specified by the codon, **GTP** and several **initiation factors** that facilitate assembly of the initiation complex.

First, the **initiation codon** (AUG) is **recognized by** the **initiation tRNA** (that **carries methionine)**. This is **facilitated by eIF-2a (**eukaryotic initiation factor-2a), which **binds to GTP** and **methioninyl-tRNA** (Met-$tRNA_i^{Met}$), and **forms a ternary complex**. Subsequently, it **requires 40S ribosomal subunit** that is **associated with eIF-3.**

Mammalian eIF-3 is a complex protein that has 8 different polypeptides. It is also called anti-association **factor,** since it blocks the association of the 40S ribosomal subunit with the 60S subunit.

A complex, comprising of the eIF-2a.Met-$tRNA_i^{Met}$.GTP, eIF-3.40S-rRNA, eIF-4c, and some more protein factors, is formed. This complex in turn binds to mRNA and forms **pre-initiation complex**. In addition, eIF-4a and eIF-4b are required to unwind the secondary structure, in mRNA. It also requires eIF-4f (also called as the cap-binding protein), that helps to place the message on the 40S subunit. During this process, a molecule of ATP is hydrolyzed and helps to locate and place the initiation sequence in mRNA.

The final **pre-initiation complex** thus, **includes 40S ribosomal subunit, eIF-2a.Met-$tRNA_i^{Met}$ GTP ternary complex**, correctly oriented **mRNA** and several **protein factors.**

Formation of this initiation complex proceeds with the involvement of the 60S subunit and eIF-5.

eIF-5, first **interacts with the pre-initiation complex, GTP is hydrolyzed,** and **eIF2a.GDP, eIF-3,** and **other factors are released. The 40S.Met-$tRNA_i^{Met}$.mRNA complex interacts with the 60S subunit and initiation factor eIF-4d to generate 80S ribosome with the mRNA and initiator tRNA,** which is correctly positioned with in the ribosome.

The eIF-2a.GDP complex so released interacts with the guanine nucleotide, eIF-2b, and GTP, to regenerate eIF-2a.GTP for another round (Fig. 17.25).

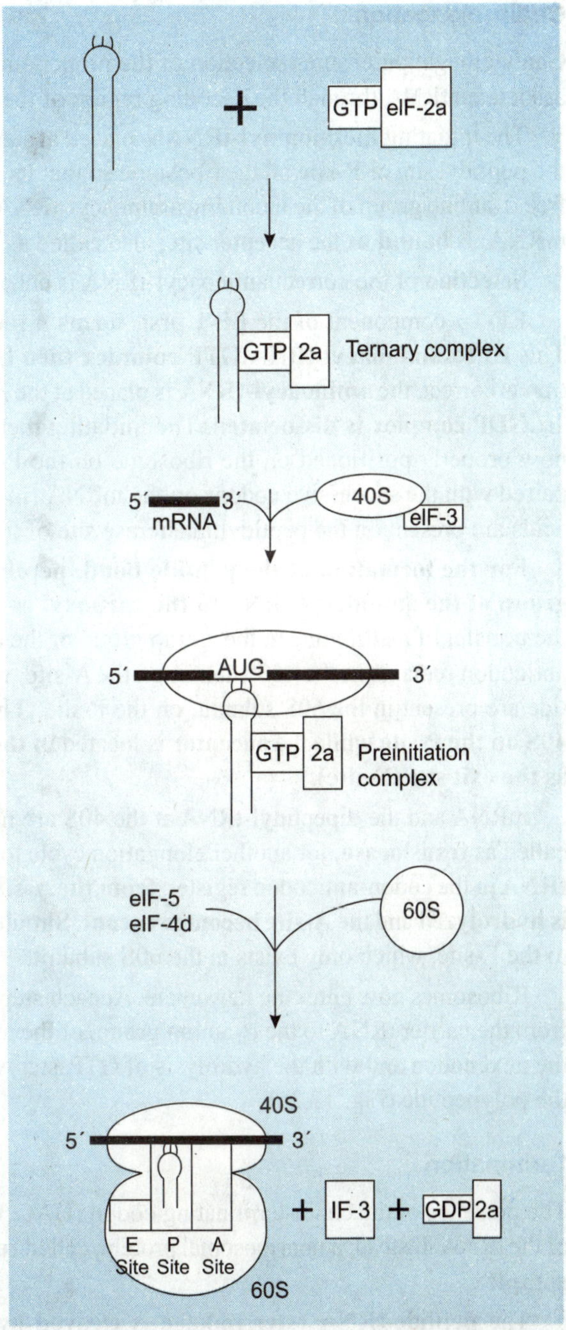

Fig. 17.25. Initiation of protein synthesis.

In *E. coli,* binding and positioning of the mRNA on the 30S ribosomal subunit, is facilitated by complementary base pairing between the pyrimidine-rich sequence of 8 nucleotides, in the 16S RNA and a purine-rich sequence of 10 nucleotides, which is designated as **Shine-Dalgarno sequence,** present on mRNA.

Chain elongation

Chain elongation ensures selection of the proper aminoacyl tRNA and movement of mRNA along with the associated tRNA through the decoding region of the ribosome.

The initiating **methioninyl-tRNA** is placed at such a position that it occupies the donor site, also called as the peptidyl site or **P-site** on the ribosome so that its methioninyl residue may be donated (transferred) to the free α-amino group of the incoming aminoacyl-tRNA. **Aminoacyl-tRNA,** specified by the next codon on the mRNA, **is bound at** the acceptor site, also called as the aminoacyl site or **A-site,** on the ribosome.

Selection of the correct aminoacyl-tRNA is enhanced by elongation factor-1 (EF-1).

EF-1α component of the EF-1 first, **forms a ternary complex with the aminoacyl-tRNA and GTP**. This **EFIα.aminoacyl-tRNA.GTP complex then binds on the ribosome** and if codon-anticodon interaction is correct, the **aminoacyl-tRNA** is placed at the **A-site.** During this process, **GTP is hydrolyzed** and **EF-1α.GDP complex is dissociated**. The initiating methioninyl-tRNA and the incoming aminoacyl-tRNA are now properly positioned on the ribosome on the P-site and the A-site, respectively. Their anticodons are paired with the successive codons on the mRNA (in the decoding region of the small subunits) while amino acids are present on the peptidyltransferase site of the large subunit.

For the formation of the peptide bond, peptidyltransferase catalyzes attachment of the α-amino group of the aminoacyl-tRNA to the carboxyl carbon of the methioninyl-tRNA. This in turn results in the transfer of methionine to the amino group of the aminoacyl-tRNA, which occupies a hybrid position. Its anticodon remains in the 40S subunit on the A-site, while the acceptor-end along with the attached polypeptide are present in the 60S subunit, on the P-site. **The anticodon of the deacylated tRNA remains in the 40S on the P-site** while the **acceptor** is located **in the 60S,** towards the upper end, which may also be called as **the exit site (E-site)**.

mRNA and the dipeptidyl-tRNA at the 40S are now repositioned by the elongationfactor-2 (EF-2), also called as **translocase,** for another elongation cycle to proceed. **EF-2 moves the mRNA and the dipeptidyl-tRNA** in the codon-anticodon register, **from the A-site to the P-site**. During this process, a molecule of **GTP is hydrolyzed** and the **A-site becomes vacant**. Simultaneously, the deacylated methioninyl-tRNA also moves to the E-site, which only exists in the 60S subunit.

Ribosomes now enter the new cycle. At each step, peptidyltransferase transfers the growing polypeptide from the carrier tRNA to the α-amino group, of the amino acid residue of the aminoacyl tRNA, specified by the next codon and with the hydrolysis of GTP, stepwise elongation of the chain results in the completion of the polypeptide (Fig. 17.26).

Termination

The presence of the chain-terminating codon (UAG, UAA, or UGA) on the A-site does not promote binding of the tRNA. Instead, a nonribosomal protein, called **releasing factor (eRF), binds the ribosome as eRF.GTP complex.**

The **peptide-tRNA ester linkage is cleaved** by the enzyme **peptidyltransferase** and polypeptide **is released from the carrier tRNA. Dissociation of the eRF from ribosome requires the hydrolysis of GTP,** and releases the **ribosome** to dissociate into two subunits, to **re-enter the cycle** at the initiation stage (Fig. 17.27).

Differences in the process of protein synthesis between prokaryotes and eukaryotes are shown in Table 17.6.

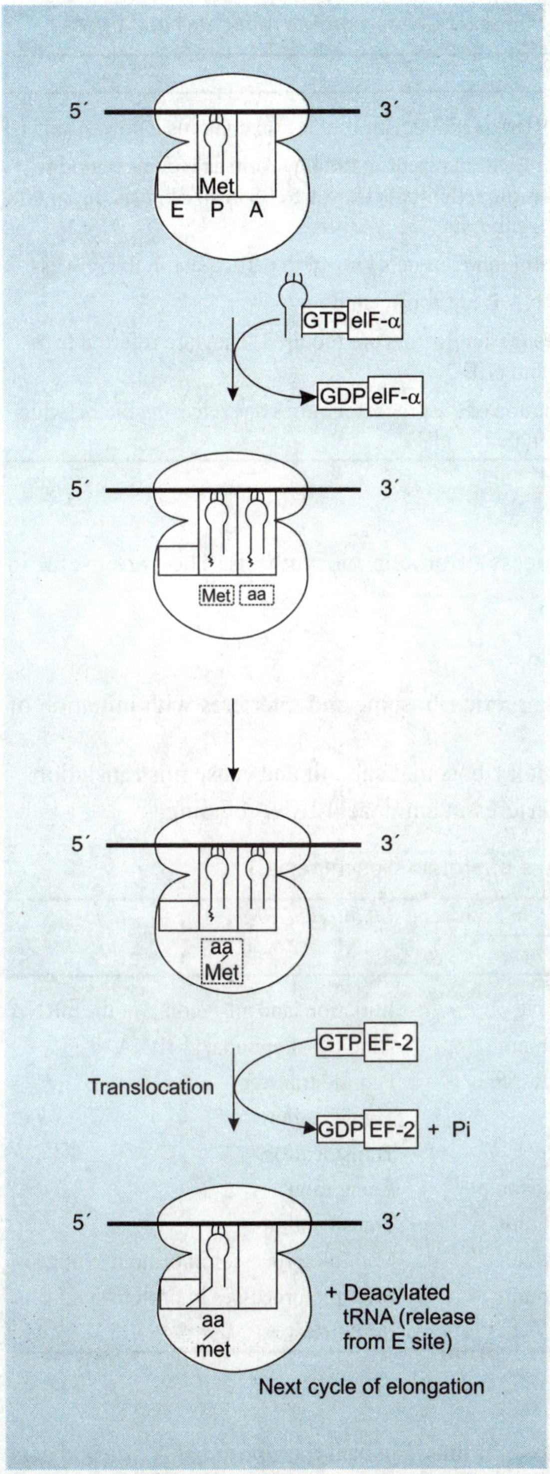

Fig. 17.26. Elongation of peptide chain.

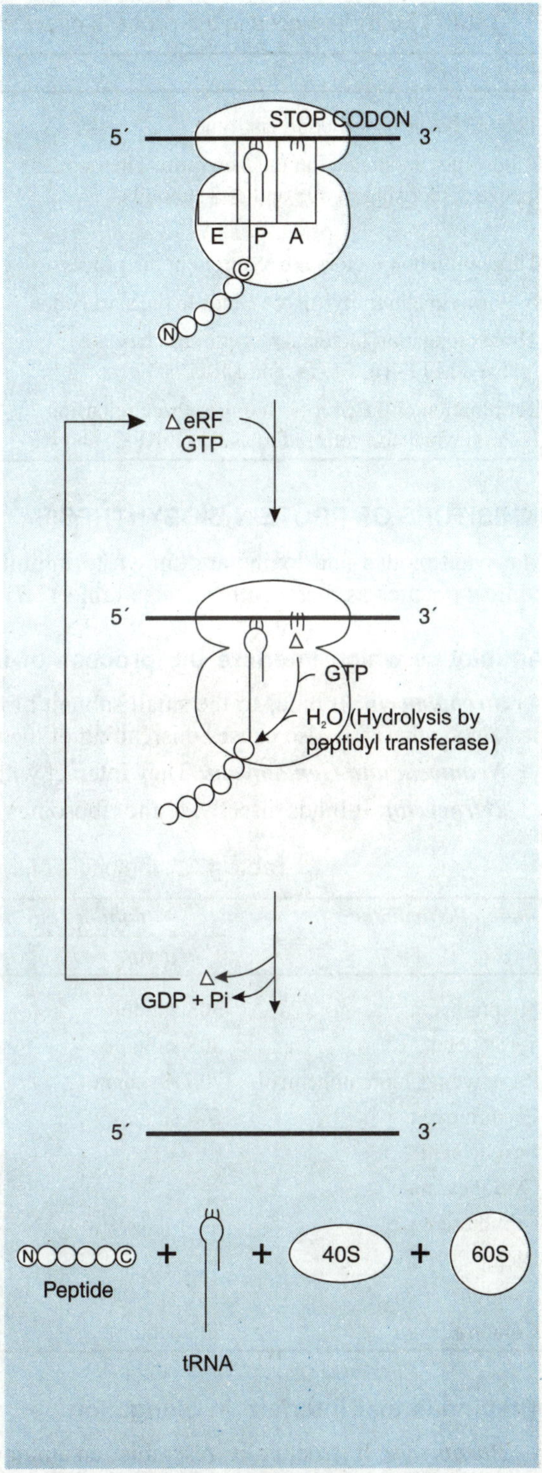

Fig. 17.27. Termination of protein synthesis.

Table 17.6. Differences in the process of protein biosynthesis between prokaryotes and eukaryotes

Prokaryotes	*Eukaryotes*
The mRNA is usually polycistronic	The mRNA is monocistronic. It also contains a poly-A tail
Ribosomes are present in the free form. They are 70S in size comprising of 50S and 30S subunits.	Ribosomes are present in the free form as well as bound to endoplasmic reticulum. They are 80S in size consisting of 60S and 40S subunits
Three initiation factors are required in the process	One initiation factors is known to participate in the process
N-Formylmethioninyl-tRNA binds to the start codon	Met-tRNA is not formylated
Three elongation factors are required. They are referred as EF-Tu, EF-Ts, and EF-G.	Two elongation factors are required. They are referred to as eEF-1 and eEF-2
Termination of the process requires three releasing factors, which are referred to as RF-1, RF-2, and RF-3	Termination of the process requires one releasing factor, which is designated as eRF

INHIBITORS OF PROTEIN BIOSYNTHESIS

Many antibiotics and toxins are known to inhibit the process of protein biosynthesis. They are useful in clinical practice as therapeutic agents (Table 17.7).

Antibiotics which interfere the process of initiation

Streptomycin: It binds to the small subunit of the prokaryotic ribosome and interferes with initiation of protein synthesis. It also causes misreading of the mRNA.

Neomycin and Gentamycin: They interact with the small ribosomal subunit and cause mistranslation.

Tetracyclin: It binds directly, to the ribosomes and interferes in aminoacyl-tRNA binding.

Table 17.7. Inhibitors of the process of protein biosynthesis

Antibiotic/Inhibitor	*Inhibitory effect in*		*Inhibits the Process of*
	Prokaryotes	*Eukaryotes*	
Streptomycin	30S subunit	—	Initiation, and misreading of the mRNA
Tetracyclin	30S subunit	40S subunit	Binding of aminoacyl-tRNA
Puromycin/Chloramphenicol	70S ribosome	80S ribosome	Peptide transfer
Erythromycin	50S subunit	—	Translocation
Fusidic acid	EF-G	—	Translocation
Cycloheximide	—	80S ribosome	Elongation
Diphtheria toxin	—	60S subunit	Translocation
Ricin	—	60S subunit	Multiple processes in protein synthesis
α-Sarcin	—	60S subunit	Multiple processes in protein synthesis
Colicin E3	30S subunit	—	Initiation

Antibiotics tnat interfere in elongation

Puromycin: It structurally, resembles an aminoacyl-tRNA. It thus, binds at the ribosomal A-site and acts as acceptor in peptidyltransferase reaction. Puromycin thus, prematurely terminates translation, leading to release of peptidyl-puromycin complex.

Chloramphenicol: It directly inhibits peptidyltransferase, by binding the transferase.

Erythromycin: It interferes with the translocation process, on prokaryotic ribosomes.

Fusidic acid: It interferes in the process of translocation, by inhibiting EF-G (GTP-dependent translocase), in prokaryotes.

Cycloheximide: It inhibits elongation process, in eukaryotes.

Diphtheria toxin: It is a protein, which is produced by *Corynebacterium diphtheriae that* inhibits the process of translocation, in eukaryotes.

Toxins that attack RNAs and inhibit protein synthesis

Ricin: It is obtained from the castor bean. It cleaves adenine from rRNA, in the large subunit and thus inactivates the ribosomes in eukaryotes.

α-Sarcin: It is a fungal toxin. It cleaves rRNA at the single site, with in the large subunit of the ribosome and inactivates the ribosome in eukaryotes.

Colicin E3: It is a toxin, which is obtained from *E. coli*. It has ribonuclease activity and cleaves 16S rRNA from the 30S ribosomal subunit, near the mRNA-binding sequence and the decoding region. It thus, inactivates small subunit of the ribosome and stops initiation of protein synthesis.

POST-TRANSLATION MODIFICATIONS

After synthesis of the polypeptide chain, several proteins undergo various changes. Since these modifications occur after translation of the process, these changes are referred as **post-translation modifications.**

Post-translation modifications include partial proteolysis of the protein chain, or **covalent modification with the addition** of one or more groups on amino acids, in the protein chain.

Partial Proteolysis of the Protein Chain

Some proteins particularly, those destined for secretion from the cell, are synthesized as the large precursors that are not functionally active, e.g. insulin, several zymogens, etc. A small portion of the protein is removed by specialized endoproteases, which in turn results in the release of a biologically active protein.

Some of them are cleaved in endoplasmic reticulum or Golgi apparatus while others in secretory vesicles, or after secretion. For example:

Conversion of preproinsulin to insulin: Insulin is synthesized as preproinsulin, which enters endoplasmic reticulum where **signal peptidase cleaves the signal peptide** and converts it to proinsulin. **Proinsulin is then transported to the Golgi apparatus** where it is **packaged into the secretory granules.** The **C-peptide** (connecting-peptide) is **removed by proteolysis** and mature **insulin is secreted** (Fig. 17.28).

Abnormally processed insulin (proinsulin) is **released into the circulation** in an autosomal dominant condition, referred to as **familial hyperproinsulinemia.**

Activation of the zymogen: Proteolysis also leads to **activation of the zymogen,** such as proteases. Inactive zymogen precursors are packaged in the storage granules and are activated by proteolysis, e.g. trypsinogen is cleaved to trypsin, or chymotrypsinogen is converted to chymotrypsin.

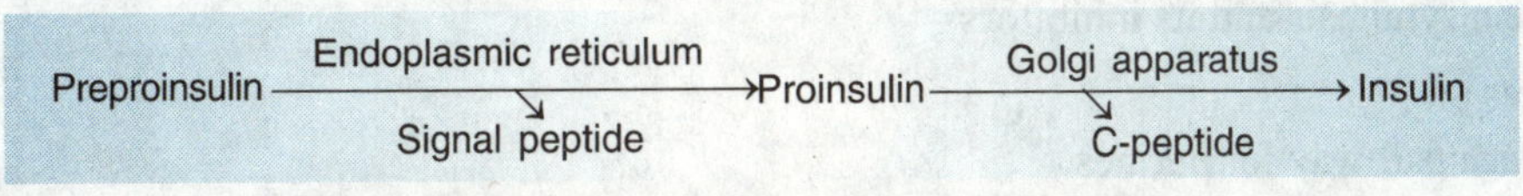

Fig. 17.28. Conversion of preproinsulin to insulin.

Covalent Modifications

Though only 20 amino acids are encoded genetically, post-translational modifications however, show the existence of many more amino acids in proteins. Modification of the amino acid may occur in several ways, such as:

Phosphorylation: Phosphorylation may occur on the hydroxyl group of serine or threonine, in a protein, e.g. reversible phosphorlyation of glycogen phosphorylase and glycogen synthase, by protein kinase and protein phosphatase, respectively.

Glycosylation: Plasma membrane proteins or some other proteins, which are to be secreted from the cell, have carbohydrate chains attached to the hydroxyl group of serine or threonine, by O-linkage or to the NH_2 group of asparagine by N-linkage. Stepwise addition of sugar molecules (glucose, galactose, mannose, fucose, etc.) occurs in the endoplasmic reticulum and Golgi apparatus. Glycosylation of the protein thus, forms a glycoprotein, such as membrane-bound glycoproteins.

Methylation: Methylation of the ε-amino group of lysine occurs in histones. This in turn modulates their interaction with the DNA.

Hydroxylation: Proline and lysine residues in collagen are extensively hydroxylated, in the endoplasmic reticulum.

SOME IMPORTANT QUESTIONS

1. Explain the process of de novo synthesis of purine nucleotides.
2. Describe the process of degradation of purine nucleotides.
3. Describe the process of de novo synthesis of pyrimidine nucleotides.
4. What is replication? Describe the process of DNA replication in prokaryotes. How does it differs from eukaryotes?
5. What are mutations? Describe different types of mutations.
6. Discuss differences between DNA polymerases found in prokaryotes and eukaryotes.
7. Describe the process of transcription in prokaryotes. How does it differ from eukaryotes?
8. Describe the process of protein synthesis, with diagram.
9. Explain significance of post-translational modifications, with examples.
10. Describe briefly:
    (i) Synthesis of IMP
    (ii) Regulation of purines biosynthesis
    (iii) Inter-conversion of purine nucleotides
    (iv) Immunodeficiency diseases associated with purines degradation
    (v) Formation of uric acid
    (vi) Primary hyperuricemia
    (vii) Secondary hyperuricemia
    (viii) Semi-conservative replication
    (ix) Salient features of the genetic code
    (x) Protein synthesis and its inhibitors
11. Write notes on:
    (i) Salvage pathway for purines
    (ii) Lesch-Nyhan syndrome

(iii) Severe combined immunodeficiency disease
(iv) Gout
(v) Hereditary orotic aciduria
(vi) DNA Polymerases
(vii) Reverse transcriptase
(viii) Replication fork
(ix) Okazaki fragments
(x) Point mutation
(xi) Frame-shift mutation
(xii) Nonsense mutation
(xiii) Silent mutation
(xiv) Promoter region
(xv) Post-transcriptional modifications
(xvi) Genetic code
(xvii) Wobble hypothesis
(xviii) Inhibitors of protein synthesis
(xix) Post-translational modifications

CHAPTER

18

Cancer

Cells reproduce by duplicating their contents and then divide into two, which is a closely regulated and complex process that is termed as cell cycle.

THE CELL CYCLE

Traditionally, cell cycle is divided into several phases (Fig. 18.1)

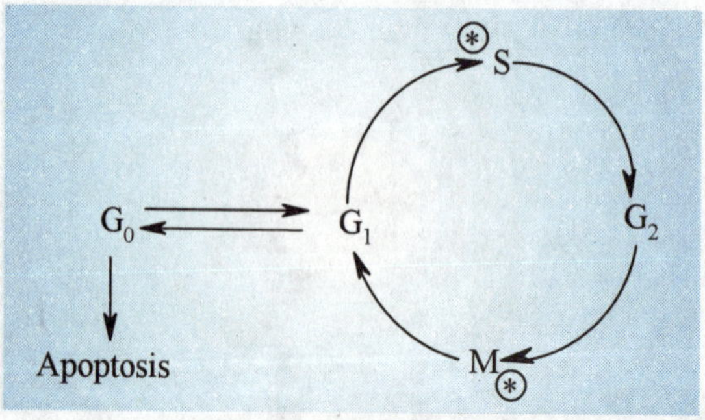

Fig. 18.1. Cell cycle.

Mitosis (M phase) is the stage of cell division. In most of the cells this takes only about an hour. The remainder of the cell cycle, during which cell growth and DNA synthesis occurs, is known as interphase. **Interphase** comprises of the G_1, S and G_2 phases. The interval **between the M phase and the S phase is called the G_1** (gap 1) phase while **interval between the S phase and the M phase is called G_2** (gap 2) phase. The G_1 and the G_2 phases determine the duration of the cell cycle and provide checkpoints at which the progress of the cell cycle may be controlled and the incorporation of DNA damage prevented, before cell division.

In mammals, the duration of the cell cycle varies greatly from one cell type to another, ranging from minutes to years. Variability in individual cell cycle timings occurs mostly during the G_1 phase. This is because cells in G_1 phase, which are not committed to DNA replication (S phase), can enter a specialized **resting state,** called **G_0 phase**, until they receive appropriate signals allowing them to progress further through the cell cycle. Time gap during G_1 phase of the cell cycle when a cell proceeds to the S phase or exits into the G_0 phase are referred to as the **restriction points.**

Various signals occur in the form of polypeptide hormones, growth factors, or cytokines.

REGULATION OF CELL CYCLE

Growth factors bind to specific cell-surface receptors and **initiate intracellular signaling cascade** that ultimately act to counter those negative controls in the resting cells, which prevent growth and block cell cycle progression.

Growth factor stimulation results in the **induction of** proteins involved in regulating the cell cycle, such as the **cyclin-dependent kinases (CDKs) and cyclins** (the regulatory proteins whose concentration rises and falls in a predictable pattern with each cell cycle). Cyclin-dependent kinases (CDKs) bind to a cyclin in order to be active. This cyclin-dependent activation of CDK regulates key steps in cell cycle progression.

The activity of cyclins is modulated by changes in their **levels of expression** both, at the mRNA level (transcriptional control) and the protein level (translational control). In contrast, the **CDKs** are expressed in relatively constant amounts and their **activities are modulated by their phosphorylation status.** A further level of control occurs by the **CDK-inhibitors** (CDKIs), which bind CDK and act as inhibitory subunits to block their catalytic activity.

Once the cell has passed through the restriction point, the remaining phases of the cell cycle through to M-phase are virtually unaffected by the extracellular signals and are committed to progress rather than to remain quiescent.

The retinoblastoma protein called Rb (a product of the retinoblastoma gene RB) controls the expression of genes, which commit cells that are at the restriction point late in G_1 phase to enter S phase of the cell cycle. Thus, in early G_1 phase, hypophosphorylated Rb represses advancement of the cell cycle, by binding to and preventing the DNA-binding activity of a family of transcription factors called E_2F, which have key roles in the G_1/S phase transition. In contrast, close to the restriction point, growth factor stimulation induces the cyclin D-CDK_4 and CDK_6 complexes and the cyclin E-CDK_2 complex to hyperphosphorylate Rb. The resulting release of inhibition of E_2F allows activation of genes, the products of which are important for its entry into the S phase.

Another protein p53 (a suppressor protein) is predominantly a DNA damage-sensing protein by which the cell monitors DNA damage throughout the cell cycle. It can halt cell cycle progression to allow DNA repair, by induction of the p21, a CDKI, which prevents the CDK-dependent phosphorylation and inactivation of Rb. Irreparable damage triggers p53-dependent programmed cell death by apoptosis.

Apoptosis (programmed cell death) is a fundamentally important biological process that is required to maintain the integrity and homeostasis of multi-cellular organisms. Whereas inappropriate apoptosis can lead to degenerative conditions, such as neurodegenerative disorders, subversion and disruption of apoptosis machinery can result in an autoimmune disease or cancer.

CANCER

Cells that undergo mutations, which disrupt the regulation of cell division, will divide without regard to the overall needs of the organism and become apparent as a tumor or neoplasm. As long as the neoplastic cells remain as an intact tumor, the **tumor is** said to be **benign**. However, if further mutations allow such tumor cell to invade and colonize other tissues, creating widespread secondary tumors or metastasis, the tumor is described as **malignant** and classified as a **cancer**. Each cancer is derived from a single cell, which has undergone some heritable mutation that allows it to outgrow its surrounding's cells. By the time they are first detected, tumors typically contain a billion cells.

Cancers are classified according to the tissue and cell types that they are derived from, viz. those derived from epithelial cells are called carcinomas, those derived from connective tissue or muscle cells are termed sarcomas and those derived from the hemopoietic system are called leukemias. About 90% of the human cancers are carcinomas, most common of these include carcinoma of the lung, stomach, breast, colon and uterine cervix.

A single mutation is not sufficient to convert a healthy cell to a cancer cell; several mutations have to occur together. For any given cancer, the incidence increases exponentially with age. Mutations that block the normal development of cells towards an undifferentiated, non-dividing cell, or a cell that would normally be programmed to die by apoptosis, have been shown to play an essential role in many cancers.

Mutations that lead to the uncontrolled proliferation of cancer cells can result either from disruption of the control of normal cell division or alternatively, from a reduction in the normal processes of terminal differentiation or apoptosis.

BASIC CHARACTERISTICS OF THE TUMOR CELLS

Many characteristics of tumor cells can be observed, in culture.

1. Cancer cells continue to grow in culture, piling on top of one another to form clumps, compared to the normal cells, which proliferate until they form a single layer. This is due to the reason that **malignant cells are not responsive to the** types of **signals** that cause their normal counterparts to cease growth and division.
2. Cancer cells **have abnormal number of chromosomes** whereas the normal cells maintain their diploid chromosomal complement as they grow and divide, i.e. cancer cells often have highly aberrant chromosome complements (aneuploidy).
3. Cancer cells **have an ability to continue to divide indefinitely**. On the other hand, normal cells, growing in culture, exhibit a limited capacity for cell division and after a definite number of mitotic divisions, they undergo an aging process and become unfit to continue grow and divide. This difference in growth potential is often attributed to the presence of telomerase in cancer cells and its absence in normal cells.
4. Cancer cells **lack responsiveness** to neighboring cells.
5. In many cases, cancer cells **depend on anaerobic metabolic pathways,** such as glycolysis and fermentation, to a much greater degree than their normal counter- parts. This may be due to their high metabolic requirements and inadequate blood supply.

CAUSES OF CANCER

Normal cells can be converted to cancer cells by treatment with a wide variety **of chemicals, ionizing radiation** and a variety of DNA and RNA-containing **viruses**. All of these agents act by causing changes in the genome of the transformed cell.

The development of a malignant tumor is a multi-step process characterized by a progression of genetic alteration that makes the cells increasingly less responsive to the normal regulatory machinery of the body and able to invade normal tissues.

Viruses

Viruses are small, obligatory intracellular pathogens that could be crystallized. They have a highly ordered well-defined structure and are vastly less complex than the simplest cells. However, they are not considered to be alive because they cannot divide directly. Viruses are responsible for dozens of human diseases, including AIDS, polio, influenza, measles and a few types of cancer.

Viruses occur in a wide variety of shapes, sizes and constructions but all of them share common properties. All viruses are obligatory intracellular parasites, i.e. they cannot reproduce unless present within a host cell. Outside a living cell, the virus exists as a particle, or **virion.** The virion contains a small amount of genetic material that depending on the virus can be single-stranded or double-stranded RNA or DNA. Some viruses have only a few (3 or 4) genes but others may have as many as several hundred genes. The genetic material of the virion is surrounded by a protein capsule, called **capsid**.

Virions are macromolecular aggregates, inanimate particles, that by them selves are unable to reproduce, metabolize, or carry on other activities associated with life. For this reason, viruses are not considered to be organisms and are not described as being alive. In many animal viruses, including the human immunodeficiency virus (HIV) responsible for AIDS, the protein capsid is surrounded by a lipid containing outer envelope that is derived from the modified plasma membrane of the host cell. Bacterial viruses called **bacteriophages** are among the most complex viruses.

Each virus also has on its surface a protein that is able to bind to a particular surface component of its host cell. For example, the protein that projects from the surface of the HIV particle interacts with a specific protein, called CD_4, on the surface of certain white blood cells, facilitating entry of the virus into its host cell. The interaction between viral and host protein determines the specificity of the virus, i.e. the type of host cells that the virus can enter and infect. Some viruses have a wide host range being able to infect cells from a variety of different organs or host species. Most viruses, however, have a relatively narrow host range.

Response of the Viral Infection

There are two basic types of responses of the viral infection:

The Lytic Response : The virus arrests the normal synthetic activities of the host and redirect the cells to use its material to manufacture viral nucleic acids and proteins, which assemble into new virions. Ultimately, the infected cell ruptures (lyses) and releases a new generation of viral particles capable of infecting neighboring cells.

The Lysogenic Response : In other cases, the infecting virus does not lead to the death of the host cell but instead inserts (integrates) its DNA into the DNA of the host cell's chromosomes. The integrated viral DNA is called a pro-virus. An integrated pro-virus can have different effects depending on the type of virus and the host cell. For example,

- Bacterial cells containing a pro-virus behave normally until exposed to a stimulus, such as ultraviolet radiation, that activates the dormant viral DNA, leading to the lysis of the cell and release of viral progeny.
- Some animal cells containing a pro-virus produce new viral progeny that buds at the cell surface without lysing the infected cell. HIV acts in this way where an infected human lymphocyte remains alive for a period, acting as a factory for the production of new virions.
- Some animal cells containing a pro-virus lose control over their own growth and division, and become malignant.

GENETICS OF CANCER

The genes involved in carcinogenesis constitute a specific subset of the genome whose products are involved in such activities as control of the cell cycle, intracellular adhesion and DNA repair.

Genes that have been implicated in carcinogenesis are divided into two broad categories, as tumor suppressor genes and oncogenes.

Tumor Suppressor Genes

Tumor suppressor genes act as brakes to the cell. They encode proteins that restrain cell growth and prevent cells from becoming malignant. The presence of these genes normally suppresses the formation of the tumor.

The first **tumor suppressor gene** identified was **RB**, which is responsible for a rare retinal tumor called **retinoblastoma.** Children with the familial form of the disease inherit one mutated copy of the gene. These individuals develop the cancer only after sporadic damage to the second allele in one of retinal cells. RB encodes a **protein** called **Rb**, which is involved in regulating passage of a cell from G_1 to S phase in the cell cycle. The unphosphorylated form of Rb interacts with certain transcription factors, preventing them from activating the genes required for certain S phase activities. Once Rb has been phosphorylated, the protein releases its bound transcription factor, which can then activate gene expression leading to the initiation of the S phase.

Another tumor suppressor gene most often implicated in human cancer is **TP53** whose protein product is **p53.** The p53 can suppress cancer formation by several mechanisms:

1. In one of its actions, p53 **acts as a transcription factor** that activates the expression of a protein p21, which inhibits cyclin-dependent kinase that moves a cell through the cell cycle. Damage to DNA triggers phosphorylation and stabilization of p53, leading to arrest of the cell cycle until damage can be repaired.
2. The p53 can also **redirect cells** that are on the path toward malignancy onto an alternate path leading **to programmed-cell death** or apoptosis.

Other tumor suppressor genes include **APC** that when mutated, predisposes an individual to develop colon cancer. **BRCA 1** and **BRCA 2** when mutated, predisposes an individual to develop breast cancer.

Oncogenes

Oncogenes arise from proto-oncogenes as the result of gain-of-function mutations, i.e. mutations that cause the gene product to exhibit new functions that lead to malignancy.

Certain RNA tumor viruses called retroviruses, such as avian sarcoma virus, carry their genetic information in the form of RNA. These **viral genes** infect the normal host cells and transform them into tumor cells.

Host cells possess a variety of genes referred to as **proto-oncogenes**, e.g. c-src (cellular sarcoma gene). After c-src (proto-oncogene) had been incorporated into the viral genome (v-src) during a previous infection, the **proto-oncogene is activated into an oncogene.**

Rous sarcoma virus (RSV), which induces the formation of sarcomas (cancers arising from connective tissues) in chickens, contains four genes. Three of these genes are essential for the viral replication whereas the fourth gene, i.e. v-src, is an oncogene that induces tumor formation. The uninfected chicken cells contain a gene, c-src (cellular sarcoma gene), which is homologous to v-src, that is highly conserved in a variety of leukocytes. Both, v-src and c-src encode tyrosine kinase. However, whereas activity of c-src is strictly regulated, the activity of v-src is under no such control and hence its presence maintains the host cell in a proliferative state.

Thus, **oncogenes are the mutated forms of proto-oncogenes, caused by some cancer causing RNA viruses.**

PROTO-ONCOGENS CAN BE ACTIVATED INTO ONCOGENES BY SEVERAL MECHANISMS:

1. **Mutation or deletion** : A mutation in the gene alters the structure and function of the encoded protein.
2. **Gene amplification** : Gene amplification results in over-expression of the gene.
3. **Chromosomal rearrangement** : A rearrangement of DNA brings a new DNA segment from a distant site in the genome into vicinity of the gene, which can either alter expression of the gene or structure of the encoded protein.

Numerous oncogenes have been identified as part of the genome of the RNA tumor viruses that have been implicated in human tumors, such as RAS, MYC, etc. (Table 18.1).

Table 18.1. Some of the Oncogenes/Proto-oncogenes that have shown to be activated in Human Tumors

Proto-oncogene	*Neoplasm*
RAS	Carcinoma of colon, lung, pancreas, genitourinary tract and acute lymphoblastic leukemia
ERBB	Squamous cell carcinoma
MYC	Carcinoma of lung, breast
BCL-2	B-Cell lymphoma

ONCOGENES ENCODE PROTEINS THAT PROMOTE LOSS OF GROWTH CONTROL AND MALIGNANCY

Oncogenes encode proteins that promote loss of growth control and malignancy, which include growth factors and growth factor receptors, cytoplasmic protein kinases, nuclear transcription factors and some other proteins that affect apoptosis.

1. Growth Factors and Growth Factor Receptors

Several oncogenes encode proteins, such as platelet-derived growth factor (PDGF) and epidermal growth factor (EGF) receptors. Malignant cells may contain a much large number of one of these growth factor receptors in their plasma membranes when compared to the normal cells. The excess receptors make the cells sensitive to lower concentrations of the growth factor and thus are stimulated to divide under conditions that would not affect normal cells.

The oncogene mutated most frequently in human tumors is RAS, which encodes a GTP-binding protein Ras that functions as an on-off switch, for a key signaling pathway, controlling cell proliferation. Oncogene RAS mutants typically encodes a protein whose GTPase activity cannot be stimulated, which leaves the molecule in an active GTP-bound form, sending continuous proliferation signals along the pathway.

2. Cytoplasmic Protein Kinases

A number of cytoplasmic protein kinases, including both, serine/threonine and tyrosine kinases are included in the list of protein products of oncogenes. For example, oncogene RAF, this encodes a protein kinase in the MAP kinase cascade. Mutations in RAS are among the most common oncogenes found in human cancers. The protein product of the RAS gene (Ras), activates protein kinase actively of Raf. If Raf remains in the activated state, it sends continuous signals along the MAP kinase pathway leading different types of proteins to perform their functions.

3. Nuclear Transcription Factors

Oncogenes, such as MYC, encode proteins that act as transcription factors. The protein product of this gene is myc. It is normally one of the first proteins to appear when a cell is stimulated to re-enter the cell cycle from the quiescent G_0 phase.

4. Protein Products that affect Apoptosis

Oncogenes, such as BCL-2, encode proteins that are involved in apoptosis. Over-expression of the BCL-2 gene leads to the suppression of apoptosis in lymphoid tissues, allowing the cells to proliferate to form lymphoid tumors.

5. Proteins involved in DNA repair

Genes that encode proteins involved in DNA repair have also been implicated in carcinogenesis. For example, the genome of patients with the most common hereditary form of colon cancer called hereditary non-polyposis colon cancer (HNPCC), contains micro-satellite sequences of abnormal nucleotide numbers. Changes in the length of a micro-satallite sequence arise as an error during replication, which is normally recognized by mismatch repair enzymes suggesting that defects in such repair systems may be responsible for cancer. HNPCC tumor cells that display DNA repair deficiencies would display a greatly elevated level of secondary mutations in tumor suppressor genes and oncogenes that would lead to increased risk of malignancy.

SOME IMPORTANT QUESTIONS

1. Illustrate cell cycle. How it is regulated?
2. What is cancer? What are its causes? Describe basic characteristics of a tumor cell.
3. Write notes on:
   (i) Oncogenes
   (ii) Proto-oncogenes
   (iii) Tumor supppressor genes
   (iv) Protein products of oncogenes
   (v) Cancer causing viruses

CHAPTER 19

Hormones

Hormones are chemical substances, which are produced and secreted by the ductless glands called endocrine glands. From the endocrine glands, they are released into circulation and reach the target tissue to exert their actions.

Hormones are synthesized and secreted in extremely minute quantities.

Normally, hormones do not exert any significant effect on the cells that produce them except the local hormones, which function at the site of their production only.

Accordingly, an endocrine hormone refers to the class of substances that arise in one tissue or gland and travel a long distance through circulation to reach the target cell, which expresses its receptors.

Glands secreting these substances are referred to as **endocrines.**

PHYSIOLOGICAL FUNCTIONS OF HORMONES

Hormones perform various functions, such as regulatory functions (homeostasis of body fluids), morphogenesis and interactive actions.

Regulatory Functions

Some of the hormones **maintain a constant chemical composition (homeostasis)** of the extra as well as the intracellular fluid for efficient physiological functions and growth of the organism. For example, maintenance of blood glucose level by insulin, calcium and phosphorus levels by parathyroid hormone, etc.

Morphogenesis

Hormones play an important **role in normal growth and development.** For example, development of male and female characteristics, under the influence of testosterone and estradiol, respectively.

Interactive Actions

A hormone may act independently or in conjunction with other hormones and **regulates several biological**

events simultaneously. For example, for the maintenance of a balance of carbohydrate metabolism, besides insulin various other hormones, such as glucagon, growth hormone, thyroxine, epinephrine as well as glucocorticoids, play an important role.

Even **a single hormone may regulate several biological functions.** For example cortisol, not only enhances gluconeogenesis in the liver but also inhibits glucose uptake and utilization by the peripheral tissues and activates lipolysis, enhances proteolysis and reduces protein synthesis in several tissues.

CLASSIFICATION OF HORMONES

According to their chemical nature, hormones are classified into three groups:

- Those containing peptide bonds, i.e. peptides/protein hormones.
- Those derived from cholesterol, i.e. steroids, and
- Those arising from amino acid tyrosine, i.e. catecholamines and thyroid hormones.

Table 19.1 shows various hormones along with their site of action and major physiological functions.

Table 19.1. Hormones along with their site of action and principal physiological functions

Hormone	*Chemical nature*	*Site of action*	*Major physiological functions*
HYPOTHALAMUS			
Growth hormone-releasing hormone (GHRH)	Polypeptide	Anterior pituitary	Release of growth hormone
Growth hormone-inhibiting hormone (GHIH)	Peptide	- do -	Suppression of GH and TSH
Luetenizing hormone-releasing hormone (LHRH)	Peptide	- do -	Release of LH and FSH
Thyrotropin-releasing hormone (TRH)	Tripeptide	- do -	Release of TSH and prolactin
Corticotropin releasing-hormone (CRH)	Polypeptide	- do -	Release of ACTH and β-Lipotropin
Prolactin-releasing factor (PRF)	Peptide	- do -	Release of prolactin
Prolactin-inhibiting factor (PIF)	Dopamine	- do -	Suppression of prolactin
ANTERIOR PITUITARY			
Growth hormone (GH)	Protein	Several tissues in the whole body	Overall growth
Follicle stimulating hormone (FSH)	Glycoprotein	Ovary	Growth of follicles
Luteinizing hormone (LH)	- do -	- do -	Ovulation, secretion of progesterone
Thyroid stimulating hormone (TSH)	- do -	Thyroid gland	Stimulation of thyroid hormone
Adrenocorticotropic hormone (ACTH)	Polypeptide	Adrenal cortex	Stimulation of hormones of the adrenal cortex
Prolactin	Protein	Mammary gland	Proliferation of mammary gland and milk secretion
β-Lipotropin	Polypeptide	—	Precursor of β-MSH and endorphins
α-Melanocyte stimulating hormone (α-MSH)	Peptide	Skin	Darkening of skin

(Contd.)

Hormone	*Chemical nature*	*Site of action*	*Major physiological functions*
POSTERIOR PITUITARY			
Antidiuretic hormone (ADH)	Peptide	Arterioles, renal tubules	Elevation of blood pressure, reabsorption of water
Oxytocin	Peptide	Smooth muscle of the uterus, mammary gland	Contraction, parturition and sperm transport, and ejection of milk
ADRENAL CORTEX			
Cortisol	Steroid	Several tissues	Metabolism of carbohydrates, proteins and lipids, resistance to infections
Aldosterone	Steroid	Kidney	Electrolyte and water balance
ADRENAL MEDULLA			
Epinephrine and norepinephrine	Amino acid derivatives	Sympathetic receptors, liver, muscle, adipose tissue	Stimulation of sympathetic nervous system, glycogenolysis and lipolysis
THYROID GLAND			
Thyroxine (T_4)	Amino acid derivative	Most of the body tissues	Stimulation of O_2 consumption and metabolic rate
Calcitonin	Polypeptide	Skeleton	Lowering of plasma Ca^{2+} and P
PARATHYROID GLAND			
Parathyroid hormone (PTH)	Polypeptide	Skeleton, Kidney, GIT	Regulation of plasma Ca^{2+} and P
PANCREAS			
Insulin	Polypeptide	Most of the cells	Regulation of blood glucose
Glucagon	Peptide	Liver	Glycogenolysis
Somatostatin	Peptide	Pancreas	Inhibition of insulin release
GIT			
Gastrin	Peptide	Stomach	Secretion of gastric acid
Secretin	Polypeptide	Pancreas	Secretion of pancreatic bicarbonate
Cholecystokinin-pancreozymin (CCK-PZ)	Polypeptide	Gall bladder, pancreas	Contraction of gall bladder
Motilin	Polypeptide	GIT	Stimulation of GIT motility
Vasoactive intestinal peptide (VIP)	Polypeptide	GIT	Neurotransmitter
Gastric inhibitory polypeptide (GIP)	Polypeptide	GIT	Inhibition of gastric secretion and motility
Bombesin	Peptide	GIT	Stimulation of release of various hormones and pancreatic enzymes
Neurotensin	Peptide	GIT and hypothalamus	Uncertain
Substance P	Peptide	GIT and brain	Sensory neurotransmitter, analgesic
KIDNEY			
1,25(OH_2).D_3 (Calcitriol)	Sterol	Intestine, bone and kidney	Regulation of serum Ca^{2+}
Erythropoietin	Glycoprotein	Bone marrow	Stimulation of red cell formation

HORMONES OF THE HYPOTHALAMUS

Hormones of the hypothalamus and the pituitary are **protein** in nature. Some of the peptide hormones may also be formed ectopically, in malignancies of the non-endocrine origin.

Hypothalamus produces a number of hormones, which control the secretion of the pituitary hormones. These include:

Growth hormone releasing hormone (GHRH): It has a dominant influence on the release of growth hormone (GH).

Luteinizing hormone-releasing hormone (LHRH): It is also called gonadotrophin-releasing hormone (GnRH). It plays a major role in the release of the luteinizing hormone (LH) as well as follicle stimulating hormone (FSH).

Thyrotropin-releasing hormone (TRH): It controls release of the thyroid stimulating hormone (TSH). It may also influence the release of prolactin.

Corticotropin-releasing hormone (CRH): It controls the release of adrenocorticotropic hormone (ACTH).

Dopamine: It acts as prolactin release inhibitory factor (PIF).

HORMONES OF THE PITUITARY

Pituitary is also known as the **master gland**. It is divided into 3 functional units, called anterior pituitary (adenohypophysis), intermediary lobe and the posterior pituitary (neurohypophysis).

HORMONES OF THE ANTERIOR PITUITARY

Hormones of the anterior pituitary include growth hormone (GH), thyroid stimulating hormone (TSH or thyrotropin), ACTH, β-melanocyte-stimulating hormone (β-MSH), corticotrophin-like intermediary peptide (CLIP), prolactin (PRL), FSH and LH. All these are single peptides except TSH, FSH and LH, which are glycoprotein in nature.

Genes for these hormones contain coding sequences for the hormone as well as the control element.

Some of the hormones of the anterior pituitary are synthesized from a large precursor referred to as pro-opiomelanocortin (POMC).

Pro-opiomelanocortin

POMC is a polypeptide that is **encoded by a single gene.** It is cleaved in the corticotropic cells of the anterior pituitary to release ACTH and β-lipotropin as the major products, which are further cleaved in the pars intermedia to release α-MSH, CLIP, γ-lipotropin and β-endorphin into the circulation.

Some of the β-lipotropin arising in the corticotrophs is further degraded to β-endorphin.

Growth Hormone

It is a protein, also called somatotropin. Although main function of this hormone is to control growth, it has various effects on different tissues.

It is a diabetogenic hormone and increases blood glucose level, by reducing peripheral utilization of glucose and promoting gluconeogenesis. GH also stimulates mobilization of fat from the depot (adipose tissue) and fatty acid oxidation in the liver. It also reduces amino acid catabolism, promotes overall protein synthesis and causes positive nitrogen balance. GH also increases DNA and RNA synthesis.

GH also increases intestinal absorption as well as excretion of calcium and helps in retaining sodium, potassium, magnesium, phosphate and chloride. It also promotes growth of the epiphyseal cartilages and stimulates osteogenesis, collagen biosynthesis and erythropoiesis.

Secretion of the hormone is regulated by GHRH, which is produced by the hypothalamus. Its secretion is also increased by arginine, estrogen, hypoglycemia, exercise and stress. Both GH as well as insulin-like growth factor-1 decreases its secretion.

Hypersecretion of GH for a prolonged period results in **gigantism** in children and **acromegaly** in adults whereas its hyposecretion leads to **dwarfism.**

ACROMEGALY

Excess of GH results in **acromegaly,** a disease associated with over-growth of the bones and the soft tissues, in adults. When GH excess develops prior to epiphyseal closure in children, it increases linear growth and leads to a condition called **gigantism.**

Patients with **acromegaly** feel weak and tired. **Basal metabolic rate** is increased, which in turn also causes increased sweating. A moist-doughy handshake, increased skin tags, acanthosis nigricans and oily skin, are some of the common features.

Insulin resistance occurs in 80% of the patients although abnormal glucose tolerance and diabetes mellitus is common.

Hypercalcemia is also frequent, apparently due to increased levels of circulating 1, 25-dihydroxyvitamin D_3.

GH also causes **increased renal tubular reabsorption** of phosphate in about one-half of the patients.

PITUITARY DWARFISM

GH deficiency may contribute to increased cardiovascular mortality in adults, with hypopituitarism.

In children, GH deficiency leads to impaired growth and short stature. It is a consequence of hypothalamic GHRH deficiency and is also referred as pituitary dwarfism.

Tropic Hormones

Hormones secreted from the anterior pituitary are referred to as tropic hormones. They influence activities of the target endocrine gland. Tropic hormones are carried to the target gland and stimulate production of their respective hormones. Tropic hormones include:

TSH: It is a glycoprotein whose production and release is controlled by the thyrotropin-releasing hormone secreted by the hypothalamus. TSH stimulates thyroid gland, increases its growth and regulates secretion of thyroid hormones. TSH also promotes synthesis of phospholipids, proteins and RNA. Besides increasing glucose oxidation by glycolysis and tricarboxylic acid cycle, TSH enhances release of free fatty acids from the adipose tissue.

ACTH: It is a polypeptide whose secretion is controlled by the corticotrophin-releasing hormone released by the hypothalamus. ACTH stimulates secretion of hormones of the adrenal cortex other than aldosterone.

It stimulates lipolysis, increases free fatty acid and cholesterol levels and ketogenesis.

Increased production of ACTH causes hypersecretion of gluco-corticoids, which in turn leads to hyperglycemia, glycosuria, muscle wasting and negative nitrogen balance, and retention of fat, Na^+ and water, and results in **Cushing's disease.**

Gonadotropic Hormones: These include follicle stimulating hormone (FSH), luteinizing hormone (LH) or interstitial cell stimulating hormone (ICSH) and prolactin.

FSH and LH are glycoprotein in nature. Their synthesis is stimulated by the gonadotropin-releasing hormone produced by the hypothalamus. FSH and LH are responsible for growth, maturation and expulsion of ova in females and stimulate spermatogenesis and production of androgens in males.

Prolactin is a protein whose secretion is regulated mainly by the hypothalamic factor called prolactin-release inhibitory hormone. Prolactin stimulates mammary gland growth and secretion of milk.

HORMONES OF THE MIDDLE LOBE OF THE PITUITARY

Middle lobe of the pituitary secretes melanocyte-stimulating hormones (MSH). They are polypeptides whose secretion is regulated by the MSH-release inhibitory hormone. Cortisone inhibits MSH secretion while catecholamines inhibit the action of MSH. MSH is essential for skin pigmentation and is involved in the deposition of melanin by the melanocytes.

HORMONES OF THE POSTERIOR PITUITARY

Posterior lobe of the pituitary secretes **oxytocin and vasopressin (ADH)** both of which are oligopeptides.

Oxytocin

Oxytocin causes contraction of smooth muscle of uterus and lactating mammary glands. It thus helps in parturition and ejection of milk. Its secretion is controlled by hypothalamus as well as by suckling.

ADH

ADH helps in reabsorption of water thereby inhibiting diuresis and results in the concentration of urine. Deficiency of the hormone leads to excretion of large volume of urine and causes **diabetes insipidus.** Secretion of ADH is influenced by various stimuli, such as trauma, increase in plasma osmotic pressure, increase in the volume of the extracellular fluid and certain drugs, e.g. morphine, nicotine, etc.

DIABETES INSIPIDUS

Diabetes insipidus refers to the excretion of large quantity of diluted urine (polyuria). It may be either due to failure of ADH release in response to normal physiological stimuli (central or neurogenic diabetes insipidus) or failure of the kidney to respond to ADH (nephrogenic diabetes insipidus).

HORMONES OF THYROID AND PARATHYROID GLANDS

Follicular cells of the thyroid gland produce thyroid hormones. Parathyroid gland secretes parathyroid hormone (PTH) while C-cells, found in these two glands, secrete calcitonin.

THYROID HORMONES

Thyroid gland secretes **thyroxine (T_4) and tri-iodothyronine (T_3)**, referred to as thyroid hormones. They are synthesized by iodination of the tyrosyl-residues of thyroglobulin. Lysosomal acid proteases hydrolyse thyroglobulin to release free hormone. TSH as well as exposure to cold environment stimulates release of thyroid hormones.

Thyroid hormones are antagonists to insulin, stimulate absorption of glucose from the intestine and increase glycogenolysis. Though these hormones also stimulate glucose oxidation via glycolysis and HMP shunt but the net effect is increased blood glucose concentration.

In physiological concentration, thyroid hormones stimulate growth and protein anabolism but when given in pharmacological doses they result in protein catabolism and negative nitrogen balance. These hormones stimulate lipolysis in the adipose tissue and thus increase plasma free fatty acid level. They also promote lipogenesis. Thyroid hormones also increase cholesterol biosynthesis as well as its degradation. Since rate of cholesterol degradation is greater than its synthesis, the net result is a decrease in serum cholesterol level in hyperthyroidism.

These hormones also exhibit calorigenic action and increase blood flow and cardiac output.

They are also essential for normal growth and skeletal maturation.

GOITER

Enlargement of thyroid gland is called **goiter**. It may be due to overproduction and excessive secretion of the thyroid hormones, called **nodular goiter,** or compensatory enlargement of the tissue as a result of iodine deficiency, called **simple goiter**. Individuals with **simple goiter** have normal thyroid functions.

Hypothyroidism is deficiency of thyroid hormones and leads to **myxedema** in adults and **cretinism** in children. Such children are dwarf and mentally-retarded. Adults complain of undue sensitivity to cold with puffiness of the face and the extremities, thick and dry skin, and hypercholesterolemia.

Hyperthyroidism is due to excessive secretion of thyroid hormones and hyperactivity of the gland, which results in **thyrotoxicosis.** It is characterized by nervousness, weight loss, heat intolerance, tremor of the outstretched fingers and hypocholesterolemia. Most common form of the hyperthyroidism is referred to as **Grave's disease** where thyroid gland is diffusely enlarged with the protrusion of the eyeballs.

PARATHYROID HORMONE

Parathyroid hormone (parathormone or PTH) is a polypeptide whose secretion is under feed back control of serum Ca^{2+}. Main function of PTH thus is to increase Ca^{2+} and reduce phosphorus (P) concentration in serum through its direct action on the kidney and bone.

In the kidney, PTH decreases reabsorption of the filtered P and increases its urinary excretion. PTH also increases reabsorption of the filtered Ca^{2+} thereby decreasing its excretion to maintain serum Ca^{2+} concentration within the normal limits. It also decreases reabsorption of K^+ and HCO_3^- by renal tubules. PTH also stimulates 1-α-hydroxylase activity and thus helps in the conversion of 25(OH).D_3 to 1, 25$(OH)_2$.D_3.

In the bones, PTH stimulates differentiation and maturation of the precursor cells to the mature osteoclasts; increases bone resorption and mobilization of Ca^{2+} and P.

Over-secretion of PTH results in **hyperparathyroidism.** It may be due to a tumor or a result of tubular damage. Serum Ca^{2+} and alkaline phosphatase levels are increased while P and Mg^{2+} levels are reduced. There is also increased osteoclastic activity of the bone, resulting in its resorption. Kidney functions are also impaired.

Decreased secretion of PTH results in **hypoparathyroidism.** Osteoclastic activity is reduced. There is decrease in Ca^{2+} and Mg^{2+} while P concentration is increased.

Decreased concentration of Ca^{2+} and Mg^{2+} also results in neuromuscular hyperexcitability leading to **tetany.**

CALCITONIN

Calcitonin is a polypepide whose secretion is regulated by serum calcium. It results in hypocalcemia as well as hypophosphatemia. It also decreases the number of osteoclasts, increases osteoblasts and inhibits resorption of bone.

It also decreases reabsorption of both Ca^{2+} as well as P, resulting in calciuria and phosphateuria. Calcitonin also inhibits 1-α-hydroxylase and thus synthesis of active vitamin D, which in turn reduces intestinal absorption of Ca^{2+}.

HORMONES OF THE PANCREAS

Endocrine function of the pancreas is present in cells of the islet of Langerhans. It has 4 types of cells, referred to as the α-cells (which secrete glucagon), β-cells for the secretion of insulin, δ-cells to secrete somatostain and F cells for the secretion of pancreatic polypeptide.

INSULIN

Insulin is a protein hormone secreted by the β-cells of the islets of Langerhans of the pancreas. It is an anabolic hormone exhibiting its main effects in the muscle, adipose tissue, liver and heart.

Insulin is composed of two polypeptide chains, which are joined together by two disulfide bridges. It is synthesized as preproinsulin and is subsequently converted to insulin. Zinc is a constituent of the stored insulin and is also required for its crystallization.

Blood glucose is an important factor in the regulation of insulin secretion. Besides glucose, certain amino acids, such as leucine and arginine, and certain gastrointestinal hormones stimulate insulin secretion while epinephrine inhibits it.

Most important function of insulin is to lower blood glucose level and increase glycogen stores. Insulin also increases glucose uptake by cells, promotes glucose oxidation by glycolysis and HMP shunt, promotes glycogenesis and inhibits neoglucogenesis and glycogenolysis.

Insulin also decreases lipolysis, enhances de novo synthesis of fatty acids and promotes synthesis of triglycerides in adipose tissue.

Insulin also increases cellular uptake of amino acids and promotes protein biosynthesis.

Insulin also stimulates growth and cell proliferation, may be in association with insulin-like growth factor I and II.

Insulin **deficiency produces diabetes mellitus.**

GLUCAGON

It is a polypeptide, which is produced by the α-cells of the islets of Langerhans of the pancreas.

Glucose and fatty acids inhibit secretion of glucagon whereas amino acids, like arginine and alanine, growth hormone, increased serum calcium concentration, exercise and stress stimulate secretion of glucagon.

Glucagon stimulates glycogenolysis and gluconeogenesis in the liver and thus increases blood glucose concentration. It also promotes lipolysis and inhibits fatty acid synthesis. Glucagon also stimulates protein catabolism and reduces protein synthesis. Since glucagon mobilizes energy stores, it thus increases heat production and BMR.

SOMATOSTATIN

It is an oligopeptide, which is secreted by the δ-cells of the islets of Langerhans of the pancreas besides hypothalamus and gastrointestinal tract.

Somatostatin inhibits secretion of both insulin as well as glucagon.

Hypothalamic somatostatin is a regulator of growth hormone and is called **growth hormone-release inhibitory hormone.**

Gastrointestinal somatostatin inhibits secretion of local hormones of the gastrointestinal tract.

HORMONES OF THE ADRENAL GLAND

Adrenal gland, also called suprarenal gland, consists of two separate parts referred to as the cortex and the medulla. **Adrenal cortex** produces various corticosteroids while **medulla** secretes catecholamines.

HORMONES OF THE ADRENAL CORTEX

Adrenal cortex is differentiated into 3 different layers, designated as zona glomerulosa, zona fasiculata and zona reticularis.

All the hormones, secreted by the adrenal cortex, are steroids and are group as gluco-corticoids, mineralo-corticoids and cortical sex hormones. Out of these gluco-corticoids and mineralocorticoids exhibit various metabolic effects.

Gluco-corticoids

A gluco-corticoid is a 21-C containing-steroid that acts predominantly on the intermediary metabolism. The principal gluco-corticoid is cortisol (hydrocortisone). Its effect is mediated by type II gluco-corticoid receptors.

Various metabolic effects of gluco-corticoids are:

1. Gluco-corticoids raise blood glucose level by acting as insulin antagonist since cortisol suppresses secretion of insulin, inhibits peripheral glucose uptake and promotes hepatic glucose synthesis (gluconeogenesis).
2. They are catabolic in nature. Increased protein breakdown and inhibition of protein synthesis results in increased amino acids from the peripheral structures, such as bone, skin and muscle. Hyperaminoacidemia facilitates gluconeogenesis.
3. Gluco-corticoids regulate fatty acid mobilization by enhancing activation of lipase.
4. Gluco-corticoids though inhibit synthesis of nucleic acids in most of the tissues but stimulate RNA synthesis in the liver.
5. Gluco-corticoids have anti-inflammatory properties.
6. These hormones also modulate immune response.
7. Cortisol also helps to regulate extracellular fluid volume by retarding migration of water into the cells and promoting renal water excretion, may be by suppression of secretion of vasopressin.
8. Gluco-corticoids also have weak mineralocorticoid like properties.
9. Cortisol also suppresses secretion of POMC and its derivative peptides, i.e. ACTH, β-endorphin and β-lipotropin as well as CRH and vasopressin from the hypothalamus.

Failure of adrenal cortex to synthesize its hormones may result in **Addison's disease.**

ADDISON'S DISEASE

Addison's disease results from progressive destruction of adrenals. It is characterized by weakness, anorexia, nausea and vomiting, weight loss, cutaneous and mucosal pigmentation, hypotension and hypoglycemia. Serum sodium, chloride and bicarbonate levels are reduced while potassium is elevated. There may be mild to moderate hypercalcemia.

Hyper-functioning of the cortex may lead to **adrenogenital syndrome,** which is a congenital disorder. Under the influence of the excessive androgens, female assumes male secondary sex characteristics.

Tumor of the adrenal cortex may lead to acquired disorders. This, in turn, may result in hyper-functioning of the gland causing **Cushing's syndrome** or adrenocortical hyperplasia, as a result of increased production of ACTH, due to pituitary effects.

CUSHING'S SYNDROME

Cushing's syndrome is due to increased production of cortisol by the adrenal cortex. Hypercortisolism promotes deposition of adipose tissue in characteristic sites, notably upper face (producing typical moon-like face), inter-capsular area (buffalo-hump) and mesenteric bed (truncal obesity).

Plasma and urine cortisol levels are variably elevated. Occasionally, hypokalemia, hypochloremia and metabolic alkalosis are present, particularly, with ectopic production of ACTH. It is also accompanied with increased hepatic gluconeogenesis and insulin resistance, which in turn impairs glucose tolerance.

Common signs and symptoms include osteoporosis, diabetes mellitus, diastolic hypertension, central adiposity, hirsutism and amenorrhea.

Plasma cortisol level at 8 A.M. is more than 140 nmol/L (5 μg/dL) after 1 mg of dexamethasone at midnight.

Mineralocorticoids

Mineralocorticoids are 21-C containing-steroids. Principal mineralocorticoid is aldosterone that predominantly, regulates metabolism of sodium and potassium. It has two important actions:

(i) It is main regulator of extracellular fluid volume; and

(ii) A determinant of potassium metabolism.

These effects are mediated by the binding of the aldosterone to type I gluco-corticoid receptors (mineralocorticoid receptors) in the target tissue. Fluid volume is regulated through a direct effect on the collecting duct.

Aldosterone causes a decrease in sodium excretion. This reabsorption of sodium, in turn, leads to a fall in transmembrane potential and enhances the flow of other cations, such as potassium, out of the cell into the lumen. Reabsorbed sodium ions are transported out of the tubular epithelium into the renal interstitial fluid and from there into the renal capillary circulation. Water passively follows sodium. Since concentration of H^+ is greater in the lumen than the cell, H^+ are also actively secreted.

Mechanisms that control release of aldosterone

Renin-angiotensin system: Renin-angiotensin system controls extracellular fluid volume via the regulation of aldosterone secretion.

Potassium: Potassium ions directly regulate aldosterone secretion, independently of the circulating renin-angiotensin.

ACTH: Physiological amounts of ACTH stimulate aldosterone secretion.

RENIN-ANGIOTENSIN SYSTEM

Diminished blood flow, reduced plasma volume, or hypotension stimulates release of enzyme renin from juxtaglomerular cells to blood. The enzyme acts on angiotensinogen (plasma α_2-globulin) and converts it to angiotensin-I. Angiotensin-converting enzyme then converts angiotensin-I to angiotensin-II, which acts on zona glomerulosa to increase the synthesis and release of aldosterone. Aldosterone, in turn, increases rate of tubular reabsorption of Na^+ as well as Cl^- and eliminates K^+. Increased reabsorption of Na^+ reduces H^+ in body fluids and results in alkalosis. Increased concentrations of Na^+, Cl^- and HCO_3^- in turn, also increase water reabsorption from tubules and result in increased extracellular fluid volume, causing edema, increased plasma volume, cardiac output and hypertension.

HORMONES OF THE ADRENAL MEDULLA

Adrenal medulla synthesizes **dopamine, epinephrine and norepinephrine.** These are collectively referred to as **catecholamines** and are synthesized from tyrosine.

Catecholamines secretion is regulated at various levels. Their synthesis is inhibited allosterically while stress and cold stimulate secretion.

The principal catecholamine is **epinephrine. It has various metabolic effects:**

1. Epinephrine produces hyperglycemia. It stimulates glycogenolysis (both in liver and muscle) and gluconeogenesis (in the liver). It also has a direct inhibitory action on insulin release.
2. It also increases lipolysis and thus release of free fatty acids.
3. Epinephrine also causes vasodilation of arterioles of the skeletal muscle and vasoconstriction of arterioles of the skin and the mucous membrane. The hormone thus, increases coronary blood flow and cardiac output, relaxes muscles of the gastrointestinal tract, causes dilation of the pupil and lowers intra-ocular pressure.

Catecholamines also have calorigenic action.

A tumor of the adrenal medulla is called **pheochromocytoma.** It is characterized by hyperactivity of the gland, showing abnormal rise in blood pressure, hyperglycemia, increased BMR and excretion of increased quantities of vanillylmandelic acid (VMA), a primary metabolite of catecholamines.

REGULATION OF SECRETION OF HORMONES

Synthesis and release of most of the hormones is under the control of hypothalamus, concentration of some of the constituents of blood as well as circadian rhythm.

Control from the Hypothalamus

Various centers present in different parts of the brain send nerve impulses to the hypothalamus and cause release of several chemical substances, such as acetylcholine, epinephrine, GABA, etc. In response to these stimuli, hypothalamus secretes various releasing factors (regulatory factors or hypothalamic neurohormones, such as corticotrophin releasing factor, thyrotropin releasing factor, etc.) as well as some inhibitory factors, which inhibit release of some hormones from the pituitary gland, e.g. prolactin release inhibitory factor.

These hypothalamic releasing factors pass to the pituitary and cause release of the specific tropic hormones (trophins or tropins). Secretions from the pituitary (the tropic hormones) control synthesis and release of hormones from the endocrine gland. For example, corticotrophin releasing factor stimulates secretion of corticotrophin (adrenocorticotropic hormone or ACTH). Similarly, ACTH stimulates production and release of corticosteroids from adrenal cortex.

By the negative feedback mechanism, circulating levels of various endocrine secretions control synthesis and release of tropic hormones from pituitary via short loop as well as of the releasing factors from the hypothalamus via long loop. Further, production of tropic hormones via short loop also controls secretion of hypothalamic releasing factors. For example, corticosteroids are secreted from the adrenal cortex and inhibit secretion of ACTH from the anterior pituitary (short-loop inhibition) as well as of corticotrophin releasing factor from the hypothalamus (long loop inhibition). Secretion of corticotrophin releasing factor is also inhibited by ACTH (short loop inhibition) (Fig. 19.1).

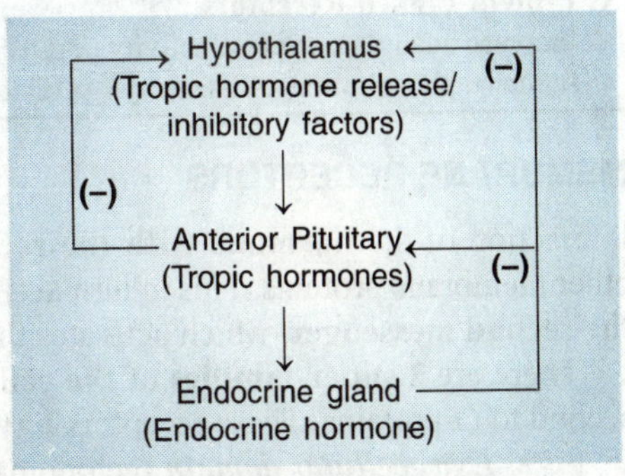

Fig. 19.1. Control of hormone secretion from the hypothalamus.

Control by Chemical Constituents of Blood

Secretion of various hormones is also under the control of some constituents of blood, e.g. synthesis and release of insulin is regulated by the concentration of glucose present in blood. Similarly, secretion of the parathyroid hormone (PTH) is stimulated by low serum calcium level.

Circadian Rhythms

Certain endocrine rhythms result from cyclic activities of biological clock, diurnal cycle, light-dark cycle, or sleep activity cycle. With a cycle periodicity of 24 hours, it is called circadian rhythm, e.g. cortisol peak is observed between 4 a.m. and 8 a.m. while growth hormone rises in early hours of deep-sleep.

MECHANISMS OF ACTION OF HORMONES

Hormones act after binding with their specific receptors, **which are located either intracellularly or on the cell membrane (extracellularly).**

Hormone receptors are **proteins** that differ by their specificity for the ligand as well as location within the cell. A **hormone-receptor complex**, usually, undergoes conformational changes, due to interaction of the receptor with the hormone.

There are several types of receptor systems, which vary in mechanism. For example, water-soluble hormones, such as the pituitary-derived proteins and glycoproteins are hydrophilic and cannot cross the lipid barrier presented by the cytoplasmic membrane. These hormones therefore interact with the receptors that are located on the **cell surface (membrane receptors)**. On the other hand, lipid soluble hormones, such as steroids and thyroid hormones, diffuse into the cell and bind to intracellular receptors, which are located either in the cytosol or in the nucleus (Table 19.2).

Table 19.2. Hormone receptors

Type of receptor	*Hormone*
Intracellular Receptors	
– Cytosolic	Steroids
– Nuclear	Calcitriol, T_3
Cell Surface Receptors	
Linked to Tyrosine Kinase	
– Intrinsic tyrosine kinase (Growth factor receptors)	Insulin, Insulin-like growth factor (IGF-1)
– Recruit tyrosine kinase	Growth hormone, prolactin
G Protein-Linked Receptors	
– Increase adenylate cyclase activity	ADH, catecholamines, epinephrine through adrenergic β-receptor, and glucagon
– Increase phospholipase C activity	Oxytocin, PTH, Ca^{2+}, calcitonin, epinephrine through α-1 receptors

MEMBRANE RECEPTORS

Interaction of the **hormone with the receptor** (cell-surface receptor) causes a conformational change in other membrane proteins. This in turn **activates enzymes inside the cell** thereby resulting in the **synthesis of the second messenger**, which activates the phosphorylating enzymes.

There are **2 super-families of the cell-surface receptors**. The first is linked to tyrosine kinase and the second to G-proteins. These receptors **have 3** clearly identifiable **domains**:

- ***Extracellular domain*** (ectodomain), which binds the hormone with a high affinity,
- ***Hydrophobic transmembrane domain*** (membrane-spanning region), which varies in structure, and

- ***Cytosolic domain***, which initiates intracellular signaling cascade. This is the effector region of the receptor, which may be linked with another membrane protein system, a set of enzymes that are guanosinetriphosphatases (GTPases). The intracellular region may also have regulatory tyrosine or serine/threonine phosphorylation sites.

TYROSINE KINASE-LINKED CELL-SURFACE RECEPTORS

They rely upon tyrosine kinase for the initiation of downstream signals. They have a relatively simple transmembrane segment and are of two types:

- **Receptor with intrinsic tyrosine kinase activity :** Tyrosine kinase activity is **located in the cytosolic domain. The most prominent member of this subgroup is the receptors for insulin and insulin-like growth factor-1 (IGF-1).**

MECHANISM OF ACTION OF INSULIN

Insulin is secreted in response to high blood glucose following a meal. It **has two primary functions in carbohydrate metabolism:**

First, insulin **reverses the actions of glucagon** in phosphorylation of protein, i.e. turning-off of glycogen phosphorylase and activating glycogen synthase, thus, promoting glucose storage.

Second, it **stimulates uptake of glucose into muscle and adipose tissue** thereby facilitating synthesis and storage of glycogen and triacylglycerol. Insulin also acts at the level of gene expression, stimulating synthesis of the enzymes involved in carbohydrate metabolism and storage and conversion of glucose into triacylglycerols.

Insulin receptors contain an intrinsic (hormone-activated) **tyrosine kinase activity**, which serves as a direct catalyst of phosphorylation reaction. Its receptor consists of two α- and two β-subunits. Its α-subunits are extracellular and contain a hormone-binding site. On the other hand, its β-subunits possess intracellular domains that contain ATP-binding sites and a catalytic kinase domain (Fig. 19.2).

Insulin binding to its transmembrane **receptor** stimulates aggregation of receptors and promotes tyrosine kinase activity in the intracellular domain of the receptor. The receptor kinase activity autophosphorylates its tyrosine residues, enhancing its protein tyrosine kinase activity as well as phosphorylating tyrosine

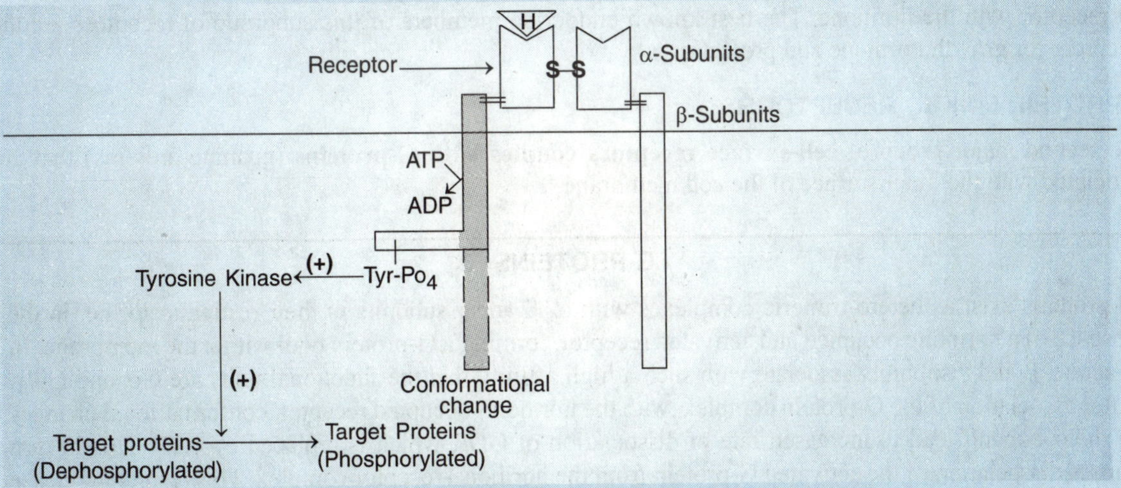

Fig. 19.2. Modulation of tyrosine kinase activity of insulin receptor.

residues of the other intracellular effector proteins, called insulin receptor substrates (IRS). Main targets of receptor tyrosine kinase are known as IRS-1 and IRS-2. When phosphorylated, these proteins interact with another set of proteins that contain two SH_2 (SH2 homology 2) domains, which become activated upon binding to IRS. As a result of different signal proteins binding to the phosphorylated IRS, several separate signaling pathways become activated. These include kinases that phosphorylate serine and threonine residues on certain proteins, such as GTPase, phosphodiesterase and phosphoprotein phosphatases. Insulin dependent activation of these proteins also checks action of glycogen. One pathway may stimulate DNA synthesis and cell division while other may activate a transcription factor that turns-on expression of insulin specific genes (Fig. 19.3).

In muscle and adipose tissue, receptor tyrosine kinase activity **induces movement of glucose transporter-4** (GLUT-4) from the intracellular vacuoles to the cell surface, thereby increasing glucose transport into cells. Glucose is then used in muscle for the synthesis of glycogen and in adipose tissue to produce glyceraldehyde-3-phosphate, which is converted to glycerol-3-phosphate for the synthesis of triacylglycerol. Hormone-receptor complex also results in internalization and degradation of receptor molecules. The process of receptor internalization provides a means of regulating the effects of insulin and effectively down regulates insulin receptors.

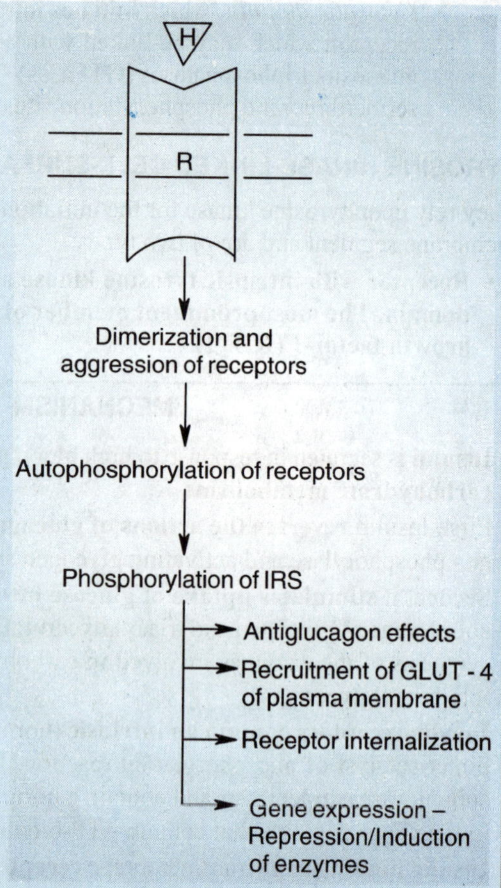

Fig. 19.3. Mechanism of insulin action.

- **Receptors that recruit tyrosine kinase activity**- They recruit tyrosine kinase activity after binding of the receptor with the hormone. The best known endocrine members of this subgroup of receptors are the receptors for growth hormone and prolactin.

G-PROTEIN LINKED RECEPTORS

The second major group of **cell-surface receptors couples with G-proteins** (guanine-proteins) that are associated with the inner surface of the cell membrane.

G-PROTEINS

G-proteins exist as hetero-trimeric complexes with α, β and γ subunits in their resting state, i.e. in the absence of a hormone occupied and activated receptor, forming a G-protein pool within the membrane. In practice, β and γ subunits associate with such a high affinity that the functional units are Gα and Gβ/γ. After association of the G-protein complex ,with the hormone-occupied receptor, conformational changes in the α-subunit lead to increased rate of dissociation of GDP, which is replaced by GTP. This in turn causes dissociation of the activated G-protein from the hormone-receptor complex. This results in release of the α-subunit from the heterotrimeric complex. GTP-activated α-subunit of the G-protein subsequently diffuses in the lipid bilayer and binds to the catalytic unit, which is either adenylate cyclase or phospholipase C.

There are four major subfamilies of Gα subunit. These are $G_s\alpha$ and $G_i\alpha$, which activate or inhibit adenylate cyclase, respectively; $G_q\alpha$, which activates phospholipase C; and $G_o\alpha$, which activates ion channels. Gα subunit can also functions as a GTPase, which cleaves phosphate from GTP, resulting in Gα- GDP. This in turn results in switching-off of the activation of the catalytic subunit and allows reassociation of Gα-GDP with the Gβ/γ, reforming new heterotrimer. The heterotrimer then returns to G-protein in the membrane and is recycled to respond to another receptor.

The most striking structural difference in G-protein linked receptor from the tyrosine kinase-linked receptor lies in the transmembrane region. The transmembrane domain has a characteristic heptahelical structure, i.e. it crosses the lipid bilayer of the plasma membrane seven times. Further, its cytoplasmic domain links the receptor to the signal traducing G-proteins. The linking G-proteins are larger members of the super family of regulatory proteins, which function as molecular switches by binding and then hydrolyzing GTP to GDP. The activated protein then undergoes major structural modifications and ultimately modulates the catalytic activity of adenylate cyclase or phospholipase C within the membrane structure. This in turn leads to the **generation of some intracellular second messenger**, such as cAMP, IP_3, etc.

SECOND MESSENGERS

Cyclic AMP

Cyclic AMP (cAMP) is a small molecule **derived from ATP** by the catalytic action of the signaling enzyme **adenylate cyclase.** It has a key role in the regulation of intracellular signal translocation leading to the conversion of glycogen to glucose.

The β-adrenergic receptor is coupled to adenylate cyclase activation by the action of the α-subunit of the **stimulatory G-protein** called G_s. $G_s\alpha$ activates membrane-bound adenylate cyclase, which catalyses the conversion of ATP to cAMP. This cyclic nucleotide acts as a potent second messenger and in turn activates cAMP-dependent protein kinase A, which modulates multiple aspects of cell function (Fig. 19.4).

G-protein coupled receptors, such as α-adrenergic receptors, which act to inhibit cAMP generation, are coupled to the inhibition of adenylate cyclase via the inhibitory G-protein called G_i. When an inhibitory G-protein binds with the receptor, it results in inhibition of adenylate cyclase and exhibits opposite effects.

Activation of Protein Kinase A by cAMP through G-protein

Inactive protein kinase A is a tetramer. It has two regulatory subunits called R and two catalytic subunits called C. The enzyme is converted to its active form with the help of four molecules of cAMP, which bind to the regulatory subunits of the enzyme and results in dissociation of its two catalytic subunits. It is the free catalytic subunit, which phosphorylates target proteins and produces various metabolic effects of the hormone (Fig.19.5).

cAMP transduces its effects on glycogen-glucose interconversion by **regulating** a key signaling enzyme **protein kinase A,** which phosphorylates target proteins on serine and threonine residues (Fig. 19.6).

Protein kinase A binds cAMP and phosphorylates and modulates activity of two key enzymes, i.e. phosphorylase kinase and glycogen synthase, which are involved in the regulation of glycogen metabolism.

Protein kinase A-mediated phosphorylation **also regulates the activity of a number of ion channels**, such as K^+, Cl^- and Ca^{2+} channels **and** that of **phosphatases** that are involved in the regulation of cell signaling. In addition, translocation of protein kinase A into the nucleus allows modulation of the activity of

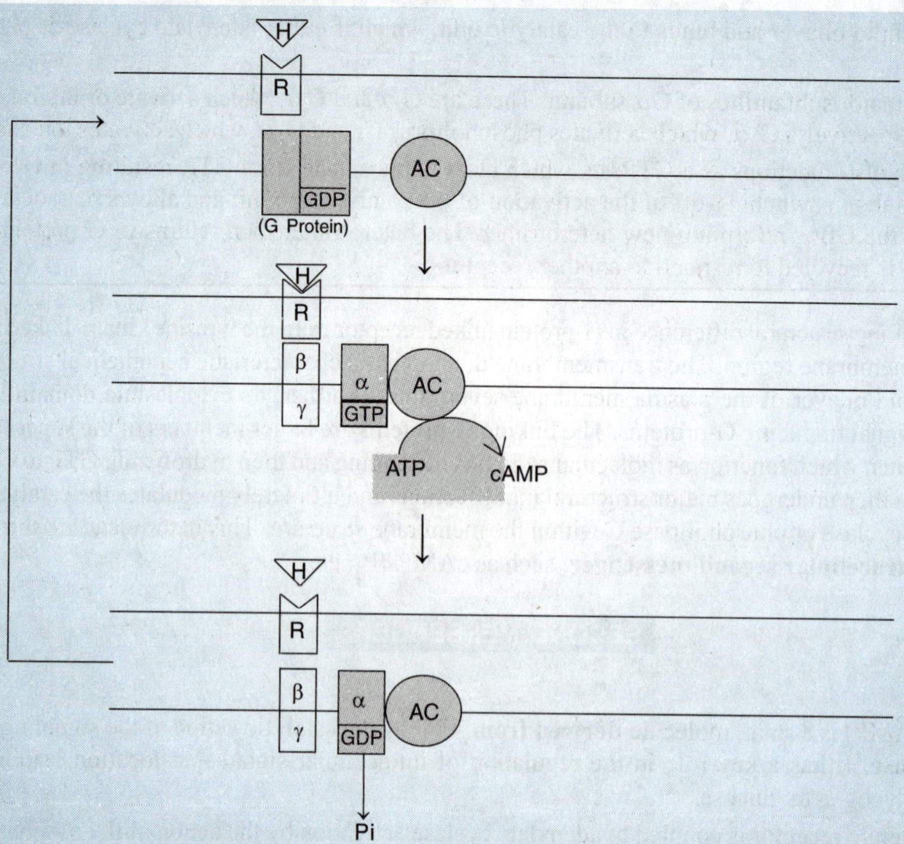

Fig. 19.4. Activation of adenylate cyclase by G. protein. (H = hormone; R = receptor; AC = adenylate cyclase)

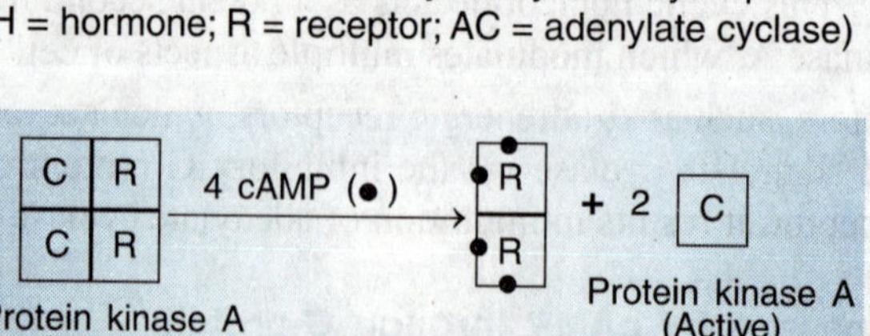

Fig. 19.5. Activation of protein kinase A by cAMP.

transcription factors, such as the cAMP responsive element-binding protein (cREB). This is then transloctaed into the nucleus where it binds a short palindromic sequence in the promoter region of the cAMP-regulated genes, referred to as CRE (cAMP response-enhancer element), and thereby has a direct effect on gene transcription.

Phosphodiesterase terminates the cAMP signal by converting cAMP to its 5′-AMP metabolite.

$$\text{ATP} \xrightarrow{\text{Adenylate cyclase}} \text{cAMP}$$

$$\text{cAMP} \xrightarrow{\text{Phosphodiesterase}} 5'-\text{AMP}$$

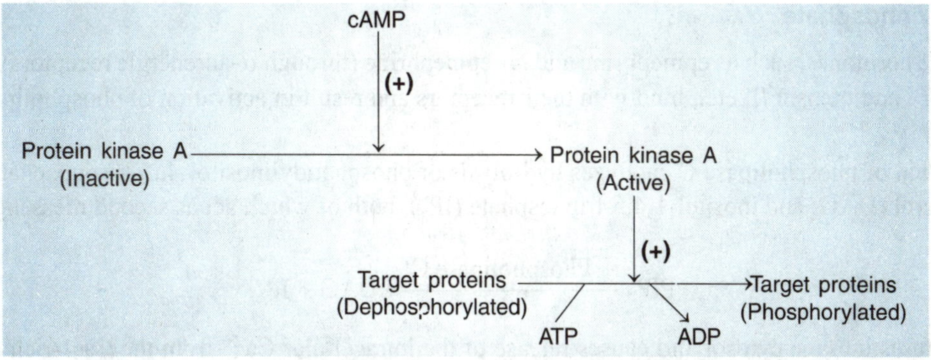

Fig. 19.6. Activation of intracellular proteins through protein kinase A.

MECHANISM OF ACTION OF GLUCAGON

Glucagon binds to its receptors on the outer surface of the target cells and stimulates breakdown of glycogen to glucose. Binding of the hormone activates adenylate cyclase on the inner surface of the membrane, leading to the production of cAMP.

cAMP in turn binds to the regulatory subunit of the cAMP-dependent protein kinase A, which phosphorylates phosphorylase kinase and glycogen synthase. It leads to the activation of phosphorylase kinase and inhibition of glycogen synthase.

The activated phosphorylase kinase in turn activates glycogen phosphorylase, which initiates glycogenolysis leading to the production of the glucose-6-phosphate that is hydrolyzed to glucose and exported to blood.

Protein kinase A also phosphorylates inhibitor-1, a protein phosphatase inhibitor protein, which in turn inhibits cytoplasmic phosphoprotein phosphatase. Other hepatic pathways, including protein, cholesterol, fatty acid, and triglyceride biosynthesis and glycolysis are also regulated by phosphorylation of key regulatory enzymes favoring metabolism in response to glycogen breakdown for the provision of glucose to blood, for the maintenance of vital body functions.

Calcium Ions

Calcium ion (Ca^{2+}) is a ubiquitous messenger and has an important role in the transduction of signals leading to a number of cellular responses.

Ligation of a wide range of hormone receptors leads to a rapid and transient increase in intracellular Ca^{2+} concentration to the micromolar range. Rapid raising and lowering of Ca^{2+} concentration is very tightly regulated and utilizes a variety of mechanisms including cell compartmentalization. For example, intracellular Ca^{2+} concentration can be lowered by sequestration of Ca^{2+} into the endoplasmic reticulum by Ca^{2+}-ATPase or into the mitochondria using energy-driven electrochemical gradient.

Ca^{2+} activates several enzymes, including protein kinases, calmodulin and some isoforms of protein kinase C.

It also activates phospholipase A_2, which liberates arachidonate from phospholipids and thereby generates eicosanoids, precursors of important chemically related signal molecules that include thromboxanes, leucotrienes, lipoxins and prostaglandins.

Ca^{2+} also activates cytosolic guanylate cyclase, an enzyme that catalyzes the formation of cGMP.

Many downstream signaling events mediated by Ca^{2+} are modulated by a Ca^{2+}-sensing and binding protein, calmodulin.

Inositol Triphosphate

Some of the hormones, such as epinephrine and norepinephrine (through α-adrenergic receptors), ADH (via V_1 receptor), angiotensin II, etc., bind with their receptors and result in activation of phospholipase C (Fig. 19.7).

Activation of phospholipase C catalyzes hydrolysis of phosphatidylinositol-4, 5-bisphosphate (PIP_2) to diacylglycerol (DAG) and inositol-1,4,5-triphosphate (IP_3), both of which act as second messengers.

$$PIP_2 \xrightarrow{\text{Phospholipase C}} DAG + IP_3$$

IP_3 diffuses into the cytosol and causes release of the intracellular Ca^{2+} from the Ca^{2+}-rich organelles, such as endoplasmic reticulum (ER). Ca^{2+} interacts with calmodulin (C) and forms Ca^{2+}-calmodulin complex (Ca^{2+}-C complex), which in turn activates calmodulin specific kinases.

DAG activates protein kinase C that generally phosphorylates a wide range of target signal–transduction proteins at several residues.

Free Ca^{2+} ions, calmodulin specific kinases as well as protein kinase C in turn may cause phosphorylation of the target protein(s) to exhibit physiological actions.

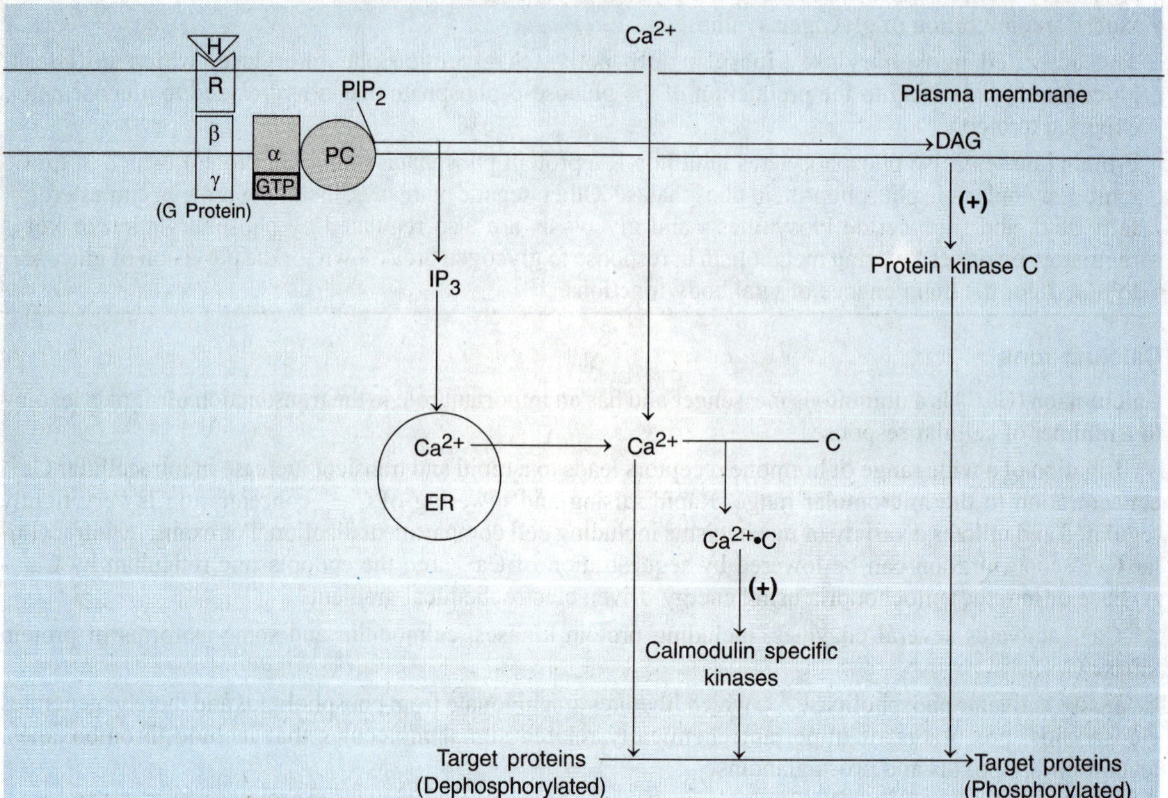

Fig. 19.7. Activation of phospholipase C by G-protein. (PC = phospholipase C; C = calmodulin; ER = endoplasmic reticulum)

MECHANISM OF ACTION OF EPINEPHRINE

Epinephrine works through several distinct receptors on different cells. The best studied of these receptors are α and β adrenergic receptors. They bind epinephrine with different affinities and work by different mechanisms.

Action on Hepatic Glycogen

Epinephrine action on hepatic glycogenolysis via β-adrenergic receptor is similar to that for glucagon, involving a plasma membrane epinephrine specific receptor, G-protein and cAMP. The epinephrine response augments the effects of glucagon during severe hypoglycemia.

Epinephrine also works simultaneously through α-receptor by a different mechanism. Binding to α-receptors also involves G-proteins but in this case the G-protein is specific for activation of an isoenzyme of phospholipase C, which cleaves phosphatidylinositolbisphosphate to diacylglycerol (DAG) and inositoltriphosphate (IP_3). Both the hydrolyzed products act as second messengers. DAG activates protein kinase C, which like protein kinase A, initiates a series of protein-phosphorylation reactions. IP_3 promotes transport of Ca^{2+} into the cytosl. Ca^{2+} then binds to the cytoplasmic protein calmodulin, which binds to and activates phosphorylase kinase, leading to phosphorylation and activation of phosphorylase, providing glucose for blood (Fig. 19.8).

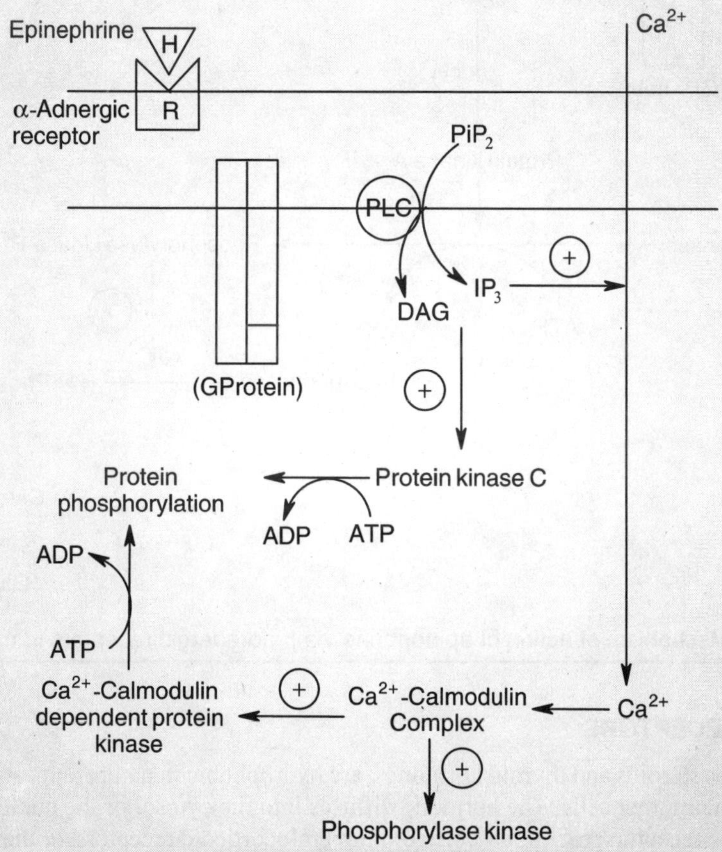

Fig. 19.8. Mechanism of action of epinephrine via α-adrenergic receptors in liver.

Ca^{2+}-calmodulin dependent protein kinase and other enzymes are also activated either by phosphorylation or by association with the Ca^{2+}-calmodulin complex. Thus, a range of metabolic pathways are activated in response to stress, causing an increase in blood glucose to support a "fight or flight" response.

Action on Glycogen in Muscle

Muscles lack glycogen receptors and glucose-6-phosphatase activity hence; muscle glycogen can not be mobilized to replenish blood glucose. Muscle glycogenolysis is activated in response to epinephrine through β-adrenergic receptor, mediated through cAMP, providing supply of carbohydrate for the energy for muscle during prolonged exercise (Fig. 19.9).

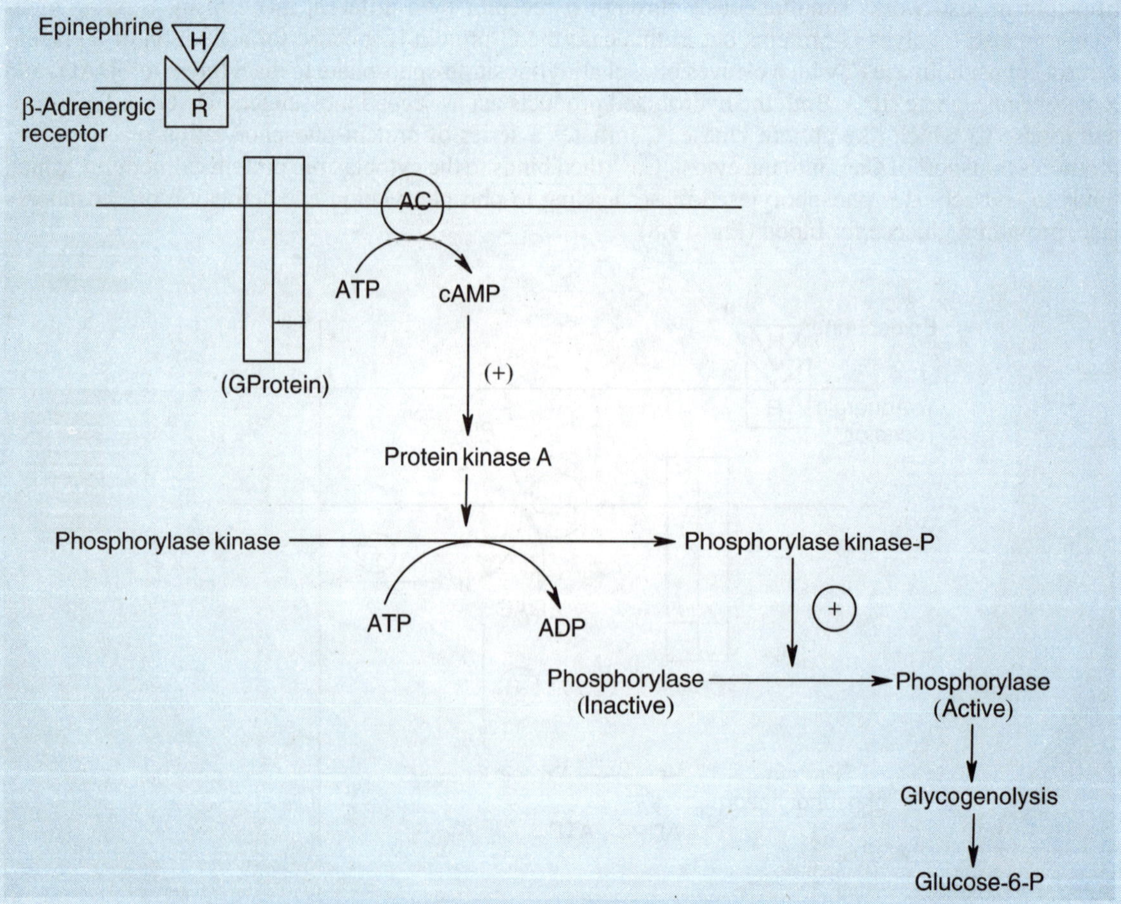

Fig. 19.9. Mechanism of action of epinephrine via β-adrenergic receptors in muscle.

INTRACELLULAR RECEPTORS

Some hormones, such as steroids and thyroid hormones, are hydrophobic in nature and can diffuse across the plasma membrane of their target cells. The hormone diffuses into the cytosol or the nucleus, where it binds either to the cytoplasmic receptors, e.g. gluco-corticoid/mineralocorticoid receptors, or the nuclear receptors, such as progesterone, estradiol, vitamin D_3 or androgen receptors. These receptors have two regions, i.e. a hydrophobic hormone-binding region and a DNA-binding region, which consists of two zinc fingers, rich in cysteine and basic amino acids.

Binding of the hormone with the receptor causes a conformational change in the receptor and activates it. The activated-receptor is thereafter translocated into the nucleus. In the nucleus, activated-receptor binds to the nuclear DNA, upstream of the specific hormone-response elements, and activates the hormone-responsive genes. This, in turn, leads to the activation/repression of the transcription of the genes.

The nonactivated receptor cannot bind to DNA because heteromeric heat-shock proteins (Hsp) block its DNA-binding site (Fig. 19.10).

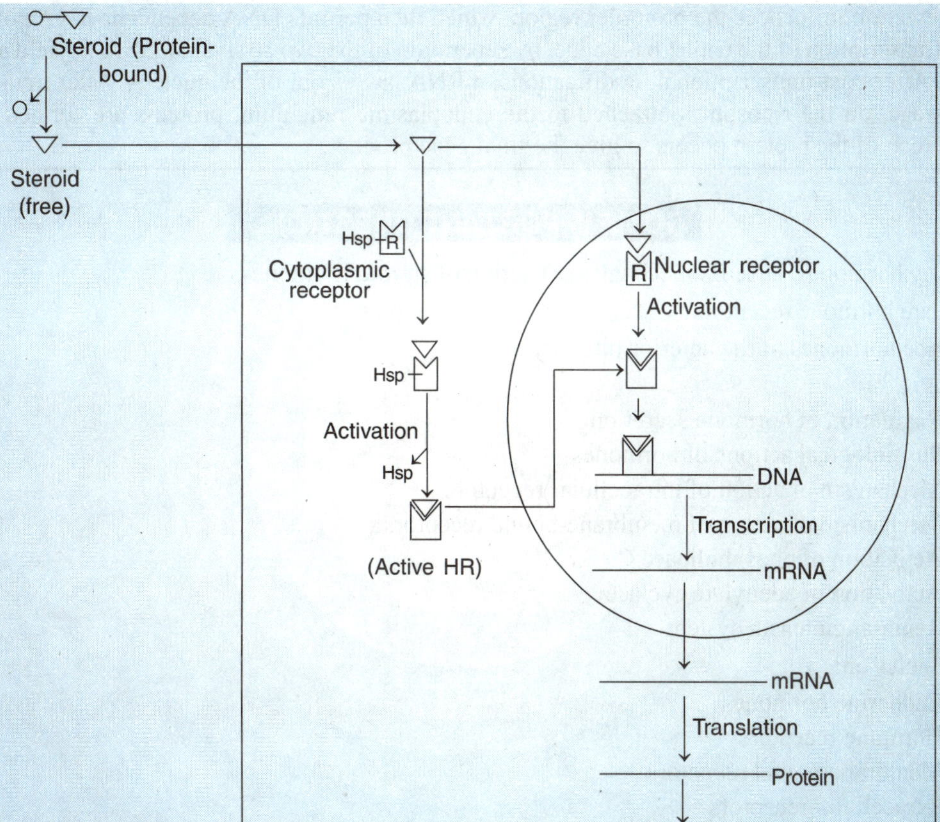

Fig. 19.10. Mode of action of hormone through intracellular receptors.

MECHANISM OF ACTION OF STEROID HORMONES

Steroid hormones have a broad range of functions in humans and are essential to normal life. They are derived from common precursor, i.e. cholesterol.

Steroids bring about their biological effects by binding to the steroid-specific hormone receptors. Steroid hormone receptors function as ligand-regulated transcription factors.

Steroid hormones diffuse across the plasma membrane and bind to their receptors, which are present in the cytosol. Hormone binding results in a conformational change that causes the hormone-receptor complex to move into the nucleus and bind to DNA at a specific response element called **steroid response element** (SRE). These SREs may be present in the promoter or enhancer regions of the hormone-sensitive genes. This interaction gives rise to an increase or decrease in the rate of gene transcription.

Free steroid is in equilibrium with that bound to serum-binding proteins and diffuses across the target cell membrane.

The hormone-receptor complex interacts with the chromatin, which is attached to the nuclear matrix structures. The hormone-receptor complex binds to a receptor site on the regulatory region of one DNA strand associated with a particular gene. This region is known as the **hormone-response element** (HRE). This interaction influences the promoter region, which then permits DNA dependent-RNA polymerase to start transcription of the triplet base code, by separation of the two strands of DNA to yield a specific mRNA. After post-transcriptional modifications, mRNA passes out of the nucleus. After translation of the message, on the ribosomes attached to the endoplasmic reticulum, proteins are formed. Finally, modification of the protein occurs to give the final gene product.

SOME IMPORTANT QUESTIONS

1. Classify hormones. Discuss mechanism of action of steroid hormones.
2. What are hormone receptors? Classify them with examples.
3. Describe hormones of the anterior pituitary.
4. Discuss :
   (i) Regulation of hormone secretion
   (ii) Physiological actions of hormones
   (iii) Mechanism of action of intracellular receptors
   (iv) Mechanism of action of membrane-bound receptors
   (v) Activation of phospholipase C
   (vi) Activation of adenylate cyclase
   (vii) Renin-angiotensin system
5. Write notes on:
   (i) Endocrine hormones
   (ii) Hormone receptors
   (iii) Membrane-bound receptors
   (iv) Intracellular receptors
   (v) G-proteins
   (vi) POMC
   (vii) Acromegaly
   (viii) Diabetes insipidus
   (ix) Gluco-corticoids
   (x) Mineralocorticoids
   (xi) Cushing's syndrome
   (xii) Addison's disease
   (xiii) Pheochromocytoma
   (xiv) Calcitonin
   (xv) Parathyroid hormone

CHAPTER

20

Acid Base Regulation

Acid is a substance **whose dissociation in water releases hydrogen ions** (H^+). An H^+ since does not contain any neutron and is essentially equivalent to a proton, **an acid** therefore is **often referred to as a proton donor. Addition of an acid to a solution thus, increases the concentration of free H^+ in the solution.** This in turn, produces a more acidic solution and results in decrease in pH.

An acid, e.g. HA, in aqueous solution reversibly dissociates into H^+ and a conjugate base (A^-). This dissociation of HA thus, can be represented symbolically, by the following equation:

$$HA \longrightarrow H^+ + A^-$$

Where, A^- represents anion (a conjugate base) and H^+ a proton. This tendency of an acid to give up H^+ depends upon its strength.

A **strong acid,** such as HCl, **completely dissociates in an aqueous solution:**

$$HCl \longrightarrow H^+ + Cl^-$$

On the other hand, **a weak acid gives up H^+ less rapidly** and **does not dissociate, completely.** A solution of a weak acid thus, contains both dissociated ions as well as undissociated molecule. **Most of the acids produced in living systems are weak acids.**

BASE

A Base releases hydroxyl ions (OH^-) in aqueous solution and decreases its H^+ concentration by accepting or binding with free H^+. **This in turn results in increase in pH of the solution.**

A strong base, such as sodium hydroxide (NaOH), dissociates completely:

$$NaOH \longrightarrow Na^+ + OH^-$$

The OH^-, so produced, accepts H^+ and results in the formation of water. This in turn, lowers the concentration of H^+ in the solution.

$$OH^- + H^+ \rightleftharpoons H_2O$$

A weak base, such as bicarbonate (HCO_3^-) can also utilize H^+ and thus lower H^+ concentration of the solution.

$$HCO_3^- + H^+ \rightleftharpoons H_2CO_3$$

Amount of an acid or a base is expressed in terms of **equivalents. One mole of HCl contains one equivalent of acid** and neutralizes one equivalent of base. On the other hand, **one mole of sulfuric acid** (H_2SO_4) **contains two equivalents of acid** since sulfuric acid can donate two H^+ and requires two moles of NaOH, to neutralize it.

AMPHOTERIC SUBSTANCES

Some substances, such as amino acids and proteins, can act as **acids as well as bases. These substances are referred to as amphoteric substances.** For example, an amino acid, such as glycine, can act as acid as well as base (an ampholyte), at physiological pH:

$$H_2N\text{–}CH_2\text{–}COOH \rightleftharpoons H_3N^+\text{–}CH_2\text{–}COO^-$$

It acts as an acid when ammonium group (NH_3^+) of glycine donates its H^+ to a base.

$$\begin{array}{c} H_3N^+ - CH_2 - COO^- \\ \big\downarrow \; OH^- \searrow H_2O \\ H_2N - CH_2 - COO^- \end{array}$$

On the other hand, glycine can act as a base when the carboxylate group (COO^-) of glycine accepts H^+ from an acid:

$$\begin{array}{c} H_3N^+ - CH_2 - COO^- \\ \big\downarrow \; H^+ \\ H_3N^+ - CH_2 - COOH \end{array}$$

pH

pH is defined as the negative logarithm to the base 10 of the molar concentration of the hydrogen ions (H^+), in a solution :

$$\text{pH} = -\log [H^+], \text{ or}$$
$$= \log (1/[H^+])$$

pH of the solution is inversely related to the free H^+ concentration, $[H^+]$. **Low pH** indicates **high H^+ concentration** while **high pH** indicates **low H^+ concentration.**

If we add a strong base, such as NaOH, to water, the OH^- will combine with H^+, supplied by the water. This, in turn, will shift equilibrium towards the undissociated water and lowers free H^+ ion concentration, thereby resulting in increase in pH.

The **scale of the pH measurement varies from 0–14. If pH of a solution is below 7,** the solution is said to **acidic;** if **equal to 7,** it is referred to as **neutral,** and if its pH is **greater than 7,** the solution is said to be **alkaline or basic** in nature.

Handerson-Hasselbalch Equation

Weak acids, when dissolved in water, do not dissociate totally but establish equilibrium between the undissociated compound and the dissociated ions, e.g.:

$$HA \rightleftharpoons H^+ + A^-$$

Concentration of the ionic species, in turn, can be determined from the equilibrium equation:

$$K'eq = \frac{[H^+][A^-]}{[HA]}$$

where, $K'eq$ is an apparent equilibrium constant, $[H^+]$, $[A^-]$ and $[HA]$ indicate concentrations of the dissociated cation (H^+), anion (A^-) and the undissociated acid, respectively. $K'eq$ is a function of temperature of the system.

Changing the concentration of any one component in the equilibrium reaction, will change concentration of all the components. For example, an increase in H^+ concentration will decrease concentration of the conjugate base with an equivalent increase in conjugate acid.

On rearranging the above equation and solving it for H^+, we get:

$$[H^+] = K'eq \times ([HA]/[A^-]), \text{ or}$$

$$[H^+] = K'eq \times ([\text{conjugate acid}]/[\text{conjugate base}])$$

Multiplying by –1, this equation becomes:

$$-[H^+] = -K'eq \times ([\text{conjugate base}]/[\text{conjugate acid}])$$

The logarithimic form of the above equation is known as **Handerson-Hasselbalch equation.**

It is derived as follows:

$$-\log [H^+] = -\log K'eq + \log ([\text{conjugate base}]/[\text{conjugate acid}])$$

Since

$$-\log [H^+] = pH, \text{ and}$$

$$-\log Ka' = pK'a$$

The above equation can be written as:

$$pH = pK'a + \log ([\text{conjugate base}]/[\text{conjugate acid}])$$

When half of the acid is present in the dissociated form, i.e. $[A^-] = [HA]$, the pH of the solution is equal to its $pK'a$.

Handerson-Hasselbalch equation thus, is a mathematical rearrangement of the fundamental equilibrium equation, which states that there is a direct relationship between the pH and the ratio of the concentration of the conjugate base to the concentration of the conjugate acid.

BUFFERS

Something **that minimizes a shock,** and **thereby promotes relative stability,** is defined as **buffer. A pH buffer minimizes change in pH when an acid or a base is added to a solution.**

A chemical buffer consists of a weak acid (HA) and its conjugate base (A^-), or a weak base and its conjugate acid, such as:

Acid		**Conjugate Base**
HA	$\rightleftharpoons$	$A^- + H^+$
H_2CO_3	$\rightleftharpoons$	$HCO_3^- + H^+$
$H_2PO_4^-$	$\rightleftharpoons$	$HPO_4^{2-} + H^+$
NH_4^+	$\rightleftharpoons$	$NH_3 + H^+$

A weak acid may be neutral, positively charged or negatively charged while its conjugate base has one less positive charge (or one more negative charge) than the weak acid, due to loss of H^+.

The effectiveness of a buffer, in minimizing changes in pH, **depends upon** two factors:

1. **The pK'a of the buffer** in relation to the desired pH, e.g. pK´a of the imidazole group of histidine in hemoglobin is close to 7.4 and thus, it is an ideal buffer in the blood.
2. The **concentration of the buffer.**

Greater the concentration of the buffer, more is its ability to bind or release H^+.

BUFFERING MECHANISMS IN THE BODY

Metabolism of food consumed in our diet, results in the production of CO_2 as well as acids, in the body. For example, most carbohydrates and fats are normally, completely, oxidized to CO_2 and water; metabolism of dietary protein results in the production of strong acids, etc.

In the pulmonary capillary blood, CO_2 reacts with water and forms carbonic acid (H_2CO_3). A zinc-containing enzyme, carbonic anhydrase, which also catalyzes the dissociation of carbonic acid to H^+ and HCO_3^-, catalyzes this reaction:

$$H_2O + CO_2 \rightleftharpoons H_2CO_3 \rightleftharpoons H^+ + HCO_3^-$$

Dissociation of H_2CO_3 or association of H^+ and HCO_3^- to form H_2CO_3 occurs, instantaneously.

Despite metabolic production of acids in the body, blood and intestinal fluid pH is maintained with in the normal limits in a healthy person. Here, **first line of defense** of pH **consists of chemical buffers that are present in the extracellular and the intracellular fluids,** while the **second line of defense is the lungs** that maintain blood pH by disposing off CO_2.

CHEMICAL BUFFERS PRESENT IN BODY FLUIDS

Blood plasma is a mixed buffer system and **has three major buffers, which are HCO_3^-/CO_2, $HPO_4^{2-}/H_2PO_4^-$, and protein⁻/H. protein.**

1. **Phosphate buffer:** Phosphate buffer has a pK of 6.8. It is a good buffer for stabilizing the pH of the blood. It is also an important buffer in the urine.
2. **Protein buffer:** A protein contains many different ionizable groups, each one of which can donate or accept H^+.

   Protein comprises of the largest amount of buffer in the body. For example, albumin acts as buffer in the blood plasma. An important example of the intracellular protein buffer is hemoglobin (Hb).
3. **Bicarbonate/CO_2 buffer:** Bicarbonate/CO_2 buffer **has special importance in buffering pH in the extracellular fluid,** due to the reason that:

(i) **The components of this buffer system,** i.e. HCO_3^- and CO_2, **are present in large quantities.** In the course of metabolism, a normal adult produces about 300L of CO_2 every day. Further, there is also an appreciable concentration of HCO_3^- in the extracellular fluid.

(ii) This buffer pair is quite effective since **it operates as an open system,** i.e. **either of its component can be removed or added**. Though CO_2, truly is not an acid but acid anhydride, since it can readily react with water and forms H_2CO_3, which ionizes to H^+ and HCO_3^-.

The sum of the two equations is:

$$CO_2 + H_2O \rightleftharpoons H^+ + HCO_3^-$$

As concentration of water, generally, does not alter much, equilibrium expression for the above reaction can be represented as:

$$K'\,eq = ([H^+]\,[HCO_3^-]/[CO_2])$$

where, $[CO_2]$ represents concentration of dissolved CO_2. Since concentration of a gas, in a solution, is directly proportional to its partial pressure, therefore, concentration of the dissolved CO_2 in the blood is proportional to pCO_2.

Two components of the buffer can be easily regulated. Whereas lungs control arterial blood pH by regulating pCO_2, the kidney controls plasma HCO_3^-.

MAINTENANCE OF ACID BASE BALANCE

Normally, lungs and **kidney** stabilize extracellular fluid pH.

REGULATION BY THE LUNGS

The **respiratory system controls partial pressure of CO_2** and **thus minimizes pH changes in the arterial blood.**

Normally, CO_2 is expired at the same rate at which it is produced and thus pCO_2 is maintained. If blood becomes acidic by the addition of the fixed acids, pulmonary ventilation is increased. **In the state of hyper-ventilation, CO_2 is flushed-out at a rate greater than the rate at which it is produced and** consequently pCO_2 falls. This reduction in arterial blood pCO_2, in turn, results in fall in H^+ concentration of the blood. The reactions are pulled to the left, which in turn lowers HCO_3^- concentration and reduces acidic shift in the blood.

$$CO_2 + H_2O \leftleftharpoons H_2CO_3 \leftleftharpoons H^+ + HCO_3^-$$

On the other hand, **if blood becomes more alkaline, changes occur in the opposite direction.** Accordingly, hypoventilation takes place, blood pCO_2 rises, and these reactions are pushed to the right, which in turn **results in a high carbonic acid concentration in the blood** and a less alkaline shift in blood pH.

$$CO_2 + H_2O \rightrightharpoons H_2CO_3 \rightrightharpoons H^+ + HCO_3^-$$

Hypoventilation, however, is limited because it causes retention of CO_2, which further stimulates venti-lation.

Buffering of acid-base disturbances by the respiratory response although is rapid but is relatively coarse. It brings blood pH close to normal but can not eliminate a fixed acid or base from the body. So, it can not restore the pH to normal.

REGULATION BY THE KIDNEY

Renal response to an acid-base disturbance though is slow but more accurate. **The kidney regulates acid-base balance by controlling bicarbonate reabsorption and secreting acid.** Both of these processes depend upon the formation of H^+ and HCO_3^- from CO_2 and H_2O, with in the tubule cells.

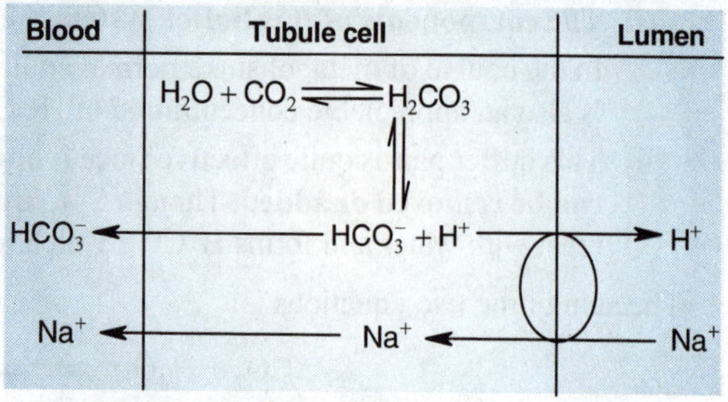

Fig. 20.1. Basic ion exchange mechanism.

Normally, H^+ formed in the reaction is actively secreted into the tubular fluid, in exchange for Na^+. Within the tubule cell, Na^+ as well as HCO_3^- is pumped out of the cell into the interstitial fluid (Fig. 20.1)

Sodium uptake by the tubular cell is partly passive, flowing down the electrochemical gradient and partly active, via Na^+-H^+ antiport system. H^+ ions that are secreted into the tubular fluid can have one of the three fates, suggesting that three processes are involved in acidification of urine:

1. Reabsorption of the filtered bicarbonate,
2. Excretion of the titratable acid, and
3. Excretion of ammonia.

All the three mechanisms involve H^+ secretion and are associated with the addition of bicarbonate to the peritubular capillary blood by the kidney tubules.

Mechanisms of H^+ secretion

Reabsorption of the Filtered Bicarbonate

H^+ ions that are secreted into the tubules (in exchange for Na^+) combine with bicarbonate that has been filtered by the glomeruli. This, in turn, leads to the formation of carbonic acid in the tubular fluid. Dissociation of this acid to CO_2 and water is catalyzed in the lumen by carbonic anhydrase. The CO_2 rapidly diffuses through the cell membrane.

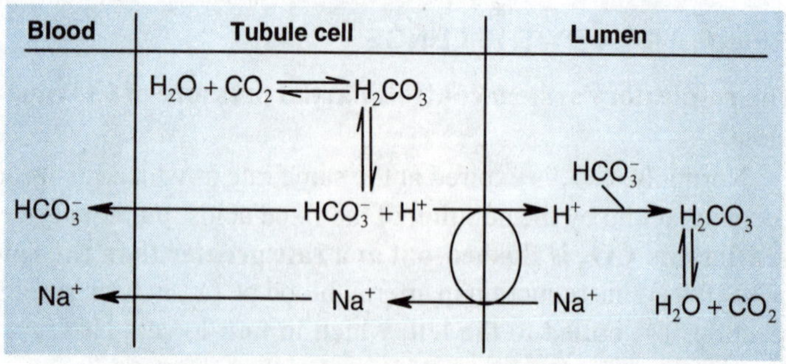

Fig. 20.2. Reabsorption of bicarbonate.

The secretion of H^+ thus, reabsorbs the filtered HCO_3^- indirectly (Fig. 20.2).

Excretion of Titrable Acid

As reabsorption of sodium bicarbonate proceeds, the tubular fluid becomes depleted of HCO_3^-, and the pH drops. Following this, **H^+ ions are taken up by the phosphate buffer**. At this stage, hydrogen ions that are secreted into the tubular fluid (in exchange for Na^+) react with the phosphate buffer:

$$HPO_4^{2-} + H^+ \longrightarrow H_2PO_4^-$$

As a result of it, basic form of phosphate (HPO_4^{2-}) is converted to acidic form ($H_2PO_4^-$). Besides phosphate, which is the most important buffer in the urine, other ions are also important in the excretion of H^+. For example, **in diabetic ketoacidosis** when pH of the urine reaches at its minimum (about 4.4), **aceto-**

acetate and β-hydroxybutyrate pass through the glomerular filtrate and appear in the tubular fluid. Under these conditions these ions **also serve as buffer.**

Excretion of titratable acids thus, not only eliminates H^+ from the body but also restores depleted plasma bicarbonate reserve since for each meq of H^+ excreted as titratable acid, a new HCO_3^- ion is added to the blood (Fig. 20.3).

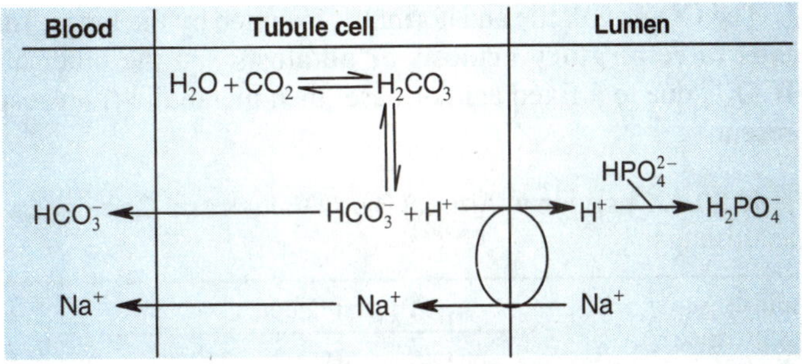

Fig. 20.3. Excretion of titrable acid.

The amount of the acid excreted (as the acid component of a urinary buffer) can be measured by the titration of the urine back to the normal pH of the plasma (to pH 7.4). The quantity of the base so required is equivalent to the quantity of the acid excreted and is referred to as **titratable acidity of urine.**

Excretion of Ammonia

The third fate of H^+ in the tubular fluid is neutralization by NH_3. Ammonia is mainly synthesized in the proximal tubule from amino acids, predominantly glutamine. It readily gets diffused through the cell membrane and combines with the secreted H^+ and forms NH_4^+. NH_4^+ is usually accompanied by an anion, e.g. chloride, in the urine. For **each H^+ excreted in the urine as NH_4^+, an equivalent quantity of HCO_3^- is added to the blood** (Fig. 20.4).

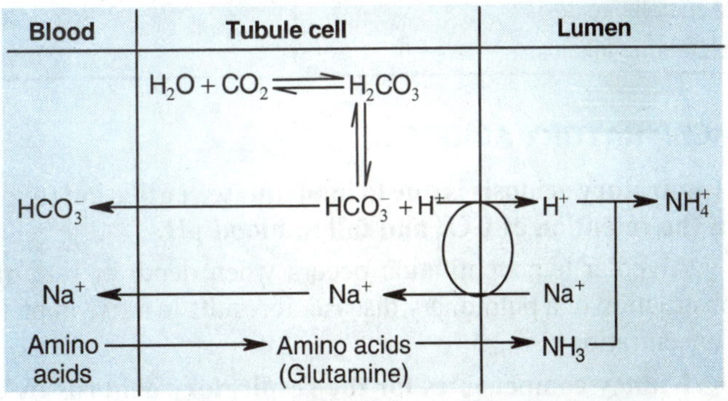

Fig. 20.4. Excretion of ammonia.

Elimination of NH_4^+ in the urine contributes to net acid excretion, as NH_4^+ is normally a major urinary acid. Nearly, one-half to two-third of our daily acid load is excreted as NH_4^+.

Ability of the kidney to synthesize NH_3, from glutamine, is increased under conditions of excess acid in the body.

The sum of the titrable acidity and NH_4^+ comprises **total acidity of urine** (total acid excretion).

DISTURBANCES IN ACID BASE BALANCE

Blood pH, compatible with life, varies between 6.8 to 7.8, while pH of the arterial blood normally varies with in a narrow range of 7.35 to 7.45 only. If arterial blood pH is acidic (pH below 7.35), it results in **acidosis** and leads to **acidemia. Acidosis may be a result of the excess of acid or deficiency of alkali in the body.**

If blood pH is more alkaline than 7.45, it results in **alkalosis (alkalemia). Alkalosis is due to excess of alkali or deficiency of acid in the body.**

There are four types of acid base disturbances (Table 20.1) :

- Respiratory acidosis,
- Respiratory alkalosis,
- Metabolic acidosis, and
- Metabolic alkalosis.

The CO_2 is volatile and normally, excreted by the lungs. **Inability of the lungs to excrete CO_2 adequately leads to respiratory acidosis or alkalosis.** On the other hand, if the problem is **an excess or deficit of HCO_3^-**, due to a fixed acid or base, then metabolic (non-respiratory) disturbances of acid base balance are present.

Table 20.1. Changes in Arterial Blood Values and Compensatory Responses in Different Types of Acid Base Disturbances

Acid-Base disturbance	Arterial Blood			Compensatory response
	pCO_2	pH	HCO_3^- concentration	
Respiratory acidosis	↑	↓	↑	Kidney increases H^+ excretion, which in turn increases plasma HCO_3^- concentration
Respiratory alkalosis	↓	↑	↓	Kidney increases HCO_3^- excretion, which in turn decreases plasma HCO_3^- concentration
Metabolic acidosis	↓	↓	↓	Alveolar hyperventilation
Metabolic alkalosis	↑	↑	↑	Alveolar hypoventilation

RESPIRATORY ACIDOSIS

Respiratory acidosis is due to inadequate ventilation (hypoventilation) **by the alveoli. This in turn results in the retention of CO_2 and fall in blood pH.**

Alveolar hypoventilation occurs when depth or rate of respiration is diminished, such as in airways obstruction or a pulmonary disease. It results in a rise in pCO_2. As pCO_2 rises, plasma pH drops, and HCO_3^- concentration rises.

Kidney compensates for the respiratory acidosis by increasing the output of H^+ in the urine. The filtered HCO_3^- in turn is reabsorbed and the increased amounts of H^+ combine with the urinary buffers and are excreted in the urine.

RESPIRATORY ALKALOSIS

Respiratory alkalosis is a result of hyperventilation, which may be caused by anxiety, central nervous system injury involving the respiratory centre, salicylate poisoning, or fever. This in turn causes **a fall in arterial blood pCO_2.** At high altitude also, due to decrease in total atmospheric pressure, alveolar pCO_2 falls and there is chronic respiratory alkalosis.

The **kidney compensates for respiratory alkalosis, by excreting HCO_3^- in the urine.** Low pCO_2 leads to decreased H^+ secretion by the tubular epithelium. This in turn results in reduced reabsorption of the filtered bicarbonate and increases its excretion in the urine. This loss of HCO_3^- in the urine results in further decrease in plasma HCO_3^- and brings plasma pH towards normal.

METABOLIC ACIDOSIS

Metabolic acidosis is characterized by the accumulation of nonvolatile acids (gain of fixed acids other than H_2CO_3) **and loss of HCO_3^-.**

The gain of metabolically produced acid may be due to several reasons, such as:

(i) Renal failure, due to reduced excretion of metabolically produced acids.

(ii) Uncontrolled diabetes mellitus, due to the production of large quantities of ketone bodies.

(iii) Inadequate circulation, due to cardiogenic or hemorrhagic shock, which in turn promotes anaerobic glycolysis and increases production of lactic acid.

(iv) Heavy exercise, resulting in the production of lactic acid, or

(v) Ingestion of certain acidifying agents, such as ammonium chloride.

Metabolic acidosis may also be due to the loss of HCO_3^- from the body, such as due to diarrhea, or abnormal excretion of HCO_3^- in the urine.

Two **compensatory mechanisms** are usually available to deal with:

1. Due to the acidic pH, respiratory system is stimulated. This in turn lowers pCO_2 and hence carbonic acid concentration in the blood. **Respiratory compensation** though is prompt but usually does not restore the blood pH to normal.
2. The other mechanism, which begins almost instantly, is the **renal compensation**. The kidney increases H^+ excretion. This, however, takes time and alone is not adequate to return HCO_3^- concentration (and the pH) to normal.

METABOLIC ALKALOSIS

Metabolic alkalosis is characterized by the intake of excess alkali, i.e. by the gain of strong base or HCO_3^-, or **abnormal loss of acid** other than H_2CO_3. For example, ingestion of excess sodium bicarbonate used in treating gastric ulcer or oxidation of organic anion, such as citrate, lactate, and acetate.

A common cause of abnormal loss of acid causing metabolic alkalosis is prolonged vomiting or gastric lavage since loss of gastric contents results in net addition of HCO_3^- to the blood. It may also be a result of rapid loss of body water, e.g. in diuresis, which in turn may result in temporary rise in HCO_3^- in the plasma and the extracellular fluid.

Characteristic **arterial blood changes include a primary increase in plasma HCO_3^- concentration, a rise in pH, and a compensatory rise in pCO_2.** Metabolic alkalosis is seldom long lasting.

In metabolic alkalosis, as a primary defect in increase in plasma HCO_3^- concentration, immediate **physiological compensation is hypoventilation, followed by increased renal excretion of HCO_3^-**.

Respiratory Insufficiency

Respiratory insufficiency is said to be present when lung function is impaired to the extent that pO_2 is reduced to usually below 8.0 kPa. There are two types of disorders. In type I, pO_2 is low with normal or low pCO_2 while in type II; pO_2 is low with high pCO_2.

Combined Respiratory and Non-respiratory Acidosis

This may occur when there is profound circulatory failure leading to severe hypoxia. pCO_2 is increased because of depressed respiration while formation of lactic acid in the tissues neutralizes bicarbonate, e.g. following cardiac stress, barbiturate over dosage, and in respiratory distress of the new born.

Combined Respiratory and Non-respiratory Alkalosis

This may develop during the treatment of a respiratory acidosis. For example in severe bronchitis, in which pCO_2 is raised and a compensatory rise in bicarbonate is present.

DIAGNOSTIC TESTS

Disturbances of acid base balance are accompanied by the characteristic changes in blood pH, pCO_2, and HCO_3^-. Normal values for these parameters in the arterial blood are, as follows:

pH	7.35 - 7.45
pCO_2	35-45 mmHg
HCO_3^- concentration	22-26 meq/L

Thus, the measurement of pH, pCO_2, and HCO_3^- concentrations in the arterial blood are the routinely used parameters of the acid base imbalance.

Besides, the above parameters, base excess and anion gap can be calculated.

Base Excess

Base excess is defined as the amount of acid, which is required to titrate the blood to the pH value of 7.4, at a pCO_2 of 40 mmHg (at 37ºC). If pH of the blood is low, base excess will be negative.

Anion Gap

Anion gap is a difference between the sum of Cl^- and HCO_3^- (anions) from the sum of Na^+ and K^+ (cations).

Anion gap thus, represents plasma anions other than Cl^- and HCO_3^-, which are not routinely measured.

$$\text{Anion gap} = (Na^+ + K^+) - (Cl^- + HCO_3^-)$$

Normal value for the anion gap is in the range of 12-16 meq/L. This is most commonly used to establish differential diagnosis for metabolic acidosis.

BLOOD GASES PROFILE IN ACIDOSIS/ALKALOSIS

Results of acid base measurements are considered in the light of the clinical findings as well as other types of investigations, such as plasma creatinine, urea, Na^+ and K^+.

Normal values for blood gases profile are shown in Table 20.2.

Table 20.2. Normal values for blood gases profile

Parameter	Normal value
pH	7.35 to 7.45
Standard HCO_3^- concentration	22.4 to 25.8 meq/L
Base excess of blood	– 2.3 to + 2.3 meq/L
Other investigations	
Total CO_2	24 to 30 mmol/L
Plasma chloride	95 to 107 mmol/L
Anion gap	10 to 20 mmol/L

SOME IMPORTANT QUESTIONS

1. Define buffer. What are the important buffers present in the body? Explain the role of various body buffers in the regulation of blood pH.
2. Define pH. How pH of blood is regulated?

3. Explain:
   (i) Role of kidney in the regulation of blood pH.
   (ii) Various mechanisms of H^+ secretion
   (iii) Disturbances of the acid base balance
   (iv) Measures of the acid base imbalance
   (v) Role of lungs in the regulation of blood pH
4. Write notes on:
   (i) pH
   (ii) Handerson-Hasselbalch equation
   (iii) Chemical buffers found in the body
   (iv) Titrable acidity
   (v) Respiratory acidosis
   (vi) Respiratory alkalosis
   (vii) Metabolic acidosis
   (viii) Metabolic alkalosis
   (ix) Base excess
   (x) Anion gap

CHAPTER 21

Electrolyte Balance

Electrolytes are **small, inorganic substances that can dissociate** or break apart **in solution and carry an electric charge**. These charged particles are called ions. In a chemical solution, the separate particles are constantly in balance between cations and anions.

Cations are ions carrying a positive charge, e.g. sodium (Na^+), potassium (K^+), calcium (Ca^{2+}) and magnesium (Mg^{2+}).

Anions are ions carrying a negative charge, e.g. chloride (Cl^-), carbonate (HCO_3^-), phosphates (HPO_4^{2-} and $H_2PO_4^-$) and sulfate (SO_4^{2-}), and organic anions, such as lactate and negatively charged proteins (mainly albumin).

A balance between the cation and anion concentrations maintains a state of chemical neutrality that is necessary for life. Electrolyte concentration in body fluids is measured in terms of meq and is expressed as meq/L.

The electrolyte concentration of the body fluid compartments is shown in Table 21.1.

EXTRACELLULAR AND INTRACELLULAR FLUID COMPARTMENTS

Body fluids are divided into two compartments, called extracellular fluid (ECF) and intracellular fluid (ICF).

EXTRACELLULAR FLUID

ECF includes interstitial fluid and plasma.

PLASMA

Plasma constitutes approximately **5% of the body volume** (about 3.5L). Most important ions in plasma are **Na^+, K^+, Ca^{2+}, Cl^-, HCO_3^- and phosphates**. In addition, glucose and urea contribute to plasma osmolality.

The total plasma concentration of cations is about 150 meq/L (mmol/L), of which **Na^+ is approximately 140 meq/L** and potassium about 5 meq/L. The most abundant plasma anions are Cl^- and HCO_3^- with average concentrations of nearly 100 and 25 meq/L, respectively.

Table 21.1. Balance of cations and anions concentrations in ECF and ICF (meq/L)

Electrolytes	ECF (meq/L)	ICF (meq/L)
Cations		
Na^+	142	35
K^+	5	123
Ca^{2+}	5	15
Mg^{2+}	5	2
Total	155	175
Anions		
Cl^-	104	5
PO_4^{3-}	2	80
SO_4^{2-}	1	10
Protein	16	70
HCO_3^-	27	10
Organic Acids	5	–
Total	155	175

Because **concentrations of Na^+, K^+, Cl^- and HCO_3^-** provide most relevant information about the osmotic status, hydration and pH of the body, they are commonly analyzed in the plasma or serum in an **electrolyte profile.**

An increase in the concentration of one anion is accompanied either by a corresponding decrease in other anions or by an increase in one or more cations or both so total the electrical neutrality is invariably maintained.

Interstitial Fluid

Interstitial fluid is essentially an ultrafiltrate of blood plasma. It accounts for **about 26%** (nearly 17L) **of the total body volume.**

Plasma is separated from the interstitial fluid by endothelial lining of the capillaries, which acts as a semipermeable membrane and allows the passage of water and diffusible solutes but not compounds of the large molecular mass, such as proteins. Oncotic pressure, exerted by the plasma proteins, determines the distribution of water between plasma and the interstitial fluid.

Intracellular Fluid

The volume of the ICF constitutes **nearly 66% of total body volume**. Composition of ICF markedly differs from that of ECF. These two compartments are separated from each other by a cell membrane, which in turn allows the composition of these fluids to differ. The composition differences are a consequence of the Gibbs–Donnan equilibrium and active and passive transport of ions. The transport of small molecules across the impermeable membrane is possible due to the existence of specific transport proteins, including ion pumps. Amongst several ionic pumps, Na^+/K^+ ATPase shows greatest transport activity.

Potassium is the main intracellular cation (about 110 meq/L). There is also a substantial amount of magnesium within the cells. The main **anions** in the ICF are **phosphates and proteins.**

REGULATION OF OSMOLALITY AND VOLUME OF ECF AND ICF

Relative volumes of ECF and ICF depend upon the amounts of osmotically active substances in each of these compartments. Under physiological conditions, average concentration of all the osmotically active substances in the ECF is nearly 290–mmol/kg water, which remains in equilibrium with the ICF.

A change in the concentration of osmotically active ions in either of the compartments creates a gradient of osmotic pressure and consequently, induces movement of water between the two compartments. Water diffuses from a compartment of low osmolality towards high osmolality until the osmotic pressure is identical in both of them, i.e. until iso–osmolality is achieved. Thus, relative volumes of ECF and ICF are reflected in the amount of osmotically active substances in these compartments.

Sodium ion is most important in the ECF. Glucose, which is normally present in plasma in a concentration of about 90 mg/dL, does not contribute much to osmolality but in very high concentrations, as in diabetes, glucose profoundly affects osmolality.

An increase in ECF osmolality leads to the movement of water from cells to ECF and results in **cellular dehydration**. On the other hand when ECF osmolality decreases, water moves from ECF into cells. This leads to expansion of the cell volume (**edema**).

Within the ECF, distribution of water between the intravascular and the extravascular compartments depends upon the concentration of plasma proteins. In the plasma, protein particularly albumin exerts **osmotic pressure** (about 25 mm Hg), which retains water in the vascular bed. It is known as the **oncotic pressure**. The **hydrostatic pressure** balances it and in turns forces the fluid out of the capillaries.

In the arterial part of the capillaries hydrostatic pressure prevails over oncotic pressure. As a result of it, water and low molecular weight substances filter out into the extracellular space. In contrast, in the venous part of the capillaries oncotic pressure prevails over hydrostatic pressure and fluid is drawn into the vascular lumen. A reduction in plasma oncotic pressure, which occurs, for instance, when plasma concentration of albumin decreases, results in movement of fluid into the extravascular space and causes edema.

SODIUM

Adult human body contains about 100 g of sodium as sodium ion (Na^+). Nearly half of it is found in the extracellular fluid while the remaining half is intracellular. Some of it is also found in bones.

Na^+ is the main extracellular cation, which exists in body in association with several anions, such as chloride, bicarbonate, phosphates, lactate and protein. Na^+, K^+–ATPase maintains high extracellular concentration of Na^+.

It is freely filtered by the glomeruli. About 70% of the filtered–sodium is reabsorbed in the proximal tubule, 15% in the loop of Henle, 5% in the distal convoluted tubule and 10% by the collecting duct.

Active reabsorption of Na^+ in the proximal tubule results in passive reabsorption of Cl^- and HCO_3^- along with water. Reabsorption of Cl^- and HCO_3^- with Na^+ helps to maintain electrical neutrality of the extracellular fluid while reabsorption of water ensures normal osmotic pressure.

Biological Functions of Sodium

1. ***Regulation of Osmotic Pressure*** – Sodium plays a dominant role in the maintenance of osmotic pressure of different body fluids and protects body against excessive fluid loss.
2. ***Regulation of Acid Base Balance*** – Sodium salts with the corresponding weak acids form chief buffer system of the extracellular fluid and thus play an important role in regulation of pH of body fluids.
3. ***Absorption of Monoscaccharides and Amino Acids*** – Na^+ also plays an important role in absorption of monosaccharides and amino acids from the small intestine.
4. ***Nerve Transmission*** – Sodium is also important in the maintenance of neuromuscular irritability and excitability.
5. ***Maintenance of Blood Viscosity*** – Sodium is also important in the maintenance of blood viscosity.

6. ***Electrolyte and Water Balance*** – Sodium is also important in the maintenance of water and electrolyte balance.

   Na^+ also acts as ***a cofactor*** for Na^+, K^+–ATPase.

Requirement

Daily requirement of sodium (as sodium chloride) varies from 5 to 15 g.

Sources

Most important source of sodium is the common salt. Meat, seafoods, milk, cheese and bread are good sources of sodium. Plant foods are usually low in sodium.

SODIUM HOMEOSTASIS

When intracellular concentration of sodium increases activity of the **sodium–potassium pump** also increases and sodium ions are extruded from the cell.

SODIUM POTASSIUM PUMP

The enzyme Na^+/K^+–ATPase, also called sodium–potassium pump or sodium pump, has a large transmembrane catalytic sub unit. It hydrolyses one ATP and the released energy drives transfer of three sodium ions from the cell to the outside and in turn two potassium ions from outside into the cell. Thus, it maintains chemical and electrical potential gradients between inside and outside of the cell, and sodium and potassium concentration gradient across the cell membrane. It also has a key role in reabsorption of sodium in the kidney tubules.

Regulation of Body Water and Extracellular Na^+ within Kidney

Regulation of water in the kidney occurs from the distal tubule through the collecting duct **under the influence of antidiuretic hormone** (ADH), also called vasopressin. When blood volume is decreased or plasma osmolality is increased, posterior pituitary, under the influence of baroreceptors and chemorectptors, releases ADH. Binding of ADH to its receptors, which are located on the membrane of tubular cells in the collecting duct, leads to the synthesis of a variety of proteins, including aquaporin–2, which facilitates passage of water through the membrane. This action of ADH in turn determines the final volume and concentration of the urine.

More than 80% of the filtered Na^+ is actively reabsorbed in the proximal tubule. The reabsorption of water and Cl^- occur passively, to maintain electrical neutrality and osmotic equivalence.

In addition, Na^+ and Cl^- are reabsorbed in the ascending limb of the loop of the Henle.

At the level of the distal tubule, different mechanism operates for the regulation of Na^+ and water. Sodium reabsorption is stimulated by aldosterone.

Regulation of Sodium Reabsorption by Aldosterone

Receptors located in the juxtaglomerular cells, sense decreased arteriolar pressure or decreased Na^+ concentration, and stimulate the production of renin.

Renin is an enzyme produced principally in the juxtraglomeular apparatus of the kidney. It is released from the secretory granules, in response to decreased renal perfusion pressure. Renin is a protease that acts on a glycoprotein angiotesinogen. It converts angiotensinogen to angiotesin I (a decapeptide). Angiotesin I is further cleaved by angiotesin converting enzyme (ACE) to angiotesin II (a potent vasoconstrictor). Angiotesin

II constricts vascular smooth muscle cells thereby increasing blood pressure and reducing renal blood flow and glomerular filtration rate. It also stimulates aldosterone secretion. This is called **renin–angiotensin system.**

Aldosterone is a major mineralocorticoid hormone in man. It stimulates distal tubules to **reabsorb Na^+ with water** following passively and secrete K^+ (and to a lesser extent H^+) to maintain electrical neutrality. Thus, when plasma Na^+ is low or when kidneys are hypoperfused (as occurs in decreased blood volume or obstruction of renal arteries), distal tubules, under the influence of aldosterone, reclaim Na^+.

DISORDERS OF SODIUM

Disorders of Na^+ homeostasis can occur due to excessive loss, gain or retention of the Na^+, or the excessive loss, gain or retention of water. It is difficult to separate disorders of Na^+ and H_2O balance due to their close relationship in establishing normal osmolality in the three body water compartments.

Hyponatremia

Hyponatremia is defined as decreased **plasma Na^+ concentration below 135 mmol/L.** Hyponatremia manifests itself clinically as generalized weakness and mental confusion. CNS symptoms are primarily due to intracellular shifting of water to maintain osmotic balance, resulting in swelling of CNS cells. Hyponatremia can occur in settings of hyperosmotic, isoosmotic or hypo-osmotic plasma.

Hyper-osmotic hyponatremia

Hyponatremia occurs in the presence of increased plasma osmolality due to increased amount of other solutes in the ECF. This in turn causes extracellular shift of water or intracellular shift of Na^+. The most common cause of hyperosmotic hyponatremia is severe hyperglycemia.

Iso-omotic hyponatremia

Iso–omotic hyponatremia occurs when measured Na^+ concentration in plasma is decreased but plasma osmolality, glucose and urea levels are normal. This can occur in the patients with severe hyperlipidemia or in state of hyperproteinemia.

Hypo-osmotic hyponatremia

Hypo-osmotic hyponatremia occurs when plasma Na^+ concentration is low and the osmolality is also low. This type of hyponatremia can be due to either excessive loss of Na^+ (depletional hyponatremia) or increased ECF volume (dilutional hyponatremia).

Depletional hyponatremia: In depletional hyponatremia, there occurs excessive loss of Na^+ accompanied by a loss of ECF water but to a lesser extent than the Na^+ loss. Hyponatremia is because of the loss of isotonic or hypertonic fluid, which can occur through either renal or extrarenal route. If urine Na^+ is low, the loss is extrarenal, such as from the gastrointestinal tract or skin. On the other hand, if urine Na^+ is elevated, there is a renal loss, such as with osmotic diuresis, thiazide diuretics, adrenal insufficiency, or potassium sparing diuretics, e.g. sprionolactone.

Dilutional hyponatremia: It is a result of excessive water retention, such as in advanced renal failure, congestive heart failure, hepatic cirrhosis or nephrotic syndrome.

Hypernatremia

Hypernatremia is defined as increased **plasma Na^+ concentration above 150 mmol/L.** It is always hyperosmolar. Hypernatremia manifests neurological symptoms due to intracellular dehydration, which include tremors, irritability, ataxia, confusion and coma. Hypernatremia can arise from:

(i) Either excessive water loss or failure to replace normal water loss (hypovolemic hypernatremia),
(ii) A net Na^+gain, in excess of water (normovolemic hypernatremia), or
(iii) Decreased Na^+ excretion (hypervolemic hypernatremia).

Hypovolemic Hypernatremia

This may occur due to the renal or extrarenal loss of hypo-osmotic fluid, leading to dehydration.

Extrarenal losses are characterized by concentrated urine with low urine Na^+, such as in diarrhea, invisible skin loss (burn or excessive sweating), or respiratory loss coupled with failure to replace the lost water.

Renal causes include osmotic diuresis or thiazide diuretics with decreased water intake. Under these conditions, urine volume is increased, urine osmolality is reduced and urine Na^+ is increased.

Normovolemic Hypernatremia

It could be due to insensible loss through lungs or skin, characterized by concentrated urine, as kidney functions to conserve water. It may also be due to water diuresis, which is manifested by polyuria. Polyuria (urine output more than 3L/d) may be a result of solute diuresis, such as in diabetes mellitus that is characterized by urine osmolality >300 mosm/L and hyponatremia. It may also be a result of water diuresis, which is a manifestation of diabetes insipidus. Dilute urine (osmolality <250 mosm/L) and hypernatremia characterize it.

Hypervolemic hypernatremia

Excess Na^+ and water retention is commonly observed in–patients receiving hypertonic saline or sodium bicarbonate. Other causes include hyperaldosteronism and Cushing's syndrome.

POTASSIUM

Potassium (K^+) is a chief cation of the intracellular fluid. Maintenance of its normal level is essential to life. Potassium is freely filtered at the glomeruli.

Biological Functions

1. Potassium helps to maintain normal osmotic pressure of different body fluids, and thus **maintains water and electrolytes balance**.
2. Potassium salts form buffer system of the intracellular fluid, and thus play an important role in the **regulation of pH of the body fluids.**
3. It is also important in the **maintenance of normal neuromuscular irritability and excitability.**
4. Bases in the alkaline digestive juices, such as pancreatic juice and bile, are derived from the **potassium salts** that are present in the blood.
5. **Storage of the cell protein** and glycogen requires retention of potassium.
6. Potassium acts as a **cofactor for several enzymes**, such as pyruvate kinase, Na^+, K^+–ATPase, etc.

Requirement

Normal daily intake of potassium has been recommended as 4g.

Sources

Potassium is widely distributed in plants and animals as chloride, phosphate, and carbonate salts of inorganic and organic acids and proteins.

Coffee, cocoa, dried beans, wheat bran, most of the vegetables, such as potato and tomato, dairy products, fish, egg, meat and fruits, like banana, peach, and orange, are good sources of potassium.

Hypokalemia

Hypokalemia (decrease of extracellular K^+) is defined as **plasma K^+** concentration less than **3.5 mmol/L.** Muscle weakness, irritability and paralysis characterize it. At levels < 2.5 mmol/L, tachycardia and specific cardiac conduction effects are apparent by ECG examination and can lead to cardiac arrest. Causes of hypokalemia can be classified as redistribution of extracellular K^+ into ICF or true K^+ deficits.

K^+ Redistribution : Fall in plasma K^+, as a result of intracellular redistribution, can occur following insulin therapy for diabetic hyperglycemia, alkalosis, catecholamines or β-adrenergic excess, etc.

True K^+ deficit : It can be a result of either decreased intake or a loss of K^+ rich body fluids (renal and non–renal losses of K^+). Hypokalemia due to decreased intake may be a result of chronic starvation or postoperative intravenous fluid therapy with K^+ poor solutions. This is based on daily excretion of K^+ in the urine. Extrarenal loss of K^+ may occur through gastrointestinal tract (diarrhea or fistula).

Urinary excretion of K^+ exceeding 25–30 mmol/L in a hypokalemic setting indicates renal loss of K^+. Renal loss of K^+ may occur during the diuretic phase of acute tubular necrosis, aldosteronism, or Cushing's syndrome. Thiazides and loop diuretics, digoxin toxicity, or hypomagnesemia can also result in loss of K^+.

Hyperkalemia

Hyperkalemia (**plasma K^+ > 5.0 mmol/L**) can be a result of redistribution, increased intake, or increased retention.

Redistribution – Transfer of intracellular K^+ into the ECF may occur in acidosis, dehydration, shock with tissue hypoxia, insulin deficiency, etc.

K^+ Retention – Decreased excretion of K^+ in acute renal disease and end–stage renal failure are the most common causes of prolonged hyperkalemia. Hyperkalemia occurs along with Na^+ depletion, as in Addison's disease. Other causes of hyperkalemia include excess administration of K^+–sparing diuretrics, e.g. spironolactone.

CHLORIDE

Chloride ion (Cl^-) is the most abundant anion in the extracellular fluid. Normal plasma chloride concentration varies between 95–107 meq/L. Its highest concentration is found in the CSF.

Biological Functions

1. Primary function of chloride is, along with Na^+ and K^+, in **maintaining normal osmotic pressure of the body fluids.**
2. It is also the major anion that participates in **maintaining the pH of the body fluids.** Hypochloremia is accompanied with metabolic alkalosis due to a compensatory increase in HCO_3^- in the plasma.
3. Chloride also plays a role in **gaseous transport of CO_2.**
4. It is also an essential **component of HCl of the gastric juice.**
5. It is also required as an **activator for enzymes**, such as salivary amylase.
6. Chloride ions help in **maintaining electrical equilibrium between intracellular and extracellular fluids.**

Requirement

Daily requirement for adults is 5–15 g.

Sources

Most important source of chloride is common table salt (sodium chloride). Seafoods, milk, meat and egg are the good sources.

Deficiency Symptoms

Decrease in plasma Cl^- concentration (**hypochloremia**) occurs in diarrhea, extreme sweating, and in certain endocrine disorders. Decreased plasma Cl^- concentration is also observed in salt–losing nephritis, e.g. chronic pyelonephritis where it is accompanied with hyponatremia. Hypochloremia is also observed in metabolic acidosis, such as in diabetic ketoacidosis and renal failure.

Persistent gastric secretion and prolonged vomiting also result in hypochloremia along with depletion of total body Cl^-.

Diarrhea and vomiting also cause considerable loss of chloride and hence result in a drop in Cl^- concentration in the blood.

Hypochloremia is also observed in–patients with Addison's disease, due to reduced renal tubular reabsorption of chloride.

Hypochloremia is also seen in respiratory alkalosis due to hyperventilation, which is turn leads to elimination of CO_2 with consequent increase in blood HCO_3^- and a compensatory decrease in Cl^-.

Hyperchloremia

Increased plasma Cl^- concentration occurs as a result of dehydration in patients with acute renal failure, renal tubular acidosis, metabolic acidosis associated with prolonged diarrhea (loss of sodium bicarbonate), diabetes insipidus, and Cushing's syndrome.

Increase in plasma chloride also occurs in patients, who develop respiratory acidosis.

ELECTROLYTE IMBALANCE

Electrolyte imbalance develops much more quickly in very young and elderly people than the other age groups. Alterations in electrolyte balance commonly develop as a result of stress, such as during strenuous physical exercise, exposure to extreme heat, use of some pharmacological agents, radiation therapy and fasting besides a variety of diseases and injury.

EDEMA

Due to the retention of water along with sodium, both sodium and water move from blood to the interstitial fluid thereby allowing the maintenance of a relatively normal blood volume. When fluid retention is observable, the condition is called edema.

Edema often takes the form of puffiness in fingers and ankles or sometimes on the entire body. Retention of sodium and water, as in patients with congestive heart failure, increases workload of the heart and precipitates acute heart failure. A serious consequence of acute heart failure may result in congestion in the lungs (pulmonary edema) and thus may lead to respiratory distress.

Dietary modifications particularly, reduced sodium intake often in conjunction with diuretic therapy is helpful in the treatment of such conditions, which are associated with the excessive retention of sodium as well as water. However, when diuretic therapy is used along with sodium restriction, special attention should be paid to the need of potassium and other minerals whose excretion is also affected by the diuretic. Use of loop diuretic, such as furosemide and thiazide, is known to cause depletion of potassium, magnesium and zinc.

Restriction of fluid intake

Though sodium restricted diet is very helpful in the prevention of fluid accumulation sometimes it is necessary to restrict both water as well as Na^+. Restricted intake of water (below 2000 ml per day) and Na^+ is collectively termed as ***fluid restriction***. In conditions, such as congestive heat failure, cirrhosis of liver with ascites or any other disease in which intravascular volume is increased, fluid restriction may be employed to promote diuresis or to prevent life–threatening hyponatremia.

Laboratory Evaluation of Water and Electrolyte Disorders

The following measurements are performed for the assessment of water and electrolyte balance:

1. Serum electrolyte concentration – it includes sodium, potassium, chloride and bicarbonate.
2. Serum creatinine and urea concentration
3. Urine volume, osmolality and sodium concentration
4. Serum osmolality

SOME IMPORTANT QUESTIONS

1. Describe disorders of sodium.
2. Write notes on:
   - (i) Anion gap
   - (ii) Sodium–potassium pump
   - (iii) Hyponatremia
   - (iv) Hypernatremia
   - (v) Hypokelmia
   - (vi) Hyperkalemia
   - (vii) Hypochloremia
   - (viii) Hyperchloremia
   - (ix) Edema

CHAPTER

22

Connective Tissue

Various types of connective tissues, including tendons, cartilage and the corneal stroma, refers to **extracellular matrix**. Major components of the extracellular matrix include **collagens, elastin, proteoglycans** and a variety of other proteins. Each of these proteins of the extracellular matrices has a modular construction composed of domains that contain binding sites for one another and for receptors on the cell surface. As a result, these various extracellular materials interact to form an interconnected network that is bound to the cell surface.

COLLAGEN

Collagens comprise a family of **fibrous glycoproteins** that are present only in extracellular matrices. Collagen is the most abundant protein in the human body. It has a long rigid structure in which **three polypeptides**, called **α-chains**, are wound around one another in a **rope-like triple helix**. Collagens are found throughout the body. Their types and organization are determined by the structural role collagen plays in a particular organ.

In some tissues, collagen may be dispersed as a gel that gives support to the structure, as in the extracellular matrix or the vitreous humor of the eye. In other tissues, collagen may be bundled in tight, parallel fibers that provide great strength as in tendons.

In the cornea of the eye, collagen is stacked so as to transmit light with a minimum of scattering. Collagen of bone occurs as fibers arranged at an angle to each other so as to resist mechanical sheer from any direction.

TYPES OF COLLAGENS

It is a superfamily of proteins, which include 27 distinct types. Although there are many differences among the members of the collagen family, all share at least two important structural features:

1. All collagen molecules are **trimers** consisting of three polypeptide chains called α-chains.
2. All **three polypeptide chains** of a collagen molecule are **wound around each other** to form a unique, **rod-like triple helix**, e.g. collagen type I is $\alpha I_2\alpha 2$, i.e. it has two αI and one α2 chains. Type II collagen is αI_3, i.e. it contains 3 αI chains, etc.

Based on their location and functions in the body, collagens are organized into 3 groups:

1. **Fibril-forming Collagens** – These are linear polymers of fibrils with characteristic bonding patterns and have rope-like triple-stranded helix, e.g. type I, type II and type III. Type I collagen fibers are found in supporting elements of high tensile strength, such as in skin, bone, tendon, blood vessels and cornea. Type II fibers are found in cartilaginous structures, such as cartilage, inter-vertebral disk and vitreous body. Type III collagens occur in more distensible tissues, such as blood vessels and fetal skin.
2. **Network forming Collagens** – They form a three-dimensional mesh, e.g. type IV and VII collagens. Type IV collagens are thin, sheet or mesh-like structures that function as semi-permeable basement membrane found in the kidney and the lung. Type VII collagens are found beneath stratified squamous epithelia.
3. **Fibril-associated Collagens** – These collagens link collagen fibrils to one another as well as to other components in the extracellular matrix, e.g. type IX and type XII collagens. Type IX collagens are found in cartilage whereas type XII collagen occurs in tendon and ligaments.

STRUCTURE AND COMPOSITION

Collagen is a fibrous protein, which has an elongated triple-helical structure. It is **rich in proline and glycine**, both of which are important in the formation of the triple-stranded helix. Proline facilitates the formation of the helical conformation of each α-chain because of its ring structure that causes kinks in the peptide chain. **Glycine** is found in **every third position** of the polypeptide chain, forming part of a repeating sequence **Gly-X-Y-**. It may be due to the reason that glycine is the smallest amino acid and fits into the restricted space where three chains of the helix come together. **X is frequently proline while Y may be proline or lysine**, which **gets hydroxylated** and occurs as hydroxyproline or hydroxylysine.

BIOSYNTHESIS

1. The polypeptide precursors of the collagen molecules are **formed in fibroblasts** (or osteoblasts of bone and chondroblasts of cartilage) and **secreted into the extracellular matrix**. The newly synthesized polypeptide precursor of α-chains contains a special amino acid sequence at the N-terminal end. This signal sequence facilitates the binding of ribosomes to the rough endoplasmic reticulum and directs the passage of the polypeptide chain into the cisternae of the RER. The signal sequence is rapidly cleaved in the endoplasmic reticulum to yield a precursor called **pro-α-chain**.
2. The pro-α-chain is processed by a number of enzymes within the lumen of the RER while the polypeptides are still being synthesized.

   Proline and lysine residues found in the Y-position **are hydroxylated** by prolyl- hydroxylase and lysylhydroxylase, respectively. This is a postransciptional modification and the hydroxylation reactions require molecular oxygen and vitamin C. Hydroxyproline is important in stabilizing the triple-helical structure of collagen because it maximizes interchain hydrogen bond formation. In case of **vitamin C deficiency**, collagen **fibers cannot be cross-linked**, greatly **decreasing the tensile strength** of the assembled fiber, such as in scurvy.

   Scurvy is a disease that results from a deficiency of vitamin C and is characterized by inflamed gums and tooth loss, poor wound healing, brittle bones, and the weakening of the lining of blood vessels, causing internal bleeding.
3. **Some hydroxylysine residues are** enzymatically **glycosylated** with glucose or glycosylgalactose.
4. After hydroxylation and glycosylation, pro-α-chains forms **procollagen**. Procollagen molecules are

translocated to the Golgi apparatus where they are **packaged in secretory vesicles**. The vesicle fuses with the cell membrane, causing the release of procollagen molecule into the extracellular space.

5. After their release, the procollagen molecules are cleaved by N- and C-procollagen peptidases, which remove the terminal propeptides, releasing **triple-helical molecules**.
6. Individual collagen molecules spontaneously associate to **form fibrils**.
7. Lysyl oxidase oxidatively deaminates some of the lysyl and hydroxylysyl residues, resulting in the **formation of allysine and hydroxyallysine**. These reactive aldehydes condense with lysyl or hydroxylysyl residues in neighboring collagen molecules to **form covalent cross-links.**

DEGRADATION

Normal collagens are highly stable molecules. However, connective tissue is constantly being remodeled, often in response to growth or injury of the tissue. Collagen fibrils are broken down with the help of specific metaloproteinases, called **collagenases**. These enzymes cleave the molecule into smaller fragments, which are further degraded to the constituent amino acids by other matrix proteinases.

ABNORMALITIES IN COLLAGEN SYNTHESIS

A large number of mutations have been identified in genes coding for collagen protein or processing enzymes. The following diseases can occur as a result of defective collage synthesis:

1. Mutations in the gene for either the pro 1- or pro 2-α chains of type I collagen can result in structurally abnormal pro-α chains that can prevent folding of the protein into a triple-helical conformation. This is called **osteogenesis imperfecta** (OI), also known as brittle bone syndrome. Extremely fragile bones, thin skin and weak tendons characterize it. It is a heterogeneous group of inherited disorders distinguished by bones that easily bend and fracture. Type I osteogenesis imperfecta, called osteogenesis imperfect tarda, is present in early infancy with fractures secondary to minor trauma. Type II osteogenesis imperfecta, called osteogenesis imperfecta congenita is more severe and patients die in utero or in the neonatal period of pulmonary hypoplasia.
2. A deficiency of any collagen processing enzyme, e.g. lysyl hydroxylase or procollagen peptidase, results in **Ehlers-Danlos syndrome**. This disorder is a heterogeneous group of generalized connective tissue disorders that result from inheritable defects in the metabolism of fibrillar collagen molecules. These patients show defects in collagen type I and type III fibrils. They have hyperflexible joints and highly extensible skin.
3. Mutation in type IV collagen gene occurs in-patients with **Alport syndrome**, an inherited kidney disease in which the glomerulus basement membrane is disrupted.

ELASTIN

Elastin is a connective tissue protein with rubber-like properties. It is the predominant protein of the elastic fibers in the extracellular matrices of blood vessels, lungs, ligaments and spine.

STRUCTURE AND SYNTHESIS

Elastin is a polymer synthesized from a precursor called **tropoelastin**. Tropoelastin is a linear polypeptide synthesized on the rough endoplasmic reticulum and secreted by the cell into the extracellular space. Tropoelastin does not undergo post-translational modifications. During the assembly process, some of the lysyl side chains of the tropoelastin polypeptides are oxidatively deaminated by lysyl oxidase, generating allysine in specific sequences. The reactive aldehyde of allysine condenses with other allysine or with unmodified lysine, from the same or on different tropoelastin polypeptide chains, to form **desmosine cross-**

link heterocyclic structures. As a result, elastin can stretch in any direction giving elasticity to the connective tissue.

Elastin is **rich in glycine, proline, lysine and valine**. One in seven of its amino acids are valine. Its primary structure consists of alternating hydrophilic and hydrophobic, lysine and valine-rich domains. Lysines are involved in intermolecular cross-linking while the weak interactions between valine residues in the hydrophobic domains impart elasticity to the molecule.

Elastin is an insoluble, polymeric, amorphous core covered with a sheath of microfibrils, the predominant constituent of which is the **glycoprotein fibriltin**.

DISORDERS OF ELASTIN METABOLISM

Mutations in the fibriltin gene results in a genetic disease of connective tissues, called **Marfan syndrome**. People with the disease have typically tall stature, long arms and legs, and long spidery fingers. The disease in a mild form causes loose joints, deformed spine, floppy mitral valves, and eye problems, such as lens dislocation. In severely affected individuals, the aorta wall is prone to rupture because of defects in elastic fiber formation.

Elastin is degraded by the enzyme **elastase**. This enzyme is a powerful protease that is released into the extracellular space and degrades elastin of alveolar walls and other structural proteins in a variety of tissues. **α_1-Antitrypsin** (α_1-AT), produced primarily by liver and other tissues, such as monocytes and alveolar macrophages, **inhibits** a number of proteolytic enzymes including **elastase**. This in turn prevents elastin degradation in the alveolar walls. A **deficiency of α_1-AT can cause emphysema,** which results from the destruction of the connective tissue of alveolar walls.

GLYCOSAMINOGLYCANS

Glycosaminoglycans, originally designated as **mucopolysaccharides,** are large complexes of negatively charged heteropolysaccharide chains associated with a small amount of protein, forming proteoglycans, which are the gel forming components of the extracellular matrices.

Glycosaminoglycans are **unbranched polysaccharides** and consist of **alternating uronic acid and hexosamine residues**. Solutions of glycosaminoglycans have slimy, mucus like consistency that results from their high viscosity and elasticity

FUNCTIONS OF GLYCOSAMINOGLYCANS

1. One of their major roles is to provide **structural support to** tissues, especially **cartilage and connective tissue.**
2. Extracellular matrix enables the tissue to **withstand torsion and shock**.
3. Cartilage provides a balance between **integrity and flexibility**.
4. They also perform **specific functions in certain organs**, such as liver, kidney, cornea, etc. Heparan sulfate mediates the attachment of hepatocytes to their substratum in the cell culture.

Changes in both the collagen and proteoglycan contents of the renal basement membrane are associated with diabetic renal disease.

Corneal clouding in macular corneal dystrophy is associated with undersulfation of keratin sulfate I.

Heparin and heparan sulfate have physiological role in binding proteins or other macromolecules, such as proteinases in mast cells, LDL, and lipoprotein lipase to the vascular wall, etc.

STRUCTURE AND CLASSIFICATION OF GLYCOSAMINOGLYCANS

Each glycosaminoglycan chain is composed of a **repeating disaccharide unit**, which comprises of **an acidic sugar and an amino sugar**, i.e. it has the structure as :

$$[\text{Acidic sugar} - \text{amino sugar}]_{n.}$$

The acidic sugar is either D-glucuronic acid or its carbon 5 epimor, called L-iduronic acid.

The amino sugar is either D-glucosamine or D-galactosamine in which the amino group is usually acetylated. It may also be sulfated on carbon 4 or 6, or on nonacetylated nitrogen.

Glycosaminoglycans are divided into **six major classes**, according to monomeric composition, type of glycosidic linkage and degree and location of sulfate units. Composition of glycosaminoglycans and their distribution are shown in Table 22.1.

Table 22.1. Composition, distribution and functions of glycosaminoglycans

Glycosamino-glycan	*Repeating disaccharide unit*	*Tissue location*	*Major functions*
Hyaluronic acid	[GlcUA-GlcNAc]	Joint and ocular fluids	Serves as excellent biological shock absorber and lubricant
Chondroitin sulfates	[GlcUA-GalNAc]	Cartilage, tendons, bone	Bind collagen and give it strength
Dermatan sulfate	[IdUA-GalNAc]	Skin, valves, blood vessels	
Heparan Sulfate	[IdUA-GlcNAc]	Cell surfaces	Initiation of signaling processes
Heparin	[IdUA-GlcNAc]	Mast cells, liver	Serves as an anticoagulant
Keratan sulfates	[Gal-GlcNAc]	Cartilage, cornea	

GlcUA – Glucuronic acid
GlcNAc – N-Acetylglucosamine
GalNAc – N-Acetylgalactosamine
IdUA – Iduronic acid
Gal – Galactose

Hyaluronic acid

Hyaluonic acid is composed of **repeating** units of **D-glucuronic acid and N-acetyl-D-glucosamine**. This polysaccharide chain is the longest of the glycosaminoglycans (GAG) and different from other types, as it is the only GAG, which is non-sulfated. It is not covalently attached to protein and is not limited to animal tissues but also found in bacteria. It is an important GAG component of **connective tissue, synovial fluid and the vitreous humor** of the eye. The visco-elastic behavior of hyaluronate solution makes them excellent biological shock absorbers and lubricants.

Chondroitin sulfates

Chondroitin sulfates contain **glucuronic acid and N-acetylgalatosamine with sulfate** on the hydroxyl group of either carbon 4 (chondroitin-4-sulfate) or carbon 6(chondroitin-6-sulfate). They are the major components of cartilage where they bind collagen and hold fibers in a tight, strong network. They are also found in **aorta, tendons and ligaments**.

Dermatan Sulfate

Dermatan sulfate is derived from chondroitin, by enzymatic epimerization of carbon 5 of glucuronate residues, to form iduronate residues. Thus, dermatan sulfate contains **L-iduronic acid** (with variable amounts of glucuronic acid) and **N-acetylgalactosamine**. It is found in **skin, blood vessels, tendon and heart valves.**

Heparan sulfate

Heparan sulfates are not constructed of identical disaccharides but exhibit structural diversity. They consist of **glucuronic or iduronic acid and glucosamine**. Some glucosamines are acetylated and may have N- and O-sulfate groups. It is a ubiquitous cell-surface component as well as extracellular substance in **blood vessel walls and brain**. Heparan sulfates, which function directly at the cell surface, interact with a variety of proteins, including important growth factors and their receptors (such as fibroblast growth factors and their receptors). The formation of ternary complexes of heparan sulfate with fibroblast growth factor and fibroblast growth factor receptor initiates signaling processes.

Heparin

Heparin consists of **glucuronic or iduronic acid and glucosamine**. Most of its glucosamine units are N-sulfated. Sulfate is also bound to the hydroxyl group on carbon 2 of the uronic acid residues and the carbon 3 or 6 of glucosamine. It is a highly charged polymer, found in the **intracellular granules of the mast cells** that occur in arterial walls, especially **in liver, lungs and skin**. Heparin is widely used, clinically, to **inhibit blood clotting**, e.g. in postsurgical patients.

Keratan Sulfates

Keratin sulfate is the most heterogeneous group of glycosaminoglycans as its sulfate content is variable and it contains small amounts of **fucose, mannose, N-acetylglucosamine and sialic acid**. The repeating disaccharide, generally, is N-acetyl- glucosamine and galactose. Sulfate content is variable and may be present on the carbon 6 hydroxyl groups. Keratan sulfates are linked to protein either by an N-linked (keratan sulfate I) or O-linked (keratan sulfate II) oligosaccharides. Keratan sulfate I is found in **cornea** while keratan sulfate II occurs in **loose connective tissue** proteoglycan aggregates with chondriotin sulfate.

SYNTHESIS OF GLYCOSAMINOGLYCANS

They are synthesized by a series of glycosyl transferases, epimerases and sulfotransferases, beginning with the synthesis of the core oligosaccharides while the core protein is still in the rough endoplasmic reticulum. Synthesis of the repeating oligosaccharide and other modifications take place in the Golgi apparatus.

The polysaccharide chains are elongated by **sequential addition of alternating acidic and amino sugars**, donated by their UDP-derivatives. UDP-glucuronic acid is produced by oxidation of UDP-glucose. After D-glucuronic acid has been incorporated into the carbohydrate chain, some of the D-glucuronic acid residues are converted to L-iduronic acid residues. Epimerization of the D- to the L-sugar is caused by the enzyme uronosyl-5-epimerase.

Sulfation of the carbohydrate chain occurs after the monosaccharide (to be sulfated) has been incorporated into the growing oligosaccharide chain. 3-Phosphoadenosyl-5′-phosphosulfate (PAPS) is the source of the sulfate, which is transferred at specific sites to cause sulfation of the carbohydrate, by sulfotransferases.

DEGRADATION OF GLYCOSAMINOGLYCANS

The glycosaminoglycan chains are degraded by the sequential action of a number of different **lysosomal acid hydrolases**. Their stepwise degradation involves exoglycosidases and sulfatases, beginning from the external end of the glycan chain. This may involve the removal of sulfate by a sulfatase, then removal of the terminal sugar by a specific glycosidase, and so on.

DEFECTS OF GLYCOSAMINOGLYCAN DEGRADATION

If one of the enzymes involved in the stepwise degradation pathway is missing, the entire degradation process is halted at that point and the undegraded molecule accumulates in the lysosome. The lysosomal storage diseases resulting from the accumulation of these undegraded molecules are known as mucopolysaccharidoses.

All the deficiencies are autosomal and recessively inherited except Hunter syndrome, which is X-linked. They are characterized by the accumulation of glycosaminoglycans in various tissues, causing varied symptoms, such as skeletal and extracellular matrix deformities and mental retardation. Children who are homozygous for one of these diseases are apparently normal at birth and then gradually deteriorate. In most severe cases, death occurs in childhood.

In general, these diseases can be diagnosed by the identification of the specific glycosaminoglycan chains in the urine, followed by the assay of the specific hydrolases in leukocytes or fibroblasts.

LYSOSOMAL STORAGE DISORDERS

Lysosomes are responsible for intracellular digestion of the extracellular and the intracellular substances. They contain a number of hydrolyzing enzymes (hydrolases) for the hydrolysis of proteins, lipids, carbohydrates, and nucleic acids. These hydrolases are most active at acidic pH and split complex molecules into simple low molecular weight compounds that can be reutilized.

In a number of genetic disorders, classified as lysosomal storage diseases, individual lysosomal enzymes are missing, leading to accumulation of the substrate of the missing enzyme. The lysosomes become enlarged with undigested material, thereby interfering with the normal cell processes. Several lysosomal storage diseases are known to exist, e.g. **sphingolipidoses, mucopolysaccharidoses**, etc.

MUCOPOLYSACCHARIDOSES

Mucopolysaccharidoses are caused by a deficiency of one of the lysosomal hydrolases, which are normally involved in the degradation of heparan sulfate and/or dermatan sulfate, e.g. **Hurler syndrome and Hunter syndrome**. These are the hereditary disorders and are characterized by the accumulation of glycosaminoglycans in various tissues, causing varied symptoms, such as skeletal and extracellular matrix deformities and mental retardation. This also results in the excretion of oligosaccharides in the urine because of the incomplete lysosomal degradation of glycosaminoglycans.

Table 22.2. The mucopolysaccharidoses

Syndrome	*Deficient enzyme*	*Product accumulated in lysosomes and excreted in urine*
Hunter syndrome	Iduronate sulfatase	Heparan sulfate and dermatan sulfate
Hurler syndrome	α-L-Iduronidase	- do -
Morquio syndromes		Keratan sulfate
A	Galactose-6-sulfatase	
B	β-Galactosidase	
Sanfilippo syndrome		
A	Heparan sulfamidase	Heparan sulfate
B	N-acetylglycosaminidase	
C	N-Acetylglucosamine-6-sulfatase	
Sly Syndrome	β-Glucuronidase	Dermatan sulfate and Heparan sulfate

SPHINGOLIPIDOSES

This is a group of lipid storage diseases caused by the deficiency of the specific lysosomal hydrolytic enzyme that causes **defects in the degradation of sphingolipids**. Usually, only a single sphingolipid, which is the substrate for the deficient enzyme, accumulates in the involved organs in each disease, such as Niemann-Pick disease, Gaucher's disease and Tay-Sach disease. These are autosomal recessive diseases that can be diagnosed by measuring enzyme activity in cultured fibroblasts or peripheral leucocytes.

Niemann-Pick disease

It results from a **deficiency of** the enzyme **acid sphingomyelinase**, which leads to accumulation of sphingomyelin in lysosomes. It is characterized by hepatosplenomegaly.

Gaucher's disease

It is a lysosomal storage disease where the enzyme **glucocerebrosidase is missing** in the afflicted individuals. It is characterized by hepatomegaly, osteoporosis of long bones and neurodegenerative involvement.

Tay-Sach's disease

It is due to **lack of** the enzyme **hexosaminidase**. It is the most common form of GM_2 gangliosidosis. Ganglion cells of the cerebral cortex become swollen due to the deposition of GM_2 gangliosides. Neurodegeration, blindness, cherry-red macula, muscular weakness, and seizures characterize it.

SOME IMPORTANT QUESTIONS

1. What is collagen? How they are synthesized? Describe some abnormalities of collagen biosynthesis.
2. What are glycosaminoglycans? Describe structure, distribution and functions of various types of glycosaminoglycans.
3. Write notes on:
   - (i) Connective tissue
   - (ii) Collagen
   - (iii) Osteogenesis imperfecta
   - (iv) Ehlers-Danlos syndrome
   - (v) Elastin
   - (vi) Marfan syndrome
   - (vii) Glycosaminoglycans
   - (viii) Hyaluronic acid
   - (ix) Heparin
   - (x) Lysosomal storage disorders
   - (xi) Tay-Sach's disease

CHAPTER

23

Bone Structure and Metabolism

BONE

Bone is a dynamic tissue that is remodeled constantly, throughout the life. It not only provides strength and density that is suitable for mobility but also acts as a reservoir for calcium, magnesium, phosphorus, sodium, and other ions.

Bone is comprised of the cellular component and **organic matrix,** and an **inorganic phase** (the mineral component).

The organic matrix

The **organic matrix** mainly consists of a collagen-like protein, referred to as **ossein**. It is a type I collagen and comprises of nearly 90-95% of the organic matrix.

The non-collagen portion of the organ matrix contains several proteins, which are derived from serum, such as albumin, α_2-HS glycoproteins, and several other proteins containing γ-carboxyglutamate (GLA) residues, e.g. the bone GLA proteins, osteocalcin, sialoproteins, etc. Some of these may also function in initiating mineralization and in the binding of the mineral phase to the matrix.

Embedded in the bone matrix are the spidery cells, referred to as osteocytes. These include osteoblasts, which secrete fibrous material and promote laying down of calcium phosphate.

The inorganic component

The **inorganic component** is made up of calcium and phosphate, and is best characterized as a poorly crystalline hydroxyapatite.

Its calcium/phosphorus ratio is less than that found in the hydroxyapatite (Fig. 23.1).

There is also a small amount of Mg^{2+}, in place of Ca^{2+}. A very small fraction of the -OH is also replaced by fluoride, which has bone-strengthening effect.

Bone also contains an amorphous phase, called as hydrated tricalciumphosphate [$3Ca_3(PO_4)_2.Ca(OH)_2$]. With increasing age, it is eventually transformed to the **crystalline apatite.**

Other salts of calcium, e.g. carbonate, citrate, chloride, and fluoride, etc., are also found but in the intercrystalline semiliquid medium, which allows free transport of materials between blood and the bone.

Two fractions of the mineral structure of bone, i.e. the crystalline hydroxyapatite and the intercrystalline fraction, are quite different from each other.

Hydroxyapatite crystals are extremely small and have enormous surface area. It is relatively stable and not easily soluble in aqueous fluid.

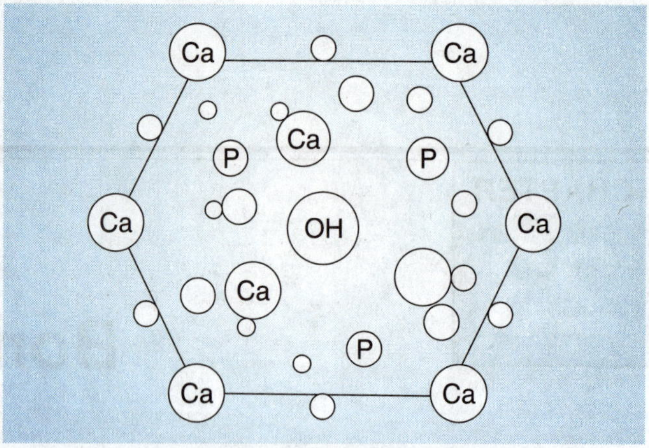

Fig. 23.1. Crystalline calcium phosphate (hydroxyapatite).

On the other hand, the **intercrystalline fraction** is small in amount than the crystalline fraction but is much more soluble. Its calcium and other elements are freely exchangeable with the blood.

Hardness and rigidity of the bone are attributable, chiefly to hydroxyapatite whereas elasticity and toughness are attributable to proteins.

Mineral phase of the bone is deposited initially, in intimate relation to collagen fibrils, and is found in the specific locations in the holes between the collagen fibrils. Formation and localization of the inorganic phase thus, are determined, in part, by the organic matrix.

FORMATION OF THE BONE

Bone formation consists of two distinct processes, i.e. the **formation of the organic matrix,** and its mineralization.

Formation of the organic matrix

Cells of mesenchymal origin, i.e. **osteoblasts, synthesize and secrete organic matrix.**

Location and morphology of the cell, presence of the specific skeletal form of alkaline phosphatase, and the receptors, characterize osteoblasts for PTH and calcitriol. They have the ability to synthesize specific matrix proteins, such as type I collagen, osteocalcin, and osteopontin. As the osteoblasts secrete matrix, which is then mineralized, they become osteocytes but are still connected through the series of canaliculi.

Vitamin C is essential for bone formation, especially **for the formation of tropocollagen. Vitamin A is also required for** normal activity of the osteoblasts, in **laying down the matrix.** Physiological concentration of **growth hormone, thyroid hormones, and androgens** are also essential. **Vitamin K** also has a role in bone metabolism. It is essential **for the carboxylation of the glutamate residues,** for their conversion into the carboxyglutamate residues, which are present in osteocalcin. Osteocalcin is a small protein that strongly binds to hydroxyapatite crystals and regulates Ca^{2+} concentration.

Mineralization of the matrix

Mineralization occurs on the organic matrix, which undergoes complex biochemical alterations, followed by crystal nucleation with calcium phosphate. For ossification, i.e. formation of bone salt, it is essential that calcium and phosphorus must exceed the saturation point, at the site of deposition. Normally, their concentration is such that product of the ionic calcium and phosphorus (Ca × P) is between 30 to 40. When concentrations of calcium and phosphorus increase beyond the saturation point, calciumphosphate is produced and changes to hydroxyapatite.

Mineralization of the matrix, largely in the osteons begins soon after matrix is secreted but it is not complete until several weeks.

Two enzymes are involved in the ossification process. These are glycogen phosphorylase and alkaline phosphatase. Phosphorylase stimulates glycogenolysis and provides energy, which is required for the mineralization process.

Alkaline phosphatase acts on sugar phosphates and pyrophosphates, and increases inorganic phosphorus concentration.

Chondroitin sulfates of the growing bone combine with calcium, to provide local surplus of the available calcium.

Carbonic anhydrase is also involved in mineralization of the bone. It makes carbonate available for the formation of bone salt, in the form of carbonate-hydroxyapatite.

REMODELING OF BONE

Remodeling (turnover) of the bone is a cyclic process. It consists of bone resorption as well as formation.

Resorption of the bone is mainly carried out by the **osteoclasts.** They are the multinucleated cells, which are formed by the fusion of the hematopoietic stem cells that are related to mononuclear phagocyte series. Resorption of the bone takes place in scalloped spaces where osteoclasts are attached through a specific ααββ integrin to the components of the bone matrix, such as osteopontin. This zone contains contractile proteins.

The resorbing end of the cell forms a specialized ruffled border. The mineral matrix is removed in this space where ruffled border is folded, and is in the control, with the bone. Proteins, including the specialized proton-pump, ATPase, are found in the ruffled-border membrane, which contributes to the production of an acid environment in the enclosed extracellular compartment that solubilizes the mineral phase. Other features of the osteoclasts include, presence of the tartarate-resistant acid phosphatase, cell-surface receptors for calcitonin, sodium pump, bicarbonate/chloride exchanger of band-3 family and the ability to resorb mineralized bone.

After bone resorption, osteoclasts undergo division and are eventually transformed to osteoblasts. After bone formation, osteoblasts become mature osteocytes, or are transformed to the undifferentiated mesenchymal cells.

Factors Affecting Bone Resorption

Bone remodeling is controlled by various factors:

1. **Serum calcium:** Bone calcium is in equilibrium with the concentration of the calcium in the blood. If serum calcium is reduced, it is derived from the intracrystalline material, which is dissolved into the surrounding fluid and enters blood. Bone calcium thus, maintains a steady concentration, by making a shift of the calcium from bone to blood, or vice versa. Calcium and phosphorus ionic product, during bone growth or healing, should be above 40.
2. **Hormones:** Transformation of the osteoprogenitor cells to the osteoclasts is stimulated by parathyroid hormone, thyroid hormones, growth hormone, and vitamin D. On the other hand, calcitonin, estrogens, and glucocorticoids inhibit the formation of osteoclasts.
   Inorganic phosphorus, calcitonin, estrogens, and growth hormone also promote conversion of osteoclasts to osteoblasts.

3. **Physical Activity:** Physical activity has a significant effect on bone composition and density.

Vigorous physical activity along with adequate dietary intake of calcium and vitamin D are required for maintenance of the dense bone in a healthy young human being.

NUTRITIONAL DISORDERS OF BONE

Osteoporosis

Osteoporosis is characterized by **loss of bone matrix** and **progressive demineralization,** primarily due to inadequate intake of calcium.

Decreased calcium intake, particularly **during menopause**, leads to **increased fragility and fractures of bones**, mainly of extremities and pelvis.

In postmenopausal woman, it can be retarded by increased supply of calcium in the food along with the estrogen therapy.

Besides calcium, vitamin D is also essential for the absorption and utilization of calcium. Vitamin C is also needed for the formation of bone matrix. Magnesium and phosphorus are also essential since they form important part of the bone structure. Vitamin K, copper, zinc, manganese, and boron are also important in bone formation.

Therefore, **an adequate diet,** sufficient in all the nutrients, **along with the regular exercise** is important for preventing osteoporosis.

Rickets

Rickets is a **bone disease of infancy** and childhood. It is a nutritional disorder, primarily, due to the deficiency of vitamin D. Besides vitamin D, exposure of the body to sunlight has both, preventive as well as curative effects.

Symptoms, such as **enlarged wrists, ankles,** and poor structural development affecting long bones are frequently seen.

Ends of the long bones become soft and bulky particularly the characteristic bowed-legs and knock-knees. There may also be extreme stunting of growth.

Deformities may also appear in bones of the skull, chest, and spine. Teeth may erupt late and are deformed.

Biochemically, in a patient with rickets, there is a **decrease** in **serum calcium** and **phosphorus** along with the **increase** in **serum alkaline phosphatase,** and **increased excretion of phosphorus in the urine.**

Product of serum calcium and phosphorus, which is normally 40 (10 mg calcium x 4 mg phosphorus), is decreased to below 30, in such children.

Osteomalacia

Deficiency of vitamin D in **adults** may result in **osteomalacia;** hence this condition might be termed as **adult rickets**. It is commonly observed in females during pregnancy and lactation, or in those who are protected from sunlight, i.e. those observing purdah. **Pelvic bones** show characteristic **deformities, which** in turn further complicates parturition.

TEETH

Teeth are important components of the facial skeleton. They are major components of the oral cavity and are essential for the start of the digestive process. Apart from their function in mastication of food, teeth add to the aesthetics, phonation, and speech.

Development of the teeth starts during sixth week of the intrauterine life. They are developed as the deciduous (primary) teeth and the permanent (secondary) teeth.

Deciduous Teeth: A child starts getting teeth from 6 months of age and are seen in the oral cavity by the two and a half years of age. Children have 10 deciduous teeth in each jaw, on each side.

Permanent Teeth: Over a period of years, 16 permanent teeth, in each jaw, gradually replace the deciduous teeth. They start erupting from the 6 years of age and the process is completed by 18-25 years.

COMPONENTS OF TEETH

Teeth are made up of three specialized tissues, called enamel, cementum, and dentin. These are the three mineralized components of a tooth.

Enamel

Enamel is an acellular mineralized tissue that covers the crown (portion that is visible in the oral cavity) of the tooth. It is highly mineralized and harder than any other mineralized tissue in the body. It consists of 96-98% of hydroxyapatite. The carbonated-calciumhydroxyapatite enamel crystals that form the enamel are arranged as rods. The enamel of an erupted tooth lacks cells and the cellular processes. Substances in the saliva, which are essential for its maintenance, influence it. The substances in the saliva that affect teeth include digestive enzymes, antibacterial enzymes, antibodies, and inorganic components.

Enamel is produced by the ameloblasts of the enamel organ, which is an epithelial formation derived from the ectodermal epithelial cells of the oral cavity. Growth and development of the enamel organ results in the stage, which consists of four cellular components, called outer enamel epithelium, inner enamel epithelium, stratum intermedium, and stellate reticulum. **Stratum intermedium** is a cell layer that develops internal to the **inner enamel epithelium.** The plasma membrane of these cells, especially at the base of the ameloblasts, contains alkaline phosphatase, the enzyme that is active in calcification.

The maturation-stage ameloblasts and the adjacent papillary cells are characterized by the numerous mitochondria. Enamel matrix is highly heterogeneous and contains proteins, which is encoded by different genes. The principal proteins in the extracellular matrix of the developing enamel are:

Amelogenins: Amylogenins are important in establishing and maintaining spacing between the enamel rods, in early stages of the enamel development.

Ameloblastins: Ameloblastins are proteins, which are produced by the ameloblasts, from the early secretary to the late maturation stages. They are believed to guide the enamel mineralization process, by controlling the elongation of the enamel crystals.

Enamelins: Enamelins are distributed throughout the enamel layer, referred to as the enamel proteinases or ameloproteases-I. They are responsible for the degradation of the amelogenins in the maturing enamel.

Tuftelins: Tuftelins are the acidic enamel proteins, which are located near the dentino-enamel junction that participates in nucleation of the enamel crystal. They are present in enamel tufts and account for hypomineralization. Enamel tufts have a higher percentage of the organic material than the remainder of the mature enamel.

As enamel matures, hydroxyapatite crystals grow and bulk of the organic matrix, mainly amelogenins and ameloblastins, are removed. Mature enamel thus, contains only enamelins and tuftelins. Maturation of the developing enamel results in its continual mineralization so that it becomes hardest substance in the body. Despite its hardness, acid-producing bacteria, acting on the food products, trapped on the enamel surface can decalcify enamel. This is the basis of the initiation of dental caries.

Cementum

Cementum covers root of the tooth. It is a thin layer of the bone-like material that is secreted by the cementocytes. Like bone, cementum is 65% mineral but unlike bone, it is avascular. Collagen fibers, that project out of the matrix of the cementum and are embedded in the bony matrix of the socket wall, form bulk of the periodontal ligament. During corrective tooth movements, the cementum is not resorbed and resynthesized.

Dentin

Dentin is a calcified material that forms most of the tooth substance. It lies deep to the enamel and the cementum. It contains less hydroxyapatite than the enamel but more than that is found in the bone and the cementum. Fully mature dentin is composed of approximately 70% of the inorganic material and 10% of water. The principal inorganic component consists of $Ca_{10}(PO_4)_6(OH)_2$, hydroxyapatite. Organic matrix accounts for 20% of the dentin, of which about 91% are collagens. Most of the collagen is of type I but there is also a minor component of type V. Noncollagenous matrix components include phosphoproteins, proteoglycans, γ-carboxyglutamate-containing proteins (gla-proteins), acidic glycoproteins, growth factors, and lipids. The elasticity of dentin provides flexibility for the overlying brittle enamel. Dentin is secreted by the odontoblasts that form an epithelial layer over the inner surface of the dentin. Circumpulpal dentin is formed after the layer of mantle dentin has been deposited and constitutes the major part of the developmental dentin.

Predentin is unmineralised organic matrix of the dentin, situated between the odontoblasts layer and the mineralized dentin, which is yet to be mineralized. Its macromolecular constituents include type I and type II trimer collagens. Noncollagenous elements consist of some unique proteins grouped as dentin sialoproteins and dentin phosphoproteins.

Dentin phosphoprotein: Dentin phosphoprotein (phosphophoryn) is a highly phosphorylated tissue specific molecule that is unique to the odontoblast cell lineage. It is produced by the odontoblasts and transported to the mineralization front. It is rich in aspartic acid and phosphoserine, and binds large amounts of calcium. It is involved in initiation of mineralization and in control of mineral size and shape.

Dentin sialoprotein: Dentin sialoprotein consists of several proteoglycans (dermatan sulfate, heparin sulfate, hyaluronate, keratan sulfate, chondroitin-4-sulfate, and chondroitin-6-sulfate), glycoproteins, glycosaminoglycans, and gla-proteins. It is rich in aspartate, serine, glutamate, and glycine. It is also involved in the mineralization process.

Dentin is the first mineralized component of the tooth, to be deposited. Mineralization of the dentin matrix commences within the initial increment of the mantle dentin. Calcium phosphate crystals begin to accumulate in the matrix vesicle, within the predentin. The hydroxyapatite crystals grow rapidly within the vesicles and in time the vesicles rupture. Apparently, matrix vesicles are involved only in mineralization of the initial layer of dentin. As the process of mineralization progresses, the advancing front projects along the collagen fibrils of the predentin matrix. Hydroxyapatite crystals appear on the surface and within the fibrils, and continue to grow as mineralization progresses, resulting in an increased mineral content of the dentin.

COMMON DENTAL DISEASES

Common dental diseases include dental caries and fluorosis.

Dental caries

Dental caries or decay, also referred to as cavity formation, is defined as chronic irreversible disease of the hard structure of the teeth. Demineralization of the inorganic components of teeth and dissolution of the organic substance of microbial etiology characterize it. Caries is a result of bacterial growth in unhygienic oral cavity. Microorganisms breed in the oral cavity, in the food debris, and produce acids (lactic, propionic, and acetic acids) by fermentation. These acids bring about demineralization of the enamel.

Dental caries is a multifactorial disease. Increasing dental plaque is viewed as a dynamic biofilm. Dental plaque contains acid producing bacteria that are born and survive at low pH. *Mutans streptococci* are believed to be the most important bacteria in the initiation and progression of dental caries. Later, following enamel cavitation, *lactobacilli* becomes increasingly important in the caries process. Once the pH in plaque drops below a critical level (around 5.5), the acids produced, begin to demineralize the enamel. Bacteria utilize fermentable carbohydrates (mainly sucrose) for energy, and the end-products of the glycolytic pathway in bacterial metabolism are acids. Bacteria can use all fermentable carbohydrates, including the cooked starches. Although any carbohydrate causes the production of acid, it is the availability of glucose that drives bacterial metabolism to produce lactic acid.

Generally, caries is initiated in the enamel but it may also begin in dentine or cementum. Saliva plays several critical roles in the caries process. In removing substrate and buffering plaque acid, saliva helps to slow the caries process and plays a critical role in remineralization, by providing a source of calcium and phosphates as well as fluoride. When salivary flow is reduced, the rate of demineralization and subsequent tooth breakdown will increase.

Diet is the single most important factor in determining caries risk. Frequency of intake is more important than the overall quantity. Grazing between meals should be discouraged. Frequent consumption of soft drinks should be avoided.

Even **low concentration of fluoride**, in the microenvironment around the teeth, inhibits demineralization and promotes remineralization of the tooth surface.

Fluorosis

Fluorosis is a crippling disorder due to the **excessive entry of fluoride in the body**. The duration required for clinical manifestations to appear, varies depending upon several factors, viz. age, hormonal status, nutritional status, efficiency of the kidney to excrete fluoride, the quantum of fluoride entry into the body, climatic conditions, and perhaps other factors presumably not so evident. Fluorosis is occurring due to drinking water contamination of fluoride. It is a slow, progressive crippling malady, affects every organ, tissue, and cells in the body, and results in health complaints having overlapping manifestations with several other diseases. Fluorosis affects young and old, men and women, rich and poor, rural and urban population. Fluoride dust and fumes are as dangerous as consuming fluoride containing foods, water, and/or drugs.

Fluoride when ingested beyond the limit of tolerance of the human body may cause three forms of fluorosis, which are referred to as the skeletal fluorosis (affecting bones), dental fluorosis (affecting teeth), and non-skeletal fluorosis (affecting soft tissues).

Skeletal Fluorosis: Excess fluoride, entering the body, mainly through drinking water, food, drugs, and cosmetics (tooth paste, mouth rinses, etc.), can cause skeletal fluorosis. It affects bones and skeletal system. Effect of fluoride on bone depends upon the type of the bone and its inorganic and organic constituents. A fluorosed bone shows:

- Increased bone mass and density,
- Exostosis at bone surfaces,
- Increased osteoid seam and resorption surfaces,
- Increased trabecular bone volume, cortical porosity and periosteocytic lacunar surface,
- Increased osteon diameter and mottling of the osteons,
- Formation of the unmineralised cartilaginous loci within the trabeculae of the cancellous bone but not in the cortical bone,
- Cartilaginous lesions will be developed in the cancellous but not in the cortical bones.
- The bone has characteristic biochemical changes,
- Reduction in collagen content,
- Reduction in hydroxylation of proline and lysine in bone collagen,
- Reduction in collagen cross-link precursors,

- Altered glycosaminoglycans and proteoglycans contents in cancellous but not in cortical bone, and
- Increased dermatan sulphate content in cancellous bone.

Skeletal fluorosis is not easily recognizable until the disease has developed to an advanced stage. Excessive fluoride tends to get distributed more in cancellous compared to cortical bone. Maximum illeffects are detected in the neck, spine and knee, pelvic, and shoulder joints. Fluoride can also damage a fetus. Abortions, stillbirths, and children born with deformities, are common in endemic areas.

Dental Fluorosis: Dental fluorosis is a qualitative defect of enamel (hypomineralization), resulting from an increase in fluoride concentration within the microenvironment of the ameloblasts, during enamel formation. Drinking water from sources having high fluoride is the cause of dental fluorosis. As the fluoride content of water increases beyond 1 ppm, the increase in severity of fluorosis is greater than the decrease in caries. Fluoride in toothpastes, mouth rinses and sodium fluoride tablets administered as prescription can contribute to the fluoride burden of the body, leading to dental fluorosis. It occurs in children during the developmental stages when the teeth are exposed to fluoride. The discoloration of the teeth may progress from white, yellow, and brown to black. The discoloration may be in spots or in streaks, invariably horizontal in orientation. The enamel will lose its luster and shine.

Calcium rich constituents of teeth, viz. enamel and dentin, have strong affinity for fluoride, during the formation of teeth. Fluoride combines with calcium, forming calcium fluoroapatite crystals, during the mineralization of teeth. Teeth commonly affected are incisors, lateral incisors, and molars of the permanent dentition. Fluorosis affects both the inner and the outer surfaces of the teeth.

Non-skeletal Fluorosis: Fluorosis may involve and damage skeletal muscle, erythrocytes, gastrointestinal mucosa, ligaments, and spermatozoa, besides kidney, liver, adrenal gland, and reproductive organs.

Besides consuming safe drinking water, nutritional intervention focusing on adequate intake of calcium, vitamin C, vitamin E, and antioxidants, are used in the management of fluorosis.

FACTORS AFFECTING DEVELOPMENT OF TEETH

Vitamins A, C, and D are necessary for proper development and calcification of teeth.

Vitamin A deficiency results in hypoplastic enamel, which is imperfectly calcified.

Vitamin C deficiency disturbs functional activities of the formative cells, thereby affecting calcification of dentine.

Vitamin D is required for the absorption of calcium, and promotes deposition of calcium and phosphorus in teeth.

SOME IMPORTANT QUESTIONS

1. Describe chemical composition of bone.
2. Describe the process of the formation of bone.
3. Write notes on:
   (i) Remodeling of bone
   (ii) Factors affecting bone resorption
   (iii) Factors affecting development of teeth
   (iv) Osteoporosis
   (v) Rickets
   (vi) Osteomalacia
   (vii) Dental Caries
   (viii) Fluorosis

CHAPTER

24

Membrane Structure and Functions

All living cells are surrounded by a highly viscous structure, called **cell membrane.** Cell membrane **in animal cells is also** referred to as **plasma membrane.**

In addition to plasma membrane, eukaryotic cells also contain **internal membrane systems,** which form specialized compartments within the cell. Such intracellular membranes separate many morphologically distinguishable organelles from each other.

COMPOSITION OF A BIOLOGICAL MEMBRANE

All **biological membranes** are **composed of** different proportions of **lipids, proteins** and **carbohydrates.**

Lipids: **Lipids form more than 50% of the total membrane constituents. Membrane lipids** comprise of both **hydrophobic** as well as **hydrophilic** regions and are termed as amphipathic molecules. Lipids have a polar head group and non-polar tail. **Fatty acids** present in the tail are **both saturated** as well as **unsaturated**.

Phospholipids form major proportion of the lipid component of a cell membrane. Besides **cholesterol and its esters, triacylglycerol** and **free fatty acids** also occur in the membrane. These are collectively referred to as neutral lipids.

There are also qualitative differences. For example, **plasma membrane has highest concentration of neutral lipids** and **sphingolipids** while **intracellular membranes,** primarily, contain **glycerophospholipids** with little sphingolipids or cholesterol.

Lipid bilayer forms the structural basis of a biological membrane.

Proteins: **Proteins** form another major portion of the membrane and play several roles, such as **structural components, transport systems, enzymes** or **recognition sites for hormones** and **other molecules**.

Protein concentration varies from about 20% in the myelin sheath to over 70% in the inner membrane of the mitochondria. Membrane proteins are present in various sizes and shapes. These are **classified** by their mode of interaction with the membrane **as integral membrane proteins and peripheral membrane proteins.**

Carbohydrates: Some of the membrane proteins and lipids have short chains of carbohydrates (oligosaccharides). Carbohydrate content of biological membranes may vary between **3-10%. Oligosaccharide** chains are normally **located on the outer surface of the membrane** or on the **terminal side of the endoplasmic reticulum.**

STRUCTURE OF A BIOLOGICAL MEMBRANE

Biological membranes have such a structure where **some proteins span the lipid bilayer** while **others are immersed partially.** This is called **fluid-mosaic model** because the membrane consists of a mosaic of proteins and lipids, which are free to drift in the fluid plane of the membrane (Fig. 24.1).

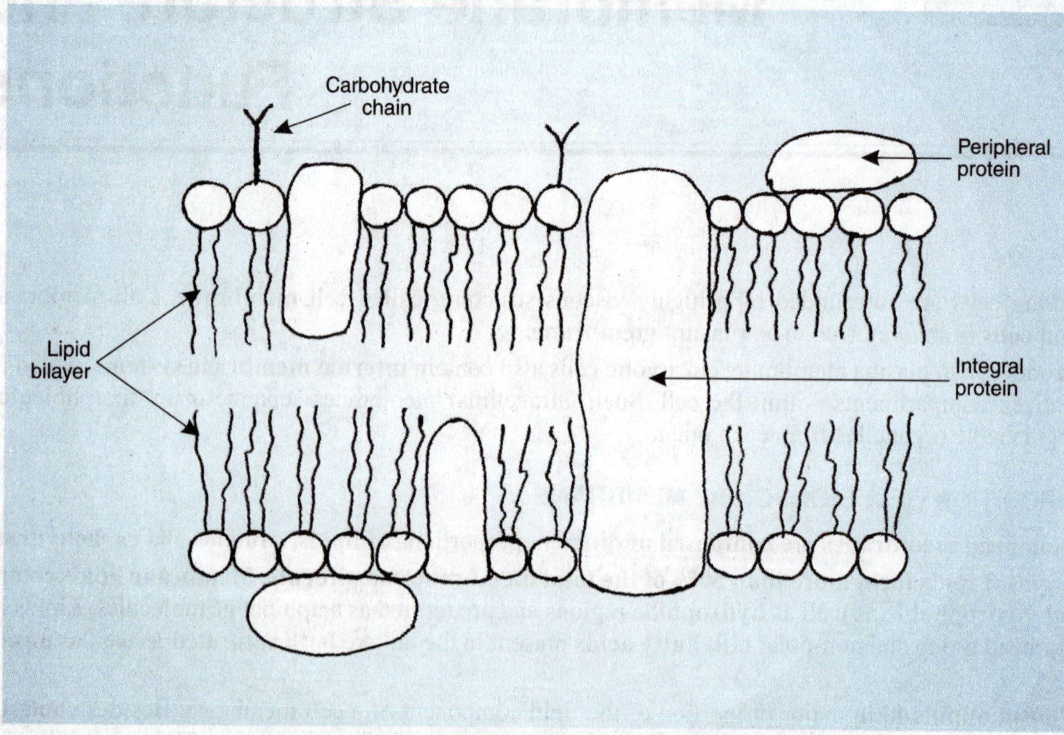

Fig. 24.1. Fluid-mosaic model of biological membrane.

In the **fluid-mosaic model** of cell membrane, **integral proteins are immersed in the lipid bilayer** and **have specific domains for ligand binding, catalytic activity** and **attachment of carbohydrates or lipids.** Some proteins also contain α-helical structure, consisting of hydrophobic amino acids. This in turn forms a transmembrane sequence which has three domains, i.e. a sequence exterior to the cell (containing the $-NH_2$ terminal end), a transmembrane sequence and a sequence extending into the cell (with the –COOH terminal end). **Peripheral proteins** have various modes of attachment. Some, apparently, **bind to integral proteins** such as an antigen. On the other hand, **some** peripheral proteins such as cytochrome b_5 have sequences of hydrophobic amino acids at one end of the peptide chain (which **serve as anchor** in the membrane lipid).

Membrane **fluidity** is due to the presence of unsaturated fatty acids. The degree of fluidity is highly dependent on lipid composition of the membrane. It changes in response to a change in the diet or physiological state of the animal. Cholesterol and Ca^{2+} decrease membrane fluidity. Fluidity of a membrane also affects its functions, e.g. it can control activity of the membrane bound enzymes, cell growth and other functions such as phagocytosis.

FUNCTIONS OF BIOLOGICAL MEMBRANES

Biological membranes serve various functions:

1. Many enzymes are associated with cell membrane, e.g. phospholipase A, Na^+/K^+-ATPase, etc. These are also used as markers of cell membrane.
2. Membrane contains specific receptors for external stimuli, such as hormones. After a hormone binds to its receptor, it generates signals and regulates cellular activities.
3. Carbohydrate component of the glycoprotein acts as recognition sites for antibodies.
4. Membrane acts as a selective barrier, preventing the loss of useful substances as well as permitting the entrance of essential nutrients.

This in turn includes the transport of both, small molecules as well as large molecules.

TRANSPORT OF SMALL MOLECULES

Transport of small molecules across the cell membrane can be described, according to the number of molecules transported, and the direction of their movement, as follows:

Uniport

Uniport transport refers to the process, which allows the **movement of one type of molecules in only one direction,** e.g. glucose transport in erythrocytes.

Cotransport

It refers to the process where **transfer of one solute depends upon the simultaneous or sequential transfer of the other**. It may be symport or antiport:

Two types of **molecules** when **move in the same direction**, it is called as **symport**, e.g. Na^+-sugar transporter or Na^+-amino acid transporter, in a mammalian cell.

Two types of **molecules** when **move in opposite directions**, it is referred to as **antiport**, e.g. Na^+, K^+-transporter or Na^+, Ca^{2+}-transporter (Fig. 24.2).

TRANSPORT SYSTEMS

There are two types of transport systems, i.e. the **non-mediated transport** and the **mediated transport**. Non-mediated transport occurs through diffusion while the mediated transport occurs through the action of specific carrier proteins. It is also referred to as carrier-mediated transport.

NONMEDIATED TRANSPORT

Some solutes and gases (O_2, N_2, CO_2, NO, etc.) transport across the cell, by diffusing down electro-chemical gradient across the membrane and do not require metabolic energy.

The direction of flow is always from a higher concentration to a lower concentration and the net movement of a molecule from one side to the other continues until concentration on each side is at chemical equilibrium.

Non-mediated transport is also called as **diffusion (passive diffusion).**

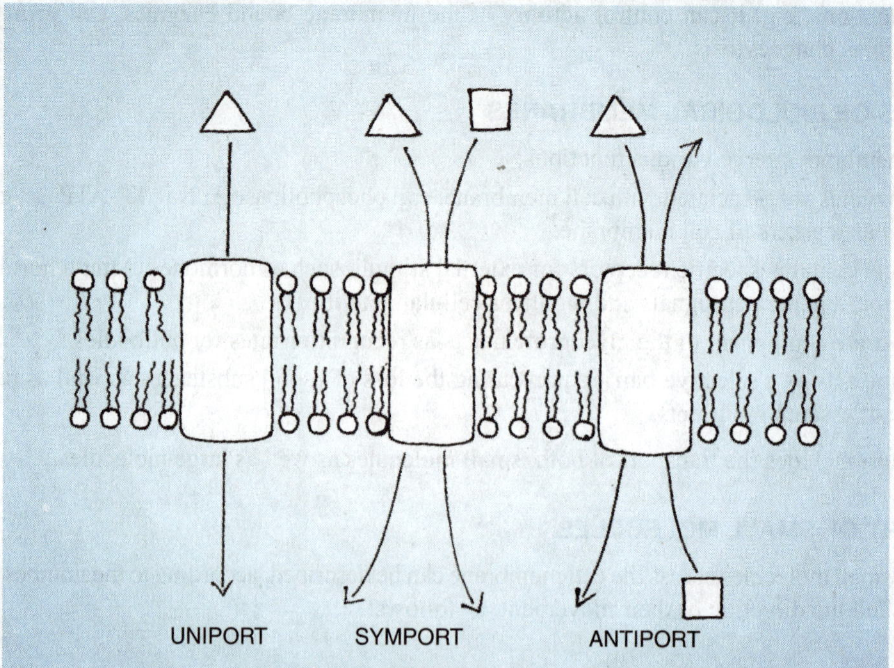

Fig. 24.2. Transport of molecules with respect to their number and direction.

CARRIER –MEDIATED TRANSPORT

Molecules that cannot freely diffuse through the lipid bilayer membrane by simple diffusion **are transported in association with a specific carrier molecule**. This process is known as mediated transport or **carrier-mediated transport.** Carrier molecules are variously designated as carriers, permeases, porters, translocases or transporters.

Carrier-mediated transport may be **passive transport** or **active transport** (Fig. 24.3)

Passive Transport: **Passive Transport, also referred to as facilitated diffusion, leads to the translocation of solutes through membrane transport proteins without the expenditure of metabolic energy.** The process can operate either unidirectionally or bidirectionally and the net flux across the membrane occur down a concentration gradient, i.e. the molecules flow from a higher concentration to the lower concentration.

Several hormones such as insulin, gluco-corticoids, growth hormone, etc., regulate facilitated diffusion by changing the number of transport proteints. Examples of transport proteins, which mediate facilitated diffusion, include glucose transporter, anion transporter, etc.

Several **transport proteins** have been identified in the plasma membrane of mammalian cells **for** the transport of D-glucose, e.g. GLUT-1, GLUT-2, etc. These are **referred** to **as glucose permeases**. They translocate several D-sugars by a uniport mechanism. Another transport protein referred to as Cl^- and HCO_3^- exchanger (anion exchanger protein) catalyzes the antiport movement of Cl^- and HCO_3^-. There are several other antiport systems in the inner mitochondrial membrane for the exchange of anions between the cytosol and the mitochondrial matrix, e.g. ATP-ADP translocase.

Active Transport: In active transport, **transport protein moves a specific molecule against the**

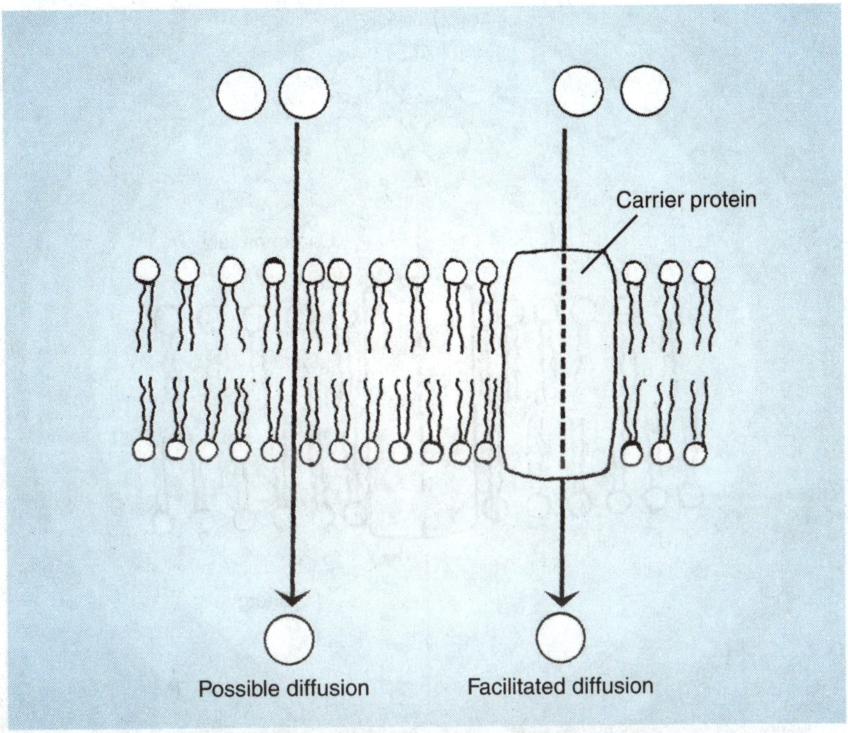

Fig. 24.3. Transport systems.

concentration gradient, i.e. from a lower concentration to the higher concentration **by a process that requires energy,** which is normally coupled to the hydrolysis of ATP (Fig. 24.4). These include :

- **Primary** active transport, and
- **Secondary** active transport

Transport proteins for **primary active transport** have same characteristics as the passive transport system but it **is an endergonic process**. Primary active transport systems are important in the maintenance of electrochemical gradient in biological systems and consume nearly one-third of the total energy expenditure of a cell. These include several membrane-bound ATPases that translocate cations. Examples of primary active transport system include Na^+, K^+-ATPase; Ca^{2+}-ATPase; H^+, K^+-ATPase; etc.

Secondary active transport is **also called** as **ion gradient-driven active transport.** In this process free energy of electrochemical gradient, generated by ion-pumping ATPase, drives the transport of another substance, such as a sugar or an amino acid, against its concentration gradient. Na^+-glucose transport system, amino acid transport system, etc., are the examples of secondary active transport system.

TRANSPORT DISORDERS

Several pathological conditions due to a defect in the membrane transport system are known. For example:

Hartnup's Disease : It is due to a decrease in the transport of neutral amino acids in the epithelial cells of the intestine and the renal tubules.

Cystinuria: Renal reabsorption of cystine and basic amino acids (arginine and lysine) is abnormal. This in turn may result in the formation of cystine stones in the kidney.

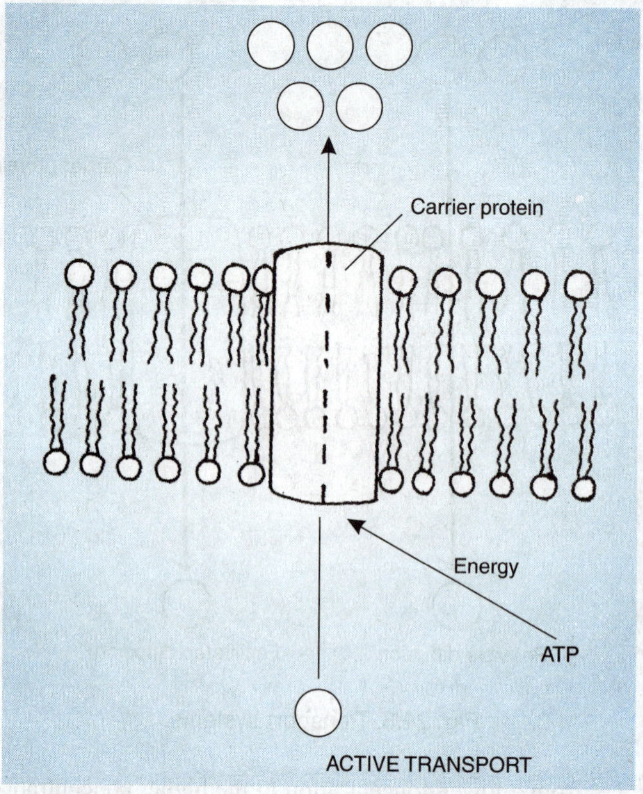

Fig. 24.4. Active transport.

TRANSPORT OF LARGE MOLECULES

Cells also transport certain large molecules (macromolecules) across the plasma membrane by the mechanism, which involves vesicle formation within or from the plasma membrane. These are referred to as **endocytosis** or **exocytosis.**

Endocytosis

Endocytosis is a mechanism for the transport of large molecules such as polysaccharides, proteins or polynucleotides into the cytoplasm (Fig. 24.5).

In the process, a region of the plasma membrane invaginates, enclosing a small volume of the extracellular fluid and its contents within a bud, and generates endocytotic vesicles. Vesicle then pinches-off, as fusion of the plasma membrane seals neck of the vesicle at the original site of invagination. The resulting small vesicle is called as endosome. It moves into the interior of the cell and delivers its contents to some other organelle, bound by a single membrane, e.g. a lysosome, by fusion of the two membranes. There are two general types of processes, i.e. phagocytosis and pinocytosis.

Phagocytosis : Phagocytosis or cell-eating occurs only in specialized cells, like macrophages and granulocytes for the ingestion of foreign particles, such as bacteria, viruses, etc.

Pinocytosis : Pinocytosis or cell-drinking, leads to cellular uptake of fluid and its contents, as a result of invagination of the plasma membrane.

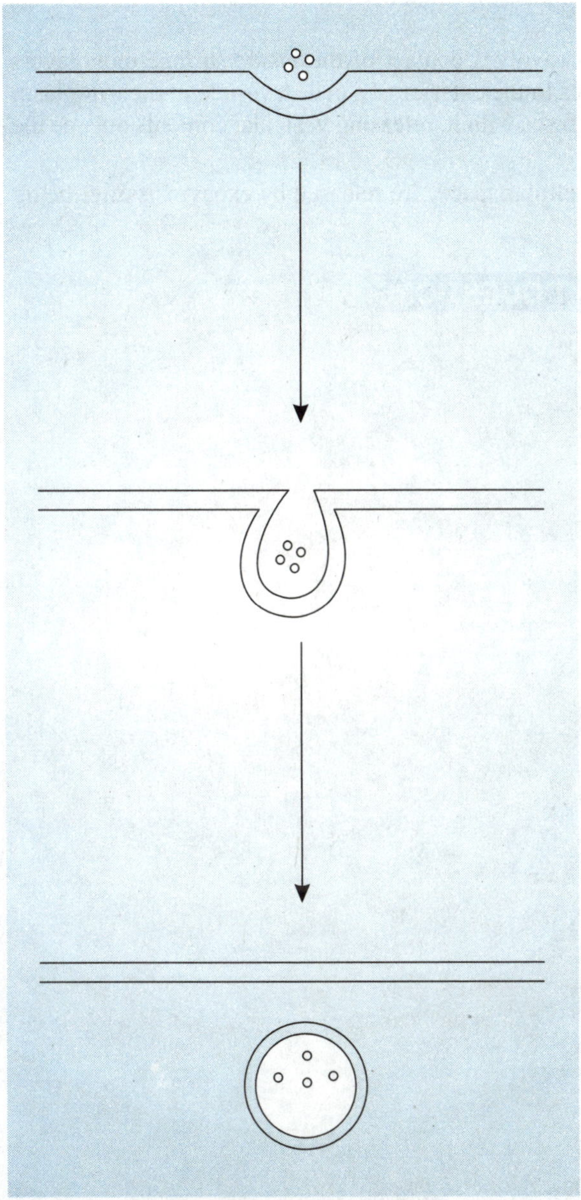

Fig. 24.5. Endocytosis.

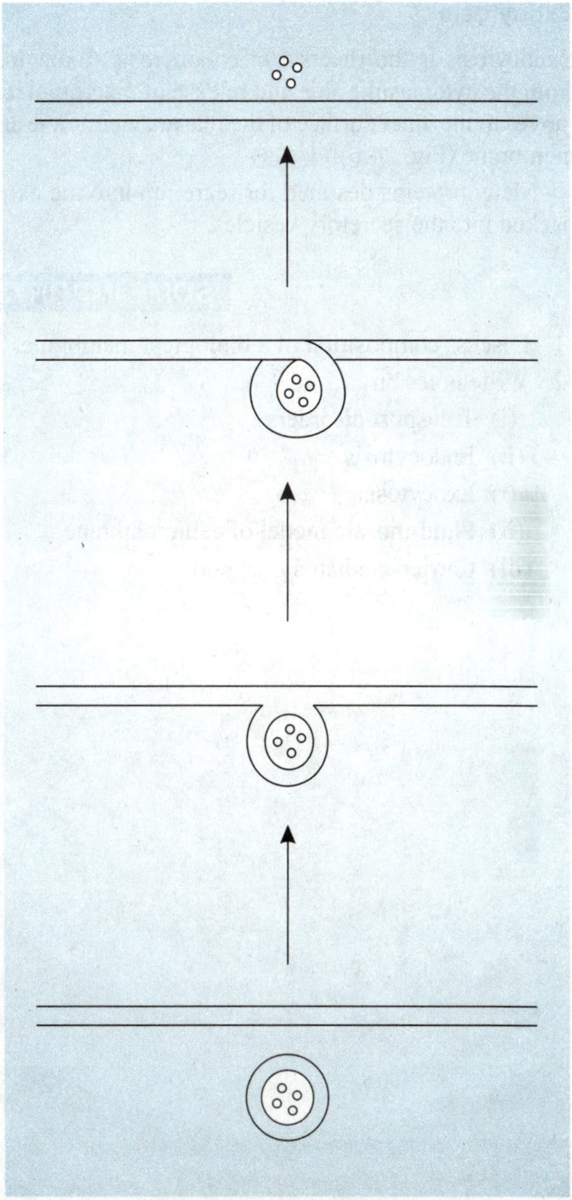

Fig. 24.6. Exocytosis.

The **receptor-mediated pinocytosis** is a selective type of pinocytosis that occurs in coated pits, lined with the protein, resulting in the formation of coated vesicles. High affinity receptors permit selective concentration of the ligand from the medium, e.g. LDL particles and its receptors are internalized by means of the coated-pits containing LDL receptors.

Several hormones are subjected to **adsorptive pinocytosis** by forming coated vesicles, called receptosomes. These coated vesicles do not deliver their contents to the lysosomes but to other intracellular organelles, such as Golgi system.

Exocytosis

Excocytosis is the reversal of endocytosis. Exocytosis involves contact of the inside surface monolayers from the cytoplasmic side and release of macromolecules to the exterior of a cell. A vesicle in the cytoplasm moves to the inner surface of the plasma membrane and fuses with it, releasing vesicular contents outside the membrane (Fig. 24.6).

Many proteins destined for secretion into the extracellular space, are released by exocytosis after being packed into the secretory vesicles.

SOME IMPORTANT QUESTIONS

1. Discuss composition of a biological membrane.
2. Write notes on:
   (i) Transport disorders
   (ii) Endocytosis
   (i) Exocytosis
   (ii) Fluid-mosaic model of cell membrane
   (iii) Carrier-mediated transport

CHAPTER

25

Cytoskeleton

Cytoskeleton is a system of protein fibers that pervades the cytoplasm with analogous functions. It is composed of three distinct types of fibrous structures referred to as **microtubules, intermediate filaments** and **microfilaments**. Each of the three types of cytoskeletal filaments is a polymer of protein subunits held together by weak, non-covalent bonds. Each **cytoskeletal element** of different non-muscle cells, such as an epithelial cell, a nerve cell and a dividing cell, has distinct properties and **perform variety of functions** (Table 25.1).

1. It provides structural support that determines the shape of the cell and resists forces that tend to deform it.
2. It functions as an internal framework that is responsible for positioning various organelles within the interior of the cell.

Table 25.1. Properties of cytoskeletal elements

Properties	*Cytoskeletal elements*		
	Microtubules	*Intermediate filaments*	*Microfilaments (actin filaments)*
Structure	Stiff, hollow tube	Tough, ropelike fibers	Flexible, helical filament
Dimensions (diameter)	25 nm (outer)	10 nm	8 nm
Subunits	GTP.$\alpha\beta$-tubulin heterodimer	Globular proteins	ATP-actin monomers
Enzyme activity	GTPase	-	ATPase
Major group of associated proteins	Microtubule associated proteins	Plectin	Actin-binding proteins
Motor proteins	Kinesins, dyneins	-	Myosins
Primary functions	Support, intracellular transport, cell organization	Structural support	Motility, contractility

3. It provides a network of tracks that direct movement of materials and organelles within cells. For example, delivery of mRNA molecules to specific parts of a cell, movement of membranous carriers from the endoplasmic reticulum to the Golgi complex, etc.
4. It functions as the force-generating apparatus that moves cells from one place to another. For example, locomotion of sperm, white blood cells, fibroblasts, etc.
5. Cytoskeletal elements make up the apparatus that is responsible for separating the chromosomes during mitosis and meiosis and for splitting the parent cell into two daughter cells during cytokinesis.

MICROTUBULES

Microtubules are stiff, hollow, tubular structures, 25 nm in diameter, that are **assembled from the protein tubulin**. In addition to cytoskeleton, they also from a part of the **mitotic spindle, centrioles,** and **core of cilia and flagella.**

Microtubules are polymers assembled from αβ-tubulin heterodimers that are arranged in longitudinal rows, termed **protofilaments**. Tubulin dimmers that are polymerized into a microtubule contain a GTP molecule that is hydrolyzed soon after its incorporation into the polymer. Tubulin thus, has GTPase activity.

Functions of Microtubules

1. **Structural Supports and Organization :** Microtubules are stiff enough to resist forces that might compress or bend the fiber. The distribution of cytoplasmic microtubules in a cell helps determine the shape of that cell. For example, in maintaining position of the membranous organelles of the biosynthetic pathway, including the endoplasmic reticulum and Golgi complex.
2. **Intracellular Motility :** The transport of materials from one membrane to another depends on the presence of microtubules since specific disruption of these cytoskeletal elements brings the movements to a halt. For example, the movement of vesicles and other material between the cell body and axon terminals of a nerve cell.

The microtubules of the epithelial and nerve cells function primarily in support and organelle transport whereas the microtubules of the dividing cells form the mitotic spindle required for chromosome segregation.

Members of a group of microtubule-associated proteins (MAP), such as tau, influence many of the properties of microtubules, including their flexibility, stability and capabilities for interaction. An abnormally high level of phosphorylation of tau has been implicated in the development of several fatal neurodegenerative disorders.

Motor Proteins

Microtubules mediate the movement of molecules by serving as tracks for a variety of proteins called motor proteins that generate the forces required for moving objects within a cell.

Kinesins and **dyneins** are the families of motor proteins, which move along microtubules. These motor proteins are able to convert chemical energy stored in ATP into mechanical energy that is used to move cellular material attached to the motor. They move materials along microtubules in opposite directions. Kinesins moves materials toward the plus end of a microtubule, cytoplasmic dynein towards the minus end.

Kinesin has been implicated in the movement of endoplasmic reticulum-derived vesicles, endosomes, lysosomes and secretory granules and is the primary motor protein mediating anterograde transport in an axon (from cell body to axon terminus).

The function of microtubule within a living cell depends on its location and orientation. The assembly of microtubules from αβ-tubulin dimmers occurs in two distinct phases. These include a slow phase of nucleation in which a small portion of the microtubule is initially formed, and a much more rapid phase of elongation.

Nucleation of microtubules takes place rapidly inside a cell, where it occurs in association with a variety of specialized structures called microtubules–organizing centers, such as centrosomes, basal bodies, etc. All microtubule organizing centers control the number of microtubules, their polarity, the number of protofilaments that make up their walls, and the time and location of their assembly.

The microtubules of the cytoskeleton are dynamic polymers that are subjected to shortening, lengthening, disassembly and reassembly. Disassembly of the microtubular skeleton can be induced by a number of agents, including colchicin, cold temperature and elevated Ca^{2+} concentration.

INTERMEDIATE FILAMENTS

Intermediate filaments are strong rope-like fibers that are approximately 10 nm in diameter. Depending on the cell type, they may be composed of a variety of different globular protein subunits, capable of assembling into similar types of filaments. Intermediate filaments are often connected by long wispy cross-bridges consisting of fibrous protein called **plectin**.

The basic unit of intermediate filament is a tetramer formed by two dimmers, which may be homodimers or heterodimers. Neither ATP nor GTP is required for its assembly. The polypeptide sub-units of intermediate filaments can be divided into five major classes, which include **keratins, vimentin, desmin, neurofilamentins and lamin proteins**, based on the type of cell in which they are found as well as biochemical, genetic and immunologic criteria.

An inherited human disease, called desmin-related myopathy is caused by mutation in gene that encodes desmin. They are resistant to tensile forces and are relatively insoluble. Phosphorylation and dephosphorylation of the subunits control assembly and disassembly of most types of intermediate filaments. Intermediate filaments provide mechanical stability to cells that may be required for specialized tissue-specific functions. Intermediate filaments include keratin filaments and neurofilaments. **Keratin filaments** constitute the primary structural proteins of epithelial cells, including epidermal cells, liver hepatocytes and pancreatic acinar cells. The cytoplasm of neurons contains loosely packed bundles of intermediate filaments, called **neurofilaments**, whose long axes are oriented parallel to that of the nerve cell axon. Intermediate filaments have tissue specific functions, which are more important in some cells then in others.

MICROFILAMENTS

Microfilaments are 8 nm in diameter and composed of a **double helical polymer of the protein actin**. Actin is one of the major contractile proteins of muscle cells. In the presence of ATP, actin monomers polymerize to form a flexible, helical filament called actin filament or F-actin. They play a key role in virtually all types of contractility and motility within cells.

Depending on the type of cell and the activity, actin filaments can be organized into highly ordered arrays, loose ill-defined networks or tightly held bundles.

Assembly of microfilament : Before it is incorporated into a filament, an actin monomer binds a molecule of ATP. The ATP associated with the actin monomer is hydrolyzed to ADP after it is incorporated into the growing actin filament, as actin has ATPase activity. The bulk of an actin filament thus, consists of ADP-actin subunits.

The molecular motors of actin filaments : Members of myosin super-family are the molecular motors of actin filaments. Myosins are generally divided into two groups, the conventional myosins (myosin type II), which were first identified in muscle tissue and the unconventional myosins.

Myosin II is the molecular motor that generates force in various types of muscle tissues and also a variety of non-muscle activities, including cytokinesis. Myosin II molecules contain a long, rod-shaped tail attached at one end to two globular heads. The head binds at one end to two globular heads. The head binds the actin filament, hydrolyses ATP and undergoes the conformational changes required for force generation. Most unconventional myosins have a single head and variable tail domains. They have been implicated in cell motility and organelle transport.

MUSCLE CONTRACTION

Muscles form a large proportion of the **active tissues** of the body. In a normal adult, though muscle mass is nearly **40% of the body weight**, metabolically it is a highly active tissue and performs more than 50% of the total metabolic activities.

Structure of Skeletal Muscle

The **voluntary muscles** which include the **skeleton muscle** have a **stariated (stripped) appearance.** Such muscles consist of **long, thin, multinucleated cells** known as **muscle fibres that** run along the length of the muscle.

The muscle fibres are nearly 0.01 to 0.1 nm in diameter and 1 to 40 nm in length. A large number of these fibres are **bound together by areolar connective tissue** and are attached via tendons to the bone **or other structures whose movement** they control. Muscle fibres are packed in an **elastic sheet** known as **sarco-lemma** which also has several **nuclei** and **mitochondria.**

The sarcolemma is an **electrically excitable membrane** and is important in the **transport of motor nerve impulses.** It **also contains** a large number of **transport ducts** called **sarcotubules.** Sarcolemma also contains **sarcoplasmic reticulum,** similar in structure and functions to the endoplasmic reticulum found in other cells.

Bundles of muscle fibres are surrounded by the **sarcoplasm** which may be called as **muscle plasma.** Sarcoplasm is **semifluid** in nature and contains **myoglobin**, similar to hemoglobin present in red blood cells.

Myoglobin transports oxygen from blood capillaries to the site of oxidation.

MYOFIBRILS

Muscle fibres contain parallel bundles of myofibrils (Greek: myos means muscle). Major features of the myofibril are that, it has a light band called as the isotropic band (I band) which contains thin filaments and a dark band, designated as anisotropic band (A band) which has a central H zone containing thick filaments and an outer segment with the over-lapping thick and thin filaments. I band is bisected by a dark zone (present in the centre of I band), called as the Z line.

The functional unit of a myofibril is known as sarcomere (Greek: sarkos means flesh). It is a region between two successive Z lines (present at the center of each I band), i.e. the region comprising of one-half of I band, the A band and one half of the next I band.

A band is formed of a large number of thick filaments whereas I band is composed of a comparable number of thin filaments which are interspaced between the thick filaments. Two sets of the filaments, in turn, are linked by cross-bridges in the area where they overlap (Fig. 25.1)

Thin filament slide over the thick filaments, as a result muscle contraction leads to a decrease in length of the sarcomere, caused by a reduction in distance between the I band and the H zone. The length of the thick filaments and the thin filaments however, remain constant. A contracted muscle thus is reduced to nearly two-third of its fully extended length (Fig 25.2)

Composition of the Skeletal Muscle

Adult muscle is 70-80% water.

Besides, muscle also contains nearly 20% proteins and 3% lipids (with variable amounts of triacylglycerol, cholesterol and phospholipids).

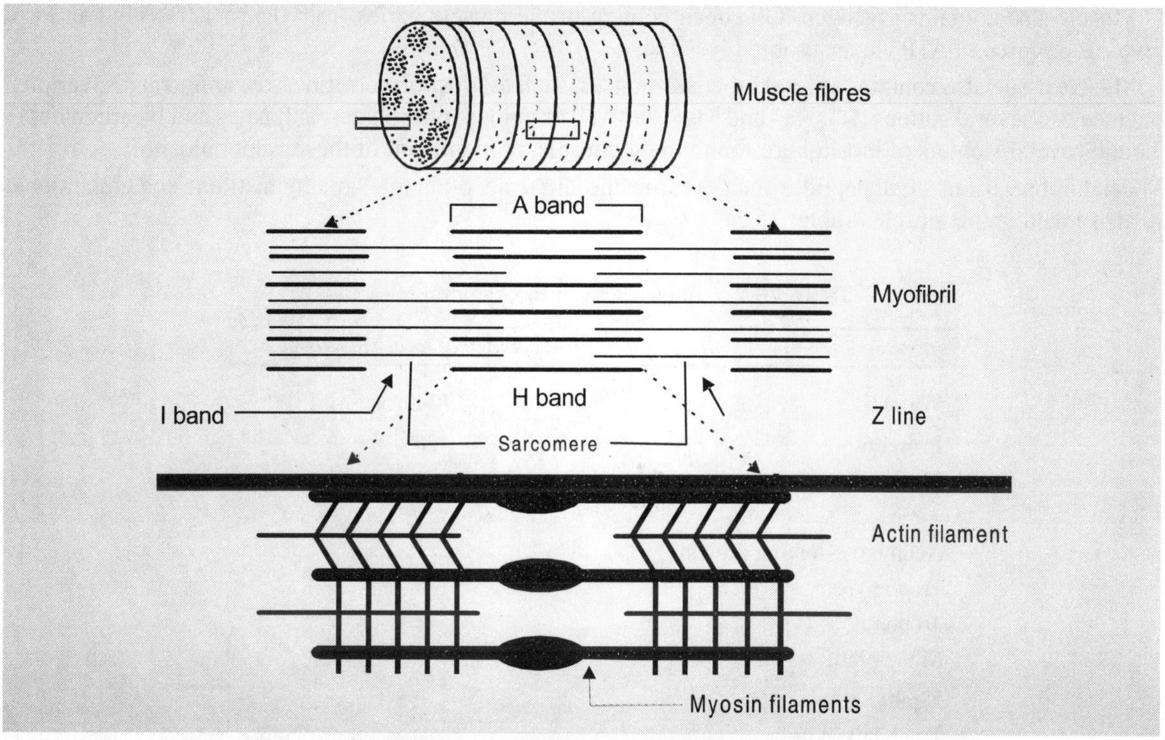

Fig. 25.1. Structure of myofibrils.

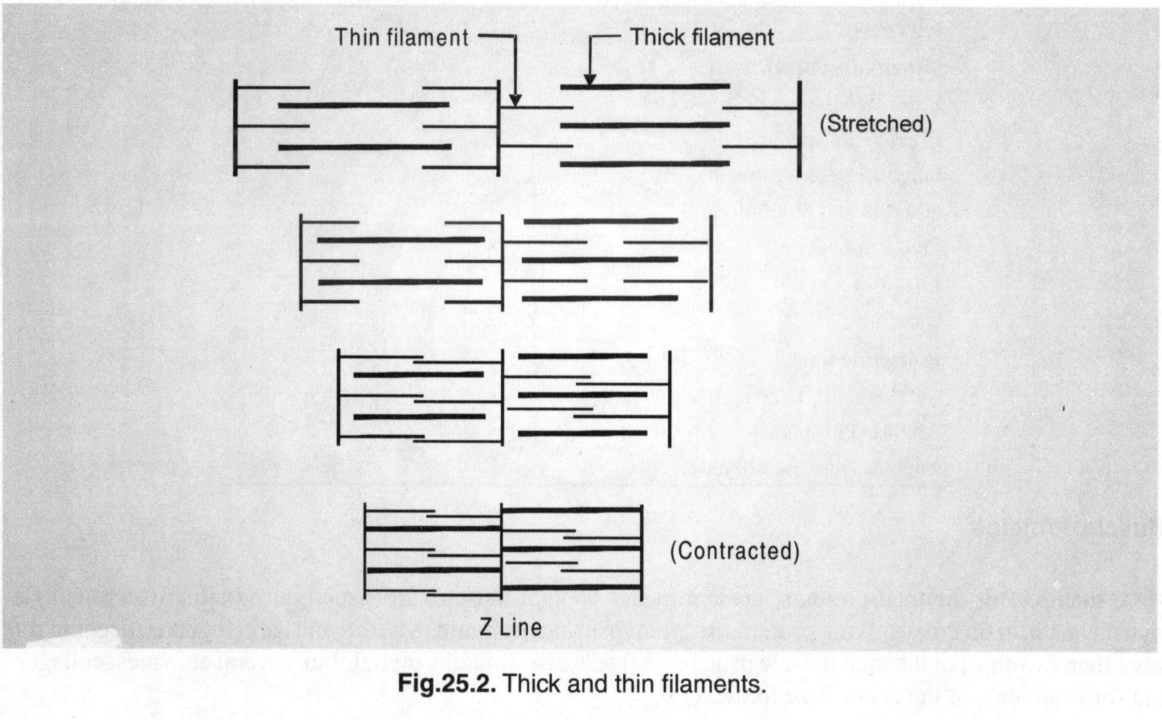

Fig.25.2. Thick and thin filaments.

Muscle also contains glycogen. Glycogen content of the muscle varies from 0.5 to 1.0%. This in turn serves as a source of ATP via anaerobic glycolysis.

Muscle tissue also contains several other substances, such as inositol, carnitine, free amino acids, various enzymes and several cations (K^+, Na^+ and Mg^{2+}) as well as anions (phosphates, sulphates and bicarbonates). Though several isomers of inositol are found in the muscle, predominant of these is myoinositol.

In addition various small peptides such as carnosine, anserine, β-alanyl-3-methylhistidine and glutathione are also found in the muscle (Table: 25.2).

Table 25.2. Composition of the skeletal muscle

Ingredients	*Percentage of total muscle mass*
Water	70-80%
Proteins	20%
Myosin	
Actin	
Actin cross-linking proteins	
Tropomyosin	
Troponin	
Myoglobin	
Lipids	3%
Triacylglycerol	
Cholesterol	
Phospholipids	
Glycogen	0.5-1.0%
Other substances	
Inositol (Myoinositol)	
Creatinephosphate	
Oligopeptides (carnosine, anserine and glutathione)	
Free amino acids	
Enzymes	
Carnitine	
Inorganic ions	
Cations (Na^+, K^+, Mg^{2+})	
Anions (Phosphates, sulphates and bicarbonate)	

Muscle Proteins

More than half of the total proteins, present in the skeletal muscle, are structural proteins which include myosin, actin, actin cross-linking proteins, tropomyosin and troponin. Myosin and actin together, account for more than two-third of the total muscle proteins. Muscle also contains myoglobin, several enzymes, collagen and some proteins of the connective tissue.

Myosin

Thick filaments are composed, almost entirely of myosin, which are placed 'end-to-end' with the light chains, striking out in the form of double heads.

Myosin consists of six polypeptide chains which include two identical heavy chains and two pairs of two different types of the light chains.

Two types of the light chains are described as regulatory light chains and essential light chains.

Each myosin head associates with an essential light chain and a regulatory light chain.

Regulatory light chains play a role in the control of muscle contraction by Ca^{2+} ions whereas the essential light chains are required for ATPase activity of the myosin head. Thus, both types of light chains are involved in the regulation of muscle contraction.

The N-terminal half of each of the heavy chain forms an elongated globular head to which one subunit, each of the two light chains binds. The C-terminal half of the heavy chain forms a long fibrous α-helical tail, two of which associate to form a left-handed coil. Taken together, a molecule of myosin, thus, consists of a long rod like segment with two globular heads (Fig. 25.3).

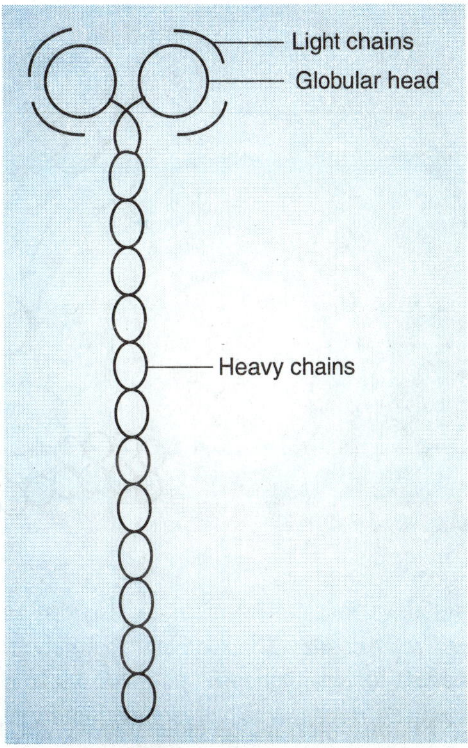

Fig. 25.3. A molecule of myosin.

Actin

Actin is a globulin and is a major constituent of thin filaments of the sarcomere. Actin exists in two forms, i.e. as G actin and as filament actin (F actin).

G actin is a low molecular weight monomeric protein (molecular weight nearly 42 kD) with a globular configuration. These monomers readily form large, elongated actin filament polymers called F actin.

For assembly of the G actin monomeric units into a polymeric F actin, Mg^{2+} ions are essential.

Besides monomeric G actin units are oriented in such a way that they acquire a pointed-region (pointed-end) and a barbed-region (barbed-end). Assembly of the monomeric units occurs at the barbed-end. A group of proteins called parafilins bind to G actin, stabilize the monomers and prevent their polymerisation.

F actin thus is a polymerized form of G actin. It contains nearly 1000 monomeric units which are organized as a string of beads. F actin filaments are made up of two strings of the G actin monomers (Fig. 25.4).

Actin is ubiquitous and is usually a most abundant cytoplasmic protein in eukaryotic cells, typically accounting for 5 to 10% of the total proteins. Though actin is most prominent in the muscle, it also exists in other tissues where it is responsible for various motile processes, such as cell locomotion, cytoplasmic streaming and cytokinesis (separation of the daughter cells, during cell division). The non-muscle actin forms fibres which are designated as microfilaments. Along with the other protein fibres, these microfilaments form elements of the cytoskeleton. Assembly of the actin monomers, into the fibres, requires ATP.

Actin Cross-Linking Proteins

There are some proteins that cross-link and stabilize actin chains. These include filamin, α-actinin and β-actinin.

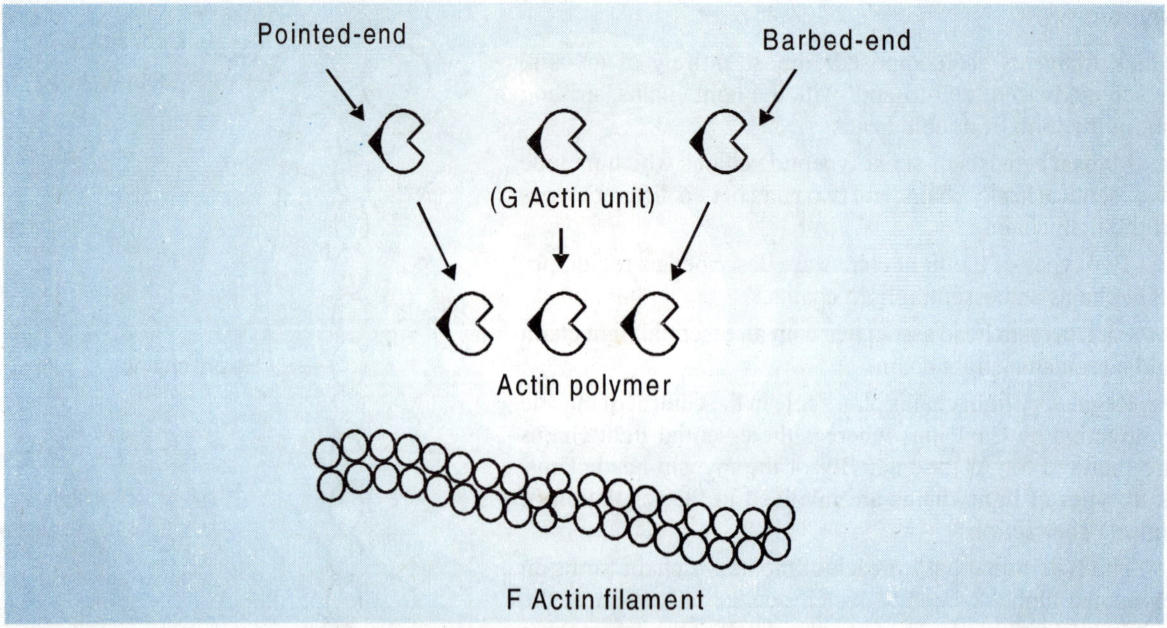

Fig.25.4. Assembly of F actin filament.

Filamin : It is a high molecular weight, flexible protein that usually exists as a dimer. It binds to actin at nearly 40 nm intervals.

α-Actinin: It is mainly located in Z line of the muscle fibres and has a role in spacing of the actin filaments.

β-Actinin: It acts as a capping protein and thus is also called as actin capping protein. It binds to the active site of the G actin monomer, so that the monomer is unable to combine with another monomer. It thus stabilises G monomers and prevents their polymerization.

Tropomyosin

Tropomyosin is a double-stranded, α-helical protein, with a molecular weight of about 70 kD. It is intervened between the two helical strands of F actin, i.e. tropomyosin molecules attach end to end and form a thin filament on each strand of the actin molecule.

One tropomyosin molecule extends over seven actin molecules whereas 300-400 actin molecules are contained in each filament of the skeletal muscle (which is about 1μm in length).

Troponin

Troponin is a spherical molecule, with a molecular weight of about 70 kD. It is positioned at regular intervals along the actin filaments.

Troponin is composed of three different types of subunits, called troponin-T, troponin-I and troponin-C.

Troponin-T : It binds the other two subunits to the tropomyosin molecules, non-covalently.

Tropmyosin-troponin complex in turn regulates muscle contraction, by controlling access of the myosin heads on the thick filaments, to their binding sites on the actin.

Troponin-I: It is the inhibitory subunit. Its function is to inhibit the interaction of the head of myosin with actin, thereby preventing contraction of myofibrils.

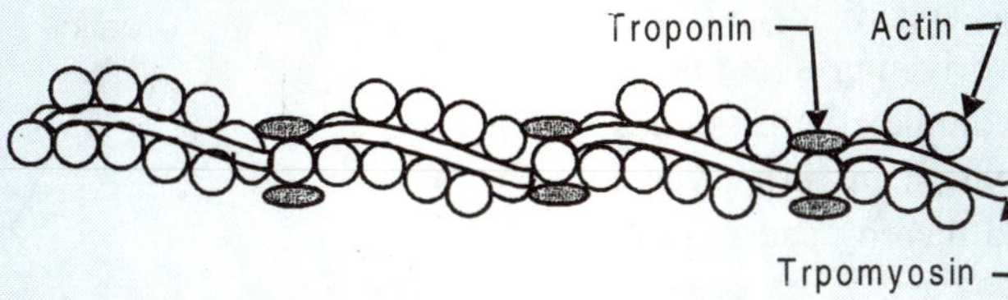

Fig.25.5. Thin filament.

Troponin-C: It is a Ca^{2+} binding protein and is rich in aspartate and glutamate.

Troponin C can also competitively bind Mg^{2+} ions.

Thin filaments consist of chains of the actin molecules with the associated tropomyosin and troponin molecules (Fig.25.5).

Biochemical Changes during Muscle Contraction

Impulses, transmitted via motor nerve (across the neuromuscular junction to the sarcolemma of the muscle fibre), initiates contraction of myofibrils. This in turn stimulates the release of Ca^{2+} ions which binds to troponin-C of the thin actin filament and produces a configurational change in it. This is followed by shift of the tropomyosin and leads to attachment of cross-bridges of the thick myosin filaments to the thin actin filaments.

ATP binds to special receptor sites on the surface of the myosin. The tendency for ATP to bind is so efficient that under normal conditions, almost every myosin head is bound to ATP. Formation of the charged myosin.ATP complex alters conformation of the protein in a manner that the charged complex has a greater tendency to bind to an actin molecule. After myosin.ATP complex binds to actin, ATP binds to a myosin head whose ATPase action causes hydrolysis of ATP. This in turn puts the myosin head into a high-energy conformation. The myosin head is now weak to bind to actin monomer that is closer to the A line. This in turn results in the release of inorganic phosphate (Pi). The release of Pi further causes a conformational shift and increases the affinity of myosin for actin. The resulting transient state is immediately followed by the power stroke; causing a further conformational shift that sweeps myosin head's C-terminal tail towards the Z line, ADP is then released, thereby completing the cycle.

Myosin heads walk or row-up the adjacent thin filaments, towards the Z line with the concomitant, contraction of the muscle, i.e. the actin filaments slide along the thick myosin filaments (which otherwise were stationary), towards the centre of the sarcomere, thereby shortening its size. These events occur so rapidly that the whole process of muscle contraction takes only 10-20 milliseconds.

At the end of the neuromusculatory phase, Ca^{2+} ions are drawn back into the sacroplasmic reticulum network and cross-bridges of the myosin retract. As a result of it, the sarcomeres and the muscle fibres relax and return to the resting state.

In the low-energy state, the complex remains intact until a new molecule of ATP is bound, usually occurring within a very short time (about 1 millisecond in a normal muscle).

The sequence continues, depending upon the supply of ATP and other components, essential for the muscle contraction.

Control of Muscle Contraction

The stimulation of a myofibril by nerve impulse, as mentioned above, results in an influx of Ca^{2+} from the sarcoplasmic reticulum. As a result of it, intracellular Ca^{2+} concentration increases. At higher concentration, additional Ca^{2+} binds to troponin C, thereby causing a conformational change in the troponin-tropomyosin complex. The movement of Ca^{2+} exposes the site on actin where myosin head binds. When myofibril Ca^{2+}

concentration is low, Ca^{2+} is specifically ejected from the myofibril, by ATP-driven protein pump. The troponin-tropomyosin complex then assumes its resting conformation which in turn blocks myosin binding to actin and thereby causing the muscle to relax.

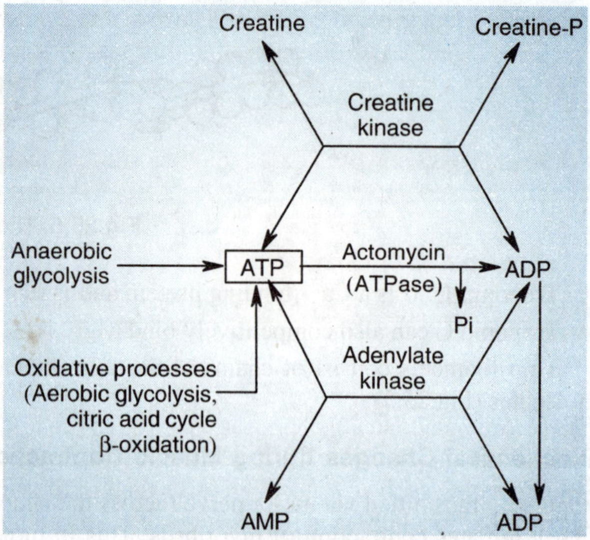

Fig.25.6. Regeneration of ATP in muscle.

Regeneration of ATP

The energy for muscle contraction, as discussed above, is provided by ATP which is hydrolysed to ADP and Pi.

ATP can be regenerated, in the muscle by several routes (Fig.25.6).

1. ***By Lohman's reaction:*** ATP can be regenerated by utilizing high-energy phosphate compound, creatine phosphate. This reation is catalyzed by creatine kinase (creatine phosphokinase or CPK) and is called as the Lohman's reaction.

$$\text{ADP + Creatinephosphate} \xleftrightarrow{\text{Creatinine kinase}} \text{ATP + Creatinine}$$

2. ***By adenylate kinase reaction:*** ATP can also be regenerated from ADP by the enzyme adenylate kinase, which is also referred to as myokinase.

$$\text{ADP + ADP} \xleftrightarrow{\text{Adenylate kinase}} \text{ATP + AMP}$$

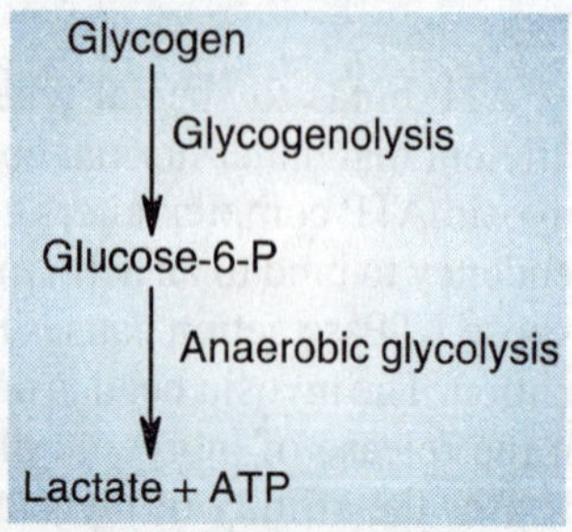

Fig. 25.7. ATP generation from anaerobic glycolysis.

3. ***From anaerobic glycolysis:*** Muscles also possess the capacity to synthesize ATP under anaerobic conditions by utilizing its glycogen stores (Fig.25.7).

   A limited supply of oxygen, i.e. a short period of strenuous exercise, in turn results in the accumulation of large amount of lactate, in the blood.

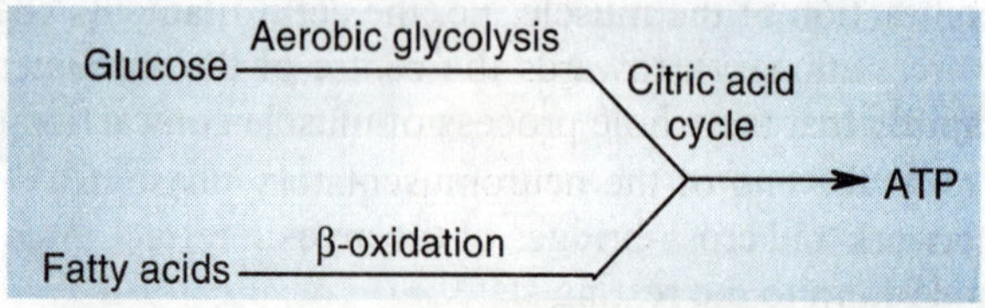

Fig. 25.8. ATP generation from oxidative processes.

4. ***By oxidative processes:*** Prolonged exercise gradually increases oxygenation of the muscle to a maximum. Thus ATP may also be produced by various oxidative processes, such as from aerobic glycolysis followed by the citric acid cycle, and from β-oxidation of fatty acids (Fig.25.8).

Types of Muscle Fibres

It is known that human muscles generally contain two types of the muscle fibres. These muscle fibres contain different isomers of the myosin molecule whose relative proportions, however, vary with the exercise, electric stimulation, thyroxine content and growth:

1. ***Type I muscle fibres:*** There are also referred as the red muscle fibres. They have a large number of mitochondria and thus have high oxidative capacity. They can regenerate ATP by aerobic metabolism of, both glucose and fatty acids. These muscle fibres are also resistant to fatigue.
2. ***Type II muscle fibres:*** These are also referred as white muscle fibres.

These muscle fibres possess very few mitochondria and thus have a low oxidative capacity. These can regenerate ATP by metabolizing glycogen stores, by the process of anaerobic glycolsis.

MUSCULAR DYSTROPHY

Muscular dystrophy refers to a group of **hereditary progressive diseases**, each with unique phenotypic and genetic features, which cripple and kill children, such as **Duchenne muscular dystrophy**.

This is an X-linked recessive disorder present at birth but usually becomes apparent between age 3 and 5. By age 5, muscle weakness is obvious by muscle testing. The disease is **caused by a mutation of the gene that encodes a protein dystrophin** and is localized to the inner surface of sarcolemma of the muscle fiber.

Serum creatine kinase (CPK) **levels are invariably elevated** to between 20 and 100 times normal. The levels are abnormal at birth but decline as the disease progresses because of inactivity and loss of muscle mass.

SOME IMPORTANT QUESTIONS

1. Describe the structure and composition of skeletal muscle.
2. Describe various functions of proteins present in the skeletal muscle.
3. Describe:
   (i) Structure of the striated muscle
   (ii) Events during muscle contraction
   (iii) Types of muscle fibres
   (iv) Regeneration of ATP in the muscle
4. Write notes on:
   (i) Sarcomere
   (ii) Actin
   (iii) Myosin
   (iv) Troponin
   (v) Control of muscle contraction
   (vi) Cytoskeleton
   (vii) Microtubules
   (viii) Microfilaments
   (ix) Muscular dystrophy

CHAPTER

26

Hemoglobin Metabolism

Hemoglobin is a globular protein, **which is** present in **high concentration in** red blood cells. A molecule of **hemoglobin consists of four heme groups along with the four-polypeptide chains,** which are synthesized separately and subsequently, bind to four heme groups. **It** binds oxygen **in the lungs and transports it to different cells in the body.**

FUNCTIONS OF HEMOGLOBIN

- Most important function of hemoglobin is the transport of gases, i.e. O_2 from the lungs to the tissues, and CO_2 from the tissues to the lungs. Binding of O_2 with hemoglobin is referred to as oxygenation while delivery of O_2 from oxyhemoglobin is designated as deoxygenation.
- **Hemoglobin also** transports CO_2 and H^+ **from the tissues to the lungs.**
- **It also** carries and releases nitric oxide (NO) in the blood vessels of the tissues.

TRANSPORT OF O_2 FROM LUNGS TO TISSUES

Each heme molecule in the hemoglobin has an atom of iron. Iron in heme is present in the ferrous (Fe^{2+}) form. It is linked to the four nitrogen atoms of the four-pyrrole rings of porphyrin. Since each polypeptide, of the globin subunit, contains one molecule of heme, which is positioned with in a hydrophobic pocket of the globin subunit, and that a molecule of **hemoglobin** has four monomeric subunits, thus, it **has four heme-binding sites for O_2.** Fe^{2+} is **also linked,** through a coordinate bond, **to one of the imidazole nitrogen of the proximal histidine** (His F8).

After O_2 binds to hemoglobin, it forms sixth coordinate bond with the Fe^{2+} atom. O_2 gets placed between the Fe^{2+} atom and to the nitrogen of the imidazole ring of another histidine, designated as distal histidine (His E7).

Binding of O_2 to the Fe^{2+} **triggers conformational change in the hemoglobin molecule.** This is **also referred to as the relaxed (R) conformational state.**

After delivery of O_2 sixth coordinate position of the Fe^{2+} atom becomes vacant (unoccupied). This is called deoxyhemoglobin. Deoxy-conformation of the hemoglobin is referred to as tense (T) conformational state.

T and R conformational equilibrium of hemoglobin **controls delivery of O_2 to the tissues and transport of CO_2 away from the tissues. This equilibrium** between the T and the R State is **regulated by H^+ concentration. H^+ is released when T conformation is converted to R.**

Thus, affinity of oxygen for hemoglobin is affected by pH. It decreases as the pH becomes more acidic.

Increase in acidity of hemoglobin (as it binds O_2), or increase in basicity (as it releases oxygen) **is referred to as Bohr Effect.** It may be expressed by the following equation:

$$H.Hb + O_2 \rightleftharpoons HbO_2 + H^+$$

It suggests that an increase in H^+ concentration favors release of oxygen from oxyhemoglobin. Conversely, oxygenation of hemoglobin lowers pH of the solution.

TRANSPORT OF CO_2 FROM TISSUES TO LUNGS

Transport of CO_2 from the tissues to the lungs (for its removal) along with the transport of O_2 from lungs to tissues is linked with protons generated Bohr effect. This is achieved by two mechanisms, i.e. isohydric transport of CO_2 as HCO_3^-, and carbaminohemoglobin.

Isohydric Transport of CO_2 as Bicarbonate

Metabolizing cells utilize O_2 and produce CO_2, which diffuses from the cells of the tissues to red blood cells. Within red blood cells, CO_2 is dissolved in water and converted to H_2CO_3, by the enzyme carbonic anhydrase. Spontaneously, carbonic acid is dissociated to HCO_3^- and H^+. H^+, which dissociates from carbonic acid, binds to deoxyhemoglobin, forcing the equilibrium from oxyhemoglobin to deoxyhemoglobin with the dissociation of O_2, which diffuses out of the red blood cells of the tissues. HCO_3^- is transported (in plasma) to the lungs (Fig. 26.1A).

In the lungs, high O_2 pressure forces the reaction in the opposite direction. It promotes conversion of deoxyhemoglobin to oxyhemoglobin. During this process, H^+ are dissociated and combine with HCO_3^- to reform carbonic acid. Carbonic anhydrase now dissociates H_2CO_3 to CO_2 and H_2O. CO_2 diffuses out of the blood, into the lung alveoli, and is expired into air (Fig. 26.1B).

About 80% of the cellular CO_2 is transported from the tissues to the lungs by this mechanism, i.e. as HCO_3^-. This is called isohydric transport of CO_2.

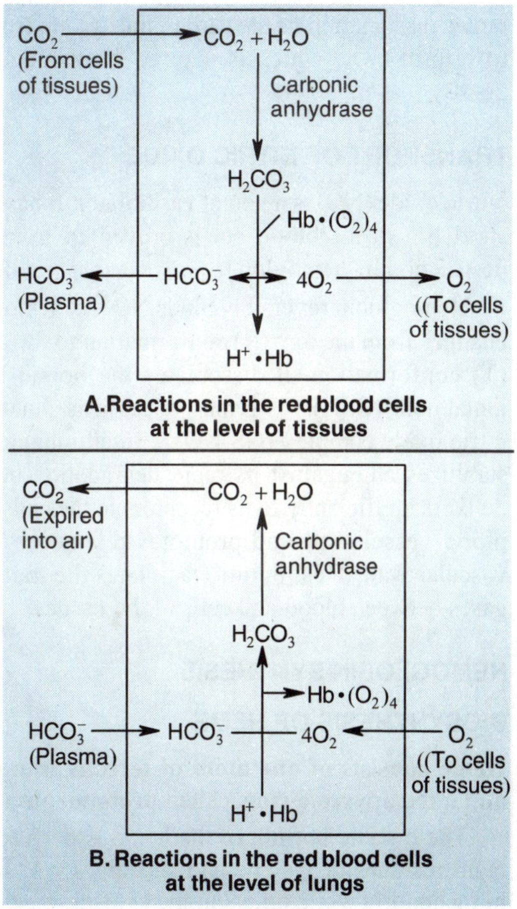

Fig 26.1. Isohydric transport of CO_2 as bicarbonate.

Transport of CO_2 as Carbaminohemoglobin

Hemoglobin also transports nearly 15–20% of CO_2 by another mechanism, referred to as carbaminohemoglobin.

From the cells of the tissues CO_2 diffuses into the red blood cells, in capillaries of tissues, and reacts with the NH_2-terminal amino groups of hemoglobin polypeptide chains forming carbaminohemoglobin (Fig. 26.2).

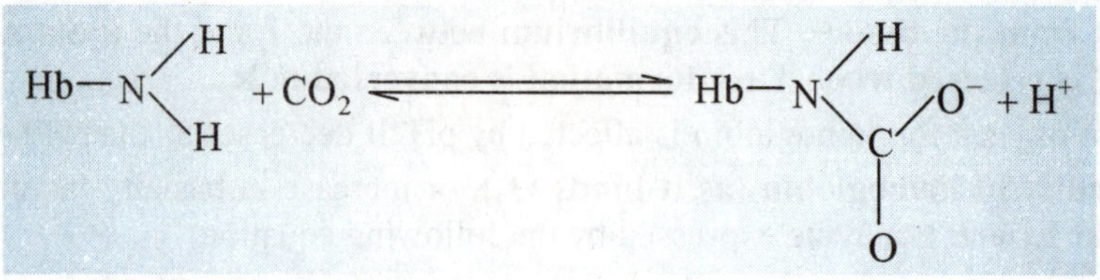

Fig. 26.2.

This reaction also produces H^+, which promotes dissociation of O_2 from hemoglobin that is diffused out of the red blood cells to the tissues (Fig. 26.3A).

In the lungs, high O_2 pressure forces these reactions in the opposite direction. This, in turn, leads to the expiration of CO_2 from lungs. Free H^+ thus, promotes dissociation of the carbamino- group from Hb, to reform CO_2, which is expired from lungs (Fig. 26.3B).

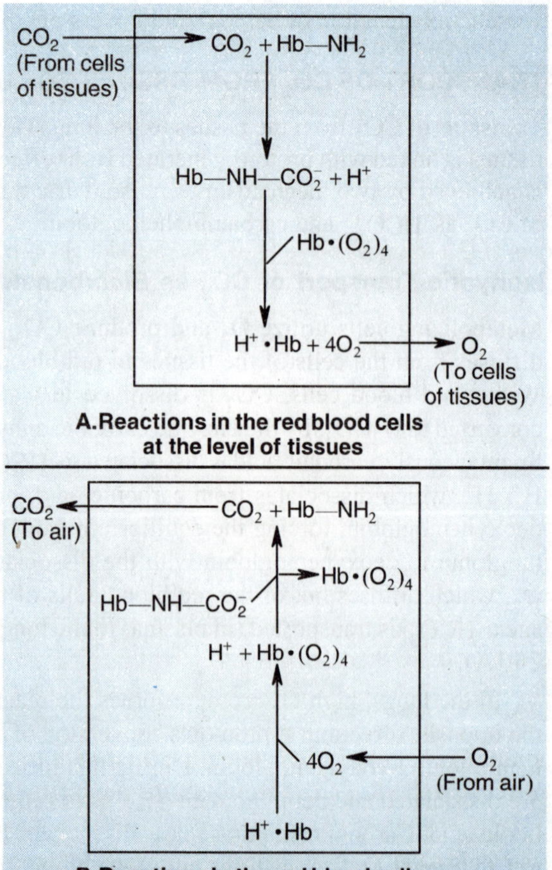

A. Reactions in the red blood cells at the level of tissues

B. Reactions in the red blood cells at the level of lungs

Fig. 26.3. Transport of CO_2 as carbamino hemoglobin.

TRANSPORT OF NITRIC OXIDE

Nitric oxide (NO) is a potent vasodilator. It has a very short life in the blood but is prevented from rapid destruction by hemoglobin.

Hemoglobin reversibly binds NO. As hemoglobin changes from the oxy (R) conformation to the deoxy-(T) conformation, it dissociates the bound NO to glutathione (GSH). NO is thus, released as glutathione-nitric oxide complex (GS-NO). Glutathione not only stabilizes NO against its rapid degradation but also delivers it efficiently to its receptors in the cells of the blood vessel wall and promotes relaxation of the vascular wall. This, in turn, facilitates the transfer of gases between blood and cells of the tissues.

HEMOGLOBIN SYNTHESIS

BIOSYNTHESIS OF HEME

Heme consists of one atom of ferrous iron (Fe^{2+}) **and a tetrapyrrole ring,** called **protoporphyrin IX.**

The organic portion of the heme is derived from eight residues of glycine and succinyl CoA. In the biosynthesis of heme, some of the reactions occur in mitochondria while others in the cytosol.

1. In the first step, **succinyl CoA condenses with glycine** and **forms δ-aminolevulinic acid** (ALA), in the mitochondria.

$$\text{Glycine} + \text{Succinyl CoA} \xrightarrow[\text{PLP} \quad \searrow \text{CoA} \quad \searrow CO_2]{\text{ALA synthase}} \delta\text{-Aminolevulinic acid}$$

This reaction is catalyzed by the enzyme δ-aminolevulinic acid synthase (ALA synthase), which requires pyridoxal phosphate (PLP) as a coenzyme. **This is the rate-limiting step of heme synthesis.**

Increased levels of ALA synthase along with the reduced levels of some enzymes of the heme biosynthetic pathway result in a group of disorders referred to as porphyrias.

Porphyria is due to abnormality in the pathway of heme biosynthesis. It may be genetic or acquired. **Six major types of porphyria have been described,** five of which are inherited as autosomal dominant (Table 26.1).

2. In the next step, **two molecules of δ-aminolevulinic acid** condense, asymmetrically, **and form porphobilinogen.**

   This **reaction is catalyzed by the enzyme aminolevulinic acid dehydratase** (ALA dehydratase).

$$\delta\text{-Aminolevulinic acid} \xrightarrow[\searrow 2H_2O]{\text{ALA-dehydratase}} \text{Porphobilinogen}$$

   ALA dehydratase is a zinc-containing enzyme, which occurs in the cytosol. It consists of eight subunits, four of which interact with the substrate.

   ALA dehydratase is sensitive to heavy metals particularly, **lead.** ALA levels increase in lead poisoning.

3. **Porphobilinogen** undergoes **deamination, by the enzyme porphobilinogen deaminase** (hydroxymethylbilane synthase or uroporphyrinogen I synthase), and is converted to a linear tetrapyrrole, called hydroxymethylbilane.

$$\text{Porphobilinogen} \xrightarrow{\text{Porphobilinogen deaminase}} \text{Hydroxymethylbilane}$$

Table 26.1. Derangement in porphyrin metabolism in different types of porphyria

Porphyria	*Enzyme defect*	*Major symptoms*	*Laboratory findings*
Acute intermittent porphyria	Increased ALA synthase, decreased porphobilinogen deaminase	Abdominal pain, neuropsychiatric symptoms	Urinary porphobilinogen (+)
Erythropoietic porphyria	Decreased uroporphyrinogen III synthase	No photosensitivity	Porphobilinogen (–), uroporphyrin (+)
Porphyria cutanea tarda	Decreased uroporphyrinogen decarboxylase	Photosensitivity	Porphobilinogen (–), uroporphyrin (+)
Hereditary coproporphyria	Increased ALA synthase, decreased coproporphyrinogen oxidase	Photosensitivity, abdominal pain, neuropsychiatric symptoms	Urinary porphobilinogen (+), urinary uroporphyrin (+), fecal protoporphyrin (+)
Variegate porphyria	Increased ALA synthase, decreased protoporphyrinogen oxidase	Photosensitivity, abdominal pain, neuropsychiatric symptoms	Urinary porphobilinogen (+), fecal protoporphyrin (–)
Hereditary protoporphyria	Decreased ferrochelatase	Photosensitivity	Fecal protoporphyrin (–), red cell protoporphyrin (+)

Decreased activity of porphobilinogen deaminase along with the increased activity of ALA synthase results in a condition called **acute intermittent porphyria.**

4. **Spontaneously, with ring closure, hydroxymethylbilane is converted to uroporphyrinogen I.**

   Alternatively, uroporphyrinogen III synthase converts hydroxymethylbilane to uroporphyrinogen III (Fig. 26.4)

   Only, type I and type III isomers are found in nature.

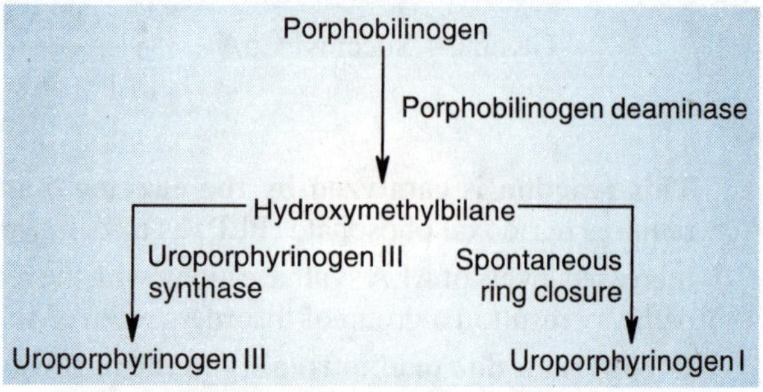

Fig. 26.4. Synthesis of uroporphyrinogens.

Porphyrins having symmetric arrangement of the substituent groups on four-pyrrol rings are designated as type I while those having **asymmetric substitutions** are referred to as **type III** (Fig. 26.5).

Under normal conditions, uroporphyrinogen formed is, almost exclusively, type III. Heme is also a type III porphyrin.

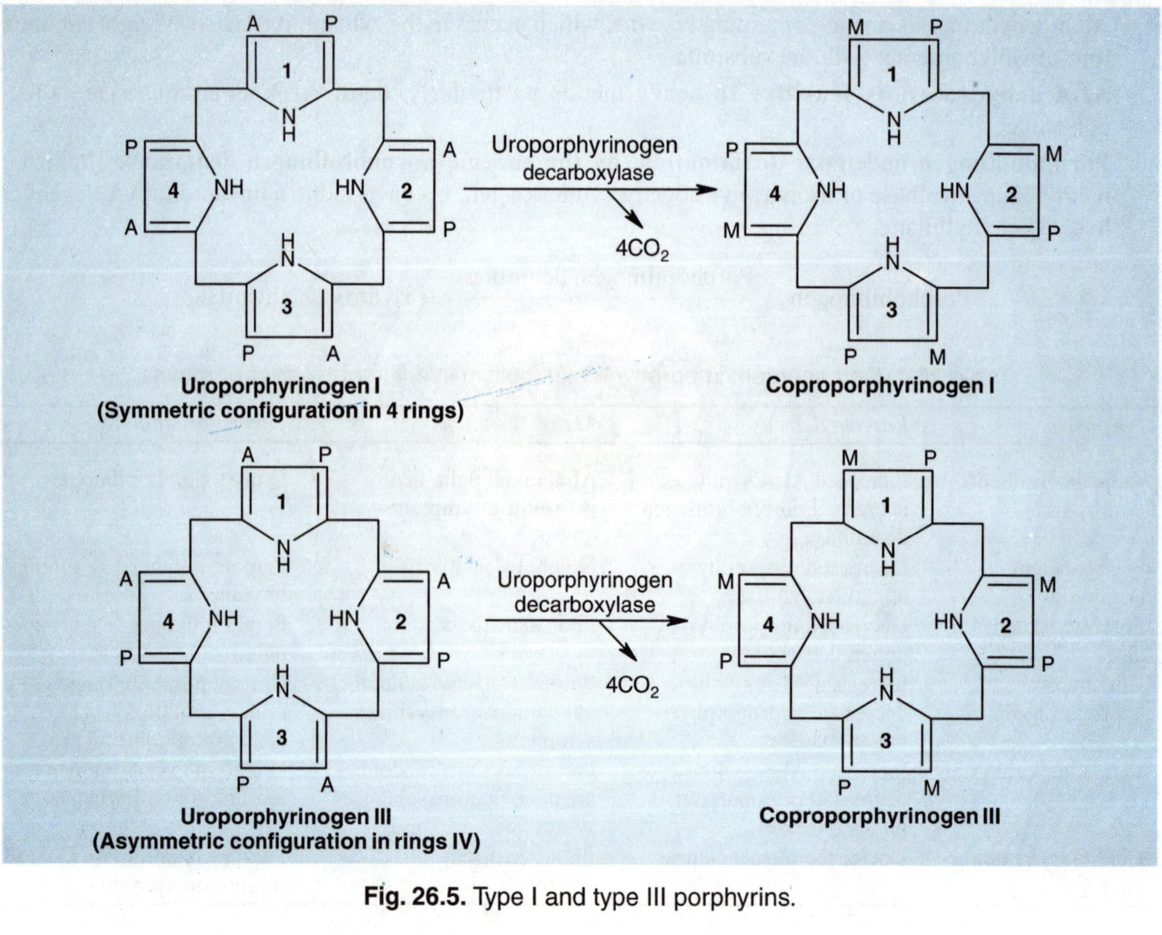

Fig. 26.5. Type I and type III porphyrins.

Abnormality of the reticulocyte uroporphyrinogen III synthase causes an inherited disease called erythropoietic porphria. It is associated with marked cutaneous light sensitization, and increased synthesis of uroporphyrinogen I and coproporphyrinogen I in the bone marrow.

5. **Uroporphyrinogen I and III are converted to the respective coproporphyrinogens by the enzyme uroporphyrinogen decarboxylase** (Fig. 26.5).

   Iron salts inhibit uroporphyrinogen decarboxylase.

   Genetic **deficiency of uroporphyrinogen decarboxylase leads to** a disease, known as **porphyria cutanea tarda,** which shows cutaneous manifestations, primarily, sensitivity to light. The manifestation is expressed in-patients who take drugs that cause an increase in porphyrin synthesis, or in individuals who consume large amount of alcohol. This, in turn, leads to accumulation of iron, which further inhibits uroporphyrinogen decarboxylase.

6. In the next reaction, **coproporphyrinogen III** enters the mitochondria and **is converted to protoporphyrinogen IX** (Fig. 26.6).

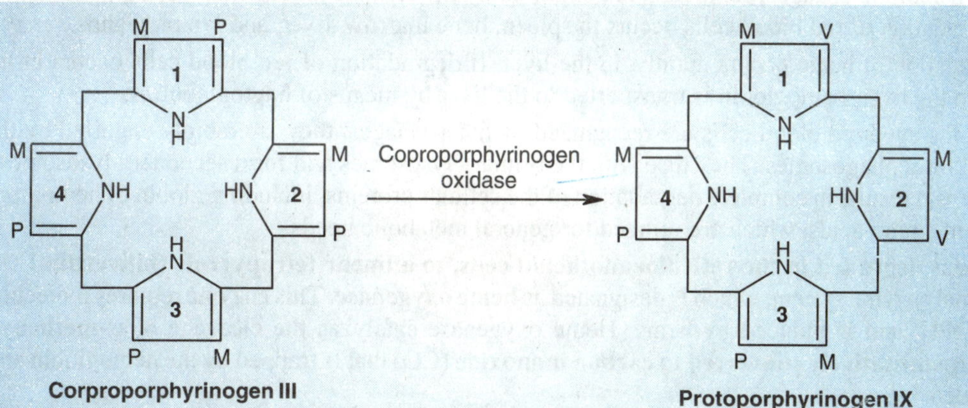

Fig. 26.6. Formation of protoporphyrinogen IX.

This reaction is catalyzed by the enzyme coproporphyrinogen oxidase, which requires molecular oxygen. This enzyme does not act on coproporphyrinogen I.

(These porphyrins are identified as IX since they were designated ninth in a series of the postulated isomers.)

Inherited **deficiency of** the enzyme **coproporphyrinogen oxidase leads to** a form of the hepatic porphyria, known as **hereditary coproporphyria.**

7. **Protoporphyrinogen oxidase acts on protoporphyrinogen IX and converts it to protoporphyrin IX,** in the mitochondria.

$$\text{Protoporphyrinogen IX} \xrightarrow{\text{Protoporphyrinogen oxidase}} \text{Protoporphyrin IX}$$

Protoporphyrin IX is water insoluble. Its excessive amounts are excreted by the biliary system into the intestinal tract. **Deficiency of the enzyme, protoporphyrinogen oxidase, leads to a condition called variegate porphyria.**

8. In the final step of heme synthesis, **ferrous iron (Fe^{2+}) is incorporated into protoporphyrin IX. This reaction is catalyzed by the enzyme ferrochelatase,** which requires some reducing substances.

$$\text{Protoporphyrin IX} \xrightarrow{\text{Ferrochelatase}} \text{Heme}$$

This enzyme is sensitive to heavy metals especially, lead. It is also sensitive to iron deprivation.

Inherited **deficiency of the enzyme ferrochelatase** results in a disease referred to as **hereditary protoporphyria.**

Regulation of Heme Biosynthesis

ALA synthase occurs in two forms. These are called **hepatic (ALA-S1)** and **erythrocytic (ALA-S2)** enzymes.

ALA-S1 controls the rate-limiting step of heme synthesis. Further, **heme acts** both, **as a repressor of synthesis of the enzyme as well as its inhibitor.**

HEMOGLOBIN DEGRADATION

Red blood cells have limited life span of approximately 100-120 days. These senescent cells are recognized by their membrane changes, removed, and engulfed by the reticuloendothelial system, at the extravascular site. Degradation of red blood cells occurs in spleen, bone marrow, liver, and lymph glands.

Degradation of heme occurs mainly, in the liver. If degradation of red blood cells occurs in the tissues other than the liver, hemoglobin is transported to the liver by means of haptoglobulins.

After the aged red blood cells are recognized by macrophages, they are rapidly engulfed by the phagocytes and form phagosomes. They fuse with the primary lysosomes and form secondary lysosomes. Lysosomal cathepsin results in complete degradation of the cellular proteins, including globin of hemoglobin, to the constituent amino acids, which are utilized for general metabolic needs.

Heme is degraded in the reticuloendothelial cells, to a linear tetrapyrrole (biliverdin IXα), by the microsomal enzyme system, which is designated as **heme oxygenase.** This enzyme requires molecular oxygen and NADPH, and is induced by heme. Heme oxygenase catalyzes the cleavage of **α-methenyl bridge,** which **is quantitatively converted to carbon monoxide** (CO) that is trapped by the hemoglobin and eventually exhaled.

Biliverdin is reduced to bilirubin by the enzyme biliverdin reductase (Fig 26.7).

One gram of hemoglobin yields about 35 mg of bilirubin.

Iron, which is released from the porphyrin ring, **is transferred from the cells** by an iron transport protein, called **transferrin, and is made available for resynthesis of hemoglobin.** Besides the senescent red blood cells, bilirubin is also derived from the turnover of the other heme containing proteins, such as cytochromes.

NORMAL AND ABNORMAL HEMOGLOBINS

Different types of hemoglobins found at various developmental stages **in normal humans** are shown in Table 26.2.

Table 26.2. Different types of human hemoglobins

Hemoglobin	Chain composition	Developmental stage
HbA_1	$\alpha_2\beta_2$	Adult
HbA_2	$\alpha_2\delta_2$	Adult
HbF	$\alpha_2\gamma_2$	Fetus
Hb.Gower-1	$\xi_2\varepsilon_2$	Embryo
Hb.Portland	$\xi_2\gamma_2$	Embryo

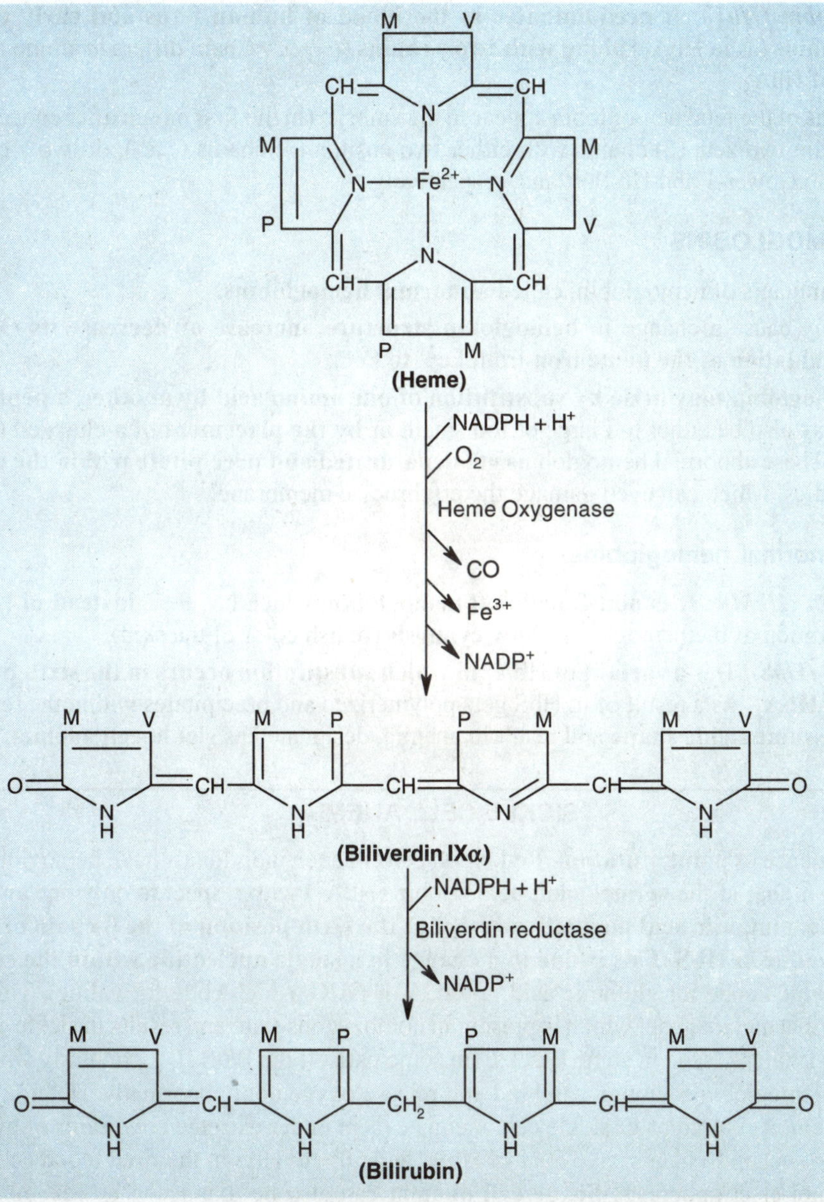

Fig. 26.7. Formation of bilirubin from heme.

Normal Hemoglobin

Hemoglobin normally found in the body that performs all the physiological functions is referred to as the normal hemoglobin. These include:

Adult hemoglobin (HbA_1): This is the major hemoglobin present in adult human beings and consists of two α chains and two β chains ($\alpha_2\beta_2$).

Minor adult hemoglobin (HbA_2): **Minor adult hemoglobin** comprises of about 2% of total hemoglobin in adults. It consists of **two α chains and two delta (δ) chains ($\alpha_2\delta_2$)**, instead of two α and two β chains present in HbA.

Fetal hemoglobin (HbF): It **predominates in the blood of human fetus and early embryo.** HbF **contains two α chains** (as in HbA_1) **along with two γ chains** ($\alpha_2\gamma_2$). γ Chain differs in amino acid sequence from the β chain of HbA_1.

Two other forms of the fetal hemoglobin appear in the embryo (in the first month after conception). These hemoglobins contain two zeta (ξ) chains with either two epsilon (ε) chains ($\xi_2\varepsilon_2$), or two γ chains, ($\xi_2\gamma_2$). These are called Hb.Gower-1 and Hb.Portland, respectively.

ABNORMAL HEMOGLOBINS

There are several mutants of hemoglobin, called **abnormal hemoglobins.**

A mutation may cause a change in **hemoglobin structure, increase or decrease its O_2 affinity,** or **increase rate of oxidation of the heme iron** from Fe^{2+} to Fe^{3+}.

Abnormal **hemoglobin may arise by substitution of one amino acid by another, a peptide chain by another,** which may also be either too large or too small, or **by the placement of a charged** (polar) **group inside a domain.** These abnormal hemoglobins get **denaturated and precipitate within the erythrocytes,** forming Heinz bodies, which can even damage the erythrocyte membrane.

Some of the abnormal hemoglobins

Methemoglobin (HbM) **: It is non-functional hemoglobin,** which has Fe^{3+} **instead of** Fe^{2+}. **Patients** with high concentration of methemoglobin **show cyanosis** (bluish color of the skin).

Hemoglobin S (HbS): **It is a variant** of HbA_1 **in which substitution occurs in the sixth position of the β-globin chain of HbA_1.** As a result of it, HbS gets polymerized and precipitates within the red blood cells. **Red blood cells assume sickle shape** and result in anemia, designated as **sickle-cell anemia.**

SICKLE CELL ANEMIA

This is a consequence of **point mutation**. Red blood cells of such individuals have hemoglobin S (HbS) which differs from that of the normal adult hemoglobin (HbA_1) with respect to only one amino acid in their β-chains, i.e. **glutamic acid normally present at the sixth position of the β chain of HbA_1 gets replaced with valine in HbS. This is due to a change in a single nucleotide within the codon** (from GAA or GAG, which code for glutamic acid, to GUA or GUG, which code for valine). This missense mutation results in a mutant gene, which is present in homozygous state and results in sickle cell disease. Such a mutation is mostly seen in some Blacks, (in some parts of the World), particularly where malaria is widespread. Hemoglobin S though can bind and release oxygen but abnormally. Heterozygous individuals do not exhibit symptoms of sickle cell anemia except under extreme conditions of hypoxia, due to the reason that such individuals have 50% of HbA_1 and 50% of HbS in their red blood cells. HbS can be detected by gel electrophoresis. **Sickle cell anemia** can also be diagnosed by recombinant DNA technique.

HEMOGLOBINOPATHIES

Patients with unstable hemoglobin **develop hemoglobinopathies** with characteristic features, such as anemia, reticulocytosis, splenomegaly and urobilinuria. Hemoglobinopathies are a **heterogeneous group of single-gene disorders.**

A mutant gene may result in the substitution of one amino acid in one type of the polypeptide chain by another amino acid, or **loss of one or more amino acid residues of a polypeptide chain.** This, in turn, **results in the formation of structurally abnormal hemoglobin**. In some cases, the change may be clinically insignificant while in others it may cause a serious disease. The **most common** hemoglobinopathy **is sickle cell disease.**

Hemoglobin C: **Hemoglobin C** is another variant of HbA_1 where glutamic acid, normally present at the sixth position of the β-chain of HbA_1, gets replaced by lysine. This, in turn, results, in the formation of aggregates and reduces survival time for red blood cells. This form of hemoglobinopathy exhibits more limited pathological effects and is commonly found among certain Black African population.

Thalassemia

Thalassemia is a family of related genetic disorders that arise **due to the deletion of one or more globin-like genes** in either the globin gene cluster or a defect in transcription, and/or processing of mRNA of the globin gene. If there is reduced synthesis or total **lack of synthesis of α-globin mRNA,** the disease is classified as α-thalassemia. On the other hand, **if β-globin mRNA level is affected, it is called β-thalassemia.**

One to four α-globin genes may be missing in the patients with α-thalassemia. If **one α-globin gene is missing, the condition is called as α-thalassemia 1** (α-thal 1). When **two α-globin genes are missing, it is called α-thal 2.** Both the conditions are associated with mild to moderate anemia. On the other hand, if **three α-globin genes are missing** it results in the synthesis of more β-globin molecules, forming a tetramer containing four β-globin sub-units. This condition is called **HbH disease.** When **all the four α-globin genes are absent, it results in** a fatal condition called **hydrops fetalis.**

β-Thalassemias also exhibits different degree of severity and can be caused by a variety of defects or deletions.

SOME IMPORTANT QUESTIONS

1. Describe the process of heme synthesis. How it is regulated?
2. What is porphyria? Describe various types of porphyrias.
3. Describe the process of heme degradation.
4. Describe:
   (i) The process of oxygenation and deoxygenation of hemoglobin.
   (ii) Isohydric transport of CO_2
5. Write notes on:
   (i) Bohr effect
   (ii) Carbaminohemoglobin
   (iii) Transport of nitric oxide
   (iv) Hemoglobin S
   (v) Sickle-cell anemia
   (vi) Hemoglobinopathies
   (vii) Thalassemia

CHAPTER

27

Immunoglobulins

Immunoglobulins form a related but enormously **diverse group of proteins** called globulin, which have **antibody activity.** They are **synthesized and secreted** by plasma cells **in response** to invasion by **an antigen.** They are **glycoprotein** in nature and are present in the serum and some tissue fluids of all the mammals. **Immunoglobulins** constitute approximately 20% of the total plasma proteins.

Some of them are carried to surface of the B cells where they act as receptors, for the specific antigens while others are found in free form in blood or lymph. Contact between B cells and the antigen is needed to convert B cells into the antibody forming cells, also called as plasma cells, which secrete large amount of antibodies.

Antibodies are highly specific for the three-dimensional conformation of the epitope.

STRUCTURAL FEATURES OF THE IMMUNOGLOBULIN MOLECULE

- A molecule of immunoglobulin has **Y-shaped structure** with two arms and a stem.
- It has **four polypeptide chains**, which are bound by –S-S-linkages. They comprise of **two small subunits** called **L chains** and **two large subunits** called **H chains.**
- Each subunit has a **variable region,** which is located towards the **N-terminal end,** and **constant region(s)** that are located towards the **C-terminal end**.
- Its two arms are called the **Fab fragments** whereas the stem is called **Fc fragment**.
- Both the **arms are linked** to the stem **by a flexible region**, called hinge region.

AN IMMUNOGLOBULIN HAS FOUR POLYPEPTIDE CHAINS

An immunoglobulin is a basic unit comprising of **four polypeptide chains**. Out of these, there are **two** identical **small polypeptides**, called **L-chains (light chains),** and **two** identical **large polypeptides**, which are designated as **H-chains (heavy chains).** They occur in light-heavy-heavy-light arrangement. Its four chains are **joined** with each other **by disulfide bonds** (–S–S–), and form, roughly, a Y-shaped molecule, which has two arms and a stem (Fig. 27.1).

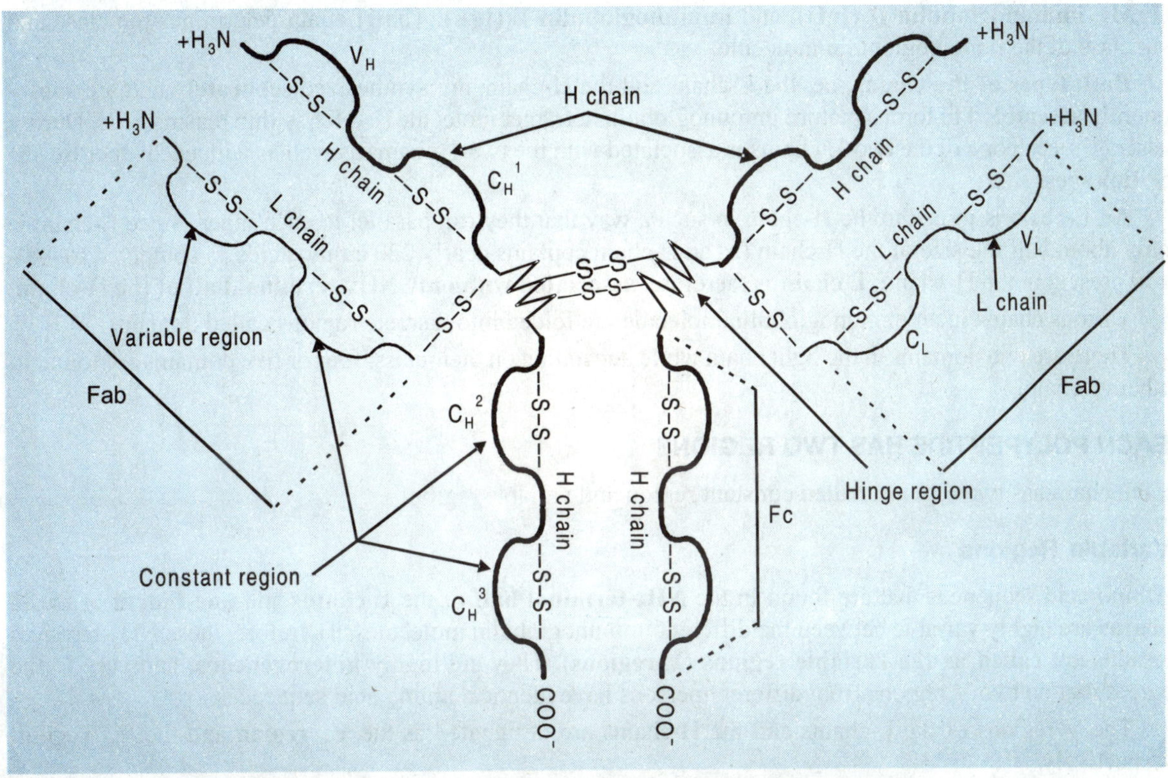

Fig. 27.1. Structure of an immunoglobulin.

Light chains

The **smaller polypeptides** (about 25 kD each) are designated as the **light chains (L-chains)**. Each L chain has approximately **220 amino acids.**

Two types of the **L chains** may occur in immunoglobulins. They are designated as **kappa** (κ-chain) and **lambda** (λ-chain).

Though any type of the L-chain may be found in an immunoglobulin molecule but, generally, an immunoglobulin has two identical chains, i.e. it has either two κ-chains (κ_2) or two λ-chains (λ_2) but never one κ-chain and one λ-chain (κλ).

These are referred to as the isotypes and are found in all the individuals.

In human immunoglobulins, κ-chains are more prevalent than the λ-chains.

Heavy chains

The **larger subunits** that are found in the immunoglobulins are called **heavy chains (H-chains).**

Five different types of the **H chains,** each containing **440-450 amino acids,** are found in immunoglobulins, in human beings. Molecular mass of an H-chain may vary from 50 to 75 kD.

Various types of the H chains are designated as **gamma (γ), alpha (α), mue (μ), delta (δ), and epsilon (ε).** Each one of the H-chain is specific to a class of the immunoglobulin. Thus, depending upon the type of the H-chain, they are called as **immunoglobulin G (IgG), immunoglobulin A (IgA), immunoglobulin M**

(IgM), immunoglobulin D (IgD), and **immunoglobulin E (IgE)**. The H-chain determines the class and subclass of the immunoglobulin molecule.

Both types of the chains, i.e. the L-chain and the H-chain, are synthesized **separately** and are subsequently **assembled** to form a mature immunoglobulin tetramer molecule (L_2H_2), within plasma cells. During assembly, each one of the two-H chains is associated with the two-L chains as well as with each other **by –S-S- linkages.**

An L-chain is joined to the H-chain in such a way that they run parallel to each other. Since L-chain is only about half the size of the H-chain (as an L-chain contains nearly 220 amino acids as compared to 440-450 present in the H-chain), **L chain** is therefore, **associated with only NH_2-terminal half of the H-chain.**

Various chains in an immunoglobulin molecule are folded into discrete regions called domains.

There are two domains in the light chain while depending on their class, four or five domains are found in a heavy chain.

EACH POLYPEPTIDE HAS TWO REGIONS

Each chain has two regions, called constant region and variable region.

Variable Regions

Amino acid sequences that are found in the **NH_2-terminal half** of the **L chains** and **one-fourth** of the **H chains** are highly variable between the different immunoglobulin molecules. Therefore, these NH_2-terminal regions are **called as the variable regions (V regions).** They are highly **heterogeneous,** and vary to the extent that no two V regions from different persons have identical amino acid sequences.

The V regions of the L-chains and the H-chains are designated as the **V_L region** and the **V_H region,** respectively.

Constant Regions

Half of the **L-chain,** towards the **COOH-terminal end** and **three-fourth** of the **H chain** towards the **COOH-terminal end** has **homologous amino acid sequences,** i.e. these segments are homologous with the same segments of the other L- or H-chains found in the same class of immunoglobulin. These regions, with a homologous primary structure, are called **constant regions (C region).** The C regions of the L-chains and the H-chains are designated as the **C_L region** and **the C_H region,** respectively.

C_H Region is further **subdivided** into **three parts,** each comprising of about 110 amino acids, and is designated as **$C_{H}1$, $C_{H}2$** and **$C_{H}3$,** respectively. Each such segment of the C_H region is **homologous to each other as well as to the C_L region**. Each of these segments (sequence repeats) contain an intra chain disulphide bond.

The μ type and ε type of the H chains have four C_H regions instead of three found in others.

V regions of the immunoglobulin is involved in **recognition and binding of the antigen with the antibody.** This ability of the antibody **resides in several short sequences,** which are located in small loops **within the V region.** These short loops are termed as ***hyper variable regions (hyper variable sequences).***

Only 5-10 amino acids in each of the hyper variable sequence **contribute to the antigen-binding site** (ab site). These hyper variable sequences (the antigen-binding sites) are **complementary to topology of the antigen,** and are **designated as complementary-determining regions. Three hyper variable sequences** are commonly found in the **V_L region. A V_H region may have three or four hyper variable sequences,** depending upon the type of the antibody.

Amino acid segments separating different hyper variable sequences from each other are referred to as the **framework regions** (Fig. 27.2).

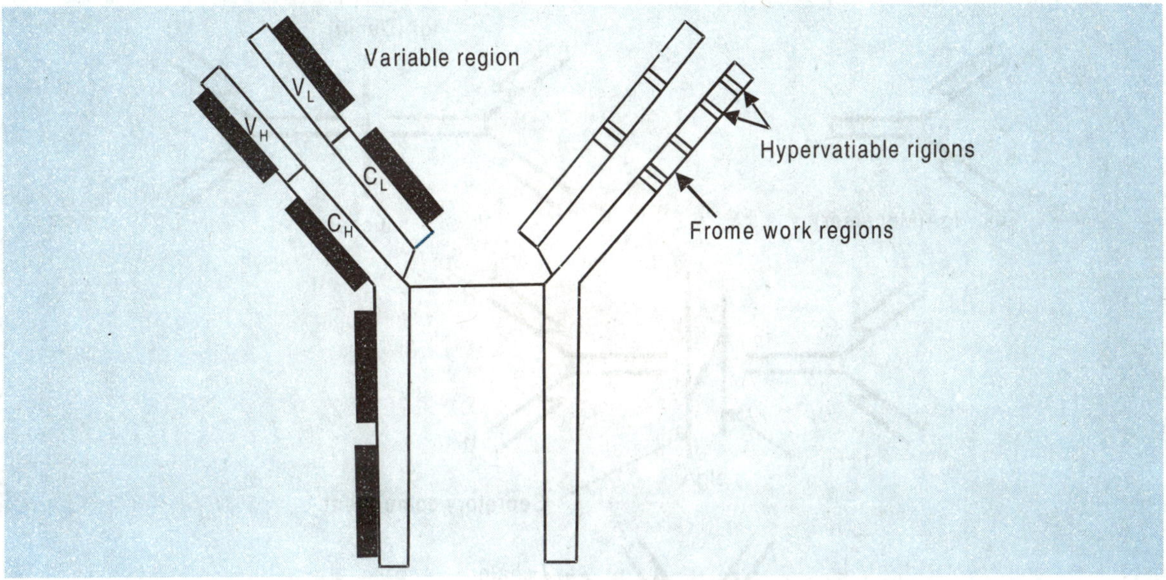

Fig. 27.2. Hypervariable sequences.

Characteristics of the C_H Region

1. C_H Region **determines the antibody class** of an immunoglobulin.
2. This region of the immunoglobulin molecule provides a **site for the binding of the complement protein.**
3. These are also the **sites**, for the antibodies, **to cross the placental membrane.**
4. Depending upon the class of an immunoglobulin, **variable amounts of carbohydrates** (2-15%) **are attached to the $C_{H}2$ region.**
5. Amino acid sequences in these C_H regions, in some cases, also promote **polymerization of the basic molecular structure** of the **immunoglobulin molecule.**

In a polymeric structure, basic molecular structures are covalently linked to each other around a peptide called joining subunit or J chain.

Immunoglobulins of the IgA class generally occur as dimmers while IgM occurs as pentamer (Fig. 27.3).

PROTEOLYTIC DEGRADATION OF AN IMMUNOGLOBULIN MOLECULE

An **immunoglobulin** molecule, such as IgG, can be **cleaved with** the enzyme **papain,** which hydrolyzes it **into three fragments** of approximately 50 kD each. **Two** of these fragments are identical and represents two arms. These are the fragments where an antigen binds and are called **Fab fragments**. The **third fragment represents the stem.** Since this fragment can be easily crystallized, it is called as the **Fc fragment** (Fig. 27.4).

Fab Fragment

Fab fragments have the **entire L-chain** and **half of the H chain** (comprising of the V_H and the $C_{H}1$ regions. Each of these two Fab fragments can bind to an antigen with the affinity similar to that of the intact antibody.

Because there are two Fab domains, a molecule of an immunoglobulin can bind two molecules of the antigen, simultaneously. Thus, an **antibody** is said to be **divalent.**

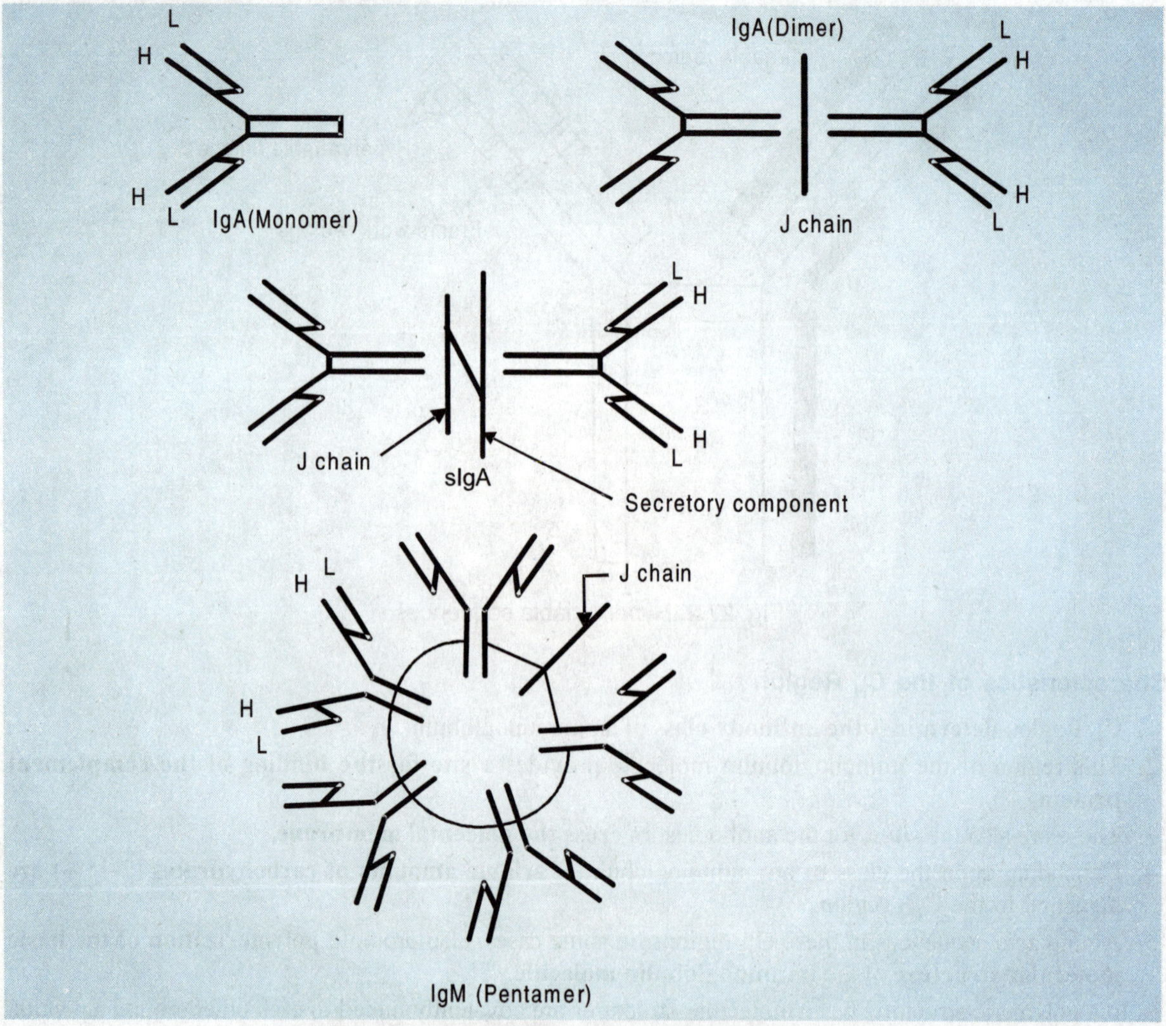

Fig. 27.3. Polymerization of immunoglobulin molecules.

Fc Fragment

The **Fc fragment** consists of the **C-terminal halves of the two-H chains**, i.e. the $C_{H}2$ and $C_{H}3$ regions, which are joined together by disulfide bridges.

All antibodies thus are bifunctional, i.e. in addition to the antigen binding, they also exhibit one or more effector functions, such as complement activation and cell binding (in the Fc region).

Hinge Region

Two **Fab fragments** of the immunoglobulin are **connected to** the **Fc fragment by a flexible region** that is referred to as the ***hinge region***. It is present between the $C_{H}1$ and $C_{H}2$ regions and confers flexibility to the molecule. This in turn allows two Fab fragments to move independently and help them to bind two antigens, simultaneously, that may be present at different distances, apart from each other. The hinge region has one or more cysteine residues, which provide **interchain disulfide bridges**. It also controls interactions between different parts of an immunoglobulin.

CLASSIFICATION OF IMMUNOGLOBULINS

There are five classes of immunoglobulins, called IgG, IgA, IgM, IgD, and IgE, each one of which differs from others with respect to the type of its H chain.

Various immunoglobulin classes have different physiological functions (Table 27.1).

Immunoglobulin G

Immunoglobulin G (IgG) is a major immunoglobulin produced by the plasma cells. It accounts for **70-75% of the total** immunoglobulins found in serum.

IgG is the most important class of immunoglobulins that occurs in secondary immune response and is distributed evenly between the intravascular and the extra vascular pools.

Antibodies of the IgG class are **produced in response to most bacteria and viruses.** These antibodies **bind to macrophages and neutrophils,** and **promote phagocytosis.**

IgG has four subclasses, which are referred to as IgG_1, IgG_2, IgG_3, and IgG_4. Structurally, these **subclasses differ** primarily, **in the hinge region**. It is the IgG_1 and IgG_3 both of which bind firmly, to Fc receptors of phagocytic cells and activate K cells (killer monocytes).

In human beings, IgG molecules of all the subclasses cross placenta and confer high degree of passive immunity to the newborn.

The major effector mechanism of the human IgG_1 and IgG_3 subclasses is the activation of the classical pathway of a complement.

Immunoglobulin A

Immunoglobulin A (IgA) accounts for about **15-20% of the total** serum immunoglobulins.

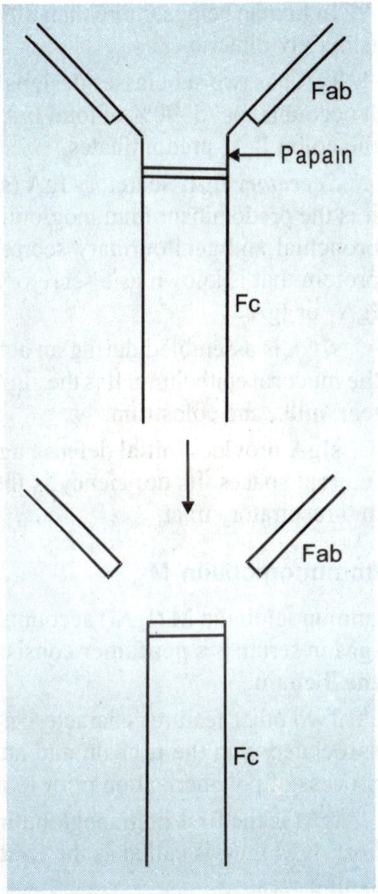

Fig. 27.4. Proteolytic degradation of immunoglobulin.

Table 27.1. Immunoglobulin (Ig) classes

Ig class	*Approximate molecular weight (kD)*	*H chain*	*Carbohydrate content (%)*	*Serum concentration (mg/dl)*	*Major physiological functions*
IgG	146	γ	2–4	800–1500	Placental transfer Provides immunity to neonates
IgA	160–380	α	5–9	150–250	Protects outer surfaces sIgA is present in mucous secretions
IgM	970	μ	8–12	70–150	First line of defense and is synthesized in neonates
IgD	160	δ	8–12	3–5	Primary function unknown, acts as B cell receptor
IgE	190	ε	10–15	0.01–0.05	Reaginic antibodies, implicated in allergic reactions Release of histamine and other vasoactive amines

In human beings, more than 80% of the IgA occurs as a monomer but in most other mammals, serum IgA is mainly dimeric.

IgA has two subclasses designated as IgA_1 and IgA_2. In human serum, IgA_1 is the predominant subclass. It accounts for 75–90% of total IgA in many secretions, such as in nasal secretions, tears, saliva, and milk. In the colon IgA_2 predominates.

Secretory IgA: Secretory IgA (sIgA) is the most important form of IgA. It is called as secretory IgA since it is the predominant immunogloulin in seromucus secretions, such as saliva, colostrums, milk, and tracheo-bronchial and genitourinary secretions. It exists, mainly in the dimeric form, in association with another protein that is known as a secretory component. sIgA may be of either of the two subclasses, i.e. it may be IgA_1 or IgA_2.

sIgA is assembled during an active transport process, as the locally produced dimeric IgA passes across the mucosal epithelium. It is the sIgA, which is found in the bronchial, nasal, and intestinal mucous **secretions,** tear, milk, and colostrum.

sIgA provides initial defense against invading viral and bacterial pathogens, prior to their entry into the internal spaces. Its deficiency is the commonest disorder, which results in recurrent infections of the sinus and respiratory tract.

Immunoglobulin M

Immunoglobulin M (IgM) accounts for nearly **5-10% of the total** circulating immunoglobulins. Most of the IgM in serum is **a pentamer** consisting of five Y-shaped monomeric molecules, which are **arranged around the J chain.**

Two other features characterize an IgM molecule, i.e. an abundance of oligosaccharide units, which are associated with the μ chain and an additional peptide chain called joining chain (J-chain), that assists the process of polymerization prior to its secretion.

IgM is the **first** immunoglobulin, which is synthesized by the cell, on introduction of an antigen into the host. IgM thus, is called as the **first line of defense**. It is the only immunoglobulin that **a neonate** normally synthesizes.

IgM is the predominant antibody in primary immune response. It is largely confined to the intravascular pool and is frequently associated with the immune response to antigenically complex blood-borne infectious organisms.

Once bound to its target, IgM is a potent activator of the classical pathway of a complement.

Immunoglobulin D

Immunoglobulin D (IgD) accounts for **less than 1% of the total** serum immunoglobulins. It is the major component of the surface membrane of many B cells and may play a role in antigen-triggered lymphocyte differentiation though its primary function is unknown.

Immunoglobulin E

Immunoglobulin E (IgE) is normally present in blood in **minute concentrations**. It is found on the surface membrane of basophils and mast cells, in all individuals.

It also sensitizes cells on the mucosal surfaces, such as conjunctival, nasal, and bronchial mucosa. It **protects** the host **against parasites** and has been **implicated in allergic reactions**. When antigen cross-links some of the attached IgE molecules, **mast cells** are stimulated to **release histamine** and other vasoactive amines, which, in turn, are responsible for vascular permeability and smooth muscle contration.

IgE is commonly associated with the **allergic diseases**, such as hay fever and asthma.

SYNTHESIS OF IMMUNOGLOBULINS

Both, **L chains** and **H chains** are synthesized independently and form an immunoglobulin molecule.

The immune system has a potential to produce large number of different antibodies that are enough to react with almost every antigen an organism encounters. A human, however, does not contain that many number of genes so that each one of it can code for an individual immunoglobulin. This is achieved by generating great diversity in the antibodies that are produced by the B cells.

Generation of such immense **antibody diversity** is achieved by recombination of a limited number of gene segments, to produce vast number of variable domains.

SOME IMPORTANT QUESTIONS

1. What are immunoglobulins? Describe the structure of an immunoglobulin.
2. Classify immunoglobulins. Describe the function of each class of immunoglobulin.
3. Write notes on:
   (i) Effect of papain on an immunoglobulin
   (ii) Hinge region
   (iii) Secretory IgA

CHAPTER 28

Liver Function Tests

BIOCHEMICAL FUNCTIONS OF THE LIVER

The liver is a multifunctional organ that is involved in a number of excretory, synthetic and metabolic functions (Table 28.1).

1. The liver has a major influence on the flow of nutrients to the rest of the body. It controls the release of absorbed material into the systemic circulation and has a central role in carbohydrate, protein and fat metabolism.
2. The liver is an important site for the storage of glycogen and for gluconeogenesis.
3. Most proteins in plasma including albumin, α and β-globulins, clotting factors and transport proteins are synthesized by the liver.
4. This is also the site for urea synthesis.
5. Fatty acids and phospholipids are also taken up from circulation by the liver and are metabolized there.
6. Cholesterol is also synthesized and esterified in the liver.
7. Liver is also a site for the detoxification of exogenous compounds (such as alcohol, drugs and toxins) as well as endogenous materials (such as bilirubin and hormones) which are excreted via the kidney or the biliary system.
8. Bile salts are synthesized in the liver.
9. Liver stores various substances, such as vitamins and minerals, and releases them as and when required.
10. Liver is also one of the biggest reticuloendothelial organs and has important immune functions.

COMMONLY USED BIOCHEMICAL TESTS FOR THE ASSESSMENT OF THE FUNCTIONS OF LIVER

Various liver function tests that are useful in the assessment of a liver disease include – the estimation of serum proteins, serum bilirubin, various enzymes and prothrombin time (Table 28.2).

Table 28.1. Important biochemical functions of the liver

Metabolism of Nutrients
• Carbohydrates
• Proteins
• Fats
Synthesis of Proteins
• Albumin
• α- and β-Globulins
• Clotting factors
• Transport proteins
Metabolism and Excretion of Exogenous substances
• Alcohol
• Drugs
• Toxins
Endogenous substances
• Bilirubin
• Hormones
Storage of Vitamins
• Vitamin A
• Vitamin B_{12}
• Folic Acid
Minerals
• Iron

Table 28.2. Commonly used biochemical tests for the assessment of liver functions

Total Proteins
Albumin
Bilirubin
Prothrombin Time
Enzymes
• GPT and GOT
• Alkaline phosphatase
• γ-Glutamyltranspeptidase (γ-GT)
• 5′-Nucleotidase
• Glutamate dehydrogenase

Serum Bilirubin

Bilirubin is an orange-yellow pigment, derived from the breakdown of red blood cells in the liver, spleen and bone marrow (Fig. 28.1).

Its daily production, in men, averages from 250-300 mg. Approximately, 85% of this is derived from the heme moiety of hemoglobin which is released from the erythrocytes that are destroyed in the reticuloendothelial cells while rest of it is formed from catabolism of other heme containing proteins, such as myoglobin, cytochromes and other heme containing enzymes.

Bilirubin, normally present in the blood, is bound to albumin and is transported to the liver.

Hepatocytes trap bilirubin by means of a specific binding protein called **ligandin. In the hepatocytes, bilirubin** gets **conjugated with UDP-glucuronate,** which is derived from the oxidation of UDP-glucose. **This reaction is catalyzed by UDP-glucuronyltransferase.**

In the normal bile, bilirubin diglucuronide is the major form of excreted bilirubin with only a small amount of the bilirubin monoglucuronide. As bilirubin diglucuronide is much more water solubie than free bilirubin, transferase thus facilitates the excretion of bilirubin, via bile duct, into the intestine.

As **bilirubin diglucuronide** is poorly absorbed by the intestinal mucosa, glucuronide residues are **released in the terminal ileum and large intestine, by intestinal β-glucuronidases and by the enzymes produced by anaerobic bacteria. It is reduced to** colorless linear tetrapyrroles, called stercobilinogen, mesobilinogen and urobilinogen. These compounds are collectively referred to as urobilinogens.

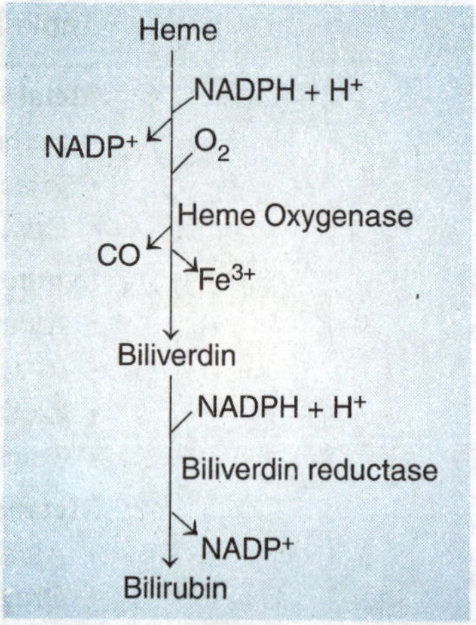

Fig. 28.1. Formation of bilirubin from heme.

A large portion of **urobilinogens are excreted in the feces.**

Majority of these re-circulating pigments are taken up by the liver and re-excreted in the bile. Some of the urobilinogens (only up to 2%) are also reabsorbed passively from the colon and return to the liver via the portal venous blood. This is referred to as **enterohepatic circulation** (Fig. 28.2).

Most of the reabsorbed urobilinogen is taken up by the liver and is re-excreted in the bile. **A small portion of urobilinogen (2-5%)** however, escapes hepatic extraction, **reaches the peripheral circulation and is excreted in the urine.**

Serum thus contains two different forms of bilirubin which are referred to as :

(i) **Unconjugated** (lipid soluble) form that is bound to albumin and is transported from the reticuloendothelial system to the liver, and

(ii) **Conjugated** (water soluble) form which is regurgitated from the liver into the plasma.

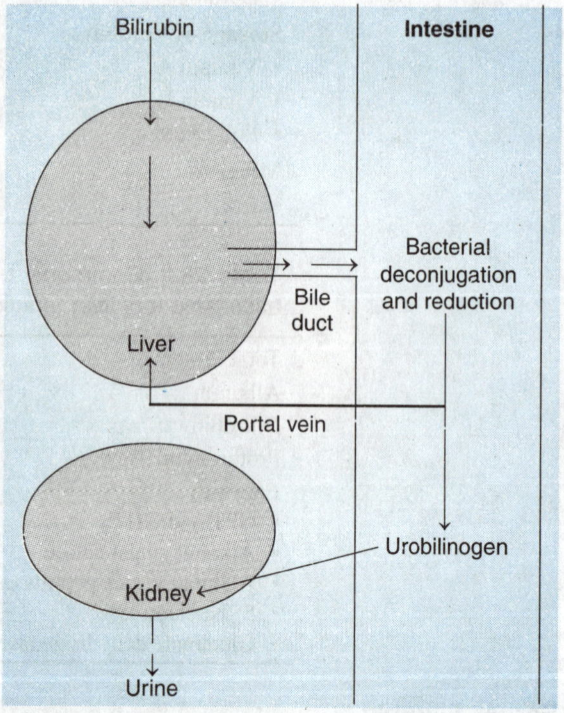

Fig. 28.2. Schematic presentation of Enterohepatic circulation of urobilinogen.

Normal value for the sum of the unconjugated and conjugated forms is 0.1-1.0 mg/100 ml of serum or plasma.

Normally, almost all the bilirubin in plasma is unconjugated.

Disorders of bilirubin metabolism lead to **hyperbilirubinemia** where serial measurement of bilirubin is helpful in knowing the severity of a liver disease.

Bilirubin fractionation is also helpful in differential diagnosis of **jaundice.**

JAUNDICE

Jaundice is a physical sign characterized by yellow appearance of the patient and is a most characteristic clinical manifestation of hyperbilirubinemia. It results from the deposition of bilirubin (bile pigment) in the skin, mucous membrane and sclera of the patient. It is apparent clinically, when serum bilirubin level is more than 2 mg/dL. If serum bilirubin is below 2 mg/dL, it is called **latent jaundice** (subclinical jaundice) since it is not detectable at this stage, clinically.

There are three types of jaundice, referred to as pre-hepatic, hepatic and post-hepatic jaundice.

Biochemical differentiation of the three types of jaundice is given in Table 28.3

Table 28.3 Differential Diagnosis of Different Types of Jaundice Based on Various Biochemical Tests

Biochemical parameter	Type of Jaundice		
	Pre-hepatic	Hepatic	Post-hepatic
Serum bilirubin	↑↑	↑↑	↑↑
Type of bilirubin	Unconjugated	Both	Conjugated
Urine urobilinogen	↑↑	N / ↑	↓ / –
Urine bile pigments	–	–	↑
Stercobilinogen	↑	↓	↓ / –
SGPT/SGOT (mainly SGPT)	N	↑↑↑	↑
Serum alkaline phosphatase	N	↑	↑↑↑
Serum 5′-nucleotidase	N	↑	↑↑↑
Prothrombin time (PT)	N	↑	↑

Pre-hepatic Jaundice

Pre-hepatic jaundice is also called as hemolytic jaundice. It is characterized by the excessive presence of unconjugated bilirubin. It may be a result of increased production of unconjugated bilirubin such as in hemolysis, decreased uptake of unconjugated bilirubin across the hepatocyte membrane as in Gilbert's syndrome or decreased biotransformation such as in neonatal jaundice, Criggler-Najjar syndrome, etc.

Hemolysis: In disorders associated with hemolysis (hemolytic anemia) rate of bilirubin production is increased which may exceed the amount that can not be removed by the liver.

Gilbert's syndrome: This is a heterogeneous group of disorders, inherited as autosomal recessive trait. Several defects include the deficiency of bilirubin glucuronyltransferase, a defect in hepatic uptake of bilirubin or a decrease in red cell survival.

Neonatal jaundice: Neonatal jaundice is also called as physiological jaundice of the newborn. Every infant exhibits some transient unconjugated hyperbilirubinemia (about 5 mg/dL) between the second and the fifth day of life, as at this stage hepatic glucuronyltransferase activity is not fully developed. Activity of the enzyme increases within 2 weeks after birth when serum bilirubin returns to normal. Neonatal jaundice is more pronounced in a premature infant.

Unconjugated bilirubin levels above 18 mg/dL lead to deposition of bilirubin in the lipid-rich basal ganglia. This is referred to as **kernicterus.**

Criggler-Najjar syndrome: This disorder is known to exist in two forms:

Type I: It is clinically more severe form of the disease. It is due to complete absence of glucuronyl-transferase.

Type II: It has moderate clinical findings and is due to partial deficiency of the enzyme. In both the conditions unconjugated bilirubin is significantly raised.

Hepatic Jaundice

Hepatic jaundice is due to a primary disease. Plasma, usually, shows elevated levels of both conjugated as well as unconjugated bilirubin, e.g. in viral hepatitis, liver cirrhosis, etc. There is also an increase in SGOT and SGPT levels.

Elevated levels of conjugated as well as unconjugated bilirubin alongwith the dark-brown pigmentation in the liver cells is also observed in a benign, autosomal recessive condition known as **Dubin-Johnson syndrome.**

Inhalation, ingestion or parenteral administration of several pharmacological and chemical agents such as carbon tetrachloride, acetaminophen, isoniazid or chlorpromazine, which result in liver injury, also lead to hepatic jaundice.

Post-hepatic Jaundice

Post-hepatic jaundice is also referred to as **obstructive jaundice** or post-hepatic cholestasis. It is caused by obstruction of the bile duct, may be due to gallstones, carcinoma of the head of pancreas or carcinoma of the bile duct. Serum of such a patient shows excessive amount of conjugated bilirubin. It is also characterized by the presence of the excessive amount of bilirubin (bile pigments) in the urine.

Urinary Urobilinogen

Normally, only about 1-4 mg of urobilinogen is excreted in the urine, in 24 hours.

Increased excretion of urobilinogen may occur when hepatocellular function is impaired. Urobilinogen excretion in the urine may also increase if there is an excess of urobilinogen in the gastrointestinal tract, which exceeds the capacity of the liver, e.g. in hemolysis, viral hepatitis, cirrhosis, etc.

In contrast, when biliary excretion of bilirubin is impaired, e.g. in cholestasis, urinary excretion of urobilinogen is decreased due to limited delivery of bilirubin to the gut and low rate of production of urobilinogen. This, in turn, results in clay-colored or chalky-white stool in patients with cholestasis jaundice.

Serum Proteins

As liver is the primary site of the synthesis of plasma proteins, a disturbance in protein synthesis occurs as a consequence of impaired hepatic function. Decreased synthesis of protein leads to a decrease in their plasma concentration. Pattern of alteration in plasma proteins, however, depends upon the type, severity and duration of the liver injury.

In a severe liver disease, hepatic synthesis of albumin is decreased. In chronic hepatocellular damage also serum albumin concentration falls.

Serum protein electrophoresis, to determine the proportion of different serum proteins, is also helpful in the diagnosis of a liver disease, e.g. α_2- and β-globulins are increased in cirrhosis due to their increased production and decreased clearance. In cholestasis, there is a small increase in serum γ-globulin with a more increase in α- and β-globulins due, in part, to increased serum lipoproteins.

Serum Enzymes

Serum levels of several enzymes are elevated in liver diseases.

SGOT/SGPT: In viral hepatitis and other forms of a liver disease, which may be associated with hepatic necrosis, serum GPT and GOT levels are elevated even before clinical signs and symptoms of the disease appear. Levels of both the enzymes may reach values as high as 100 times the upper normal limit. Peak values occur between day seven and day tweleve. Thereafter, their activities gradually decrease and reach toward normal by third to fifth weak of recovery.

Five to ten fold increases in both the enzymes occur in patients with primary metastatic carcinoma of the liver. Although serum levels of both GPT and GOT are elevated in a liver disease, however, GTP levels are comparatively more elevated, as it is more liver specific.

Alkaline phosphatase: Serum alkaline phosphatase levels are important in a hepatobiliary disease as well as in bone diseases that are associated with increased osteoblastic activity.

As biliary obstruction results in induction of the enzyme, rise is more marked in extrahepatic obstruction than in intrahepatic obstruction.

Glutamate dehydrogenase: Glutamate dehydrogenase (GDH) is found in the liver, heart, muscle and kidney. It is present only in traces in normal serum but increased activity is observed in a liver disease with hepatocellular damage.

5′-Nucleotidase: 5′-Nucleotidase (5′-NT) activity is increased by two to six fold, in some of the hepatobiliary diseases. It may be due to extrahepatic causes such as stone or tumor, obstructing the bile duct or in intrahepatic conditions, e.g. cholestasis that may be caused by chlorpromazine, malignant infiltration of the liver or biliary cirrhosis.

Gamma-glutamyltransferase: Gamma-glutamyltransferase is also referred to as γ-glutamyltranspeptidase or γ-GT. It is present in high concentration in the serum in intra-hepatic or post-hepatic biliary obstruction.

Elevated levels of γ-GT are also observed in the sera of people who are heavy drinkers.

This enzyme has been shown to be of significance in the detection of an alcohol-induced liver disease.

PROFILES OF LIVER FUNCTION

A useful combination of tests, which can be done to determine whether a liver disease is present and to given some indication of the aetiology, include **serum bilirubin, glutamate pyruvate transaminase (SGPT or alanine aminotransferase), alkaline phosphatase, γ-glutamyltranspeptidase (γ-GT) and albumin.** Examination of the **urine for** the amount of **urobilinogen** can also be done. Additional tests, which study some liver function tests, such as galactose tolerance test and the hippuric acid synthesis test can be done in doubtful cases.

In Jaundice Patients

In jaundice patients, **unconjugated hyperbilirubinemia** is usually due to hemolysis or Gilbert's syndrome. In hemolysis, **bilirubin is absent from the urine** and **urinary urobilinogen** concentration **is increased**.

In conjugated hyperbilirubinemia (increase in both conjugated and unconjugated bilirubin) large **increase in SGPT** suggests hepatocellular damage, which may be caused by drugs, toxic agents (like alcohol), or infection (viral hepatitis).

On the other hand, marked **elevation in γ-GT and alkaline phosphatase** suggests alcoholic liver disease and **cholestasis** (obstruction).

Plasma γ-GT concentration provides a fairly good index of the **progress of a chronic liver disease.**

Normal values of the various parameters are shown in Table. 28.4.

Table 28.4. Normal serum concentration of some of the liver function test parameters, which are done routinely

Parameter	*Normal value*
Plasma albumin	3.6–5.0 g/dl
SGOT activity	Up to 40 U/L
Alkaline phosphatase activity	80–300 U/L
Total bilirubin	< 1.0 mg/dl
γ-GT activity	5–35 U/L

SOME IMPORTANT QUESTIONS

1. Describe hepatic function tests. How will you use these tests for differential diagnosis of different types of Jaundice?
2. Describe the role of bilirubin as a liver function test to differentiate between different types of jaundice.
3. Write notes on:
   (i) Jaundice
   (ii) Neonatal jaundice
   (iii) Biochemical functions of the liver.

CHAPTER 29

Kidney Function Tests

Various metabolic processes occurring in the body produce a number of substances, many of which, such as CO_2, water, nitrogenous compounds and inorganic salts, are waste products. If not regularly removed from the body, these toxic metabolites may severely affect normal health. The kidneys excrete most of the water as well as organic and inorganic substances whereas CO_2 is expired through lungs. Besides, kidney performs several other biochemical functions (Table 29.1).

- Excretion of waste products
- Regulation of water and electrolytes
- Acid-base balance, and
- Synthesis and activation of hormones

1. EXCRETION OF WASTE PRODUCTS

Urine is an ultrafiltrate of plasma. It is formed in the kidney, a paired-organ, which is meant for filtration, concentration and reabsorption of various constituents.

Each kidney has nearly one million basic filtration units called nephrons. A **nephron** consists of the **glomerulus** and the **tubule.**

The **glomerous** is a **network of arteriolar afferent and efferent capillaries** and is **surrounded by** a double-walled epithelial sac called **Bowman's capsule.** Bowman's capsule leads to the **tubule,** which is **divided into proximal convoluted tubule, loop of Henle and distal convoluted tubule.**

Table 29.1. Important functions of the kidney

- Filtration of blood and preparation of ultrafiltrate fluid as urine
- Reabsorption of useful substances such as glucose, amino acids, electrolytes, etc.
- Homeostasis of the extracellular volume
- Maintenance of the acid-base status, water and electrolytes
- Endocrine functions and activation of hormones such as synthesis of erythropoietin, activation of vitamin D, etc.

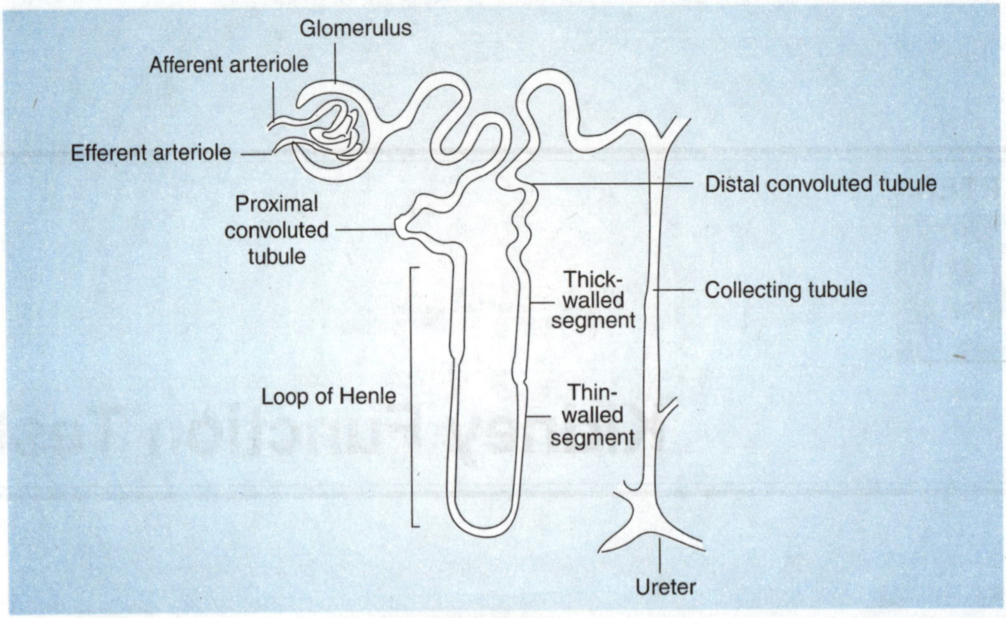

Fig. 29.1. Nephron.

Loop of Henle consists of the descending limb, a thin segment and the ascending limb. Proximal convoluted tubule has its **opening into the descending limb of the loop of Henle,** which **continues into the thin segment from where ascending limb arises. It continues into the distal convoluted tubule, which finally opens into the collecting duct** (Fig. 29.1).

Filtration is carried out in the nephron through glomeruli. As blood passes through the glomeruli, **non-colloidal substances** (usually of low molecular weight), **filter through capillaries, with the retention of protein,** which is not normally found in the urine.

Total amount of the filtrate formed per minute, by all the nephrons of both the kidneys, is known as **glomerular filtration rate** (G.F.R). Under **normal** physiological conditions, **G.F.R. is 125 ml/min.**

About 150-200 L of the ultrafiltrate passes through the glomeruli in 24 hrs. **Reabsorption** of water and solutes in various regions of the tubule reduce its volumes to nearly 500-1800 ml per day, as urine.

In the proximal tubule, nearly 60-80% of the ultrafiltrate is absorbed in an obligatory fashion, along with Na^+, Cl^-, HCO_3^-, Ca^{2+}, HPO_4^{2-}, and other ions. Glucose is reabsorbed almost completely, predominantly in the proximal tubule by a Na^+-dependent passive process. Uric acid is also reabsorbed in the proximal tubule. When blood level of creatinine increases above normal, creatinine is secreted in this region.

In the loop of Henle, Cl^- and more of the Na^+ but without water are reabsorbed, resulting in diluted urine. Water reabsorption is then regulated in the distal tubule and collecting duct by antidiuretic hormone (ADH or vasopressin).

In the distal tubule, **secretion** is the prominent activity as organic ions; K^+ and H^+ are transported from the blood in the efferent arteriole into the tubular fluid. This region also secretes H^+ and reabsorbs Na^+ and HCO_3^-.

Substances, which are reabsorbed by the renal tubule, are divided into two groups, according to their threshold value:

High Thresh-hold Substances: These compounds are vital for life and body can not afford to loose them. Such substances are completely reabsorbed by the renal tubule, e.g. glucose, amino acids, etc.

Glucose is reabsorbed in the tubular epithelial cells.

Sodium, potassium, amino acids and other substances are reabsorbed, apparently by specific transport mechanisms.

Transfer of **carbon dioxide and bicarbonate** is controlled by carbonic anhydrase.

Low Thresh-hold Substances: These compounds are not required by the body and are reabsorbed to a very small extent only, e.g. urea, creatinine, etc.

At the same time, certain solutes are added to the fluid by an excretory function of the tubule. These include hippuric acid and other organic waste products.

Urine thus carries off:

1. Water and salts in such amounts so as to maintain normal equilibrium between extracellular and intracellular fluids,
2. Acids or bases, to maintain a normal acid base balance,
3. Waste products,
4. Toxic and detoxified substances, and
5. Other substances that are present in the blood in excessive amounts.

2. REGULATION OF WATER AND ELECTROLYTES

Regulatory functions of the kidney have a major role in homeostasis, by maintaining constant optimal chemical composition of the blood as well as interstitial and intracellular fluids.

REGULATION OF WATER

The kidney plays an important part in regulating water balance. If excessive amount of water (fluid) is ingested, kidney excretes the same. On the other hand if intake is low, kidney excretes more concentrated urine.

Water homeostasis is intrinsically linked to renal urea handling. Only 40-50% of the filtered load of urea is reabsorbed.

Most of the glomerular filtrate is reabsorbed through tubule cells.

About 90% of water is reabsorbed as a result of the difference in pressure. Of the remaining 10% of water is reabsorbed actively, by tubular cells, as a result of the action of ADH.

In the absence of ADH little water and urea are reabsorbed, and a large amount of water is excreted. On the other hand, in the presence of ADH only 1.0-1.5 L of the filtrate is excreted as urine.

Regulation of ADH excretion is thus of vital importance to fluid homeostasis.

REGULATION OF ELECTROLYTES

The kidney plays an important role in the maintenance of electrolyte balance. Salts are either excreted or conserved by the kidney by tubular reabsorption, depending upon dietary intake and physiological need.

Plasma electrolytes pass through the glomerulus but some potassium leaves the blood by way of tubules, by active secretion.

Sodium and Chloride

Sodium and chloride ions predominate in the glomerular filtrate as in plasma. As the glomerular filtrate flows through tubule, these electrolytes are absorbed into the blood.

Reabsorption of Na^+ is required for the reabsorption of water, Cl^-, glucose, HCO_3^-, and amino acids.

The proximal tubule is highly permeable to Na^+. Approximately 80% of the Na^+ entering tubular cells do so in exchange for H^+ secretion, which in turn leads to the entry of both Cl^- and HCO_3^- into the cells.

Sodium transport is regulated by many factors:

- Protein kinase-dependent phosphorylation
- Aldosterone
- Na^+, K^+–ATPase
- Na^+–H^+ exchanger, and
- H^+–ATPase

Calcium and Phosphorus

Approximately 98% of filtered Ca^{2+} is reabsorbed. Out of which 65–75% in the proximal tubule, 20–25% in the thick ascending limb of the loop of Henle, 10% in the distal tubule and a small amount in the collecting duct.

A passive process that is linked to active Na^+ reabsorption predominantly absorbs calcium. However, in the distal tubule Ca^{2+} reabsorption is an active process catalyzed by Ca^{2+}-ATPase.

Reabsorption of Ca^{2+} is increased by the action of PTH and calcitonin.

Normally, less than 20% of the filtered load of phosphorus is excreted in the urine. Its excretion is directly related to the filtered load when plasma phosphorus concentration is above normal.

Reabsorption of phosphorus though is dependent on Na^+ reabsorption, is regulated by:

- Protein kinase C-dependent phosphorylation
- PTH
- Active vitamin D
- Calcitonin, and
- Dopamine and serotonin

3. ACID-BASE BALANCE

Oxidation of various metabolites in the living organism results in the formation of a variety of acids as well as bases. For example, protons are generated from ionization of various substances such as organic acids (produced during metabolism of glucose, fatty acids and amino acids), uric acid (from purines), sulfates (from sulphur containing amino acids) and carbonic acid (from CO_2).

Similarly, bases arise during catabolism of various metabolites such as ammonia (from amino acids), bicarbonate, phosphates, acetate and citrates.

All these substances enter blood plasma and other extracellular fluids for disposal. Inspite of the entry of these acids and bases, pH of the blood does not alter much and remains within the normal limit of 7.35–7.45. This is due to the presence of various defense mechanisms, which include:

1. Buffer systems of the blood, tissue fluids and cells,
2. Excretion or retention of CO_2 by lungs,
3. Excretion of an acid or alkaline urine, and
4. Formation and excretion of ammonia as well as organic acids.

PRINCIPAL BUFFERS OF THE BLOOD

Buffer pairs in the first line are those present in the plasma and the extracellular fluid. These include:

- Bicarbonate/CO_2

- Na_2HPO_4/NaH_2PO_4, and
- $Protein^-/H.Protein$

In the second line of defense are the buffer pairs that are found in the red blood cells. These include:

- HCO_3^-/CO_2,
- $Hb^-/H.Hb$, and
- K_2HPO_4/KH_2PO_4.

Though respiratory system serves as a mechanism for rapid adjustment of the acid-base balance, by regulating the concentration of carbonic acid in the blood and other body fluids, maintenance of a constant level of blood pH is mainly done by the kidneys by reabsorbing, secreting and excreting acidic or basic substances, as the need may be. Besides, phosphates are also concentrated by the kidney. It is the principal buffer in the urine, e.g. in acid urine there is a relative excess of $H_2PO_4^-$. On the other hand, there is a relative excess of HPO_4^{2-} in the alkaline urine.

Four reactions are mainly involved in the **regulation of acid-base balance** by the kidneys (Fig. 29.2).

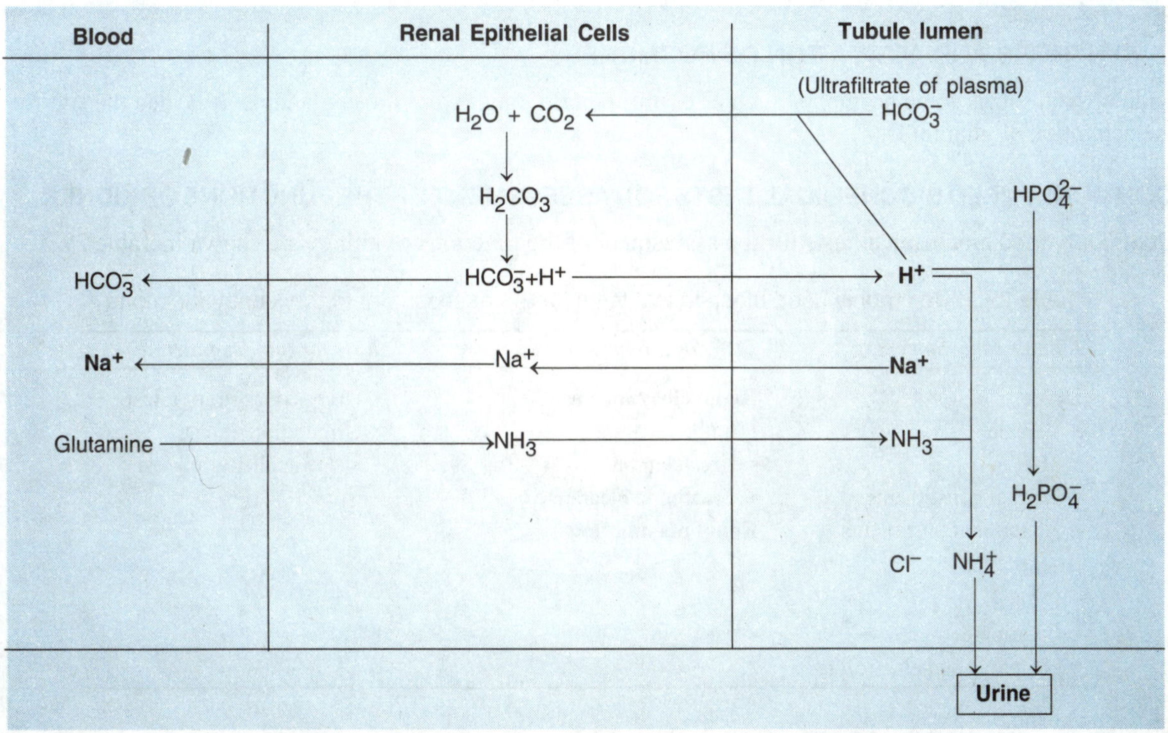

Fig. 29.2. Regulation of acid-base balance by the kidney.

1. ***Exchange of H^+ for Na^+:*** Na^+ that is present in the lumen of the renal tubule, i.e. in the ultrafiltrate of plasma, is exchanged for H^+, which is formed in the tubular epithelial cells from CO_2 and H_2O. Na^+ is transported from the epithelial cells into the blood plasma for recycling. This transport of Na^+ is mediated by sodium pump.

   In the presence of carbonic anhydrase, CO_2 and H_2O form carbonic acid, which is dissociated into H^+ and HCO_3^-. HCO_3^- diffuses from the epithelial cells into the blood plasma as the accompanying ion to Na^+ and thus HCO_3^- is conserved.

2. ***Reabsorption of HCO_3^- from the tubular urine:*** The H^+ that is exchanged into the tubular urine, reacts with HCO_3^- in the plasma ultrafiltrate and forms H_2CO_3. This is dissociated to CO_2 and H_2O from where CO_2 diffuses back into the epithelial cells.
3. ***Formation and excretion of NH_3:*** Glutamine is extracted from the renal blood plasma of the peritubular capillaries and is deaminated by glutaminase in the tubular epithelial cells, to release NH_3 and glutamate.

   NH_3 so formed is diffused into the tubular urine and binds with H^+ to form NH_4^+.
4. ***Excretion of H^+:*** The H^+ ions that are exchanged for Na^+ bind to HPO_4^{2-} to form $H_2PO_4^-$ (titratable acid). Both $H_2PO_4^-$ and NH_4^+ are thus excreted in the urine. The accompanying ions are predominantly, Na^+ and Cl^-, respectively.

Kidney thus participates in the regulation of acid-base balance, primarily, by maintaining the HCO_3^- concentration in the plasma.

In the event of acidosis, excretion of both $H_2PO_4^-$ and NH_4^+ are increased in the urine while the reverse occurs in alkalosis, until acid-base balance is restored.

4. SYNTHESIS AND ACTIVATION OF HORMONES

Kidney synthesizes some hormones such as erythropoietin, rennin and prostaglandins. It is also the site for the activation of vitamin D.

COMMONLY USED BIOCHEMICAL TESTS FOR ASSESSMENT OF THE FUNCTIONS OF KIDNEY

Commonly used biochemical tests for the assessment of the functions of kidney are shown in Table 29.2

Table 29.2. Commonly used biochemical tests for the assessment of the kidney functions

Routine laboratory tests	*Tests for glomerular functions*	*Tests for tubular functions*
Urine	**Renal clearance test**	• Urine concentration test
• Volume	• Inulin clearance	• Urine dilution test
• pH	• Urea clearance	• Urine acidification test
• Normal constituents	• Creatinine clearance	
• Abnormal constituents	**Renal plasma flow**	
Blood		
• Urea		
• Creatinine		
• pH, gases and electrolytes		

ROUTINE LABORATORY TESTS

EXAMINATION OF THE URINE

Physical Characteristics of Urine

Volume

Volume of the urine varies from person to person and time to time. Average volume of urine, excreted by a normal individual, over a period of 24 hours, is **1000-1500 ml**. It is influenced by diet, particularly, ingestion of fluids. Strenuous physical exercise, hot weather and fever diminish urine output.

Certain pathological conditions alter urine output. If 24 hours volume is increased, the condition is called **polyuria**, such as seen in diabetes and early renal failure.

When urine output is decreased, it is termed as **oliguria** such as seen in acute renal failure, dehydration (diarrhea and vomiting), edema and urinary obstruction.

In acute renal failure and shock, urine may not be formed. This condition is called **anuria.**

Color

Normal urine is usually pale, straw-yellow colored, due to the presence of urochrome, uroerythrin and urobilin.

Change in color may be due to some pathology, secondary to the intake of some drug, or a particular type of food.

In fever it is usually dark in color, if there is blood in the urine (due to hemorrhage in the kidney or the urinary tract), urine becomes red in color. In jaundice urine may be dark-yellow or green due to the oxidation of bilirubin to biliverdin.

General Appearance and Odor

Freshly excreted urine is normally clear and transparent, as all the substances are present in the soluble form. On standing, it becomes turbid due to precipitation of phosphates.

Pathological urine may be turbid due to the presence of fat globules or pus cells.

Odor of the urine is usually aromatic, due to the presence of volatile acids. On standing urine may develop pungent odor due to formation of ammonia from urea because of its decomposition by bacteria.

In acidosis and diabetes mellitus, urine has a peculiar sweet smell due to the presence of acetone.

Specific Gravity

Specific gravity of urine normally varies between 1.010–1.030.

Volume has a great influence on specific gravity of urine. Low values (up to 1.003) are observed after large water intake, on diuretic therapy or excretion of large amount of acetone. High values (up to 1.040) are seen in dehydration or due to the presence of large amount of glucose.

Specific gravity of urine is measured by means of hydrometer, known as urinometer. Mark on the urinometer, in contact with surface of urine, indicates specific gravity of the sample.

pH (Reaction)

Under normal circumstances urine is slightly acidic in reaction, with a **mean pH of about 6.0 (ranging from 4.8-8.0)**

The pH of urine varies widely depending upon the nature of the food taken. High protein diet leads to acidic urine while alkaline urine is excreted after a vegetarian diet, particularly after large intake of vegetables and fruits.

Following meals, pH of the urine becomes alkaline due to the production and secretion of HCl by the stomach.

Alkaline urine is seen in patients with systemic alkalosis since body attempts to conserve H^+ ions and remove fixed bases. Strongly acidic urine is seen in patients with systemic acidosis, e.g. diabetes mellitus due to the excretion of large amount of ketone bodies.

An increase in pH, greater than 8.0, indicates urinary tract infection by an organism that splits urea to ammonia.

The pH of urine is routinely checked with the help of pH paper. Its reaction can be tested with the help of litmus paper.

CHEMICAL CONSTITUENTS OF THE URINE

NORMAL CONSTITUENTS

Major constituents of normal urine are shown in Table 29.3.

Normally, 50–60 g of solids are excreted in the urine over a period of 24 hours. About half of the total solids is urea. It comprises of nearly 80–90% of total organic substances. Other organic constituents of normal urine include creatinine, uric acid, hippuric acid and ethereal sulfates.

Major inorganic substance excreted is chloride (as sodium chloride). It constitutes about 25% of the total solids excreted in 24 hours. Other inorganic constituents normally excreted in the urine include ammonia, phosphates and sulfates.

In certain pathological conditions these constituents may be excreted in abnormal amounts.

Table 29.3. Normal constituents of urine

Constituents	*Daily excretion (g/24 hours)*
Water	1000–1500
Total solids	50–60
Organic Substances	30–35
Urea	25–30
Uric acid	0.5–1.0
Creatinine	1.0–1.8
Free amino acids (as amino acid N)	0.15–0.20
Inorganic substances	20–25
Chloride (as NaCl)	10–15
Total sulfates (as sulfur)	0.7–1.0
Total phosphates (as inorganic phosphorus)	0.8–1.1
Ammonia	0.5–0.7

Organic Substances

Urea

Urea is a principal end product of protein catabolism in mammals. An adult man excretes 25–30 g of urea under normal conditions in 24 hours.

Urea excretion is increased on high protein diet or in protein catabolic states such as fever.

On low protein diet urea excretion is reduced. Decrease in urea excretion is also observed in disorders, which are associated with impaired liver function, such as cirrhosis, as well as in a kidney disease, such as nephritis.

Uric Acid

Uric acid is derived from nucleic acids by the oxidation of purine bases. It is found in urine to the extent of 0.5 to 1.0 g/24 hours. Its daily excretion however varies, depending upon the diet and several other factors.

On a purine-free diet, uric acid output may be reduced up to 0.1 g/24 hours. On a high purine diet, uric acid excretion may be increased up to 2.0 g/24 hours.

Pathologically, uric acid excretion is increased in gout and leukemia.

Creatinine

Creatinine (a waste product) is anhydride of creatine. Creatinine is present in considerable amount in muscle, in the form of creatine phosphate. Very little of creatine is found in the urine.

On the other hand, about 1.0 to 1.8 g of creatinine is excreted by an adult in 24 hours. Excretion of creatinine is related to the amount of body creatine, i.e. muscle mass. Daily excretion of creatinine is therefore fairly constant and is used to check the accuracy of 24 hours urine collection.

Creatinine content of urine is increased in conditions associated with increased muscular activity.

A decrease in creatinine excretion may be observed in disorders, which are associated with muscular weakness as well as in a kidney disease.

Amino Acids

Due to high threshold, normally only small amounts of free amino acids are found in the urine. Their daily excretion (as amino acid nitrogen) is about 150-200 mg. Infants excrete more amino acids as compared to adults. During pregnancy excretion of amino acids is increased.

Amino aciduria may be prominent in certain liver diseases and after poisoning by chloroform or carbon tetrachloride.

In certain metabolic diseases increased excretion of some of the amino acids may be observed, such as arginine, cystine, lysine and ornithine in cystinuria.

Inorganic Substances

Chloride

Chloride is a major inorganic constituent of the normal urine. Its excretion is dependent upon chloride content of the food. On an average daily output of chloride (expressed as sodium chloride) varies between 10–15 g. Fasting as well as excessive perspiration decreases its urinary output.

Pathologically, its excretion may be decreased in chronic nephritis, fever, burn, diarrhea and vomiting.

Phosphates

Phosphates are present in the urine in various forms, e.g. **alkaline phosphates** such as sodium, potassium and ammonium phosphates, which are derived from the ingested inorganic phosphate or **earthy phosphates** such as phosphates of calcium and magnesium. These are insoluble phosphates and get precipitated in alkaline urine.

Excretion of phosphorus is dependent upon diet but on an average nearly 1.0 g of phosphate (as inorganic phosphorus) is excreted in 24 hours.

Urinary phosphorus is increased in acidosis and certain bone diseases, e.g. rickets and osteomalacia.

Phosphorus excretion is reduced in pregnancy, renal and infectious diseases as well as in hyperparathyroidism.

Sulfates

Sulfates arise in the urine from the oxidation of sulphur, which is obtained from the sulphur containing amino acids. Only a small amount of the ingested sulphur is excreted.

Sulfates are present in the urine in various forms, e.g. **inorganic sulfates** such as sodium, calcium and magnesium sulphates; **etheral sulfates** which are mostly the detoxification products, and **neutral sulfates** e.g. cystine, taurine, etc.

Under normal conditions about 1.0 g of sulfates (as sulfur) are excreted in the urine daily.

Ammonia

Tubular cells of the kidney form ammonia. Precursor for ammonia is the amide nitrogen of glutamine. A decrease in blood pH speeds up ammonia production.

Normally, about 0.5-0.7 g of ammonia is excreted in 24 hours. Although very little of it is present in a fresh sample of the urine, its level increases on standing, due to bacterial decomposition of urea.

Ammonia excretion is decreased in a kidney disease while its excretion is increased in acidosis such as in diabetic ketoacidosis.

ABNORMAL CONSTITUENTS

In the process of filtration of plasma through glomeruli, large molecular weight substances such as proteins are retained while small molecular weight substances, which are useful for the body, are reabsorbed. Normally, their amounts are so low that they are not detectable, by the routine laboratory tests.

Under certain pathological conditions, when either their metabolism is disturbed or a tubular damage occurs, large quantities of these substances are excreted in the urine. Hence these substances are called **abnormal constituents of urine.** These include sugar (glucose), ketone bodies, protein (albumin), blood, bile salts and bile pigments (Table 29.4).

Table 29.4. Abnormal constituents of urine

Constituent	*Conditions in which excreted*
Sugar (glucose)	Diabetes mellitus, renal glycosuria
Ketone bodies	Prolonged starvation, low-carbohydrate high-fat diet, diabetic ketoacidosis
Protein (albumin)	Nephrotic syndrome, glomerulonephritis
Blood	Hematuria, hemoglobinuria
Bile salts/bile pigments	Different types of jaundice

Sugar

Excretion of, readily detectable amount of sugar in the urine is known as **mellituria** or **glycosuria** whereas excretion of glucose is referred to as **glucosuria**.

When blood glucose concentration exceeds 180 mg/100 ml such as in diabetes mellitus, reabsorptive capacity of the tubule is reduced and glucose appears in the urine. Glucose may also be found in the urine in hyperthyroidism, hyperpituitarism, hyperadrenalism or I-cell disease of the pancreas.

Glucosuria may also be observed in a proximal tubular disease that impairs reabsorptive mechanism. This is known as **renal glucosuria.** In this condition, glucose utilization as well as blood glucose level may be normal.

Besides glucose, other sugars that may be excreted in the urine include lactose, galactose, fructose or pentoses.

Lactosuria may be observed in lactating women.

Fructose may be present in the urine after ingestion of large quantity of honey. Essential fructosuria is an inborn error of metabolism due to the deficiency of the enzyme fructokinase.

Pentoses may be found after ingestion of large quantities of fruits like plums and cherries. Pentosuria, referred to as L-xylulosuria, is an inborn error of metabolism due to the deficiency of xylitol dehydrogenase.

Galactosuria may be observed in infants suffering from congenital galactosemia. Galactosuria may also be seen in infants as well as adults with a liver disease.

Ketone Bodies

Ketone bodies (acetoacetate, β-hydroxybutyrate and acetone) are formed in considerable amount when fat is metabolized, excessively. Their accumulation in the blood is called **ketonemia** while their excretion in the urine is referred to as **ketonuria.** Ketonemia and ketonuria occur in a condition, which is referred to as **ketosis.**

Ketosis may occur during prolonged fasting or carbohydrate deprivation. Pathologically, ketone bodies appear in the urine in diabetic ketoacidosis.

Proteins

Normal urine contains only traces of protein, which can not be detected by routine procedures. When readily detectable amount of protein is seen in urine, this condition is called **proteinuria.** Since it is mainly the albumin that is detected abnormally, hence, proteinuria may also be referred to as **albuminuria.**

Proteinuria or albuminuria may be physiological (benign albuminuria) or pathological (renal albuminuria).

Physiological proteinuria is usually transitory. There is no evidence of kidney damage but proteinuria may be observed after severe exercise, high protein diet, pregnancy or postural effect (when an individual assumes an upright position for a long period). The later is called **orthostatic** or **postural proteinuria.**

Pathological proteinuria may be classified as:

- Pre-renal proteinuria
- Renal proteinuria, or
- Post-renal proteinuria

Pre-renal proteinuria: Pre-renal proteinuria may be observed in conditions that are primarily not related to the kidney, e.g. a cardiac disease, by affecting the circulation of the kidney, may lead to proteinuria. Besides, fever, convulsions, anemia and a liver disease may also result in proteinuria.

Renal proteinuria: Renal proteinuria may be observed due to inflammation of the kidney (nephritis) or kidney damage (nephrosis). Proteinuria due to a glomerular disease can lead to nephrotic syndrome where large amount of protein is excreted.

Acute tubular necrosis and pyelonephritis also lead to proteinuria, which is generally mild.

Post-renal proteinuria: Post-renal proteinuria may occur due to some inflammatory, degenerative or traumatic lesions of the pelvis of the kidney, ureter, bladder, prostate or urethra.

BENCE-JONES PROTEIN

It is a specific type of protein that appears in the urine of patients who are suffering from multiple myeloma, leukemia and Hodgkin's disease. Bence-Jones proteins are small molecular size subunits of γ-globulin (macroglobulin).]

They have a peculiar property of getting coagulated between 50-60°C and dissolve on heating above 60°C. They again reappear on cooling.

Blood

Either intact red blood cells or hemoglobin may be present in the urine.

Presence of red blood cells in the urine is referred to as **hematuria.** It can be confirmed by the presence of red blood cells by microscopic examination of the urine. RBCs may be seen in acute glomerulonephritis or trauma to the urinary tract.

Hemoglobinuria may be observed due to intravascular hemolysis. This, in turn, results in the liberation of the hemoglobin which is filtered in the glomerulus and appears in the urine. Hemoglobinuria may occur under various pathological conditions such as mis-matched transfusion of blood, hemolytic jaundice, typhoid or malaria.

Bile

Bile is produced in the liver. It is secreted through biliary tract and enters duodenum. It is alkaline in reaction and bitter in taste. Its colour varies from yellowish-brown to dark green. Important constituents of the bile are bile salts, bile pigments, lipids particularly phospholipids and cholesterol, proteins like mucin, urea and certain inorganic salts such as sodium chloride and bicarbonate.

Bile salts are the sodium and potassium salts of glycocholic and taurocholic acids.

Cholic acid has the basic ring structure of cyclopentanoperhydrophenanthrene, like cholesterol. In glycocholic acid, glycine is conjugated with cholic acid through a peptide linkage. Similarly, in taurocholic acid, taurine is conjugated with cholic acid. Bile salts are essential for the digestion of fat. Since fat is insoluble in water, it is not digested in the absence of bile salts. Bile salts emulsify fat by lowering surface tension of water and help to bring fat in intimate contact with the lipase.

Bile pigments are the degradation products of hemoglobin. When hemolysis of red blood cells takes place, hemoglobin is dissociated into heme and globin. Globin is hydrolyzed to amino acids by the proteolytic enzymes, while heme looses its iron, which is reutilized for heme synthesis. The tetrapyrrole ring (protoporphyrin) is broken down to biliverdin which is further oxidized to bilirubin. Bilirubin is predominant in human bile. When it enters the intestine, further changes take place due to bacterial action and a number of pigments are formed. Some of these are reabsorbed into blood through the intestine, modified and excreted through urine.

Urobilinogen

Urobilinogen is an important constituent of the freshly voided normal urine. Following its oxidative degradation, it disappears quickly. Increased amount of urobilinogen may be seen in the urine of patients with hemolytic jaundice.

ESTIMATION OF THE CONSTITUENTS OF BLOOD

Blood Urea

Urea is a major nitrogenous metabolic product of protein catabolism in man, accounting for more than 75% of the nonprotein nitrogen which is eventually excreted. Urea is freely filtered by the glomeruli. In a normal kidney, 40-70% urea moves passively out of the renal tubule into the interstitium.

Measurement of blood urea is widely used as a test of renal function. However, a number of non-renal factors influence circulating urea concentration. For example, urea production and consequently blood urea concentration are increased on a high protein diet, in protein catabolic states, gastrointestinal hemorrhage, treatment with cortisol, in some cases of chronic liver disease and with decreased perfusion of the kidney. Blood urea also depends upon the state of hydration of the patient.

Blood urea level, in a normal individual, may vary between 15-35 mg/dl. In patients with untreated chronic renal failure blood urea level may be increased to 100-150 mg/dl.

Serum Creatinine

Creatine is synthesized in the kidney, liver and pancreas. A portion of free creatine in muscle is spontaneously and irreversibly converted to its anhydride, i.e. creatinine. Free creatinine thus is a waste product of creatine. Its daily production is related to muscle mass and does not vary greatly from day to day. Hence, its level in the blood remains fairly constant. Creatinine is freely filtered at the glomerulus. Although it is not reabsorbed to any great extent by renal tubules but a small amount of it is secreted. Its secretion is increased with the increasing level of plasma creatinine.

Normal serum creatinine concentration varies between 0.8–1.5 mg/dl.

Meal, containing meat may increase serum creatinine concentration. Certain drugs, e.g. salicylates, cimetidine, etc., also increase serum creatinine level.

Serum creatinine values are lower in children than in adults, in women than in men, and during pregnancy. Determination of serum creatinine gives a useful indication of the degree of renal failure.

An increase in serum creatinine, due to fall in GFR is observed when:

1. There is decreased renal perfusion, e.g. reduced blood pressure, fluid deprivation or renal arterial stenosis,
2. There is a loss of functional nephrons, e.g. in acute and chronic glomerulonephritis, and
3. Pressure is increased on the tubular side of the nephron, e.g. in urinary tract obstruction due to prostate enlargement.

Blood pH, Gases and Electrolytes

Diminished capacity of the kidney to excrete H^+ results in metabolic acidosis, the severity of which may be assessed by measuring arterial H^+, HCO_3^- and pCO_2 concentrations.

Estimation of plasma sodium, potassium, calcium and phosphorus are also of value in certain kidney conditions, e.g. chronic renal failure or metabolic acidosis accompanied by hyponatremia, hyperkalemia, hypocalcemia and hyperphosphatemia.

TESTS FOR THE ASSESSMENT OF GLOMERULAR FUNCTIONS

Renal Clearance

Clearance is defined as **the volume of plasma that is cleared-off a particular substance by two kidneys in one minute.**

It can be calculated by the following mathematical relationship:

$$C = \frac{U \times V}{P}$$

where:

C = Clearance of the substance (ml/min)

U = Concentration of the substance (mg/dl) in urine

V = Rate of flow of urine (ml/min)

P = Concentration of the substance (mg/dl) in plasma, blood or serum

Markers of Renal Clearance

Suitable marker of renal clearance should meet the following criteria:

1. It should be freely filterable at the glomerulus.
2. It should not be reabsorbed by the tubules.
3. It should not be secreted by the tubules, and
4. It should be present at a stable plasma concentration.

For this purpose either an exogenous substance such as inulin or an endogenous substance like urea or creatinine is used.

Inulin clearance: Inulin is a polymer of fructose. It is filtered by the glomeruli but is neither reabsorbed nor secreted by the tubule. Inulin clearance therefore, is nearly equal to GFR.

Normal value for GFR, as per inulin clearance, found in adults is about 125 ml/min.

Although inulin meets most of the criteria for measuring GFR, it is not suitable for routine use as it is an exogenous substance and has to be administered intravenously.

Urea clearance: Urea clearance depends upon the rate of flow of urine. Accordingly, it has to be calculated as **standard urea clearance** or **maximum urea clearance.**

Standard urea clearance is calculated with standard rate of urine flow, i.e. when urine volume is below 2 ml/min.

$$\text{Standard Urea Clearance (ml/min)} = \frac{U}{B} \times \sqrt{V}$$

where U and B are concentrations of urea (mg/100 ml) in urine and blood, respectively, while $\sqrt{V}$ is square root of the volume of urine excreted (ml/min). Mean value for standard urea clearance is 54 ml/min.

Maximum urea clearance is calculated when volume of urine excreted is 2 ml/min or more. It is calculated by putting the actual value of V in the above equation, instead of $\sqrt{V}$. Mean value for maximum urea clearance is 75 ml/min.

Urea clearance is not preferred to estimate GFR as it depends upon the rate of urine flow. Besides blood urea concentration is also affected by dietary protein.

Creatinine clearance: Creatinine is produced endogenously from creatine and gains access to the urine by glomerular filtration. As the volume of urine flow does not affect it, it is preferred as a measure of GFR.

Creatinine clearance (per 1.73 m^2 surface area) is low at birth (35–40 ml/min) and reaches the normal adult value (80–120 ml/min) by 6 months of age. It further declines with age.

Creatinine clearance is increased by 20% during pregnancy.

Renal Plasma Flow

By measuring excretion rate of a substance, which undergo both, glomerular filtration as well as tubular secretion, e.g. p-aminohippuric acid, we can measure renal plasma flow (PAH).

As determined with PAH clearance, renal plasma flow for normal adult male is 700 ± 130 ml/min.

TESTS FOR THE ASSESSMENT OF TUBULAR FUNCTIONS

Urine Concentration Test

Urine concentration test is done by measuring osmolality (number of solute particles per kg water) of the specimen of urine after water deprivation or administration of vasopressin (ADH).

Restriction of water results in maximum stimulation of ADH secretion, in a normal subject. Since ADH acts on collecting tubules and promotes reabsorption of water, it results in concentrated urine.

For the test, the subject is not given water or any other fluid for 8 hours. Thereafter, osmolality of the urine is measured which should be 800 mosm/kg. Specific gravity of this sample should be 1.022. If the urine sample has less osmolality or specific gravity, it indicates impaired renal concentrating power of the kidney either due to a tubular defect or decreased ADH secretion.

Urine Dilution Test

Urine dilution test is done to assess ability of the kidney to eliminate excessive amount of water.

After an overnight fast, the subject is asked to empty the bladder and given 1000 ml of water to drink within 20 minutes. In a normal subject 750 ml of it is excreted within 4 hours. During this period, urine samples are collected after every one-hour. Specific gravity of one of the specimen should be 1.003 while its osmolality should be less than 100 mosm/kg. If renal function is impaired, quantity of water eliminated in 4 hours will be reduced. Moreover, specific gravity of the urine will be 1.010 or higher.

The test is not advisible in patients with adrenal insufficiency.

Urine Acidification Test

Ability of the kidney to produce acidic urine is also an important function of the tubule.

For this test, person is asked to empty the bladder and given ammonium chloride (0.1 g/kg body weight, in a gelatin capsule). Thereafter, urine samples are collected each hourly, for 8 hours. The pH of the urine during this period should be between 4.6-5.0.

In patient with renal tubular acidosis, pH of the urine does not fall below 5.3.

UREA, URIC ACID AND CREATININE PROFILE IN KIDNEY DISORDERS

UREA

Over 75% of the non-protein nitrogen is excreted as urea, mainly by the kidneys, and failure of the kidneys to excrete urea may lead to increase in blood urea. Hence, urea measurement is widely accepted as a measure of renal function.

Estimation of plasma urea concentration, however, is a less valuable test of renal function than plasma creatinine concentration. This is due to the reason that nearly 50% of the urea, filtered at the glomerulus, is passively reabsorbed through the tubules and this fraction increases if urine flow rate increases, such as in dehydration. Plasma urea concentration is also more affected by diet than plasma creatinine.

Low blood urea concentration may be observed in several situations, such as reduced synthesis, e.g. on a low protein diet or in an acute liver disease. Blood urea level may also fall as a result of water retention.

High blood urea concentration may be due to several causes, which may be subdivided into pre-renal, renal and post-renal:

Pre-renal causes of increase in blood urea concentration include increased production by the liver (such as on a high protein diet), haemorrhage into the upper gastrointestinal tract, or in protein catabolic states (e.g. due to trauma, major surgery, or starvation). It may also be due to impaired renal perfusion (e.g. extracellular fluid loss, cardiac failure, hypoproteinemia, etc.).

Renal causes of increase in blood urea concentration include acute or chronic renal failure with reduction in glomerular filtration.

Post-renal causes include obstruction to urine flow, such as stone, benign prostatic hypertrophy, malignant stricture, or obstruction.

CREATININE

Serum creatinine concentration is a more precise measurement than creatinine clearance and is usually sufficient for following the progress of patients with renal disease. Because:

1. Plasma creatinine concentration normally remains fairly constant throughout adult life whereas creatinine clearance declines with advancing age.
2. Plasma creatinine concentration correlates well with GFR as does creatinine clearance in patients with renal disease.
3. Measurement of plasma creatinine concentration is as effective in detecting early renal disease as creatinine clearance, and
4. Sequential plasma creatinine concentration measurements enable the progress of renal disease to be followed with better precision than creatinine clearance.

Reduced plasma creatinine concentration is found in subjects with a small total muscle mass. Thus, a lower value is found in children. Values are, on average, normally lower in women than in men. Abnormally low values may be found in wasting diseases (reduced muscle bulk) and starvation, and in patients on steroid therapy, due to their protein catabolic effect. Plasma creatinine concentration is also usually low in pregnancy.

Increased plasma creatinine concentration may be observed in several non-renal situations. For example:

1. High meat intake can cause temporary rise in plasma creatinine level.
2. Transient small increase in plasma creatinine level may occur after vigorous exercise.
3. Some drugs, e.g. salicylates, cimetidine, etc., reduce tubular secretion of creatinine hence, exhibit elevated plasma creatinine concentration.
4. High concentration of certain compounds, such as acetoacetate or cephalosporin antibiotic exhibit analytical interference and result in its overestimation.

An increased plasma creatinine concentration indicates a fall in GFR. Renal causes of increased plasma creatinine level include:

1. A disease, in which there is impaired renal perfusion, e.g. reduced blood pressure, fluid depletion, renal artery stenosis, etc.,
2. Diseases in which there is loss of functioning nephrons, e.g. glomerulonephritis,
3. Urinary tract obstruction due to prostatic enlargment.

URIC ACID

An increase in serum uric acid is found to correspond roughly with the increase in urea. With increasing renal failure, serum uric acid is markedly increased. However, estimation of uric acid is of little use in renal disease; it may be due to the reason that several other factors also influence uric acid level.

SOME IMPORTANT QUESTIONS

1. Describe various functions of the kidney.
2. Describe various kidney function tests.
3. What are normal constituents of urine? Describe conditions in which their levels are increased.
4. What are abnormal constituents of urine? Discuss various conditions in which they are excreted.
5. Discuss briefly :
   (i) Excretory functions of kidney
   (ii) Water and electrolytes homeostasis
   (iii) Acid-base balance
   (iv) Blood buffers
6. Write notes on :
   (i) Polyuria
   (ii) Abnormal constituents of urine
   (iii) Renal glycosuria
   (iv) Ketonemia
   (v) Ketonuria
   (vi) Physiological proteinuria
   (vii) Bence-Jones proteins

CHAPTER 30

Specimen Collection and Normal Values

SPECIMEN COLLECTION

Collection of Blood for Various Biochemical Tests

Blood may be obtained from veins, arteries or capillaries. Venipuncture is mainly used for obtaining venous blood, preferably from the median cubital vein. In infants, skin puncture is done to obtain capillary blood. Arterial puncture is used mainly for blood gas analysis, preferably, from the radial artery in the wrist.

For most of the investigations, in biochemistry either serum or plasma can be used. For investigations, such as bilirubin, calcium, cholesterol, creatinine, electrolytes (sodium and potassium), phosphorus, protein, uric acid as well as many enzymes, e.g. acid and alkaline phosphatases, amylase, SGOT/SGPT, LDH, etc., 3 to 5 ml of blood is collected in plain vial.

For glucose, 2 ml of fluoride-oxalated, heparinized or plain blood is collected. For urea 2 ml blood may be collected either in a plain vial or with fluoride/fluoride and oxalate.

For triglycerides 3–5 ml blood is collected in a plain vial, essentially after 12 hours of fasting.

For blood gases, 1–2 ml of arterial blood is collected in a syringe with heparin, without any air bubble. It should be immediately transported to the laboratory for analysis.

Collection of Urine

For the quantitation of creatinine, protein, 17-ketosteroids or VMA in urine, 24 hours sample is collected, in 2 litres bottle, with few crystals of thymol.

For calcium 10 ml of 6 N HCl is added in the bottle.

First morning and midstream urine sample (about 25-30 ml) is collected for Bence Jones protein as well as urobilinogen.

NORMAL VALUES OF SOME IMPORTANT CONSTITUENTS OF BLOOD, URINE, C.S.F. AND GASTRIC JUICE

The range of normal values of some important constituents of blood, urine, C.S.F and gastric juice are shown for male adults, in the fasting state, in conventional units in Table 30.1–30.4.

Table 30.1. Normal values of some constituents of blood

Constituent	*Normal range*
Common Constituents	
Bilirubin (total)	0.2–0.8 mg/dL
Calcium (total)	9–11 mg/dL
Cholesterol (total)	140–220 mg/dL
Creatinine	0.8–1.3 mg/dL
Glucose (fasting)	60–100 mg/dL
Phosphorus (inorganic)	3.0–4.5 mg/dL
Urea	15–40 mg/dL
Uric acid	3–7 mg/dL
Proteins	
Total serum proteins	6.0–8.3 g/dL
Serum albumin	3.5–5.2 g/dL
Serum globulins	2.5–3.5 g/dL
A/G Ratio	1.1–1.7
Lipid Profile	
Serum triglycerides	50–160 mg/dL
Total cholesterol	140–220 mg/dL
HDL-Cholesterol	30–60 mg/dL
LDL-Cholesterol	60–160 mg/dL
VLDL-Cholesterol	upto 32 mg/dL
Electrolytes	
Sodium	136–145 meq/L
Potassium	3.5–5.0 meq/L
Chloride	98–107 meq/L
Enzymes	
Acid phosphatase	1–3.5 KA Units/dL
Alkaline phosphatase	3–13 KA Units/dL
Amylase	60–180 Somogyi U/dL
LDH	100–190 U/L
SGOT	upto 40 U/L
SGPT	upto 40 U/L
CPK (total)	20–90 U/L
Hormones	
Cortisol	5–25 μg/dL (8 AM)
T_3	70–200 ng/dL

(Contd.)

Constituent	*Normal range*
T_4	5–12 ng/dL
TSH	0–5 µU/ml
Acid-base analysis and blood gases	
pH	7.35–7.45
Total CO_2	22–28 mmol/L
Bicarbonate (actual)	22–26 mmol/L
pCO_2	31–45 mm of Hg
pO_2	85–95 mm of Hg
Oxygen saturation	96–100%
Anion gap $[(Na^+ + K^+)-(Cl^- + HCO_3^-)]$	10–20 mmol/L
Base excess	–2 to +3 mmol/L

Table 30.2. Normal values for some constituents in urine

Constitution	*Normal excretion*
D-xylose	1–2 g/5 hrs
Total nitrogen	10–20 g/24 hrs
Creatinine	1.0–2.0 g/24 hrs
Calcium	0.1–0.7 g/24 hrs
Chloride	110–250 meq/24 hrs
Sodium	40–220 meq/24 hrs
Potassium	25–125 meq/24 hrs
Phosphorus	0.6–1.5 g/24 hrs
Urea	20–35 g/24 hrs
Uric Acid	0.5–1.0 g/24 hrs

Table 30.3. Normal values for some constituents in C.S.F

Constitution	*Normal concentration*
Total protein	15–40 mg/dL
Glucose	50–75 mg/dL
Chloride (as NaCl)	700–750 mg/dL (118-132 mmol/L)

Table 30.4. Normal values for some parameters in gastric juice

Parameter	*Normal Range*
Volume	2–3 L/24 hrs
pH	1.6–1.8
Titrable acidity (fasting sample)	15–35 meq/L
Basal acid output	
Males	1.0–5.0 meq/hrs
Females	0.2–3.8 meq/hrs
Maximal acid output (after histamine/pentagastrin)	
Males	18–28 meq/hrs
Females	11–21 meq/hrs

CHAPTER

31

Practical Exercises

I. QUALITATIVE ANALYSIS OF CARBOHYDRATES

Several tests are done for the detection of a carbohydrate. The unspecific tests include Molisch's test, which is based on the formation of a furfural or its derivatives in the presence of concentrated acid. Other tests, e.g. Fehling's test, Benedict's test, etc., are based on their reducing properties. Complex formation, such as the formation of phenylhydrazone crystals, is also used as a specific test for some of the carbohydrates. For testing polysaccharides, iodine is commonly used.

MOLISCH TEST

Take about 2 ml of a carbohydrate solution in a test tube. Add a drop of the Molisch reagent and mix cautiously. Continuously pour down about 1 ml of concentrated H_2SO_4 so that two distinct layers are formed (the bottom layer being that of the acid). A reddish-violet zone appears at the junction of the two layers.

Molisch reagent is 10% solution of α-naphthol in ethanol.

This reaction is due to the formation of the furfural or its derivatives (Fig. 31.1).

Furfural and furfural derivatives are highly reactive substances. They react with a number of compounds to produce complex-colored products.

It is not a specific test for a carbohydrate. It is, however, an indication of the presence of a carbohydrate.

TESTS FOR A REDUCING SUGAR

Due to the presence of a free aldehyde or ketone group, carbohydrates are readily oxidized and behave as reducing agents. Only the reducing sugars therefore, will give a positive reaction. Non-reducing sugars like sucrose will respond to these reactions after its hydrolysis to glucose and fructose.

The following tests are based on the reducing properties of a sugar.

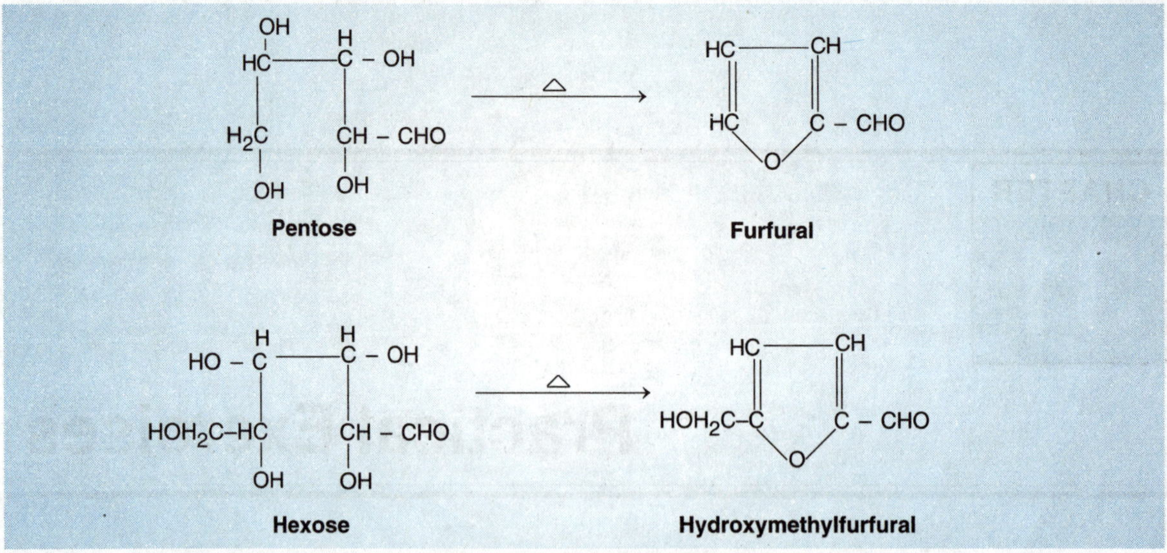

Fig. 31.1. Formation of furfural/furfural derivative from a carbohydrate.

Fehling's Test

Add 1 ml of a sugar solution (a few drops at a time) to 4 ml of warm Fehling solution and heat the mixture. Red precipitate indicates the presence of a reducing sugar.

Fehling solution is a mixture of copper sulfate and sodium-potassium tartarate. The two solutions are mixed afresh in equal volumes. This test is obtained due to the reduction of copper sulfate ($CuSO_4$) to cuprous oxide (Cu_2O) in an alkaline medium.

Benedict's test

Add 5 ml of the Benedict reagent (qualitative Benedict reagent) to 0.5 ml of a sugar solution in a test tube. Mix and heat the contents. In case of a reducing sugar, there is the appearance of a red precipitate.

Benedict qualitative solution is prepared by dissolving sodium citrate and sodium carbonate in water. Copper sulfate solution is slowly added with constant stirring to the citrate-carbonate mixture. In the presence of a reducing sugar, a red precipitate is observed.

This test is routinely used in the examination of urine, for the detection of a reducing sugar.

Benedict test is more specific for a reducing sugar than the Fehling test. In the Fehling test, reduction of $CuSO_4$ takes place in a strong alkaline medium, where even a small quantity of a reducing substance gives red precipitate while in the Benedict test reduction occurs in a weak alkaline medium. Hence, Fehling test is more sensitive but less specific whereas Benedict test is less sensitive but more specific.

Barfoed's Test

Mix 5 ml of the Barfoed reagent with 0.5 ml of the carbohydrate solution in a test tube and heat in a boiling water bath for 5 min. Appearance of the red precipitate within 5-min indicates the presence of a monosaccharide. If red precipitate is seen after 5 min, it confirms the presence of a reducing disaccharide (lactose or maltose).

Barfoed reagent is prepared by dissolving neutral copper acetate in water, thereafter glacial acetic acid is added to it. Barfoed test is also a copper reduction test. It however, differs from the Fehling or the Benedict tests. In Barfoed test, reduction of copper sulfate occurs in acidic medium, instead of the alkaline medium in the other two tests.

When a sugar solution is boiled with the Barfoed reagent, a disaccharide is hydrolyzed by the acetic acid present in the reagent and the monosaccharides give a positive test. Hence, monosaccharides respond quickly than a disaccharide.

TEST FOR PENTOSES

Take 3 ml of the orcinol reagent and add 0.5 ml of the sugar solution to it. Boil the contents. Presence of a deep-green color indicates the presence of a pentose.

Orcinol reagent contains orcinol and ferric chloride in concentrated HCl.

Pentoses react with HCl to form furfural, which then reacts with a phenol compound, such as orcinol, and forms a deep green colored complex.

TEST FOR GALACTOSE

Take 2 ml of the sugar solution in a test tube. To it, add 2 ml of concentrated HCl and 1 ml of fluoroglucinol solution. Boil slowly. A red color confirms the presence of galactose. This test is referred to as Tollen's test.

Galactose forms a red colored complex with fluoroglucinol in concentrated HCl.

Lactose, after hydrolysis in hot acid reagent, also gives the positive test due to the presence of galactose.

TEST FOR A KETO SUGAR

To 0.5 ml of the sugar solution, add 5 ml of the Saliwanoff's reagent. A blank (containing water) is prepared without the sugar solution to judge for the color. Place the test tube in a boiling water bath for 1 min. Red color indicates the presence of a keto sugar such as fructose. This test is called Saliwanoff test.

Saliwanoff reagent is resorcinol in concentrated HCl.

A ketose gives a fiery-red color. Aldoses such as glucose may also give the weak test. If boiling is prolonged, the positive test may be obtained with glucose due to its partial conversion to fructose.

This test may also be given by sucrose, which is hydrolyzed during the course of the test, yielding fructose as one of the products. However, the test will be positive after 1 min.

OSAZONE TEST

Take about 200–300 mg (nearly 2–3 spoonfull) of phenyl hydrazine mixture in a test tube. Add few drops of glacial acetic acid and about 5 ml of the sugar solution. Shake well and heat the content in a boiling water bath for 15–30 min. Remove the test tube and allow it to cool, slowly. Yellow crystals of phenylhydrazine, called osazone crystals, appear. This test is called phenylhydrazine test or osazone test.

Crystals of the maltose and the lactose appear only on cooling and not in the hot solution while that of glucose appear even when the tube is in the water bath.

Collect some of the crystals by a pipette, transfer them to a glass slide, and examine under microscope.

Fine needle-shaped yellow crystals are characteristic of a monosaccharide. Glucose, mannose, and fructose give identical osazones. This is due to the reason that except first two carbons (which are identically involved in the formation of osazones), the remaining four carbons have the same configuration in the three sugars.

Sucrose does not form osazone because of not having a free reducing group available for its reaction with phenylhydrazine.

Crystals of lactose are puff-shaped while those of maltose are petal-shaped.

Phenylhydrazine mixture is prepared by mixing equal quantities of the phenylhydrazine hydrochloride with anhydrous sodium acetate.

TEST FOR POLYSACCHARIDES

Take 5 ml of starch solution in a test tube. Add a drop of dilute iodine solution and note the presence of blue color. This test is called iodine test.

Heat the test tube. The blue color disappears but reappears on cooling. Blue colored substance is an adsorption complex between the starch and the iodine. Since this complex dissociates on heating therefore, the color subsequently disappears on heating.

The complex is formed under neutral or acidic conditions. Under alkaline conditions I_2 reacts with NaOH so blue color disappears. If alkali is neutralized with acid, I_2 is released and blue color reappears. Color formed by iodine test depends upon the length of the unbranched (linear) chain of the molecule.

Amylose gives deep blue color; amylopectin (branched chain compound) gives a purple color while glycogen (highly branched structure) gives a reddish brown color. Dextrin that is formed by the partial degradation of the starch gives brownish red color, as the linear chain length becomes smaller. On extensive degradation of the starch, the dextrin is formed, which may not give any color.

IDENTIFICATION OF AN UNKNOWN SOLUTION OF CARBOHYDRATE

The presence of a particular carbohydrate can be identified in an unknown solution by the Molisch's test. Fehling's and Benedict's tests confirm the presence of a reducing sugar. A non-reducing sugar may be a polysaccharide or sucrose.

Iodine test confirms the presence of a polysaccharide. If iodine test is negative, the non-reducing sugar is sucrose.

A reducing sugar may be a monosaccharide or a disaccharide. Barfoed's test confirms the presence of a disaccharide, which can be further identified by the phenylhydrazine test.

The orcinol test, Tollen's test, or the Saliwanoff's test may confirm the presence of pentoses, galactose, or fructose, respectively (Fig. 31.2).

II. COLOR REACTIONS OF PROTEINS AND AMINO ACIDS

PROTEIN PRECIPITATION

Precipitation by Salts

Proteins are the large molecular weight substances that can be easily precipitated by the addition of a salt solution. This process is known as **salting out**. Highly soluble salts like NaCl and $(NH_4)_2SO_4$ are used for this purpose.

For the ***precipitation of globulin*** from egg white, add **equal** volume of saturated solution of **ammonium sulfate** to **egg white** solution. Mix and wait for 10–15 minutes. Filter the precipitate. Residue on the filter paper contains **globulin**.

For the ***precipitation of albumin***, which is half-saturated **with ammonium sulfate**, add ammonium sulfate power to the filtrate so as to **saturate it completely**. **Albumin** is precipitated.

This shows that albumin is more soluble in water than globulin. Since, at full saturation albumin precipitates whereas at half saturation only globulin precipitates.

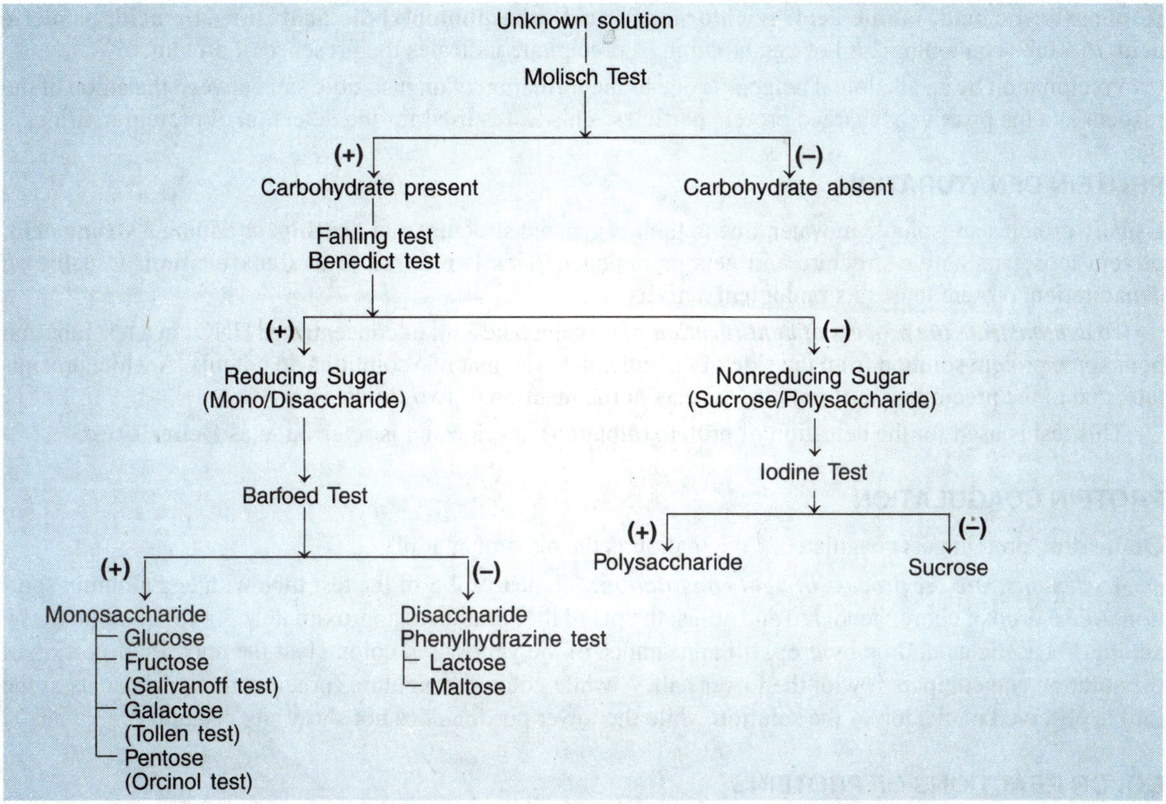

Fig. 31.2. Scheme for the identification of an unknown carbohydrate.

Precipitation of protein by a salt solution is, apparently, due to the neutralization of charge as well as dehydration of the molecule. Protein, which has been precipitated by a salt solution, remains native and usually gets redissolved when again, put in the solvent.

Precipitation by the Non-aqueous Solvent

Since proteins are not soluble in organic solvents, they can be easily precipitated with the addition of non-aqueous solvents, like **alcohol, acetone**, etc.

For the ***precipitation of protein*** from egg albumin ***by an organic solvent***, add 5 ml of **alcohol** to 3 ml of egg albumin solution. A white precipitate indicates that protein has been precipitated.

Precipitation by Heavy Metals

Most commonly used metals as protein precipitants, include metal salts such as **lead acetate, mercuric chloride, barium chloride,** or **zinc sulfate.**

For the ***precipitation of protein by a heavy metal***, add few drops of a salt solution of some heavy metal to 2 ml of egg albumin solution. A white precipitate indicates precipitation of protein.

Protein gets precipitated due to adsorption of the metallic cation by the negatively charged colloidal particles of the protein.

Precipitation by the Alkaloid Reagents

To see the ***precipitation of protein by an alkaloid solution***, add few drops of an alkaloid reagent, such as

sulphosalicylic acid, tannic acid, trichloracetic acid, phosphomolybdic acid, tungstic acid, or **picric acid,** to a tube containing 2 ml of egg albumin. A precipitate indicates the presence of protein.

Precipitation by an alkaloidal reagent is due to the formation of an insoluble salt between the anion of the reagent and the positively charged protein particles. This test is used for the detection of protein in urine.

PROTEIN DENATURATION

Usually proteins are soluble in water, due to their organized structure. On **heating,** or adding a **strong acid**, protein looses its native structure and gets precipitated. This is referred to as **denaturation**. Usually, on denaturation, protein **looses** its **biological activity**.

To ***demonstrate the process of denaturation*** of protein, take 3 ml of concentrated HNO_3 in a test tube and pour some protein solution from the side of the tube, in a way that two solutions do not mix. A white precipitate, due to the precipitation of protein, appears at the junction of two fluids.

This test is used for the detection of protein (albumin) in urine and is referred to as **Heller's test.**

PROTEIN COAGULATION

On heating protein gets coagulated. Coagulation is the maximum at pI.

To ***demonstrate the process of heat coagulation***, fill, nearly, 2/3 of the test tube with egg albumin solution. Add a drop of chorophenol red and adjust the pH of the solution to approximately 5.4 (pI of albumin) by adding 1% acetic acid, drop by drop, till appearance of the yellow-red color. Heat the upper-half portion of the solution and compare it with the lower half. A white colored coagulum (precipitate, which floats at the top) is observed on the top of the solution while the lower portion does not show any coagulum.

COLOR REACTIONS OF PROTEINS

A number of tests can be performed for the detection of proteins. These tests are either based on the presence of **peptide bonds,** such as **biuret test,** or indicate the presence of some **specific amino acid** in the protein, e.g. **xanthoproteic test, Millon's test, Hopkin-Cole test, Sakaguchi test,** or **lead acetate test.**

TEST BASED ON THE PRESENCE OF PEPTIDE BONDS

Biuret Test

To perform biuret test, take 2 ml of some **protein solution** in a test tube, add 2 ml of the qualitative **biuret reagent,** and mix. Depending upon the nature of the protein, **bluish-violet** to pink **color** is obtained.

In a separate tube, mix 2 ml of water with 2 ml of the biuret reagent for comparison.

To prepare **biuret reagent**, sodium potassium tartarate is dissolved in NaOH. Thereafter, $CuSO_4$ is added and the contents are mixed, until dissolved. Then add potassium iodide to it.

Principle of the Biuret Test: Peptide bonds (–CO–NH–), which are present in the protein, are responsible for the biuret test. A minimum of two consecutive peptide linkages give a positive test; i.e. minimum of a tripeptide (having two peptide linkages) gives the positive test. This test is called as the biuret test because biuret, which is formed on heating urea, also gives the test (Fig. 31.3).

$$\underset{\textbf{Urea}}{2NH_2-CO-NH_2} \xrightarrow[\searrow NH_3]{} \underset{\textbf{Biuret}}{NH_2-CO-NH-CO-NH_2}$$

Fig. 31.3. Formation of biuret.

Intensity of the color depends on the nature of the protein. Proteoses and peptones (partially degraded proteins) give a distinct pink color while gelatin (obtained by partial hydrolysis of collagen, which is present in the connective tissues, bones, etc.) gives blue color.

TESTS BASED ON THE PRESENCE OF SPECIFIC AMINO ACIDS

Xanthoproteic Test

To perform xanthoproteic test, ***heat 2 ml of a protein solution with 1 ml of concentrated nitric acid. Cool and add few drops of 10% NaOH. Orange color is obtained, which indicates the presence of aromatic amino acids.***

This reaction is due to the presence of benzene ring that gets nitrated in the presence of concentrated nitric acid, and forms nitrobenzene derivatives, which are yellow in color.

Among the 20 amino acids, which occur in most of the proteins, only 3 have a benzene ring. They are tyrosine, phenylalanine, and tryptophan. These amino acids are referred to as **aromatic amino acids.**

Millon's Test

To perform Millon's test, take 3 ml of some protein solution in a test tube, and add 3 to 4 drops of Millon's reagent. Mix, and heat the contents of the tube, over a flame so as to bring the solution to boiling. Usually, protein is precipitated under this condition (at high temperature, in the presence of a strong acid). A white precipitate is obtained, which is slowly turned to red, on heating. This indicates the presence of tyrosine.

Millon's reagent is prepared by dissolving Hg metal in fuming HNO_3, with gentle heating. Thereafter, 2 parts of water are added to it.

Tyrosine, due to the presence of the phenolic group, gives positive test with Millon's reagent.

Hopkin-Cole Test

To perform Hopkin-Cole test, take 3 ml of some protein solution, add 2 ml of the Hopkin-Cole reagent, and mix. Then, cautiously, pour down about 1 ml of concentrated H_2SO_4, so that the two layers do not mix together. A violet ring is formed at the junction of the two fluids, indicating the presence of tryptophan.

Hopkin-Cole reagent is an aqueous solution of glyoxylic acid. It is prepared by mixing magnesium powder with water. The mixture is shaken, cooled, and thereafter, cold saturated oxalic acid is added to it. The mixture is then thoroughly shaken and filtered.

Indole derivatives, such as **tryptophan,** give colored condensation products when treated with an aldehyde, like glyoxylic acid in the presence of H_2SO_4 or HCl.

Sakaguchi Test

To perform Sakaguchi test, take 3 ml of some protein solution and add 1 ml of 5% of NaOH, 2 drops of 1% alcoholic solution of α-napthol, and 1 drop of 10% sodium hypochlorite solution to it. Mix well. A bright-red color is observed due to the presence of arginine, an amino acid containing a guanidine group.

Lead Acetate Test

To perform lead acetate test, heat 1 ml of some protein solution with 1 ml of 40% NaOH. Thereafter, add few drops of 10% lead acetate solution, and again heat. A black precipitate is observed due to the formation of PbS, indicating the presence of sulphur containing amino acids.

III. SALIVA

Saliva is a **mixture of secretions from salivary glands.** Salivary glands are three pairs of bilateral glands, referred to as **the parotid, the submendibular, and the sublingual glands.** They are located along the jaw, from the base of the ear to the chin.

Secretion of one set of glands differs from that of the other. Secretion from the **parotid gland** is a serous fluid and contains an enzyme, referred to as **amylase. Sublingual glands** secrete a mucoid type of fluid, which contains mucous while secretion of the **submandibular gland** is **seromucous.**

COMPOSITION OF SALIVA

Saliva, a mixture of three different secretions, is a colorless, slightly opalescent, and viscous fluid with a specific gravity of 1.002–1.008. Its pH may vary from 6.4–7.3 whereas the resting salvia is slightly acidic (pH 6.4–6.9), salvia secreted under the influence of a stimulus is neutral to slightly alkaline (pH 7.0–7.3).

On an average, saliva contains nearly 99.4% water and 0.6% solids. Primary secretion is isotonic with plasma and contains both **organic** and **inorganic substances.** Nearly 65% of the total solids are organic substances while the remaining are inorganic salts (Fig. 31.4).

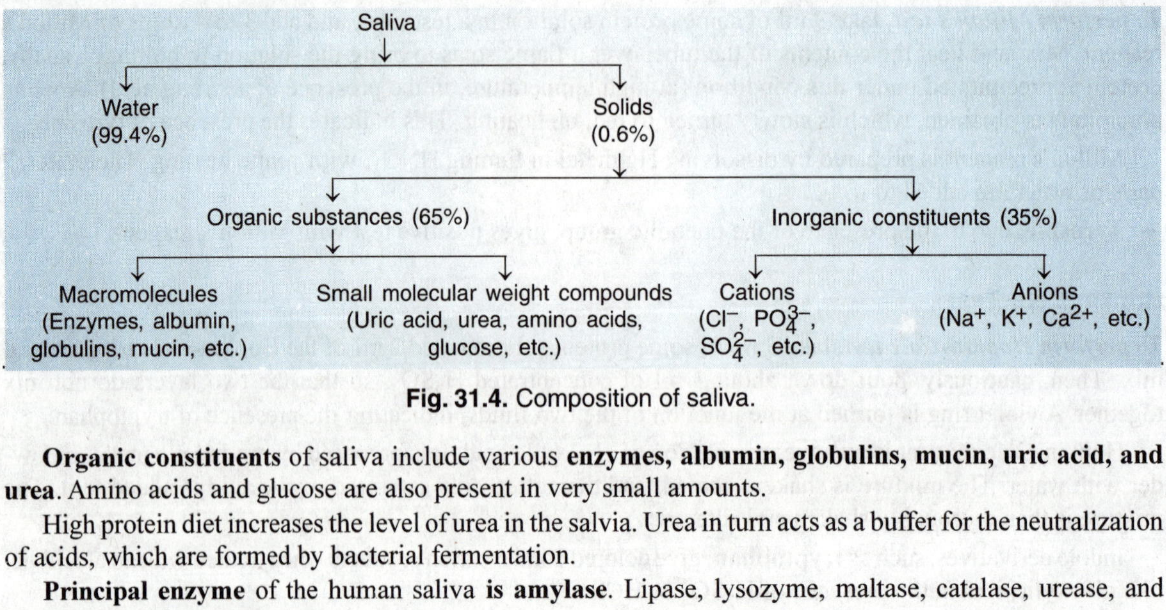

Fig. 31.4. Composition of saliva.

Organic constituents of saliva include various **enzymes, albumin, globulins, mucin, uric acid, and urea**. Amino acids and glucose are also present in very small amounts.

High protein diet increases the level of urea in the salvia. Urea in turn acts as a buffer for the neutralization of acids, which are formed by bacterial fermentation.

Principal enzyme of the human saliva **is amylase**. Lipase, lysozyme, maltase, catalase, urease, and proteases are also present in traces.

SALIVARY AMYLASE

Salivary amylase (the **S-type enzyme)** is a most important enzyme present in saliva. It is secreted chiefly, by the parotid glands. It is also referred to as **ptyalin**.

Salivary amylase is an **α-amylase**. It has an important role in the **digestion of polysaccharides** and hydrolyses polysaccharides, **like starch, glycogen, and dextrin, into glucose, maltose, maltotriose,** and a mixture of branched oligosaccharides or dextrins. Action of salivary amylase occurs mainly, in the mouth for a short period only (5-6 min, i.e. till the food gets mixed with the gastric juice). **Salivary amylase is a α-1, 4-glycosidase** because of its specific hydrolytic action on α-1,4-glycosidic bonds. **Optimal pH** for the enzyme **is 6.8.**

Lesions in the salivary gland, such as those caused by infections, irradiation, obstruction, surgery, or tumor, produce **hyperamylasemia**. Mumps and maxillary surgery may cause two-fold elevation while salivary gland irradiation can produce 9–10 fold elevation of serum amylase. Increased levels of salivary amylase also occur in biliary tract diseases, such as in cholecystitis, intra-abdominal events, e.g. ruptured ectopic pregnancy, peritonitis, and acute appendicitis.

LINGUAL LIPASE

The lingual serous glands secrete lingual lipase. It is of particular importance **in neonates** where it **hydrolyses dietary fats.**

LYSOZYME

Lysozyme is a polysaccharidase, which **hydrolyses complex polysaccharides** that are present in the bacterial cell wall. Its activity in saliva, is nearly equal to that of the blood, and is only about 1% of that present in tears.

MUCIN

Mucin is a **mucoprotein, secreted** chiefly **by the sublingual and submandibular pairs**. It is mainly responsible for giving viscosity to saliva. It acts as a lubricant and **facilitates swallowing of food.**

INORGANIC SALTS

Chief inorganic ions, present in the saliva, are **K^+, PO_4^{3-}, and Cl^- with small amounts of Na^+, Ca^{2+}, and SO_4^{2-}**. Of these, Ca^{2+} helps to stabilize salivary amylase while Cl^- acts as an activator for it.

Ionic concentration of saliva varies with its rate of flow. Under resting conditions, concentrations of Na^+ and Cl^- are lower than that of the plasma while those of K^+ and HCO_3^- are higher than the plasma.

Some of these inorganic ions may combine and form insoluble precipitates such as $Ca_3(PO_4)_2$, or $CaCO_3$. This is turn may lead to the formation of **salivary calculi.**

REGULATION OF THE SECRETION OF SALIVA

Total flow of saliva in an adult man is nearly **1.0–1.5 L/day**. It may vary widely, depending on the intake of water and food, character of food, and the process of chewing. Under resting conditions, about **0.5 ml** of the saliva is secreted **per min**. The presence of food in the mouth may increase rate of secretion of saliva up to 8 ml/min. Rate of secretion of saliva is entirely under the control of the nervous system.

A variety of **stimuli**, by reflex stimulation, cause **increased rate of flow**. These include:

1. **Psychic stimuli,** such as **sight, smell, or thought of the palatable food**, increase salivary secretion by conditioned reflex mechanism,
2. **Mechanical stimulation,** such as **chewing of food,** and
3. **Chemical stimulation**, e.g. **contact of sugar, salt, acid, or spices on the taste buds**.

Stimulation of certain taste receptors, e.g. sour food, causes more profused secretion than other types of taste receptors.

Aging causes atrophy of the cells in the salivary glands, resulting in decreased salivary flow and changes its composition.

Decreased salivary flow leads to **dryness of mouth**, called **xerostomia**. Lack of saliva causes dryness of the oral mucosa and makes chewing and swallowing more difficult. It **also increases the incidence of dental caries**. Chewing stimulates salivary flow and helps in prevention of xerostomia.

PHYSIOLOGICAL FUNCTIONS OF SALIVA

Various physiological functions of saliva are shown in Table 31.1.

Table 31.1. Important physiological functions of saliva

• Formation of food bolus • Hydrolysis of starch • Bactericidal ac.ion • Protection of teeth and gums against decay • Excretion of toxic substances • Perception of taste • Speech • Helps in absorption of vitamin B_{12}

1. During mastication, saliva gets mixed with the **food** and **changes** it **into a semisolid form**, called **bolus**, which can be easily swallowed.
2. Due to the presence of α-amylase, **digestion of starch** starts in the mouth. This role of salivary amylase, however, is limited since as bolus reaches the stomach and mixes with the gastric juice, acidic pH stops its action.
3. Saliva **contains** buffering substances, e.g. **bicarbonate, phosphates, and mucin**. It thus keeps the mouth at neutral pH and **protects teeth from decalcification**. Saliva also contains several proteolytic enzymes and antibodies that have **bactericidal action.** Saliva thus, has a **protective effect on** the development of **dental caries.**
4. Normally, tooth enamel is continuously bathed in saliva. As there is an exchange of nutrients, particularly minerals, between the enamel and the saliva, it contributes to the **resistance to tooth decay**. Adequate saliva production is therefore essential to maintain integrity of teeth as well as other oral structures.
5. Saliva also has **excretory functions.** It acts as a channel for **excretion of toxic substances**, such as lead and mercury, which enters mouth along with the food material.

   Some of the **waste products of metabolism**, such as urea, uric acid, ammonia, and other detoxified products, e.g. thiocyanate, are also, partially excreted in the saliva.

   Iodine, which is produced as a result of deiodination of thyroxine in the parotid and submaxillary glands, is also excreted via saliva.

   Some of the **drugs**, such as morphine and alcohol, may also be excreted through saliva.
6. Saliva also **serves as a solvent** for the transport of molecules so that they reach **taste** receptors, in the taste buds.
7. Saliva also **helps in speech** by keeping the mouth, lips, and tongue moist.
8. Saliva also helps in **absorption of vitamin B_{12}.**

At low pH of stomach, most of the cobalamin is temporarily bound to a salivary protein called R-protein (R refers to rapid electrophoretic mobility). This complex reaches duodenum where R-protein is degraded by the pancreatic proteases so that vitamin B_{12} can bind to the intrinsic factor (IF). IF-B_{12} complex is resistant to proteolysis and directly passes into the distal ileum, which is the site of vitamin B_{12} absorption.

DIAGNOSTIC SIGNIFICANCE OF SALIVA

Estimation and/or isolation of the various substances from saliva is helpful in clinical evaluation of certain diseases (Table 31.2):

1. Most of the **steroids** of clinical interest can be measured in saliva. For some of the steroids, such as cortisol, estriol, and progesterone, measurement of **their salivary level is a reliable indicator of their free concentration in plasma.**

   Measurement of cortisol in saliva is a more practical and convenient approach for assessing the concentration of free hormone. Salivary cortisol measurement reflects concentration of nonprotein-bound cortisol in blood, which is independent of salivary flow rate.

   Morning salivary cortisol concentration is decreased in adrenal insufficiency (Addison's disease) while evening values are increased in hyperactivity of the adrenal gland (Cushing's syndrome).

   Salivary **testosterone concentration** also correlates well with the free testosterone level in plasma. It has been suggested as an indicator of the androgen status.
2. Saliva is tested for **secretary IgA** in infantile hypogammaglobulinemia and β-macroglobulinemia, in Sjogren's syndrome.
3. Measurement of a drug in the saliva can be used as an estimate of free and pharmacologically active **concentration of the drug** in the serum.
4. Saliva can also be used for the **isolation of viruses,** such as mumps virus, rabies virus, Epstein-Barr virus, or Herpes simplex virus.
5. Saliva can also be used for identifying a suspect in a **forensic** laboratory.

Table 31.2. Diagnostic significance of saliva

• Estimation of steroids
• Estimation of proteins, including antibodies, in a diseased condition
• Estimation of drugs
• Isolation of viruses
• Forensic applications

ARTIFICIAL SALIVA

Certain conditions, such as radiation during the treatment of head and neck cancer, damage salivary glands and reduce salivary secretion. At this stage, a substitute of saliva (artificial saliva) can be used to avoid dryness of mouth.

Mineral content of the artificial saliva resembles the natural saliva. This, in turn, helps in relieving soft tissue discomforts and reduces the incidence of dental caries.

EFFECT OF SALIVARY AMYLASE ON THE HYDROLYSIS OF STARCH

Salivary amylase catalyses hydrolysis of α-1,4-glucosidic linkages, which are present in amylose and amylopectin (two components of starch), and glycogen, randomly. Hydrolysis of starch yields polysaccharides of gradually diminishing molecular size.

Various stages of the hydrolysis of starch include:

Starch (Blue)
↓
Amylodextrin (Violet)
↓
Erythrodextrin (Red)
↓
Achrodextrin + Maltose (No color)

Time taken by the enzyme to hydrolyze starch, to the stage of achrodextrin, i.e. when it fails to change the color of iodine is referred to as **achromic point**. Normally, it is 8–10 minutes.

To demonstrate the effect of salivary amylase on the hydrolysis of starch, and to find out the achromic point, saliva is collected. It is mixed with the reaction mixture containing starch, NaCl, and buffer. The mixture is thereafter, periodically added to iodine and the change in color of iodine is observed.

COLLECTION OF SALIVA

Take about 15–20 ml of water in mouth and chew it for about 2–3 minutes. Collect the secretions in a beaker.

Procedure

Take **5 ml of starch** in a test tube. Add **2 ml of phosphate buffer** (pH 6.8) and **1 ml of NaCl** solution (5%) to it. Incubate this **reaction mixture** at 37ºC for 4–5 min.

Take 0.5 ml of iodine solution in 10–12 tubes and place them in a rack at room temperature.

Thereafter, add 2 ml of the salivary amylase (collected salivary secretion) to the tube containing the above reaction mixture, which is kept in a water bath, at 37ºC. Mix the contents and take a drop from the mixture. Add it to one of tubes containing iodine. Starch gives blue color. Thereafter, repeat the same, after every one-minute by adding a drop of the reaction mixture, each time to a new tube containing iodine, and continue up to 10–15 minutes. Decrease in blue color gives the idea of starch hydrolyzed by the enzyme. Note the time required for achieving the achromic point.

FACTORS AFFECTING ENZYME ACTIVITY

Several factors are known to affect enzyme activity, such as pH, temperature, etc.

EFFECT OF pH ON ENZYME ACTIVITY

Amylase has optimum pH of 6.8–7.0. Its activity is reduced with the change in pH.

To demonstrate the effect of pH on salivary amylase, take 2 test tubes. Mark them as control and test, and add various solutions, as follows:

Solution	*Control*	*Test*
Starch solution	5 ml	5 ml
Buffer	2 ml (pH 6.8)	2 ml (pH 5.0)
NaCl solution	1 ml	1 ml
	Mix and incubate at 37ºC for 3–4 min.	
Saliva (Enzyme)	2 ml	2 ml

Mix the contents and incubate at 37ºC. Take one drop from each of the above two tubes containing reaction mixtures, after every one min and add to two separate tubes containing iodine solution.

Note the achromic point for each tube. Compared to the control tube (pH 6.8), achromic point is prolonged in the tube, containing buffer of pH 5.0 (test).

It demonstrates that low pH reduces enzyme activity.

EFFECT OF TEMPERATURE ON ENZYME ACTIVITY

Optimum temperature for salivary amylase is between 37–40ºC. When temperature is increased beyond 50ºC, its activity is reduced. On boiling, enzyme gets denatured and its activity is lost.

To demonstrate that enzyme is destroyed on boiling, take 2 ml of saliva (enzyme) in a tube, boil it over the flame (to denature the enzyme) and cool it.

Take 2 test tubes and mark them as control and test. Add various solutions to them, as follows:

Solution	*Control*	*Test*
Starch solution	5 ml	5 ml
Buffer (pH 6.8)	2 ml	2 ml
NaCl solution	1 ml	1 ml
	Mix and incubate at 37ºC for 3-4 min.	
Saliva (Enzyme)	2 ml (normal enzyme)	2 ml (boiled enzyme)

Mix the contents and incubate at 37ºC. Add a drop from each of the two tubes containing reaction mixtures, to separate tubes containing iodine solution. Repeat after every one-minute. Note the achromic point for the control tube.

Continue with the other tube, labeled as test for about 10 more minutes. Achromic point is not observed in this tube as the enzyme has been denatured on boiling and lost its activity.

EFFECT OF ACTIVATOR ON ENZYME ACTIVITY

Chloride ions (Cl^-) act as activator for salivary amylase whereas fluoride, oxalate, citrate, or EDTA act as inhibitor for the enzyme

To demonstrate the effect of (Cl^-) as activator for salivary amylase, take 2 test tubes, and label them as control and test. Add various solutions to these tubes, as follows:

Solution	*Control*	*Test*
Starch solution	5 ml	5 ml
Buffer (pH 6.8)	2 ml	2 ml
NaCl solution	1 ml	–
Distilled water	–	1 ml
	Mix and incubate at 37ºC for 3-4 min.	
Saliva (Enzyme)	2 ml	2 ml

Mix the contents and incubate at 37ºC. Add a drop of the reaction mixture from each of the above two tubes, to separate tubes containing iodine solution. Repeat after every one-minute till achromic point is reached.

Achromic point is prolonged in the tube, which contains distilled water instead of NaCl. It demonstrates that Cl^- ions are required as activator for salivary amylase.

IV. MILK

During recent years, although dried milk foods are being used extensively for feeding infants, human milk is regarded as the ideal food for feeding infants during the early months of life, universally.

COMPOSITION OF MILK

In general, milk contains **80–90% water**. Amongst the various nutrients, **lactose, fat,** and **proteins** are the major constituents of milk.

Milk contains **three types of proteins**, called **casein,** albumin, and globulins. The later are also referred to as **lactalbumin** and **lactglobulins**.

Casein is a phosphoprotein and has high biological value. It can be precipitated at pH 5.4, by the addition of acid. After the precipitation of casein, lactalbumin and lactglobulin remain in the filtrate. **Lactglobulin provides immunity** to the child.

Milk fat contains **triglycerides, short and medium chain fatty acids, phospholipids** (particularly lecithin) and small amount of **cholesterol**. In addition, milk also contains large amounts of **calcium, phosphorus, vitamin A** and **riboflavin**. Thiamin, vitamin C, vitamin D, and iron are present in small amounts.

COMPOSITION OF MILK FROM DIFFERENT SOURCES

Milk from different species differs in the relative amounts of protein, fat, lactose, minerals, and vitamins. They also differ in digestibility. For example, human milk contains more lactose compared to cow's milk while cow's milk contains more protein, calcium, and phosphorus.

Data regarding chemical composition of human milk as compared with those from some other species are shown in Table 31.3.

Table 31.3. Composition of milk from different sources (values are per 100 ml of milk)

Nutrients	*Human milk*	*Cow milk*	*Buffalo milk*	*Goat milk*
Calories (Kcal)	71	69	100	76
Protein (g)	1.2	3.3	3.8	3.3
Fat (g)	3.8	3.7	7.5	4.1
Lactose (g)	7.0	4.8	4.4	4.7
Calcium (mg)	33	125	210	130
Phosphorus (mg)	15	96	130	106
Vitamin A (mg)	48	47	60	36
Riboflavin (mg)	40	180	100	120

Colostrum: Milk secreted during the first few days after delivery is known as colostrum. It is comparatively more yellowish and contains more proteins. There is a steady fall in protein content of milk with the advancement of lactation.

Modification of the Animal Milk for Infant Feeding

Milk from animal source is modified for infant feeding by adjustment of some of the nutrients by dilution, boiling, and adding sugar. This is also referred to as humanization of the animal milk.

Dilution and boiling: Dilution with water is essential to reduce its protein and mineral contents. Animal milk is generally diluted with equal amount of water for feeding infants (1–2 months of age). As an infant grows, proportion of water is gradually reduced.

Boiling also brings physico-chemical changes in milk and improves it digestibility.

Adjustment of fat: Animal milk, particularly from buffalo, should be partially skimmed, to reduce its fat, to about 3.5%.

Addition of sugar: Sugar is added to bring its level to about 5%, after dilution.

ANALYSIS OF MILK FOR ITS CHEMICAL CONSTITUENTS

Milk contains large amount of casein, which is first precipitated at its isoelectric point (pH 5.4) and thereafter removed by filtration. The precipitate and the filtrate are thereafter tested separately, as follows:

1. Precipitate for fat and protein (casein). Since casein is a phosphoprotein, test for phosphorus will also be positive with the precipitate.
2. Filtrate for lactose, proteins (lactalbumin and lactglobulin), Ca^{2+} and phosphorus.

PRECIPITATION OF CASEIN

Take 1 test tube full of milk and transfer it to a beaker. Thereafter, add 1 test tube of water and 1 test tube of 1% acetic acid. Keep for 5 min and centrifuge/filter.

TESTS WITH THE PRECIPITATE

Test for Fat

Take a small amount of the precipitate in a test tube and add 2 ml of alcohol. Heat the contents to solubilize lipids. Add a few drops of water. Fat droplet appears. Shake and put a drop on a paper. A greasy-spot is observed on the paper.

Tests for Protein

To confirm the presence of casein, biuret test for protein and color reactions for various amino acids are done with the precipitate after its suspension in water.

Biuret test: Take a small amount of the precipitate in a test tube and suspend it in 2 ml of water. Add 3 ml of qualitative biuret reagent. Purple color indicates the presence of protein.

Ninhydrin test: Heat the suspension of casein with 2–3 drops of ninhydrin. Deep blue color is observed due to the presence of free amino groups of amino acids in the protein.

Xanthoproteic test: To 2 ml of suspension of casein in a test tube, add 1 ml of concentrate nitric acid. Boil and add 2–3 drops of NaOH solution. Orange color is observed due to the presence of aromatic amino acids in the protein.

Millon's test: To 2 ml suspension of casein in water, add 1–2 drops of Millon's reagent. Boil and cool the contents and add 1 ml of sodium nitrite. Red color confirms the presence of tyrosine in the protein.

Hopkin's cole test: To 2 ml water suspension of casein in a test tube, add 2–3 drops of Millon's reagent and 2-3 drops of formalin. Mix and add concentrate H_2SO_4 along the side of the test tube. Violet colored ring indicates the presence of tryptophan in the protein.

Sakaguchi test: Take 2 ml of water suspension of casein in a test tube. Add 1 ml of 10% NaOH and 2-3 drops of alcoholic solution of α-naphthol. Mix and add 2–3 drops of sodium hypobromide solution. Red color confirms the presence of arginine in the protein.

Lead acetate test: Take 2-ml water suspension of casein in a test tube. Add 1 ml of 40% NaOH and 2–3 drops of lead acetate solution. Black precipitate is seen due to the presence of sulphur containing amino acids in the protein.

TESTS WITH THE FILTRATE

Tests for Lactose

Lactose may be determined either by Benedict and Barfoed's test or with the KOH reduction test.

Benedict 's test: Take 5 ml of the qualitative Benedict's reagent in a test tube. Add 0.5 ml of the filtrate to it and boil. Red precipitate appears due to the presence of a reducing sugar.

Barfoed's test: Take 5 ml of Barfoed's reagent in a test tube. Add 0.5 ml of the filtrate to it. Mix and place the t[illegible] a boiling water bath. Appearance of the red precipitate after 5 min confirms the presence of a reducing disaccharide.

KOH reduction test: Take 5 ml of the filtrate in a test tube. Add 2 ml of ammonium hydroxide and few drops of 15% KOH solution. Mix and place the tube in boiling water bath. Orange color indicates the presence of lactose.

Tests for Lactalbumin

Heat coagulation test: As the isoelectric pH for albumin is 4.6 hence it does not get precipitated at the isoelectric pH of casein (5.4) and appears in the filtrate.

Take a test tube nearly 2/3 filled with the filtrate. Add a drop of chlorophenol red. Yellow color is observed. Add 1% acetic acid drop by drop to lower the pH from 5.4 to 4.6 (isoelectric pH for albumin), till the solution turns pink. Heat upper half of the solution, a white coagulum appears due to coagulation of lactalbumin at its pI.

Color reactions for the presence of various amino acids: Perform following tests, with the filtrate:

- Biuret test
- Ninhydrin test
- Xanthoproteic test
- Millon's test
- Hopkins cole test
- Sakaguchi test, and
- Lead acetate test

Test for Calcium

Take 2 ml of filtrate in a test tube and add 2–3 drops of potassium oxalate solution to it. White precipitate of calcium oxalate is observed due to the presence of Ca^{2+} in the filtrate.

Test for Phosphorus

Take 2 ml of filtrate in a test tube. Add 2 ml of concentrate sulfuric acid and 2–3 drops of concentrate nitric acid. Heat the contents and add 2–3 drops of ammonium molybdate reagent. Yellow precipitate of phosphomolybdate indicates the presence of phosphorus.

This is referred to as **Neumann's reaction.**

V. GASTRIC JUICE

Gastric juice consists of water (99.4%), hydrochloric acid, mucin, and enzymes, such as pepsin, carbonic anhydrase, and lipase.

1. Hydrochloric acid is secreted by the parietal cells.
2. Pepsin in secreted, as pepsinogen, by the chief cells. HCl activates it to pepsin.
3. Renin is secreted in the fourth stomach of calf and young ruminants, and in infants. It clots milk, by converting casein into caseinogen.
4. Gastric mucin comprises of mucoid, mucoprotease, and glandulary mucoprotein. Mucoprotein is the main carrier of the intrinsic factor that is necessary for the absorption of vitamin B_{12} (which is referred to as the extrinsic factor).

FACTOR AFFECTING SECRETION OF GASTRIC JUICE

The secretion of gastric juice is increased reflexly, in response to various stimulants:

1. Psychic stimuli such as thought, sight, smell and taste of food;
2. Mechanical stimuli, e.g. presence of food in the stomach;
3. Chemical substances like histamine, alcohol, etc.; and
4. Hormone gastrin secreted by gastric mucosa, in response to the food present in stomach;

Secretion of gastric juice may be inhibited by fat and HCl.

CONTENTS OF THE GASTRIC JUICE

HYDROCHLORIC ACID

Parietal cells secrete iso-osmotic solution of HCl, with a hydrogen ion concentration of about 150 meq/L (pH near 0.9–1.0).

It is practically free of ions other that H^+ and Cl^-. It is due to the reason that parietal cells contain high concentration of carbonic anhydrase.

HCl performs several functions:

1. HCl of gastric juice initiates conversion of pepsinogen to pepsin.
2. It has some physical action on proteins and make them more easily digestible.
3. It also converts the colloidal ferric hydroxide, which is found in the foodstuffs, to ferric ions that can be more readily reduced to ferrous ions by ascorbic acid, cysteine, and sulfhydryl groups of proteins of the food.

Gastric acidity may be decreased by various factors:

- Variations in the rate of parietal secretion.
- Dilution by the secretions of other cells, particularly mucus.
- Dilution and buffering by food.
- Dilution and buffering by the swallowed saliva.
- Regurgitation of the duodenal fluid and bile.

PEPSIN

Pepsin is present in the chief cells, as the zymogen (pepsinogen). Pepsinogen is converted to the active enzyme (pepsin) by the acidity of gastric juice and also autocatalytically by pepsin itself.

Acetylcholine and peptides stimulate secretion of HCl by the parietal cells, and thus play an important role in the activation of pepsin as well as maintenance of acidic pH, which is required for its optimal activity.

Pepsin content is high in patients having peptic ulcer. In pernicious anemia, cirrhosis of the liver and in various chronic gastric ailments pepsin content is low.

COLLECTION OF THE GASTRIC JUICE

The gastric fluid is obtained by aspiration, through a gastric tube (such as Ryle's tube).

The patient should be seated with the head titled slightly forward. Place the tip of the tube on the tongue, hold well and push it towards the throat or introduce the tube along the floor of the nose until it is felt that the top turns down into the pharynx. Thereafter, the patient is asked to swallow it quickly until it is passed to the desired length.

EXAMINATION OF THE GASTRIC RESIDUE

The content of the stomach after nearly 12 hours of fast is referred to as **gastric residue (residuum).** It is examined for its physical characteristics, chemical constituents, and free and total acidity.

Physical Characteristics

Color: Resting gastric content is usually colorless. It may be slightly yellow or green due to the regurgitation of bile. It may be dark-red or brown due to the presence of blood.

Volume: Total volume of the resting gastric residue normally varies from 20–50 ml. Volume above 100–200 ml may be considered as abnormal. It may be due to hypersecretion, retention or regurgitation from the duodenum. Other causes include pyloric obstruction, duodenal ulcer or Zollinger-Ellison syndrome.

Consistency: Resting gastric juice is a fluid of low specific gravity. It may be viscous due to the presence of mucus. Food particles may be present in carcinoma of the stomach.

Chemical Constituents

Bile: A small amount of bile may regurgitate into the stomach during intubation. Increased amount may be a result of intestinal obstruction or ileal stasis.

Mucus: Small amount of mucus is normally found. Excessive amount may be due to excessive amount of saliva in the gastric juice. Increased amount may also be seen in gastritis and gastric carcinoma.

Blood: Normally, blood is not present in the gastric juice. Accidental trauma to the gastric mucous membrane during the passage of the tube may result in traces of blood. Increased amount of blood may be present due to lesion such as gastric carcinoma or gastric ulcer.

Organic Acids: Lactic acid and butyric acid may be present in large amounts in hyperacidity, achlorhydria and carcinoma of the stomach.

In the absence of free HCl, organic acids are formed in increased amounts by bacterial fermentation of food, as food is retained in the stomach for longer period.

Pepsin: Absence of pepsin is seen in a condition called **achylia gastrica.**

Decreased levels of pepsin are seen in diseases such as atrophic gastritis and gastric carcinoma.

Increased pepsin activity may be observed in diseases associated with increased gastric output or in patients with gastrinoma, Zollinger-Ellison syndrome, duodenal ulcer and gastritis as well as after omeprazole administration.

FREE ACIDITY

HCl is the main acid in the gastric juice, which is a strong mineral acid and accounts for free acidity. It is secreted by the parietal cells at a concentration of about 55 mmol/L (meq/L) with a pH of less than 1.0. As parietal secretion gets mixed with other gastric constituents, concentration of hydrogen ions usually reaches less than 40 meq/L, with pH between 1.5–2.5.

Free acidity concentration in the gastric residue, in a normal individual, varies from 10–40 meq/L.

Increase in free acidity (more than 45 meq/L) is referred to as **hyperchlorhydria.** It occurs in duodenal and gastric ulcers, Zollinger-Ellison syndrome, etc.

Decreased secretion of HCl is called hypochlorhydria. It is observed in gastric carcinoma, chronic gastritis, constipation, and anemia.

Complete absence of HCl in the gastric juice is called **achlorhydria**. It occurs in pernicious anemia. Achlorhydria may also be seen in tuberculosis, gastric carcinoma and atrophic gastritis.

In the absence of HCl, bacterial fermentation of food is increased, which in turn, leads to the formation of lactic acid.

TOTAL ACIDITY

Total acidity in the gastric residue is due to hydrogen ions occurring as free HCl, mucoproteins, and organic acids, such as lactic acid and butyric acid. Total acid concentration in a normal state is usually between 10–50 meq/L.

STIMULATION OF GASTRIC SECRETION

Many compounds or processes such as test meal, alcohol, caffeine, gastrin, pentagastrin or insulin stimulate gastric secretion and thus secretion of HCl.

Alcohol: Fifty to hundred ml of 7% ethyl alcohol (3.5 ml of ethanol in 50 ml of water) is administered through syringe that is attached to Ryle's tube.

Caffeine: Caffeine sodium benzoate (500 mg in about 200 ml of water) is administered into the stomach through a gastric tube.

Histamine: Histamine is a powerful stimulant for the secretion of gastric juice. It causes secretion of increased volume of highly acidic gastric juice with low pepsin content.

Two types of histamine tests are carried out.

Standard histamine test: Subcutaneous injection of histamine (0.01 mg/kg body weight) is given and gastric contents are removed. Absence of free HCl in gastric secretion, after giving histamine indicates **achylia gastrica.**

Augmented histamine test: A large dose of histamine (0.04 mg/kg body weight) is given. In pernicious anemia, no free HCl is secreted but in other forms of achlorhydria some amount of free HCl may be secreted after augmented histamine test.

Sometimes high dose of histamine may cause a severe reaction. Under such conditions, injection of some antihistaminic (100 mg) may be given, intramuscularly. Administration of antihistamine does not interfere in gastric stimulation.

Insulin: Intravenous injection of insulin (0.1–0.2 U/kg body weight) may be given for the stimulation of gastric secretion and samples are withdrawn after every 15 min. This is called as **Hollander's Test.**

Insulin stimulation is helpful to ascertain the effectiveness of vagotomy, in patients with duodenal ulcer where concentration of free HCl may be as high as 100 meq/L. After successful vagotomy since there is no response to insulin, gastric acidity remains at a low level of 15–20 meq/L before as well as after insulin administration.

This test is not preferred, as insulin results in hypoglycemia (within 30 minutes).

Gastrin and Pentagastrin: **Gastrin** is a powerful stimulus for HCl secretion. It is administered in a single subcutaneous dose of 2 mg/Kg body weight.

Pentagastrin is a synthetic pentapeptide with physiologically active part of gastrin. It is also a potent stimulus for HCl secretion and is commonly used now a day.

ESTIMATION OF FREE ACIDITY BEFORE AND AFTER STIMULATION

Fasting content of stomach is aspirated. Secretions are collected at 15 minute intervals, up to 1 hour, pooled and volume is measured. This is termed as **basal acid output (BAO).**

Pentagastrin is, thereafter, given 6 mg/kg body weight, subcutaneously and post stimulation secretions are again collected at 15 min intervals, up to next one hour. This acid output is termed as **maximal acid output** (MAO).

This test is useful in differentiating the diagnosis of achlorhydria and hyperchlorhydria.

ESTIMATION OF FREE AND TOTAL ACIDITY IN GASTRIC JUICE

Principle

Acids present in the gastric juice are titrated with a strong alkali. During titration with alkali (0.1 N NaOH),

HCl is completely neutralized at about pH 3.5, whereas weak acids are neutralized in the alkaline range (at about pH 8.0). Thus titration is done by using Topfer's reagent as indicator, during titration for free acidity while phenolphthalein is used for titrating total acidity.

Topfer's reagent has a pH range of 2.9 (red) to 4.0 (yellow). On the other hand, phenolphthalein works in the pH range of 8.2 (colorless) to 10.0 (pink).

Procedure

Fill 0.1N NaOH solution in a burette. Take 10 ml gastric juice in a conical flask or china dish and add a drop of Topfer's reagent to it. If initially, on adding the indicator, yellow color is seen, no free acid is present. Titrate this sample only for total acidity.

If initially red color appears, titrate it with 0.1N NaOH till salmon pink color appears. At this stage, the initial red color becomes yellow. Note the volume of NaOH used. This gives the value of free acidity.

Add a drop of phenolphthalein and again titrate with 0.1N NaOH. Note the change in color from salmon pink to colorless, which further turns pink. Note down total NaOH used for titration. This gives the value for total acidity.

Calculation

$$\text{Free acidity (meq/L)} = \frac{\text{ml of 0.1 N NaOH required to titrate 10 ml}}{\text{of gastric juice with Topfer's reagent (A)}} \times \frac{100}{10}, \text{ or } = A \times 10$$

$$\text{Total acidity (meqL)} = \frac{\text{ml of 0.1N NaOH required to titrate 10 ml}}{\text{of gastric juice with phenolphthalein (B)}} \times \frac{100}{10}, \text{ or } = B \times 10$$

The result may also be expressed in terms of **clinical units.**

One clinical unit is defined as the **amount of 0.1N NaOH required to neutralize** the amount of acids present in **100 ml of gastric juice.**

Normally, free HCl is 0–30 meq/L. Concentration above 50 meq/L may be suggestive of hyperacidity.

Total acidity includes free HCl and combined acidity.

Combined acidity includes organic acids (mainly lactic acid) and H^+ bound with proteins. Total acidity is up to 10 meq/L more than free acidity.

VI. ESTIMATION OF BLOOD GLUCOSE

There are several photometric oxidation-reduction methods, besides the enzymatic method to measure blood glucose concentration. Some of these are relatively nonspecific and result in falsely increased values.

COLLECTION OF SAMPLE AND USE OF PRESERVATIVE

In methods for self-monitoring of glucose though whole blood can be used, in most of the clinical chemistry laboratories plasma or serum is used for glucose determination.

Fasting whole-blood glucose concentration is nearly 10–15% lower than plasma. This is due to lower water content with in red blood cells.

During fasting, capillary blood glucose concentration is nearly 3–5 mg/dl higher than the venous blood.

In a normal blood sample, serum glucose concentration is decreased by 5–7% in 1 hour, at room temperature. In separated non-hemolysed sterile serum, glucose concentration is generally stable for nearly 8 hours at 25°C and up to 72 hours at 4°C.

Glycolysis in the red blood cells reduces blood glucose value by nearly 5% each hour, at room temperature. To prevent this loss, most commonly, the sample is collected in a vial containing a mixture of sodium fluoride (2 mg/dl) and potassium oxalate (2 mg/dl). Alternatively, either the sample should be analyzed within 30 min of its collection or an inhibitor of glycolysis such as sodium fluoride should be added. Sodium fluoride (NaF) prevents glycolysis by inhibiting enolase.

OXIDATION-REDUCTION METHODS

Many procedures for measuring glucose are based on its property of acting as a reducing agent, in a hot alkaline solution.

The principle of these methods is that in a hot alkaline solution, aldehyde group of glucose readily reduces cupric ions (Cu^{2+}) to cuprous ions (Cu^{+}), which is turn form cuprous oxide (Cu_2O).

Standard solution is also analyzed in the same manner as protein free filtrate due to the reason that this reaction is dependent on the alkalinity, the time and temperature of heating, and the concentration of reagents.

Thereafter, phosphomolybdic or arsenomolybdic acid is added which in turn is reduced by the cuprous ions and form molybdenum blue (the compound with lower oxidation state of molybdenum and is blue in color). The intensity of which can be measured colorimetrically.

Most commonly used oxidation-reduction methods include Folin-Wu method and Somogyi-Nelson method.

Folin-Wu Method

As in some the laboratories it is still being used, its details are given below.

This is based on the reducing property of glucose and may over estimate blood glucose value by 15–20%. This is due to the presence of other reducing substances such as glutathione, vitamin C, other sugars, etc., in the blood.

Principle: In Folin-Wu method, proteins are precipitated with tungstic acid and the clear protein-free filtrate is used in the reaction with cupric ions. Re-oxidation of cuprous ions by oxygen from the air is prevented, by using a specially designed constricted tube referred to as the Folin-Wu tube. The cuprous oxide, so formed, is treated with phosphomolybdic acid solution. Blue color is formed whose intensity is compared with the standard.

Preparation of protein free filtrate: Take 3 test tubes and label them as blank (B), Standard (S) and test (T). Add distilled water, standard, blood and other solutions as follows:

	B	*S*	*T*
Distilled water	3.4 ml	3.2 ml	3.2 ml
Standard (0.1 mg/ml)	–	0.2 ml	–
Blood	–	–	0.2 ml
10% Sodium tungstate	0.3 ml	0.3 ml	0.3 ml
2/3N H_2SO_4	0.3 ml	0.3 ml	0.3 ml

Mix the contents and centrifuge/filter after 5 min to obtain a protein-free filtrate.

Procedure: Take 3 Folin-Wu tubes and label them as blank (B), standard (S) and test (T). To each Folin-Wu tube, add 2 ml of filtrate/supernatant, from the above respective tubes. Thereafter, add 2 ml of alkaline copper reagent to each tube. Mix and keep the tubes in a boiling water bath for 6 min. Cool and add 2 ml of phosphomolybdic acid solution to each tube.

Mix and dilute the contents of each tube to 25 ml mark, with distilled water. Mix and read optical density at 420 nm, against water.

Calculations

$$\text{Blood sugar (mg/dl)} = \frac{OD_{T-B}}{OD_{S-B}} \times \text{Concentration of standard, or}$$

$$= \frac{OD_{T-B}}{OD_{S-B}} \times 100$$

Reference value of blood sugar for fasting venous blood by this method is 80–120 mg/dl. Out of this, reducing substances other than glucose constitute nearly 20–30 mg/dl of whole blood.

Somogyi-Nelson Method

In Somogyi-Nelson method, proteins are precipitated by the addition of barium hydroxide [$Ba(OH)_2$] and zinc sulfate ($ZnSO_4$). In this method, besides proteins, sulfhydryl compounds, such as glutathione, are removed as zinc salts while other reducing substances like uric acid and creatinine, etc., are precipitated and adsorbed on barium sulfate ($BaSO_4$). The resultant filtrate is thus free of non-sugar reducing substances.

O-Toluidine Method

Principle: An aldohexose, such as glucose, when heated with O-toluidine in acidic medium, forms a condensation product glycosylamine, and subsequently a Schiff's base, which has blue-green color.

O-Toluidine reagent: O-Toluidine reagent contains O-toluidine, glacial acetic acid and thiourea.

Preparation of protein-free filtrate: Take 0.2 ml of blood/serum, in a test tube. Add 1.8 ml of 4% trichloracetic acid, mix and centrifuge/filter, after 10 min.

Procedure: Take 3 test tubes and mark them as blank (B), standard (S) and test (T). Add distilled water, standard, protein-free filtrate and O-toluidine reagent, as follows:

	B	*S*	*T*
Distilled water	0.5 ml	–	–
Standard (0.1 mg/ml)	–	0.5 ml	–
Protein free filtrate	–	–	0.5 ml
O-Toluidine reagent	2.5 ml	2.5 ml	2.5 ml

Mix and keep in a boiling water bath for 10 min. Cool under tap water and read the optical density at 630 nm, against blank.

Calculation

$$\text{Blood glucose} = \frac{OD_T}{OD_S} \times \text{Concentration of standard}$$

$$= \frac{OD_T}{OD_S} \times 100$$

GLUCOSE OXIDASE METHOD

It is based on the principle that glucose is oxidized by glucose oxidase. This in turns leads to the formation of H_2O_2 and gluconic acid. With the addition of the second enzyme, i.e. peroxidase, and a chromogenic oxygen acceptor, such as O-dianisidine or 4-aminophenazone, a colored compound is formed, intensity of which is directly proportional to the concentration of glucose.

This is also referred to as glucose oxidase-peroxidase (GOD/POD) method.

Normal value: Normal values for glucose, by methods other than Folin-Wu, vary between 60–90 mg/dl of whole blood or 70–100 mg/dl of serum or plasma in adults.

In neonates, blood glucose concentration varies between 30–60 mg/dl of serum/plasma, which is still lower in premature neonates.

Blood glucose concentration increases with age by about 2–3 mg/dl, per decade.

Glucose concentration in the cerebrospinal fluid (CSF) is nearly 60–65% of the serum/plasma level.

GLUCOSE TOLERANCE TEST

Glucose tolerance test (GTT) determines the ability of an individual to tolerate an extra load of glucose.

Oral GTT is helpful in-patients who have fasting blood glucose concentration in the upper normal limit, those with transient or sustained glycosuria without the symptoms of diabetes or those with family history of the disease, etc.

Procedure

For GTT, fasting venous blood sample (after 12–16 hours of fast) is drawn, in a fluoride-oxalate bottle.

Thereafter, 75 g of glucose (about 1 g/kg body weight) is given, in nearly 200–300 ml of water, to drink. Blood samples are again drawn after every 30 minutes, till 2 to 2½ hours.

Urine specimens are also collected, simultaneously.

Each sample is analyzed and glucose tolerance curve is plotted.

Interpretation of the Glucose Tolerance Curve

Fasting blood glucose, maximum value of glucose, rate at which it returns to the fasting value and glycosuria give idea about the disease.

For a normal individual, fasting blood glucose value is within the normal limit. It is increased by more than two-fold within 60 min and thereafter returns to normal after about two hours of the ingestion of glucose. Moreover, glycosuria is not observed in any of the sample (Fig. 31.5).

Any deviation from the above is referred to as abnormal glucose tolerance curve. In a patient with diabetes mellitus fasting blood glucose level is above the normal and/or curve is raised as well as prolonged. This is also accompanied with glycosuria.

In a patient of renal glycosuria, glucose tolerance curve is normal but there is glycosuria.

GLUCOSE TOLERANCE TEST PROFILES

Recently, International Committee of Diabetologists has recommended simplifying the glucose tolerance test to require only an overnight fasting measurement and 2 hours sample after 75 g oral glucose load.

An oral glucose tolerance test is normal if the fasting venous plasma glucose value is less than 100 mg/dl and the 2-hours value falls below 140 mg/dl.

A fasting value of 126 mg/dl or higher, or 2 hours value of greater than 200 mg/dl is diagnostic of diabetes mellitus.

Values between the upper limits of normal and those diagnostic of diabetes (fasting between 100–125 mg/dl and 2-hour value between 140–200 mg/dl) refers to impaired glucose tolerance (Table 31.4).

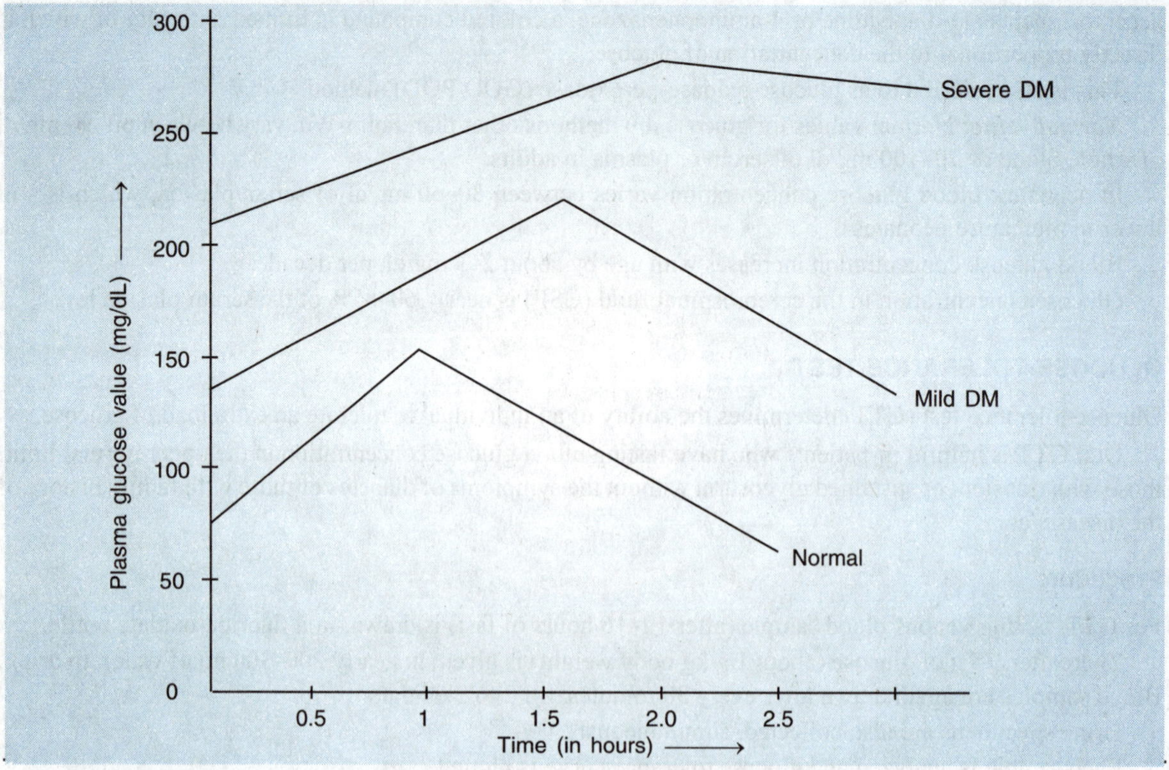

Fig. 31.5. Glucose Tolerance Curve.

Table 31.4. Criteria for evaluating the standard and abnormal glucose tolerance test

GTT	*Fasting plasma glucose (mg/dl)*	*Two hours after 75g glucose (mg/dl)*
Normal	< 100	< 140
Impaired GT	100–125	≥ 140–199
Diabetes Mellitus	≥ 126	≥ 200

Hypoglycemia (plasma glucose concentration below 40 mg/dl) is a common and potentially dangerous complication of insulin treatment, particularly in tightly controlled diabetes. Insulinoma (benign adenoma of pancreatic islets) can also cause hypoglycemia. Estimating plasma insulin concentration, which is raised during fasting, can make its diagnosis.

VII. SERUM PROTEIN ESTIMATION

Routinely, total protein estimation in serum is done by the biuret method.

BIURET METHOD

It is referred to as the biuret method since biuret, which is obtained on heating urea, gives same color with cupric ions as some protein. Besides biuret, this reaction can occur with any compound containing at least two peptide bonds. Free amino acids and dipeptides do not give this test. Intensity of the color is directly proportional to the number of peptide bonds that are present in the protein.

Either serum or plasma may be used but serum is preferred. A fasting specimen is not essential but may be preferred. Lipemia interferes with the test as it results in turbidity in the final reaction mixture. Hemolysed sample should not be used since hemoglobin interferes in this reaction.

Sample is stable for 1 week at room temperature, or for 1 month at 2–4°C, if stored in a tightly stoppered bottle.

BIURET REAGENT

Biuret reagent, which is used for the quantitative estimation of protein in serum, is referred to as quantitative biuret reagent. It has copper sulfate, sodium potassium tartarate, potassium iodide, and sodium hydroxide.

PRINCIPLE OF THE METHOD

Proteins and peptides (containing at least two adjacent peptide bonds) react with cupric ions (Cu^{2+}) in an alkaline solution and form violet colored complex, which has absorption maxima at 540 nm.

The complex is formed between the Cu^{2+}, and the carbonyl oxygen and amide nitrogen of the peptide bond.

Procedure

Take 3 test tubes and label them as blank (B), standard (S), and test (T).

Add distilled water, standard solution of albumin, serum, and biuret reagent, as follows:

	B	*S*	*T*
Distilled Water	2.5 ml	–	2.4 ml
Standard protein solution (2.8 mg/ml)	–	2.5 ml	–
Serum	–	–	0.1 ml
Biuret reagent	3.5 ml	3.5 ml	3.5 ml

Mix the contents and place the tubes for 10 min at 37°C or for 15 minutes at room temperature (if below 37°C). Read the optical density at 540 nm.

Calculation

$$\text{Serum protein (g/dL)} = \frac{OD_T}{OD_S} \times \text{Concentration of the standard, or}$$

$$= \frac{OD_T}{OD_S} \times 7$$

Total protein concentration in a normal serum varies between 6.0–8.3 g/dl.

OTHER METHODS

FOLIN-CIOCALTEU METHOD

Folin-Ciocalteu method is also referred as Lowry's method. It is based on the principle that tyrosine and tryptophan residues present in a protein reduce phosphotungstic-phosphomolybdic acid reagent (Folin-Ciocalteu reagent) and form blue colored complex.

In this method, protein, first reacts with the Cu^{2+} in the alkaline solution, to form a copper-peptide bound protein complex. After Folin-Ciocalteu reagent is added, copper-protein complex joins with the tyrosine and tryptophan residues, in the reduction process. Most of the color produced depends upon the Cu^{2+} complex, absorbency of which can be measured between 650–750 nm.

Detection limit of this method is 100 times lower than the biuret reaction. Thus, it is more suitable for the estimation of very low concentration of protein in a sample.

It is widely used in research, to measure tissue protein and enzyme concentrations, in the purified preparations. This is, however, not satisfactory for measuring total protein concentration in urine or CSF because reagent reacts nonspecifically with the non-protein compounds.

KJELDAHL METHOD

It is based on the principle that acid digestion of a protein (after heating a protein in the presence of a strong mineral acid) converts protein nitrogen to ammonium ions (NH_4^+), concentration of which is evaluated by titration or nesslerisation. This value of ammonia nitrogen is multiplied with 6.25 (considering the average nitrogen content of the protein as 16%) to get the concentration of protein in the sample.

It is a very accurate method but time consuming and inconvenient in practice. So, it is not used, routinely. It is, however, used for the standardization of the reference material for the biuret method.

REFRACTOMETERY

It is a quick alternative to chemical analysis for serum total protein when a rapid estimation is required. Refractometery is based on the principle that refractive index of water at 20°C is 1.33. When a solute is added to water, the refractive index value of the solution is increased linearly, proportionately to the concentration of the solute.

Clinical refractometers are pre-calibrated for total solids and the concentration of protein in the sample is directly expressed in g/dl.

Large positive errors occur with azotemia and hyperglycemia. At protein concentration less than 3.5 g/dl, results are not very accurate.

ESTIMATION OF SERUM ALBUMIN

Serum albumin is estimated by dye binding method.

Dyes, such as bromocresol green (BCG), bind very specifically to albumin. On addition of alkali, color of BCG is changed from green to blue, intensity of which is proportional to the amount of albumin present in the serum.

ALBUMIN: GLOBULIN RATIO

Albumin: globulin ratio (A: G ratio) can be calculated by estimating albumin and then subtracting its value from the value of the total serum protein.

Globulin = Total serum protein – albumin

$$\text{A:G ratio} = \frac{\text{Concentration of albumin (g/dl)}}{\text{Concentration of globulin (g/dl)}}$$

Normal value for A: G ratio varies between 1.5:1 to 2.5:1.

SEPARATION OF PLASMA PROTEINS BY ELECTROPHORESIS

Electrophoresis is a technique for the separation of the charged particles by means of electric current. A charged particle, when placed in an electric field, migrates either towards the anode or the cathode, depending upon the net charge carried by the particles.

Different molecules migrate at different speeds depending upon their charge, particle size, and shape. Their movement occurs in a liquid medium (a buffer), supported on an inert material, like filter paper, cellulose acetate strip, agar gel, starch gel, or polyacrylamide gel.

PAPER ELECTROPHORESIS

In **paper electrophoresis**, a strip of filter paper is dipped in a buffered solution (barbitone buffer, pH 8.6) and is laid on a platform. Two ends of the strip are dipped in the buffer. Entire apparatus is covered with a sheet, to minimize evaporation. Two electrodes are also dipped in two compartments containing buffer. Current is supplied through a power supply, which either supplies constant current and/or voltage. Current is carried by the charged particles, and depending upon the charge, protein migrates towards either anode or cathode.

PROCEDURE

About 10 μl of serum is applied along a thin line, near the cathode. Since at pH 8.6, all the proteins carry a net negative charge and tend to migrate towards the anode, thus, on passing a constant current (about 1-2 mA per strip), different proteins migrate at different rates. At the end, their positions are revealed by some dye, such as bromophenol blue, which stains proteins. Different proteins form separate bands on the paper strip.

In the normal serum five bands are observed. Since albumin carries largest number of the negative charges, it moves fastest while γ-globulin has less negative charges and moves the least. Starting from anode, these bands are designated as albumin, α_1-globulin, α_2-globulin, β-globulin, and γ-globulin.

Pattern of serum protein, on electrophoresis, may be used in the diagnosis of a disease, e.g. multiple myeloma (Fig. 31.6).

ALTERATIONS IN SERUM TOTAL PROTEIN

Alterations in serum total protein may be observed due to a change either in plasma water or concentration of a specific plasma protein (albumin or globulin).

HYPOPROTEINEMIA

Decrease in total protein concentration in serum below normal, is referred to as hypoproteinemia.

Increase in plasma volume (hemodilution) is reflected as relative hypoproteinemia. Hemodilution may occur with water intoxication or salt retention during massive intravenous infusion, or physiologically, when a recumbent position is assumed. The later in turn decreases total protein concentration by 0.3 to 0.5 g/dl.

Hypoproteinemia is consistently related to low concentration of albumin (hypoalbuminemia), which may be a result of:

1. Decreased protein intake, such as kwashiorkor,
2. Decreased synthesis of albumin, e.g. in a chronic liver disease (hepatitis, cirrhosis, etc.),

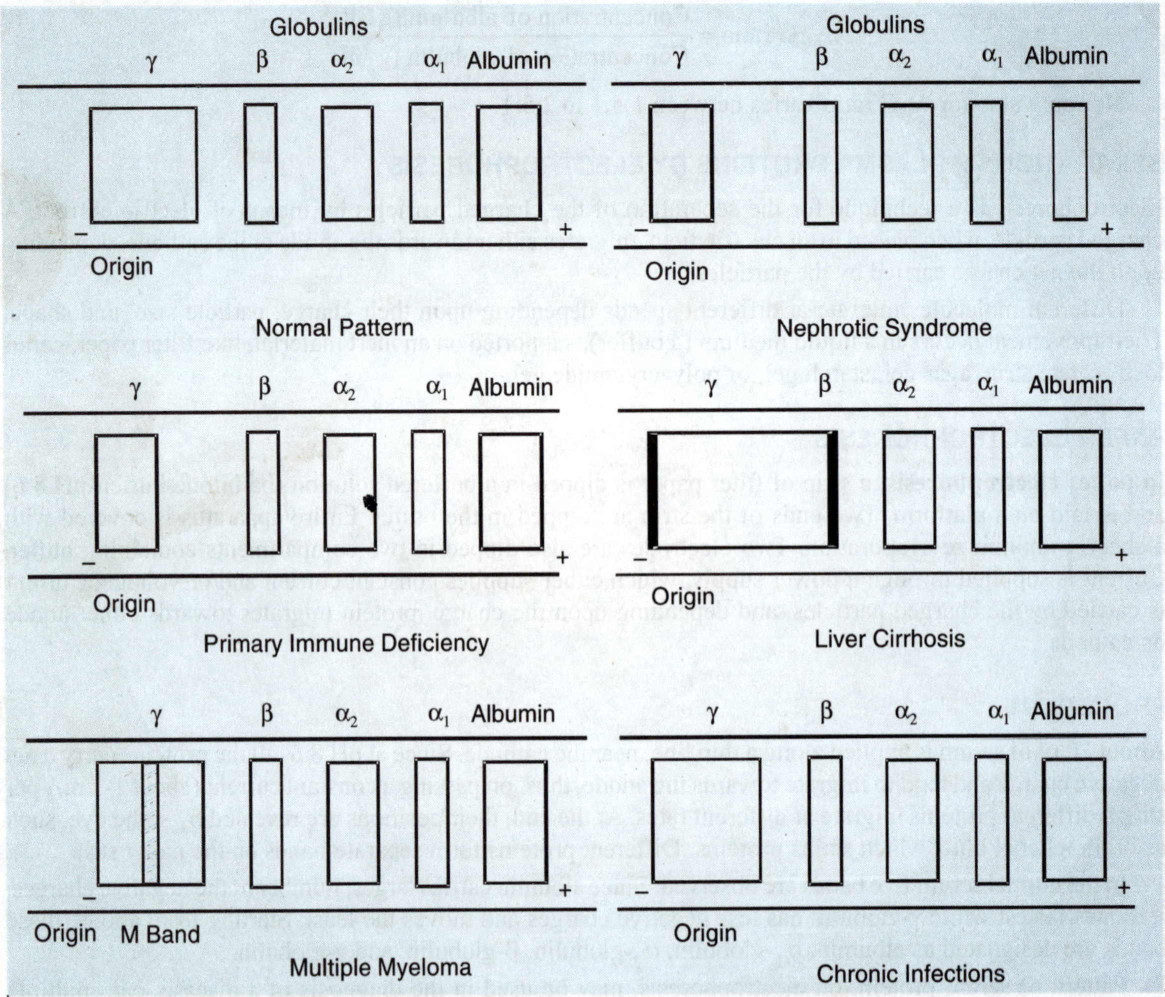

Fig. 31.6. Separation Patterns of Serum Proteins by Electrophoresis.

3. Increased loss of albumin from body, e.g. in protein losing enteropathy, or a renal disease, such as nephrotic syndrome, or
4. In a protein catabolic state, like high-grade fever or acute infections such as tuberculosis.

HYPERPROTEINEMIA

Increase in total protein concentration in serum above normal, is referred to as hyperproteinemia.

It may be a result of:

1. ***Hemoconcentration***: Hemoconcentration (decrease in volume of plasma water) is reflected as relative hyperproteinemia, e.g. in burns (above 20%). It may also be observed in dehydration due to either inadequate intake of water or excessive water loss, such as severe vomiting, diarrhea, Addison disease, diabetic acidosis, etc.
2. ***Hyperglobulinemia:*** High levels of the monoclonal immunoglobulins produced in multiple myeloma and other malignant paraproteinemia may cause marked hyperproteinemia.

VIII. ESTIMATION OF CREATININE

The amount of creatinine, which is produced daily, is related to muscle mass and does not vary greatly. Thus its level in the blood remains fairly constant.

Free creatinine is a waste product of creatine. It is present in all body fluids and secretions. Creatinine is freely filtered by the glomerulus. Although it is not reabsorbed, a small amount of it is secreted by renal tubules. Hence, its clearance is measured as an indicator of GFR.

Principle: Estimation of creatinine is based on the reaction with alkaline picrate, first described by **Jaffe**. In this reaction, creatinine reacts with picrate ions, in alkaline medium to yield an orange-red-complex.

Estimation of Serum Creatinine

For the estimation of creatinine in serum, a protein-free filtrate is prepared.

Preparation of protein-free filtrate: Take 1 ml of serum in a test tube. Add 1 ml each of distilled water, sodium tungstate and sulfuric acid (2/3 N). Mix the contents and filter/centrifuge after 10 min to obtain protein free filtrate.

Procedure: Take 3 test tubes and mark them as blank (B), standard (S) and test (T).

Add distilled water, standard, protein free filtrate and other reagents, as follows:

	B	*S*	*T*
Distilled water	4 ml	3 ml	2 ml
Standard creatinine solution (0.01 mg/ml)	—	1 ml	—
Protein-free filtrate	—	—	2 ml
NaOH	1 ml	1 ml	1 ml
Picric acid	1 ml	1 ml	1 ml

Mix the contents and read optical density at 520 nm, after 15 min.

Calculation

$$\text{S. creatinine (mg/dl)} = \frac{OD_T}{OD_S} \times \text{Concentration of standard, or}$$

$$= \frac{OD_T}{OD_S} \times 2$$

Normal value for serum (plasma) creatinine is 0.8–1.5 mg/dl.

Value slightly increases in elderly individuals due to its decreased excretion. Serum level is lower in women than in men. Serum creatinine is increased in renal failure and obstruction to urine outflow.

Estimation of Urine Creatinine

Since the concentration of creatinine in urine is very high as compared to serum, hence urine is diluted 1:100 times with distilled water and the diluted urine is treated in the same way as the protein free filtrate by the same method, as above.

IX. URINE ANALYSIS

NORMAL COSTITUENTS OF URINE

INORGANIC SUBSTANCES

Chloride

To demonstrate the presence of chloride in urine, take 5 ml of urine in a test tube. Add few drops of concentrate nitric acid and 2-3 drops of silver nitrate solution. A white precipitate, due to the formation of silver chloride is observed, indicating the presence of chloride in urine.

Nitric acid is added to prevent precipitation of phosphates, urates, and other organic radicals, which may be present in the urine.

Phosphates

To demonstrate the presence of phosphates **take 3 ml of urine in a test tube and add few drops of concentrate nitric acid. Then add 3 ml of 5% ammonium molybdate solution to it. A yellow precipitate of ammonium phosphomolybdate is seen, which indicates the presence of phosphates in urine.**

Sulfates

To demonstrate the presence of sulfates **take 5 ml of urine in a test tube and add 2–3 drops of concentrate hydrochloric acid. Add few drops of barium chloride solution. A white precipitate of barium sulfate is observed, indicating the presence of sulfates in urine.**

Hydrochloric acid is added to prevent precipitation of phosphates and other salts of barium.

AMMONIA

To demonstrate the presence of ammonia, take 5 ml of urine in a test tube. Cautiously add, dilute sodium hydroxide until the mixture is faint pink. Dip a glass rod in the solution of phenolphthalein. Boil the contents of the tube and hold the glass rod on the top of it. Phenolphthalein turns pink, due to vapors of ammonia.

NONPROTEIN NITROGENOUS SUBSTANCES

Urea

Presence of urea in the urine can be shown by the alkaline hypobromite test where urea is decomposed, under the influence of sodium hypobromite, and liberates CO_2 and N_2. CO_2 is absorbed by sodium hydroxide and the effervescences are observed due to evolution of nitrogen.

To demonstrate the presence of urea in urine, take 5 ml of urine in a test tube and add 3–4 drops of the hypobromite reagent. Effervescences are observed due to the evolution of N_2, which is liberated from urea thereby showing the presence of urea in urine.

Hypobromite reagent is prepared by mixing equal volume of concentrated sodium hydroxide solution with bromine water.

Uric Acid

Using Benedict's uric acid reagent (alkaline phosphotungstic acid solution), uric acid can be detected, qualitatively. Uric acid reduces this reagent and leads to formation of tungsten blue, producing blue color.

To demonstrate the presence of uric acid in urine, take 2 ml of urine in a test tube. Make it alkaline by adding a pinch of sodium carbonate. Add few drops of uric acid reagent and mix the contents. Deep blue color is observed, confirming the presence of uric acid in urine.

Creatinine

Creatinine is detected by alkaline picric acid solution. This is known as Jaffe's reaction.

To demonstrate the presence of creatinine in urine, take 5 ml of urine in a test tube and add 1 ml of saturated picric acid solution. Make this mixture alkaline with the addition of 1 ml of 10% sodium hydroxide solution. A reddish-orange color, due to the formation of creatinine picrate is observed, indicating the presence of creatinine in urine.

ABNORMAL CONSTITUENTS OF URINE

Sugar

Presence of sugar in the urine can be detected by **Benedict's test.**

Take 5 ml of qualitative Benedict's reagent in a test tube and add 0.5 ml (8–10 drops) of the urine sample. Contents of the tube are boiled for 1–2 min and allowed to cool thereafter. In the presence of a reducing sugar, red colored precipitate of cuprous oxide is seen.

Depending upon the quantity of sugar in the sample, contents of the tube may be seen as green, yellow, orange, or red. This intensity of the precipitate can also be indicated by arbitrary signs as +, ++, +++, or ++++.

This test not only indicates the presence of sugar in the urine but also gives its approximate concentration indicating that it is a semiquantitative test (Table 31.5).

Table 31.5. Semi-quantitative nature of the qualitative benedict test

Color of the Solution (with precipitate)	*Arbitrary sign (unit)*	*Approximate concentration of sugar (g/dl of urine)*
Green	+	Up to 0.5
Yellow	++	About 1.0
Orange	+++	About 1.5
Red	++++	2.0 or above

KETONE BODIES

Ketone bodies may be detected by **Rothera test,** using sodium nitroprusside.

Take 5 ml of urine in a test tube and saturate it with ammonium sulfate powder, by shaking. Add 2–3 drops of 5% sodium nitroprusside solution. Mix and add few drops of liquid ammonia (ammonium hydroxide) from the side of the tube. Development of purple/violet color indicates the presence of ketone bodies.

PROTEIN

Presence of protein in the urine can be confirmed by various tests such as **sulphosalicylic acid test, heat coagulation test or nitric acid test.**

Sulphosalicylic acid test: To 2 ml of urine, add few drops of 20% sulphosalicylic acid solution. White precipitate (turbidity), due to denaturation of albumin by sulphosalicylic acid, indicates the presence of protein in urine.

Heat coagulation test: Fill two third of test tube with the urine and adjust its pH to 4.6 (the isoelectric pH of albumin). It may be done by adding a drop of chlorophenol red, followed by few drops of either dilute acetic the red color is discharged) or dilute sodium carbonate (till pink color appears). Gently heat the upper part of the fluid to boiling. Turbidity indicates the presence of protein or phosphates.

Add few drops of dilute acetic acid. Phosphates are dissolved. If turbidity persists, it is due to coagulation of albumin.

Nitric acid test: Take 5 ml concentrate nitric acid in a test tube. Slowly add urine along the side of tube so that it forms a separate layer, above the acid. A white ring, due to precipitation of protein by nitric acid is observed. This is referred to as **Heller's test.**

Test for Bence-Jones proteins: Take 5 ml urine in a test tube. Heat it carefully by immersing in a beaker of warm water. Urine becomes turbid at 40°C and shows a precipitate up to 60°C. On increasing the temperature above 60°C precipitate disappears. It again reappears on cooling.

BLOOD

Benzidine test or O-toluidine test can show presence of blood (hemoglobin) in the urine.

Take 3 ml of benzidine/O-toulidine reagent (saturated solution of benzidine or O-toulidine in glacial acetic acid) in a clean and dry test tube. Add 3 ml of hydrogen peroxide, mix and pour one-half of it to another tube. To one of the tubes add few drops of water (to serve as control). To the other tube add few drops of urine. Fluid rapidly acquires a deep blue color due to the presence of hemoglobin.

The principle of the test is that hemoglobin acts as pseudoperoxidase and decomposes hydrogen peroxide. Oxygen is liberated, which in turn, oxidizes benzidine/O-toulidine and forms blue-colored complex. On exposure to air, blue color rapidly changes to brown within few minutes.

BILE

Bile Salts

Bile salts are surface-active agents. They form a layer on the surface of water and lower its surface tension.

This principle is used to detect the presence of bile salts in the urine and is referred to as **Hay's sulphur test**.

Fill the test tube with urine and sprinkle powdered sulphur on the top of it. Sulphur powder sinks.

When similar test is repeated with water, sulphur does not sink.

Due to surface tension (unbalanced force at the surface) sulphur powder floats on the surface. When bile salts are present, they lower surface tension and sulphur goes down.

Bile Pigments

Bile pigments are the degradation products of heme. On oxidation, heme forms a series of colored compounds such as biliverdin (green) and bilirubin (yellow).

Following tests are commonly performed to show to presence of bile pigments in the urine:

Gmelin test: Take 3 ml of fuming HNO_3 in a test tube and add 3 ml of urine (without disturbing the HNO_3 layer). Gently rotate the tube. At the junction of the two fluids, multicolored rings are formed due to the oxidation of bilirubin by HNO_3. Starting from the acid layer to the bile layer the color is yellow, red, violet, blue, and green.

Fauchet test: Take 5-ml urine in a test tube and acidify it by adding 1–2 drops of acetic acid. Add 5 ml of 10% barium chloride solution and 2–3 drops of the saturated solution of ammonium sulfate. Mix; allow to stand for 5 min and filter. Collect the precipitate.

Bilirubin is adsorbed on the precipitate of barium sulfate, giving it a yellow color. Unfold the filter paper, allow extra water to drain (by laying on dry filter papers) and carefully add 1 drop of Fauchet reagent on the precipitate. Blue-green color indicates the presence of bile pigments.

Fauchet reagent consists of trichloracetic acid and ferric chloride.

Ammonium sulfate and $BaCl_2$ react to form the precipitate of $BaSO_4$, which adsorbs bile pigments. They are released by trichloracetic acid and react with $FeCl_3$, which oxidizes bilirubin (blue) to biliverdin and gives green color.

UROBILINOGEN

Presence of urobilinogen can be tested by **Ehrlich test**.

One ml of the Ehrlich's reagent is added to 10 ml of urine in a test tube. A deep red color is seen. Color remains light red with the normal sample. Rapidity and intensity of the color gives the idea about the quantity of urobilinogen in urine.

Ehrlich's reagent is prepared by dissolving p-dimethylaminobenzaldehyde in hydrochloric acid.

DRY CHEMISTRY

In clinical practice presence of an abnormal constituent can also be detected in the urine by the use of strips, called dipsticks. A dipstick is a thin strip of plastic with one or more cellulose pads fixed on it. Each pad is saturated with buffer and certain chemicals, which are present on the pad in the dry form. Hence, this technique is called **dry chemistry.**

Dipsticks are also referred to as **uristicks (uristixs)** since they are used for the analysis of urine.

Principle: Various chemicals, fixed on the pad, get activated when they soak water (from the urine sample). These reagents then react with the test component of the urine and change the color. Presence of an abnormal constituent in the urine can thus be detected and its approximate concentration can be found by comparing the color with the chart provided by the manufacturer.

Table 31.6 lists basic principle of each test with the use of dipsticks.

Table 31.6. Basic principle of urine analysis with dipsticks

Test	*Principle*	*Reagent used*
pH	Double indicator	Methyl red and bromothymol blue
Protein	Protein error of indicators	Citrate buffer (pH 3.0), bromophenol blue, and protein absorbent
Glucose	Double sequential enzyme reaction	Glucose oxidase-peroxidase and buffer
Ketone Bodies	Sodium nitroprusside	Sodium nitroprusside and glycine buffer
Blood	Pseudoperoxidase activity of hemoglobin	O-toulidine, H_2O_2, and buffer
Bile pigments (bilirubin)	Diazo reaction	Diazo reagent
Urobilinogen	Ehrlich reaction	Buffered p-dimethylaminobenzaldehyde

Various types of dipsticks are commercially available. Some of these are specific for a particular test and have a single pad whereas others have two or more pads and are used for various test combinations.

Precautions: There are a number of precautions, which should be observed for the successful use of these dipsticks:

1. As reagents (most of them enzymes) have a fixed shelf life, dipsticks should not be used after the date of expiry.

2. Dipsticks should be properly stored in an area free from moisture, as moisture may inactivate the chemicals.
3. Test area of the strip (pad) should not be physically touched.
4. The test strip should be immersed in the sample only for a very short period (2–5 seconds) and should be tapped thereafter to remove the excess of water. Immersion for longer time may dissolve chemicals and wash the pad.
5. Allowable time, before color comparison, as per manufacturer should be strictly complied with.

DETERMINATION OF TITRATABLE ACIDITY IN URINE

To measure titratable acidity, a suitable volume of fresh urine (10 ml) is titrated with 0.05 N sodium hydroxide to pH 7.4, with neutral red or phenol red as indicator.

Titratable acidity for a normal person, on an ordinary diet, varies between 20 to 30 meq. Increased values are observed in severe diabetic acidosis. Titratable acidity is reduced in alkalosis.

DETERMINATION OF AMMONIA IN URINE

To estimate ammonia in urine, Berthelot reaction is commonly used. In this method, ammonia is allowed to react with alkaline hypochlorite solution in the presence of phenol reagent.

Take 3 test tubes and mark them as blank, standard and test. Add 2 ml of the phenol reagent to each test tube. Then add 40 µl of diluted urine (1:5) to the test and 40 µl of standard ammonium sulfate solution (1meq/l) to the standard tube. Thereafter, add 2 ml of alkaline-hypochlorite solution to each tube. Place the tubes at 37°C for 20 minutes. Read the intensity of the color against the blank at 630 mm.

The normal daily output of ammonia is 30-50 meq, on an average diet. There is an increase when acid-forming foods are taken and a decrease with alkali-producing foods.

There is a marked increase in the acidosis in diabetes and starvation.

INDEX

Index

Reader's Notes

Reader's Notes